Clinical Child Psychiatry, Second Edition

Clinical Child Psychiatry, Second Edition

Editors

William M. Klykylo and Jerald L. Kay
Wright State University School of Medicine, Dayton, Ohio, USA

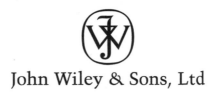

John Wiley & Sons, Ltd

DEDICATION

To our teachers, our students, our patients, and our families.

Contents

Preface To Clinical Child Psychiatry, Second Edition

In the preface to the first edition of this work, we stated that the changes in child psychiatry occurring then would have been barely imaginable 15 years earlier. *Pari passu*, we could not have predicted then how much the whole world would change thereafter. Yet a world in crisis has only intensified the demands placed upon child and adolescent psychiatry. We have ever-growing demands for service to our patients, whose stressors and pathology become more severe and pervasive. We are fortunate that our understanding of disease and our armamentarium of treatments also continue to increase. Regrettably, the resources allocated for those treatments have not always grown apace; and so we must continue to do more with less and do so ever more quickly and efficiently.

The welcome growth of knowledge in our field has effected changes in clinical practice and created a need for an update of this book. Like its predecessor, *Clinical Child Psychiatry*, Second Edition, is presented neither as a comprehensive textbook covering the entire field, nor as a brief introduction. It still attempts to serve as a focused study of major problems, challenges, and practices commonly encountered in clinical work. It remains directed toward experienced clinicians encountering new areas of practice, as well as to students and residents entering the field. We especially hope that pediatricians and family physicians, who in the United States now provide the preponderance of child psychiatric services, will find this volume useful. We also wish it to be informative to professionals outside of medicine as an overview of what child psychiatry can – and should – do today. As always, but in these times especially, we must work together as best we can.

Whatever its merits, *Clinical Child Psychiatry*, Second Edition, is the product of the many individuals' efforts. We have been well served by our publisher John Wiley and Sons, Ltd, and especially by our consultants Charlotte Brabants, Deborah Russell and Andrea Baier. They bring to their work an enviable combination of knowledge, experience, patience, and good humor that has encouraged and sustained us. We could not have assembled this book without the support of our staff at Wright State University, most notably Edward Depp. David Rube, who served as co-editor of the first edition, was able to assist us as an editorial consultant as well as the contributor of two chapters. Our contributors are the ultimate source of this volume's content and value, and we are in their debt. Finally, our families continue to support us with their affection and patience.

William M. Klykylo
Jerald L. Kay

Contributors

Pamela J. Beasley, Harvard Medical School and Department of Psychiatry, Children's Hospital of Boston, Hunnewell 121, 300 Longwood Ave, USA

Rick T. Bowers, 1331 Talon Ridge Court, Kettering, OH 45440, USA

Christina C. Clark, University Psychological Services Association, Inc., 1020 Woodman Drive, Suite 225, Dayton, OH, USA

Barbara J. Coffey, Child Study Center, New York University School of Medicine, 577 First Avenue, New York, NY 10016, USA

Edwin H. Cook, Jr, University of Chicago, Department of Psychiatry, MC 3077, 5841 South Maryland Avenue, Chicago, IL 60637, USA

Antoinette S. Cordell, 5045 N. Main Street, Dayton, OH 45415, USA

G. Oana Costea, Queen's Children's Psychiatric Center, 74-03 Commonwealth Blvd, Bellrose, NY 11426, USA

Jacqueline Countryman, 74th MDOS/SGOHC, 4881 Sugar Maple Drive, Wright Patterson AFB, OH 45435, USA

Jennifer Couturier, University of Western Ontario, London Health Centre, 800 Commissioners Road East, Room E1-605, London, Ontario, Canada

Sergio Delgado, Children's Hospital Medical Center, 3333 Burnet Avenue, Cincinnati, OH 45229-3039, USA

David Ray DeMaso, Harvard Medical School and Department of Psychiatry, Children's Hospital of Boston, Hunnewell 121, 300 Longwood Ave, USA

Craig L. Donnelly, Section of Pediatric Psychopharmacology, Dartmouth-Hitchcock Medical Center, One Medical Center Drive, Lebanon, NH 03756-0001, USA

Martin J. Drell, LSU Medical School, 1542 Tulane Ave, Room A 328, New Orleans, LA 70112-2822, USA

Sidney Edsall, Department of Psychiatry, Stanford University, 401 Quarry Road, Palo Alto, CA 94305

Daniel J. Feeney, Pediatric Psychiatry Services, Willford Hall Medical Center (WHMC), 59th Medical Wing, 2200 Bergquist Drive, Lackland AFB, TX 78236, USA

Dorothyann Feldis, College of Education, 341 Teacher's College, University of Cincinnati, Cincinnati, OH 45221-0002, USA

Pamela A. Gulley, Greene County Educational Service Center, 360 E. Enon Road, Yellow Springs, OH 45387-1499, USA

Scott D. Grewe, Tri-Cities Neuropsychology Clinic, 303 Bradley Blvd., Suite 100, Richland, WA 99352-4497, USA

Jerald L. Kay, Department of Psychiatry, Wright State University School of Medicine, P.O. Box 927, Dayton, OH 45401-0927

Niranjan S. Karnik, Department of Psychiatry and Behavioral Sciences, Stanford University Medical Center, 401 Quarry Road, Palo Alto, CA 94305, USA

Bryan H. King, Professor of Psychiatry and Behavioral Sciences, University of Washington and Children's Hospital and Regional Medical Center, Seattle, WA

William M. Klykylo, Department of Psychiatry, Wright State University School of Medicine, 627 S. Edwin C Moses Blvd, P.O. Box 927, Dayton, OH 45401-0927, USA

Bennett L. Leventhal, University of Chicago, Department of Psychiatry, BH 440, 5841 South Maryland Avenue, Chicago, IL 60637, USA

James Lock, Department of Psychiatry and Behavioral Sciences, Stanford University School of Medicine, 401 Quarry Road, Palo Alto, CA 94305-5719, USA

Arthur Maerlender, Dartmouth-Hitchcock Medical Center, One Medical Center Drive, Lebanon, NH 03757, USA

Jill D. McCarley, Department of Psychiatry, Wright State University School of Medicine, 627 S. Edwin C Moses Blvd, P.O. Box 927, Dayton, OH 45401-0927, USA

Brian J. McConville, Department of Psychiatry, University of Cincinnati College of Medicine, MSB 7258, ML 0559, Cincinnati, OH 45267-0559, USA

Deborah V. McQuade, Section of Child and Adolescent Psychiatry, Dartmouth-Hitchcock Medical Center, One Medical Center Drive, Lebanon, NH 03756, USA

Douglas Mossman, Division of Forensic Psychiatry, Wright State University School of Medicine, East Medical Plaza, First Floor, 627 S. Edwin C. Moses Blvd., Dayton, OH 45401-1461, USA

Susan Mumford, Department of Psychiatry, Wright State University School of Medicine, 627 S. Edwin C Moses Blvd, P.O. Box 927, Dayton, OH 45401-0927, USA

Tom Owley, University of Chicago, Department of Psychiatry, 5841 South Maryland Avenue, Chicago, IL 60637, USA

George Realmuto, Department of Psychiatry, University of Minnesota, F256/2B West, Riverside Avenue, Minneapolis, MN 55454-1495, USA

David M. Rube, Queen's Children's Psychiatric Center, 74-03 Commonwealth Blvd, Bellrose, NY 11426, USA

Dorothy Reddy, Queen's Children's Psychiatric Center, 74-03 Commonwealth Blvd, Bellrose, NY 11426, USA

Lori A. Sansone, Premier Health Net, 6611 Clyo Road, Suite D, Centerville, OH 45459, USA

Randy A. Sansone, Sycamore Primary Care Center, 2115 Leiter Road, Suite 300, Miamisburg, OH 45342-3659, USA

Cyvia A. Scharf, Center for Research in Sleep Disorders, 1275 East Kemper Road, Cincinnati, OH 45237, USA

Martin B. Scharf, Center for Research in Sleep Disorders, 1275 East Kemper Road, Cincinnati, OH 45237, USA

Rachel Shechter, Child Study Center, New York University School of Medicine, 577 First Avenue, New York, NY 10016, USA

Jamie Snyder, 3500 S. 91st Street, Lincoln, NE 69520-1429, USA

Michael T. Sorter, Cincinnati Children's Hospital Medical Center, 3333 Burnet Avenue, Cincinnati, OH 45229, USA

Matthew W. State, Department of Psychiatry, Wright State University School of Medicine, 627 S. Edwin C Moses Blvd, P.O. Box 927, Dayton, OH 45401-0927, USA

Hans Steiner, Division of Child Psychiatry and Child Development, Stanford University School of Medicine, 401 Quarry Road, Palo Alto, CA 94305-5719, USA

Christina G. Weston, Department of Psychiatry, Wright State University, School of Medicine, PO Box 927, Dayton, OH 45401-0927, USA

Keith Owen Yeates, Department of Psychology, Children's Hospital, 700 Children's Drive, Columbus, OH 43205, USA

Section I
The Fundamentals of Child and Adolescent Psychiatric Practice

1

The Initial Psychiatric Evaluation

William M. Klykylo

This chapter serves as an introduction both to this textbook and to the approach of patients and families in child and adolescent psychiatric practice. Child and adolescent psychiatrists should be broadly trained clinicians able to address a variety of somatic, psychologic, and social needs of the patient and family. Their approach should combine the caution and competence required of a physician treating an individual patient with a broad concern for that patient's development in the context of family, school, and society. This textbook provides an overview of child and adolescent psychiatric practice while focusing on the more common areas of clinical practice. As such, it should serve the established practitioner as a rapid and accessible introduction to unfamiliar areas by taking into account the ever-expanding breadth of clinical practice. For general readers or students in professions other than medicine, this book will serve as an introduction both to the assessment and management of some commonly encountered clinical entities and to the range and standards of practice expected of a contemporary child and adolescent psychiatrist. There are currently about 6000 child psychiatrists in some sort of clinical practice in the United States, whereas there are between 7 and 12 million children with psychiatric illnesses, as identified by DSM-IVTR criteria [1,2]. Most of these children will not see a child and adolescent psychiatrist and, in many instances, the parents, teachers, and other professionals attempting to serve them may be unaware of the contribution that child and adolescent psychiatry can make to the child's care.

The traditional roles of child and adolescent psychiatrists are those of diagnostician, therapist, and consultant. First, child and adolescent psychiatrists should offer a child and family a comprehensive diagnostic assessment that addresses the medical condition of the child; delineates the child's emotional, cognitive, social, and linguistic development; and identifies the nature of the child's relationship with his or her family, school, and social milieu.

Second, child and adolescent psychiatrists, like all physicians, treat illnesses, bringing to bear an armamentarium of somatic treatments and the more traditional skills of individual, family, and group psychotherapists. Because of the breadth of training they receive, child and adolescent psychiatrists should have special skill in appreciating the interaction among these therapies and their effects on one another and on the child and family.

Finally, in many cases, child and adolescent psychiatrists will serve as consultants. This role is more developed in our specialty than in most other areas of medicine because of the constant disproportion between the number of patients and the number of clinicians. Inevitably, we consult and collaborate with parents, educators, and other professionals who may see the child and family more frequently and intensively than we do; because of the breadth of our training, we should offer a special competence in coordinating these efforts. Concurrent with this role, we often must serve as advocates for children and their families in today's environment of great clinical needs and comparatively limited resources.

Referral Sources

Because of the broad responsibility shared by child and adolescent psychiatrists, our evaluations must address not only a narrow consideration of clinical diagnosis but also a larger set of issues that are truly biopsychosocial and require a more than casual competence in each of these areas. We must therefore address the specific needs and questions posed by each referral source. Children are today served by a variety of individuals and agencies, each possessing their own

Clinical Child Psychiatry, Second Edition. Edited by W.M. Klykylo and J.L. Kay
© 2005 John Wiley & Sons Ltd.

particular agendas and separately approaching physicians and other consultants. These agendas must be recognized and served, given today's consumer-oriented society. At the same time, we have a responsibility to those individuals seeking our professional services to educate them with the wider range of concerns that may be affecting a given child's or family's life.

In today's environment, we frequently receive referrals from, or may be employed in contractual relationships with, various social and legal agencies such as courts and departments of human services. Each of these agencies has a particular agenda, generally mandated by legislation or its charters, to determine the eligibility of children for various services or proceedings. The agencies frequently approach their duties with an intense dedication to children but an incomplete familiarity with the knowledge and assumptions that inform our practice. Referrals may also come from teachers or schools. These referrals may be a result of the child's behavioral disruptions or eccentricities, his or her academic difficulties, or simply the distinct – if at times uncertain – perception of a dedicated teacher that something is wrong. Referrals may come to us from other physicians. In today's atmosphere of comprehensive primary practice, these physicians may have already begun the diagnosis and treatment of mental illness in a child, and established an ongoing relationship with this child and his or her family. Such referrals require a balanced response of both expertise and respect. Finally, many referrals come directly from parents, who are generally very concerned about their child's impaired functioning and suffering. They may bring to the process a mixed heritage of concern, guilt, and shame, frequently fearing that they will be judged as they seek help. Concurrent with this are often ambivalent feelings of love and frustration toward a difficult child. The task of child and adolescent psychiatrists is to recognize all these needs and address them in a fashion that is not only authoritative but also tactful and empathetic.

Elements of the Evaluation

This section provides an overview of the elements of a comprehensive child and adolescent psychiatric evaluation in the context of contemporary knowledge and patient needs. More detailed considerations of the process of the clinical interview are also available [3–6]. The assessment of particular disorders as well as laboratory, psychologic, and educational assessments is covered in other chapters of this book.

Collateral and Preliminary Information

Today, most children who are seen by child and adolescent psychiatrists have already received a great deal of attention from other professionals. To fail to gather information from these people prior to a formal evaluation is a serious mistake, leading to wasted time and frustrated relationships. If at all possible, it is usually most efficient to speak directly with a referring professional. This is especially true in the case of primary care physicians, who may have a long-standing relationship with the child and family. Other mental health professionals referring a child usually have conducted their own evaluation. Children's school records can be a rich source of information about their cognitive and emotional development. Examination of all these data can enrich an evaluation; similarly, failure to do so can lead to embarrassing lapses.

Clinicians may at times be tempted to assess a child while deliberately ignoring collateral information, presumably to evolve an unbiased assessment. There may be certain unusual situations in which this tactic is indicated. More often than not, however, this approach ignores the reality of the lives of children, who live in asymmetrical relationships with adults and agencies, both of whom have considerable knowledge and power over them. In general, this approach is a departure from best practices.

Encounters with Referring Professionals

Often a child and adolescent psychiatrist's first personal encounter in assessing a patient is with another professional – a clinician, educator, or case worker who has sought the evaluation. The enormous value of their information has already been addressed. The clinician must also recognize the sensitivities of these people: they may be grateful for the opportunity to meet with the psychiatrist and eager in their anticipation of the evaluation, perhaps even to an unrealistic degree. At the same time, the act of seeking a consultation may, at least unconsciously, signify to them a failure on their part. They may be concerned that their relationship with the child or family will in someway be disrupted or supplanted, or that they will be criticized by the psychiatrist.

Parents

Parents bringing their child to a child and adolescent psychiatrist come with a rich and often contradictory mix of feelings. Frequently they reach the psychiatrist at the end of a long, complicated process of evaluations and treatment attempts. They are almost invariably concerned and anxious over their child's condition and prospects. In a way that may be difficult for those who are not parents to understand fully, they may have many fears about the consequences of a psychiatric referral, as do referring professionals. They may feel that they will be judged or, in extreme cases, that their children will be removed from their care. In a more subtle way, they may also worry that their relationship with their child will be supplanted or superseded. They may be concerned about the moral and philosophic basis of the psychiatrist's approach, fearing that parental ethical standards and religious beliefs will in some way be contradicted. Sometimes, simultaneously, they may have unrealistically optimistic or hopeful fantasies of 'absolution' of unconscious guilt, or of quick cures. More often than not, in my experience, parents have no idea of the specifics of psychiatric assessment or treatment. Their opinions have been formed by mass media and public prejudice. Before any specific information can be gathered or plans made, the above issues must be addressed, in the interest of time and efficiency as well as of engagement. Simply put, the child and adolescent psychiatrist needs to understand how the parents feel about the referral and what they expect to gain from it.

A great deal of information should be collected from parents, since they know the child best. The details of this data collection, including various outlines for its organization, are described elsewhere in this book. Most child and adolescent psychiatrists today use a traditional medical format to organize their data, with headings such as Chief Complaint, History of Present Illness, Past Medical History, Family History, and Review of Systems. More often than not, the specifically medical aspects of these data are already available. Not infrequently, however, child and adolescent psychiatrists encounter families that have not received regular primary pediatric care. In these cases, it is incumbent on the psychiatrist as physician to take a comprehensive medical history in addition to acquiring other information. In all these areas of questioning, psychiatrists collect data as do all other physicians, usually attempting to delineate and organize the information in a chronological fashion. What is unique about a psychiatric evaluation is that physicians pursue not only the specific data but also their affective implications. In other words, they seek to find out not only what specifically happened but how it made the child or family members feel and what consequences it had on their lives.

Another area of inquiry of particular importance to physicians treating children, and perhaps especially to

child and adolescent psychiatrists, is the developmental history. Child and adolescent psychiatrists must be absolutely familiar with normal developmental patterns, milestones, and expectations. Psychiatrists often approach these phenomena informed by traditional theories of psychosexual, social, and cognitive development. Although these theories frequently hold great importance for their heuristic value, the clinician must remember that they are, at best, models or theories and not immutable facts. Thus, the clinician must also be aware of contemporary empirical data about normal development and its variations. The developmental history secured by a child and adolescent psychiatrist should in many ways be similar in depth and breadth to that obtained by a developmental pediatrician. At the same time, as psychiatrists we should focus special emphasis on the social and affective consequences of developmental phenomena. In other words, we should be concerned not only about what age a child reached a given milestone but how the occurrence of that milestone affected that child and his or her family. We must recognize that some developmental processes or stages may inherently be more or less comfortable for some parents, and that there is a wide range of variation in the degree of comfort and discomfort that development engenders. Finally, we must recognize the great variations in developmental patterns and expectations found among different cultures. Summaries of typical developmental sequences are found in the Appendix.

A detailed consideration of family dynamics and therapeutics is beyond the scope of this textbook. We know from the contributions of clinicians with approaches as diverse as those of Satir [7], Whitaker [8], Minuchin [9], and Haley [10] that the family has an immense and profound influence on the development of each of its members and may be viewed as a distinct entity. It is therefore invaluable, as part of a comprehensive psychiatric observation, to spend some time in the company of the entire family. Frequently, families referred to us have already been assessed in this fashion by competent family therapists, and the child and adolescent psychiatrist may not need or have the opportunity to pursue extensive family treatment. Nonetheless, the opportunity to observe firsthand how the members of a family act with each other can be enriching for a clinician attempting to understand the consequences of each family member's behavior on the others. In addition, if this observation is done early, it may serve as a more comfortable entrance to the evaluation process for a shy or otherwise recalcitrant child or other uncooperative family member.

Meeting the Child

In practice, most clinicians develop a somewhat personal style of interaction usually formed by psychodynamic and interactional approaches and also more structured, empirical techniques. Clinicians in any setting soon realize that, outside of the specific requirements of a structured interview instrument, they need to be flexible in their approach. The schemes that we use for reporting an interview are generally best conceived as devices for retrospective organization rather than templates for an interview. This is of particular importance with children. Any pediatrician knows that in the course of a physical examination one does what one can when one can. Similarly, in the psychiatric interview with the child, one must be flexible and mobile both verbally and physically.

The most important element of an initial psychiatric interview with the child is the establishment of a productive relationship – in other words, 'making friends.' The clinician must keep in mind how children feel in the context of an interview. Children may share or reflect the same complicated and ambivalent mixture of fear, shame, hope, and misapprehension that their parents bring to the process, and they often have not been fully prepared by the parents or others for the interview. Such preparation, if it can be done by parents prior to bringing the child in, can be helpful. Many children, in my experience, have been told nothing at all, other than 'Come along, we are going to see someone.' Or they may have been told that they are going to see a doctor, which can convey fears of injections and manipulations. Some children may have been led to assume that the evaluation is part of a punitive process. Others may feel that by virtue of referral they have been singled out in some way as 'weird' or 'crazy.' Concurrently, the child may expect to see the physician as some sort of remote, distant, punitive, or bizarre figure. All these issues must be promptly investigated and addressed in a developmentally appropriate fashion for a productive interview to ensue.

How one deals with the above issues is affected by one's own personality and training, and by the circumstances of the child and family. Preschool children are seldom able to sustain any type of formal interview, although they may answer some questions during play activities or while 'on the run.' Their preoperational style of cognition makes the standard interview format, with its attention toward consequence and chronology, irrelevant. One assesses these children through observation and interaction. By contrast, the school-age child will have some comprehension of the psychiatrist's role. It may help to introduce one's self as a 'talking doctor' or 'problem doctor' who deals with the problems that many children have (generalization may make the child feel less singled out) through conversation as well as traditional somatic treatments, and who does not give injections in the office setting. Older children and adolescents can often be asked directly about how they were brought to evaluation, as well as their opinions about its necessity and desirability. With school-age children, an initial request about what sort of problems they may have encountered in their life may be met with diffidence or avoidance. In this instance, simply playing together at some mutually acceptable activity may be an important first step. Older children and adolescents may at this time be able to tolerate tactful questions or the mention of other material or information. They will still benefit from the opportunity to talk or interact about areas that they like, perhaps later in the interview. A frequent icebreaker employed by child and adolescent psychiatrists is drawing. Children who are seated in the waiting room while their parents are being interviewed can be given the opportunity to draw a picture of their family or some other subject of interest to them. Such a drawing can serve as both a projective device and a conversation starter later in the process. Of course, children can also be encouraged to draw at other times during the interview.

In many instances, children do not respond to a standard, direct, complaint centered line of questioning, even after several attempts by the clinician. The clinician is then best advised to relent and ask the child to talk about more general aspects of his or her life. The patient can be encouraged to tell the physician about his or her family, including each individual member and relationship, and school, including academic and social–behavioral aspects and social life in general. In doing so, the clinician can often assemble a broad picture of the child's life as well as specific medical information about phenomenology. Some areas may need to be more directly pursued, usually later in the interview when a presumably more trusting relationship has been established. These include items that are considered part of the mental status examination, such as the presence of affective symptomatology (including suicidal ideation or plans) and psychotic phenomena (including hallucinations, delusions, or ideas of reference). Not every child needs to be asked about these things, since for some children, merely inquiring in an initial interview can be disruptive or fearsome. Nonetheless, these issues must be pursued if there is any indication of a disorder in the given area. Suicidal ideation in particular must be pursued in the context of any affective disorder. Other important behavioral areas such as sexual behavior, using drugs, and health risk behavior may also need to be pursued.

The issue of confidentiality warrants special consideration. Child and adolescent psychiatrists must use their clinical skill to moderate two conflicting demands: the child's right to confidentiality as a patient versus the right of parents and, in some instances, agencies or institutions to be aware of the child's needs and requirements. In my experience, most parents want to know what their child is experiencing; concurrently, most children want their parents to understand them, although they may prefer to conceal some specific details. Younger children may be told they have a right to hold secrets, but that their parents also have a right to know what in general is going on in their lives. Adolescents and their parents may be told that in general they have a right to confidentiality, but that some information involving a serious risk to themselves or others could be shared. Conflicts over confidentiality often overlie larger family issues that, if addressed, make the confidentiality issues moot or irrelevant.

Child and adolescent psychiatrists have traditionally been encouraged to pursue children's fantasies in the course of an assessment. The various approaches to this tend to be highly personalized by each clinician and may include asking a child for three wishes, positive or negative animal identifications (what animal would you like or not like to be), story completion, response to fables, or other techniques. Few if any of these approaches, as used idiosyncratically in an unstructured interview, have ever been validated. They should not be treated as sources of empirical data in and of themselves. They can, however, be important probes to seek other information that can be validated and, more importantly, that relate to specific emotional concerns of an individual child or adolescent.

Frequently nonmedical professionals refer to the psychiatric evaluation as the 'mental status exam,' but in fact this examination is not always used in evaluating children and adolescents – certainly a formal mental status examination must be pursued when there is evidence of a thought disorder. In these instances, the type of examination used with adults generally suffices for adolescents as well. In younger children, the mental status examination is often a list of observations that is retrospectively organized from the content of the interview thus far described. (The outline of this examination is summarized in Lewis's article [6] and in Table 1.1). In most child and adolescent psychiatric assessments, these parameters are not all specifically cited but are mentioned as part of the narrative or may be drawn from inference by the reader. When the

Table 1.1 Mental status examination outline.

1. Physical appearance
2. Separation from parent
3. Manner of relating
4. Orientation to time, place, and person
5. Central nervous system functioning
6. Reading and writing
7. Speech and language
8. Intelligence
9. Memory
10. Thought content
11. Quality of thinking and perception
12. Fantasies and inferred conflicts
13. Affects
14. Object relations
15. Drive behavior
16. Defense organization
17. Judgment and insight
18. Self-esteem
19. Adaptive qualities
20. Positive attributes
21. Future orientation

Adapted from Lewis ME, King RA: Psychiatric assessment of infants, children and adolescents. In: Lewis ME, ed. *Child and Adolescent Psychiatry: A Comprehensive Textbook, Third Edn.* Baltimore, MD: Williams & Wilkins, 2002:531.

patient in question possibly has a major thought or affective disorder, however, specific adherence to this outline may be useful.

Other Aspects of Psychiatric Evaluation

Standardized Assessment Instruments

Structured interviews, rating scales, and questionnaires have become increasingly used in child and adolescent psychiatry in recent years, although their primary venue remains in research settings. In many cases, a comprehensive evaluation can be conducted and reported without resort to these instruments; and some instruments may require a degree of time and expense unavailable outside a research setting. However, as diagnostic categorization under the DSM system has become more standardized and reproducible, clinicians are more frequently using validated instruments to clarify or affirm impressions that come from their personal evaluations. Thienemann has produced a thoughtful commentary on the process of combining these elements in a fashion that is both dynamically sensitive and empirically valid:

Ideally, using intuition and experience, the psychiatrist blood-hound will use clinical senses to sniff out clues to diagnosis at first encounter. On picking up a diagnostic scent, he or she will doggedly follow it into a specific diagnostic room to gather details, thereby determining a diagnosis' presence and clarifying its severity. Integrating this reliable diagnostic information with clinical observations, the clinician will be better positioned to engage patients and their families with effective treatments. [11]

Many clinicians use initial screening or parental report instruments such as the Achenbach Child Behavior Checklist (CBCL) [12] to aid in the early collection of data. Other instruments such as the Conners questionnaires used by parents or teachers [13,14] may be useful in the ongoing assessment for management of specific disorders such as attention-deficit hyperactivity disorder (ADHD).

The Children's Interview for Psychiatric Syndromes (ChiPS) [15] is a screening tool that addresses some 20 Axis I entities. Respondent-based instruments rely upon responders to identify the presence or absence of symptoms. Besides the Conners scales, these include the DISC [16], the computer-assisted (but not the live version) DICA [17], and the pictorial DOMINIC-R [18] which is used with children under the age of 11 years. The specific utility of these instruments is discussed by Myers *et al.* [19] and in Chapters 2 and 8.

Psychologic and Educational Evaluation

Psychologic and educational evaluation are both discussed in subsequent chapters. Along with psychiatric evaluation, they stand as distinct and useful procedures that cannot be substituted for each other. Today, many patients who come to a child and adolescent psychiatrist have already been given psychologic testing; the results, as noted, can be useful information. Far fewer of these children have received an educational evaluation or prescription, which may be an extremely useful part of the child's assessment and rehabilitation, especially as psychiatric treatment progresses. In both cases, psychiatrists should present these assessments as opportunities to better understand a patient's assets and liabilities. Parents should not be led to believe that either the psychologic or educational assessment will produce some sort of miraculous answer to chronic problems or that seeking them implies some failure or inadequacy on the part of them or the physician. Rather, these assessments are specialized procedures that hold unique value in understanding a child's cognitive structure, learning style, and educational needs. Projective testing can be useful in obtaining a deeper understanding of the patient's emotional substrate, especially early in the treatment of withdrawn or verbally inhibited children.

Laboratory Assessment

Laboratory assessment has become a much more frequent part of psychiatric evaluation in recent years (see also Chapter 3). Many patients of child and adolescent psychiatrists will have already undergone a comprehensive laboratory assessment, even including neuroimaging, by their referring physicians; the burden of further assessment of these patients is thus not borne by the psychiatrist.

Conversely, some patients will have had little if any laboratory workup, and such assessments may be indicated in an orderly, stepwise fashion. For example, patients might receive standard hematologic and chemical screenings prior to more exotic endocrinological and nutritional assessments. Similarly, it is seldom appropriate to seek an expensive and complicated neuroimaging procedure in a patient who has not yet received a neurologic examination.

Given both the immense progress in neuroimaging and the intense media coverage devoted to this progress in recent years, some patients and families will assume that procedures such as computed tomography (CT) or magnetic resonance imaging (MRI) scanning are an essential part of the psychiatric examination. This, of course, is frequently not the case. Clinicians may be best advised to deal with these demands by recognizing the underlying motivations of concern, anxiety, or entitlement that evoke these requests. At the same time, as physicians, child and adolescent psychiatrists must be aware of the infrequent but poignant circumstances in which gross central nervous system pathology, such as vascular malformations and space-occupying lesions, may manifest themselves.

Outcome of the Evaluation

Presentation of Findings and Recommendations to Parents and Referring Sources

In the past, some psychiatrists, perhaps out of a specialized conception of confidentiality, have been reluctant or even reclusive in sharing their findings with others. In some instances, this practice has even been directed to parents who may have been told merely to continue bringing their child for treatment. Such positions were, thankfully, relatively unusual, and current demands for consumer orientation and accountability have since made them utterly untenable. Parents or guardians and referring professionals or agencies are entitled to a concise and comprehensible statement of findings and recommendations. The manner in which this information is delivered depends on the needs of the child and the relationship of the child to these individuals or agencies.

As noted earlier, parents approach psychiatric evaluation with a rich mixture of concerns, hopes, and fears, which often come to a head at the time of the counseling or informing interview. I have met parents who could give me a verbatim account of their contact years earlier with a professional regarding their child's status; the affective intensity of this moment sears it into memory. The fashion in which this powerful circumstance is addressed can profoundly affect the subsequent conduct of the patient's treatment. It is a truism that at such moments, parents may hear only the first thing told them. Indeed, it often may be enough in one interview to convey a single major piece of information and attempt thereafter to address its affective consequences. If a diagnostic impression or therapeutic recommendations are at all complicated, parents may need a frequent restatement of this content, perhaps accompanied by written or audiovisual supplements and aids. Many parents may require a series of contacts to fully understand and process this information. Given the restrictions in contact imposed by some care-management agencies, it may be helpful to incorporate into this process case managers or other professionals who have a relationship with the family. In my experience, however, the ultimate responsibility as well as the ultimate effectiveness in dealing with these issues for families resides with the diagnosing physician. It is therefore absolutely incumbent on child and adolescent psychiatrists to deal first and foremost with the affective consequences of whatever information is being presented. To fail to do so is not only inhumane but is likely to seriously compromise the subsequent physician–family relationship and the family's compliance with treatment recommendations. It should go without saying that all these considerations must also be addressed, in a developmentally appropriate fashion, in explaining the findings and recommendations to the child or adolescent as well.

Many psychiatric disorders of children have been addressed with varying degrees of accuracy in the public media, for example, conveying both conscious and unconscious expectations to parents. The child and adolescent psychiatrist must thus explore the specific meaning and implication of any diagnosis for a given family. Specific treatment recommendations may carry with them certain implications, any or all of which may amplify or exaggerate a parent's feelings of inadequacy or incompetence. Fears may arise in connection with specific treatment recommendations. The use and misuse of psychopharmacology has been pursued in excruciating detail and with variable accuracy by the media. In addition, certain religious and political groups have publicly pursued an agenda opposing psychopharmacology, often in an ill-advised and misinformed fashion. All this information can be on parents' minds. Concurrently, however, they or their children may see medication as a means of control or as a source of some sort of magical improvement.

Although many parents may see psychotherapy as a more benign intervention than somatic treatment, they may still have concerns or misconceptions about it. The usual recommendation for family involvement or family therapy may be interpreted by some parents as an indictment of their own actions. Psychotherapy, and the fashion in which it helps or cures, may also be a mystery to parents. A careful, thoughtful, and concise explanation of the rationale for psychotherapy should always be given. The explanation should include the indications for psychotherapy, the options of therapeutic methods and approaches applicable to a given situation, the manner in which psychotherapy can be expected to help, the role of the family in this therapy, and an estimate of duration and cost.

Treatment Planning

Treatment planning is considered in greater detail in Chapter 6. It is informed by a variety of considerations, including the specific disorders of the patient or family; the preferences, hopes, fears, and fantasies of the patient or family; and systemic availability and limitation of resources. A treatment plan must be developed that is both appropriate for the disorder under treatment and realistic in the context of patient and family wishes and resource limitations. In today's environment of care management for fiscal ends and with limited resources, clinicians may frequently be tempted to offer treatment plans that are suboptimal or even inadequate for the patient's needs. It is the professional and ethical responsibility of any physician, certainly including child and adolescent psychiatrists, to provide patients and families with a clear indication of the most clinically effective treatment recommendations – even if they are not economically feasible. McConville (see Chapter 6) offers a model of treatment planning that places interventions on separate continua of directivity and restrictiveness and allows for a sequential arrangement of multiple interventions.

Sharing Information with Other Physicians, Schools, and Agencies

Since many patients come to seek child and adolescent psychiatrists as a result of a referral from physicians, schools, or other agencies, information must frequently be shared regarding the patient's condition, prognosis, and treatment. It is axiomatic that information on any patient cannot be released without the expressed (and usually written) permission of the patient or, in the case of a minor, the patient's parents or legal guardian. Both the content of shared information and the manner in which it is communicated are matters of clinical judgment and practical wisdom and should be discussed in advance with patients, families, or guardians. Information should be distributed only as requested, and psychiatrists should avoid automatic release of entire reports or clinical notes. These issues of confidentiality are especially complicated by third-party reimbursement. Many patients and families routinely authorize unlimited release of clinical information for the purpose of reimbursement, and in fact may be forced to do so. Unfortunately, this information can then become accessible to an almost unlimited number of individuals and organizations.

In general, referring sources should not be given detailed information about members of the family other than the patient This is especially critical in educational settings, since many school records are virtually public documents. Much of the time, these dilemmas can be claimed or resolved before any records or reports are released by conversing with the professional or agency requesting information. The type of information shared with a referring physician may be very different from that shared with the school, however, in both content area and detail.

Referral sources sometimes pursue psychiatric evaluation of a child or adolescent in a conscious or unconscious attempt to gain information about the parents or other family members. Such requests, even when made with good intentions, are usually ethically indefensible. They are also logically suspect, since they seek information that arises from hearsay and surmises. An extreme example of this situation is when the child and adolescent psychiatrist is asked to comment on the fitness for child custody of a parent whom the psychiatrist has never met. Complying with such a request can embroil the psychiatrist in conflicts that make further engagement with the family impossible, while the child has been done no substantive good. The psychiatrist should be ready to discuss the specific needs of a child, however, irrespective of the particulars of physical setting.

Consultation, Collaboration, and Advocacy

Children's needs are addressed in our culture by a wide variety of people: parents, professionals, and educators, among others. Even in the case of the child with a major mental illness whose psychiatric needs may be paramount, it is usually impossible for a child and adolescent psychiatrist to function alone. The psychiatrist will therefore be asked to consult with other professionals and educators. (The manner of these consultations is discussed in Chapters 4, 5, 29, and 30.) Such consultation may be an intermittent advisory relationship, or it may involve ongoing collaboration wherein child and adolescent psychiatrists and other professionals interact in discipline-specific roles.

In today's environment of competition for social and educational resources, and of active intervention in the lives of children and families who are in danger, the child and adolescent psychiatrist has a special role of advocacy. This role may develop as a result of a request by a patient and family or the psychiatrist's perception that some special intervention or communication is required. Despite the changing and challenged role of physicians in our society, the child and adolescent psychiatrist can still be an important and potent agent in the workings of educational, social, and legal systems.

Conclusion

The child and adolescent psychiatrist has a unique role within medicine, providing diagnostic assessment, therapeutic services, consultation, and advocacy for children and their families. In a broad biopsychosocial context, child and adolescent psychiatrists attempt to best meet the needs of children and families by providing these services in a fashion informed by scientific rigor, personal sensitivity, and social responsibility. An encounter with the child and adolescent psychiatrist should provide clinical clarification, personal reassurance, and practical direction.

Appendix

Biological Development
0–24 months

0–2 months

Increasing organization of sleep patterns
Quantitative changes in brain developmet

18–20 months

Density of dendritic spines
   dercreases
Cerebral glucose metabolic rates
   reach adult levels
Increasing lateral and anterior-
   posterior cerebral specialization
   of language centers

2–6 months

Rapid growth of synapses
Rapid increase in cerebral glucose metabolism
Social smiling emerges
Diurnal sleep–wake cycles emerge

7–9 months

Growth in head circumference with rapid cerebral growth
Myelination of limbic system
Enhanced associative pathways
Improved inhibitory control of higher centers

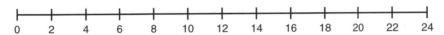

Figure 1.1 Biological development during the first two years of life.

Cognitive Development
0–24 months

0–2 months

Rapid development of olfactory and auditory recognition
Emergence of cross-modal fluency
Recognition of maternal face

18–20 months

Development of
   symbolic representation
Emergence of personal pronouns
Pretend play is progressively
   other directed

2–6 months

Emergence of classical and operant conditioning
Development of habituation

7–9 months

Means-ends behavior develops
Demonstration of object permanence
Stranger reaction and separation protest appear
Exploration of novel properties of objects
Emergence of mastery motivation and symbolic play
Emergence of the discovery of intersubjectivity

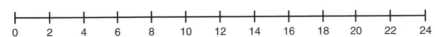

Figure 1.2 Cognitive development during the first two years of life.

Emotional Development
0–24 months

0–2 months

Maternal recognition of contentment
Maternal recognition of interest
Maternal recognition of distress

2–3 months

Differentiation of joy from contentment
Differentiation of surprise from interest
Differentiation of sadness, disgust, and anger

7–9 months

Affect attunement
Emergence of instrumental use of emotion
Emergence of social referencing

9–24 months

Discriminates emotions by facial expressions
and vocalizations

18–20 months

The Rapprochment crisis occurs
Emergence of embarrassment,
empathy, and envy

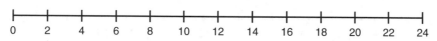

Figure 1.3 Emotional development during the first two years of life.

Social Development
0–24 months

0–2 months

Interactive communication
occurs
Stimulates social responses

2–3 months

Vocalizations become social
Emergence of turn taking in vocalizations
Emergence of mutual limitation
Emergence of sound localization
Recognition of verbal affect

2–7 months

Eye to eye contact begins
Emergence of the social smile
Emergence of social interaction
Diminished crying

7–9 months

Increasing evidence of intersubjectivity
Responds to caregiver empathy
Emergence of separation protest and
stranger reactions

18–20 months

Words used for social functions
Language development
enhances relatedness
Increased evidence of
social relationships

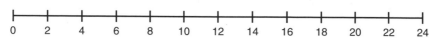

Figure 1.4 Social development during the first two years of life.

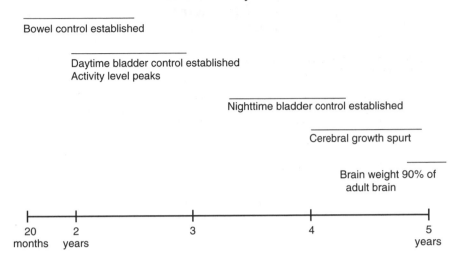

Biological Development
20 months–5 years

Bowel control established

Daytime bladder control established
Activity level peaks

Nighttime bladder control established

Cerebral growth spurt

Brain weight 90% of
adult brain

| 20 months | 2 years | 3 | 4 | 5 years |

Figure 1.5 Biological development during the preschool years (20 months–5 years).

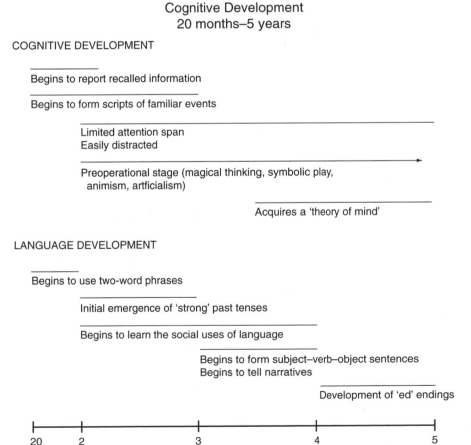

Cognitive Development
20 months–5 years

COGNITIVE DEVELOPMENT

Begins to report recalled information

Begins to form scripts of familiar events

Limited attention span
Easily distracted

Preoperational stage (magical thinking, symbolic play,
   animism, artficialism)

Acquires a 'theory of mind'

LANGUAGE DEVELOPMENT

Begins to use two-word phrases

Initial emergence of 'strong' past tenses

Begins to learn the social uses of language

Begins to form subject–verb–object sentences
Begins to tell narratives

Development of 'ed' endings

| 20 months | 2 years | 3 | 4 | 5 years |

Figure 1.6 Cognitive development during the preschool years (20 months–5 years).

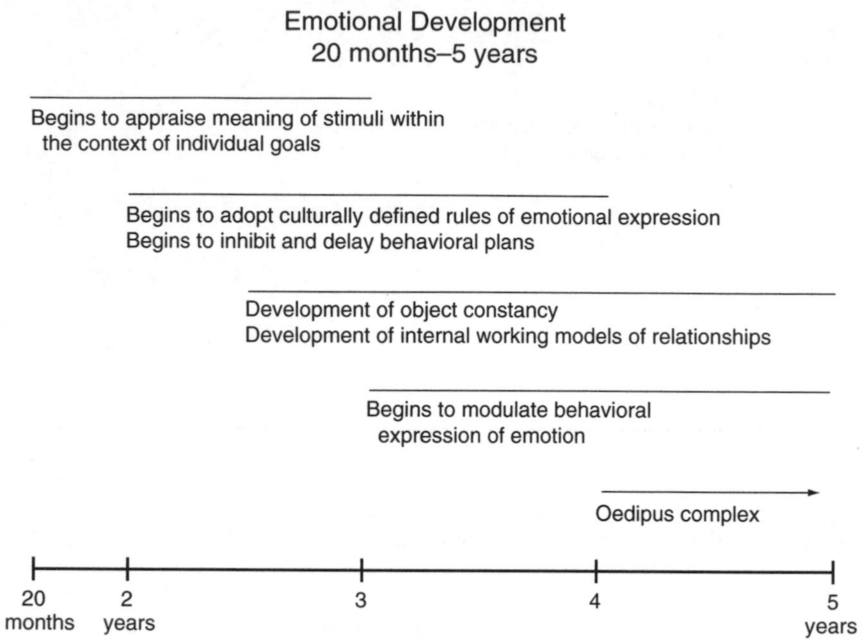

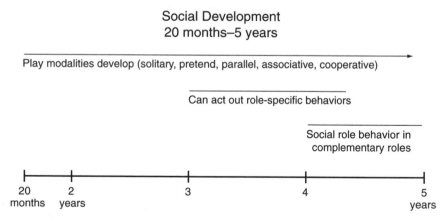

Figure 1.7 Emotional development during the preschool years (20 months–5 years).

Figure 1.8 Social development during the preschool years (20 months–5 years).

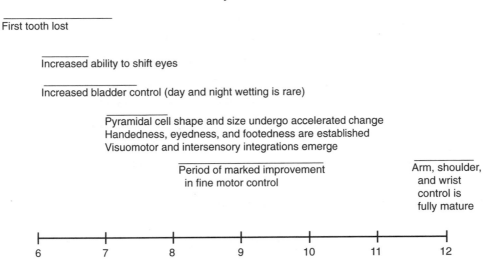

Figure 1.9 Biological development in the school-age child (6–12 years).

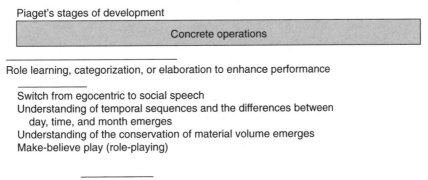

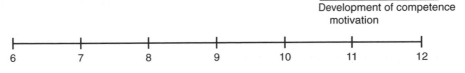

Figure 1.10 Cognitive development during the school-age child (6–12 years).

Emotional Development
6–12 years

Emergence of emotional control
Vacillates from one emotional extreme to another

Increasing sensitivity to attitudes of others

Decrease in 'sensitivity'
Increasing feeling of anticipation and impatience

Becomes more independent, dependable, and obedient
Development of a sense of empathy

Increased mood variation
and 'moodiness'

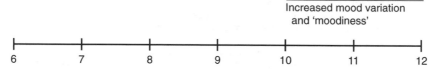

```
6       7       8       9       10      11      12
```

Figure 1.11 Emotional development during the school-age child (6–12 years).

Social Development
6–12 years

Understands that people can have multiple roles
Likes some social routines

Interested in secrets, collecting, and organized games and hobbies
Off-color humor emerges
Primarily unisex friendships
Explains actions by referring to events of immediate situation

Redefines status relationships with friends
Same-sex groupings prominent
Punchlines emerge in humor
Focus on peoples' physical appearances as opposed
   to their personality dispositions

Adoption of group's values, speech patterns, and manners
Strong peer group affiliation

Rise in social consciousness with
   respect to what is 'in'
Increased self-regulation
Best friends rise in importance

Understands that emotions have
   internal causes
Recognizes that people can have
   conflicting feelings and can sometimes
   mask true feelings

Relates actions to
   personality traits and feelings
Sees friends as people who
   understand each other and
   share thoughts and feelings

```
6       7       8       9       10      11      12
```

Figure 1.12 Social development during the school-age child (6–12 years).

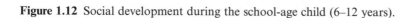

Cognitive Development
13–18 years

Formal operations: Development of logical reasoning, including combinatorial system, ability to understand combinations of objects and new propositional combinations, appreciation of inversion, reciprocity, and symmetry.

Abstract thinking first emerges

Acquisition of processing capacity
Development of mutual perspective taking

Resolution of adolescence:
Attain a personal value
system respecting the needs
of others and the needs of self

Refinement of processing capacity
Elaboration of skills for handling and processing information, including scanning skills,
    flexible use of learning strategies, control or monitoring of information processing
Expansion of informational and factual catalog

Development of mutual perspective taking

Growing recursive thought

Formal operational thought

```
|----------|----------|----------|----------|----------|
13         14         15         16         17         18
```

Figure 1.13 Cognitive development during the adolescent period (age 13–18 years).

Emotional Development
13–18 years

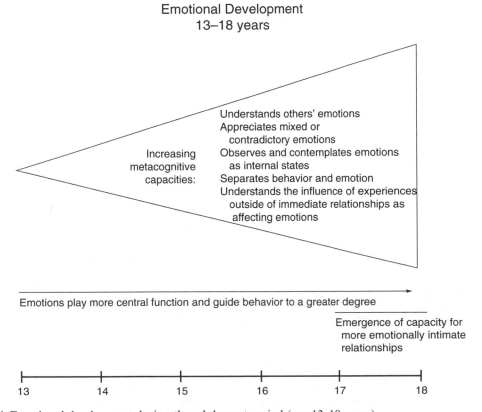

Increasing
metacognitive
capacities:

Understands others' emotions
Appreciates mixed or
    contradictory emotions
Observes and contemplates emotions
    as internal states
Separates behavior and emotion
Understands the influence of experiences
    outside of immediate relationships as
    affecting emotions

Emotions play more central function and guide behavior to a greater degree

Emergence of capacity for
more emotionally intimate
relationships

```
|----------|----------|----------|----------|----------|
13         14         15         16         17         18
```

Figure 1.14 Emotional development during the adolescent period (age 13–18 years).

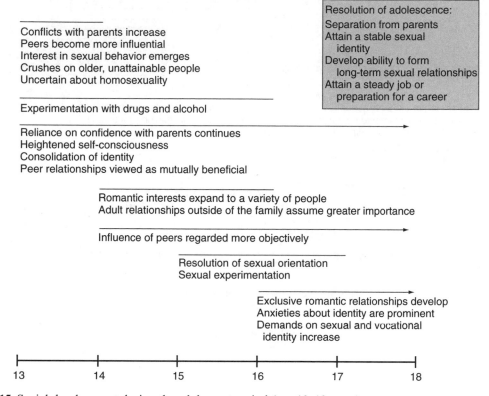

Figure 1.15 Social development during the adolescent period (age 13–18 years).

References

1. Costello EJ, Pantino T: The new morbidity-Who should treat it? *Dev Behav Pediatr* 1987; **8**:288–291.
2. US Public Health Service (1999): *Mental Health: A Report of the Surgeon General*. Rockville, MD: US Department of Health and Human Services, National Institutes of Health, National Institute of Mental Health.
3. Greenspan SI, Greenspan NT. *The Clinical Interview of the Child*. Washington, DC: American Psychiatric Press, 2003.
4. Kestenbaum CJ: The clinical interview of the child. In: Wiener JM, ed. *Textbook of Child and Adolescent Psychiatry, Second Edn*. Washington, DC: American Psychiatric Press, 1997:79–88.
5. King RA, Schowalter JE: The clinical interview of the adolescent. In: Wiener JM, ed. *Textbook of Child and Adolescent Psychiatry, Second Edition*. Washington, DC: American Psychiatric Press, 1997:89–94.
6. Lewis ME, King RA: Psychiatric assessment of infants, children and adolescents. In: Lewis ME, ed. *Child and Adolescent Psychiatry: A Comprehensive Textbook*, 3rd ed. Baltimore, MD: Williams & Wilkins, 2002:525–543.
7. Satir V: *Conjoint Family Therapy: A Guide*. Palo Alto, CA: Science and Behavior Books, 1964.
8. Whitaker C: My philosophy of psychotherapy. *J Contemp Psychother* 1973; **6**:49–52.
9. Minuchin S: *Families and Family Therapy*. Cambridge, MA: Harvard University Press, 1974.
10. Haley J: Conducting the first interview. In: Haley J, ed. *Problem-Solving Therapy*. San Francisco, CA: Jossey Bass, 1976; 9–47
11. Thienemann M: Introducing a Structured Interview Into a Clinical Setting. *J Am Acad Child Adolesc Psychiatry* 2004; **43**(8):1057–1060.
12. Achenbach TM, Edelbrock CS: *Manual for the Child Behavior Checklist and Revised Child Behavior Profile*. Burlington, VT: University of Vermont Press, 1983.
13. Conners CK, Siarenios G, Parker JD, Epstein JN: The Revised Conners' Parent Rating Scale (CPRS-R): Factor structure, reliability, and criterion validity. *J Abnorm Child Psychol* 1998; **26**:257–268.

14. Conners CK, Sitarenios G, Parker JD, Epstein JN: Revision and restandardization of the Conners Teaching Rating Scale (STRS-R): Factor structure, reliability, and criterion validity. *J Abnorm Child Psychol* 1998; **26**:279–291.

15. Weller E, Weller R, Fristad MA, *et al.*: Children's Interview for Psychiatric Syndromes (ChIPS). *J Am Acad Child Adoles Psychiatry* 2000; **39**(1):76–84.

16. Shaffer D, Fisher P, Lucas C, Dulcan MK, Schwab-Stone ME: NIMH Diagnostic Interview Schedule for Children Version IV (NIMH DISC-IV): Description, differences from previous versions, and reliability of some common diagnoses. *J Am Acad Child Adolesc Psychiatry* 2000; **39**(1):28–8.

17. Reich W: Diagnostic Interview for Children and Adolescents (DICA). *J Am Acad Child Adolesc Psychiatry* 2000; **39**(1):59–66.

18. Valla JP, Bergeron L, Smolla N: The Dominic-R: A pictorial interview for 6- to 11-year-old children. *J Am Acad Child Adolesc Psychiatry* 2000; **39**(1):85–93.

19. Myers K, Winters N: Ten-Year Review of Rating Scales. I: Overview of scale functioning, psychometric properties and selection. *J Am Acad Child Adolesc Psychiatry* 2002; **41**(2):114–122.

2

Psychological Assessment of Children

Antoinette S. Cordell

Effective diagnosis and treatment planning requires a flexible approach to child assessment that includes data from multiple sources as well as parental involvement. Mooney and Harrison reported that those psychologists who see many children for school-related concerns address cognitive–academic or personality issues but provide much less information on social influences and the context of the children's lives [1]. The most frequently used means of gathering information include the Wechsler, Rorschach, and Bender Gestalt tests, the Thematic Apperception Test (TAT), achievement tests, and drawings. There are limitations to the strictly intrapersonal perspective, however, since children should be understood within the context of their lives [1]. Assessment techniques should be broad and should include measures that draw on the child 'in action.' Psychological techniques suggested for this type of assessment include parent/teacher questionnaires, intelligence and achievement testing, drawings, projective testing, child questionnaires, behavioral assessment, play observations, and family interaction (Appendix 2.1).

Parent/Teacher Questionnaires

The Eyberg Child Behavior Inventory is a straightforward 36-item questionnaire that can be completed by parents of children who are 2–7 years of age. The Eyberg is relatively simple to fill out and yields information on a wide variety of behavioral problems [2] including dawdling, defiance, and opposition, seeking attention and difficulty concentrating.

The Parenting Stress Index (PSI) by Abidin is filled out by parents of children ranging in age from 1 month to 12 years [3]. (A short form is available.) The PSI provides Child Domain scores for the following categories: distractibility/hyperactivity, adaptability, reinforcement of parents, demandingness, mood, and accept-ability. In the Parent Domain, the categories include competence, isolation, attachment, health, role restriction, depression, and relationship with spouse. The Total Stress score combines both domains and allows for an analysis of the source of stress. This index, then, can be used to assess the degree to which the child's behavior is stressful versus the difficulty the parents have in adjusting to their parenting roles. PSI results are also helpful in communicating with parents; the clinician can report, for example, that the parents provided the information that they feel depressed or that they are experiencing communication barriers with their spouse. Parents are less likely to be defensive, and the clinician can be more reflective and understanding rather than intrusive (Figure 2.1).

The same authors headed by Sheras (1998) developed the Stress Index for Parents of Adolecents (SIPA), a questionnaire for parents which applies to teens 11–19 years of age [4]. Categories in the Adolescent Domain (AD) include: Moodiness/Emotional Lability (MEL); Social Isolation/Withdrawal (ISO); Delinquency/Antisocial (DEL); and Failure to Achieve or Persevere (ACH). In the Parent Domain, the following categories are assessed: Life Restrictions (LFR); Relationship with Spouse/Partner (REL); Social Alienation (SOC); and Incompetence/Guilt (INC). The Adolescent–Parent Relationship Domain (PRD) assesses the parents' view of the quality of the relationship that the parent has with the adolescent. Additional scales include the Life Stressors scale (LS) and an index of Total Parenting Stress (TPS). Like the PSI, this tool is useful in assessing the parental perspective in raising an adolescent. The parent is able to provide information on their teen's behavior, their own assessment of their parenting, and the relationship between them.

The Child Behavior Checklist is completed by parents or teachers of children aged 4–16 years [5,6].

Clinical Child Psychiatry, Second Edition. Edited by W.M. Klykylo and J.L. Kay
© 2005 John Wiley & Sons Ltd.

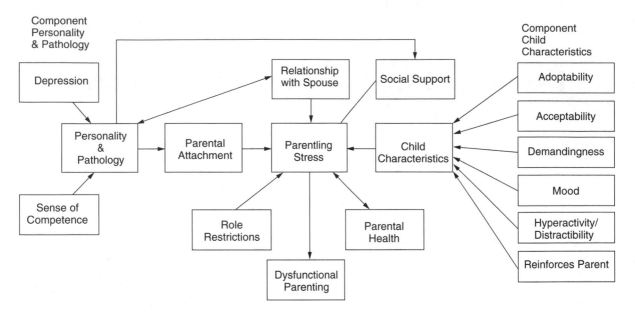

Figure 2.1 Reproduced by special permission of the Publisher, Psychological Assessment Resources, Inc., 16204 North Florida Avenue, Lutz, Florida 33549, from the Parenting Stress Index Professional Manual by Richard R. Abidin, Ed.D., Copyright 1983, 1990, and 1995 by PAR, Inc. Further reproduction is prohibited without permission of PAR, Inc.

The accompanying Youth Self-Report Scale is completed by youngsters from 11 to 18 years of age. These questionnaires have the advantage of providing a behavior profile which gives information on the following dimensions: Withdrawn; Somatic Complaints; Anxious/Depressed; Social Problems; Attention Problems; Delinquent Problems; and Aggressive Behavior. Separate forms are used for boys and girls aged 4–5, 6–11, and 12–16 years. The Child Behavior Checklist-Direct Observation form can also be used for structuring behavioral observations. There is also the Caregiver–Teacher Report Form for preschoolers 18 months to 5 years of age to be filled out by the preschool teacher or caregiver in a daycare setting. This tool provides the clinician working with young children an additional perspective on the child's behavior and emotional needs in a structured setting outside of the home [7].

The Conners' Rating Scales-Revised provide teacher- and parent-rating scales and an adolescent self-report scales [8]. A new empirically based attention deficit hyperactivity disorder (ADHD) index can be used to assess children at risk for ADHD. In addition, the McCarney Attention Deficit Disorders Evaluation Scale condenses the three subscales of inattentiveness, impulsivity, and hyperactivity to two scales: inattentiveness and impulsivity/hyperactivity [9]. It is useful to have a measure of both of these characteristics in child evaluations since they have different implications for treatment. These scales can also be used to assess improvements from the use of psychoactive medication.

The Attachment Disorder Questionnaire developed by E. M. Randolph allows an assessment of the more problematic behaviors and traits of children who have reactive attachment disorder [10]. Items include statements such as 'My child uses his/her "cuteness" or charm to get others to do what he/she wants'; 'My child goes up to strangers and becomes overly affectionate with them or asks to go home with them'; 'My child is cruel to animals or other people.' This questionnaire can be helpful in identifying the nature and severity of the child's symptoms.

Cognitive Assessment

Kaufman and Ishikuma presented a model for intelligence and academic testing that allows the clinician to combine test administration with an in-depth understanding of human development [11]. The goal is to assist individuals in addressing their problems and to improve their functioning, rather than to limit them via labeling or diagnosing.

Intelligence testing is both overrated and underrated. Many people place too much emphasis on intelligence quotient (IQ) scores per se. It is important to realize that psychological tests provide a wide range of information regarding strengths, weaknesses, learning style, and needs. There are many personal qualities that intelligence tests do not measure, however, such as creativity, determination, and persistence over a period of time. As a result, many individuals who score high on IQ tests perform below this level of expectation, and others who score at more modest levels nonetheless accomplish many fine and far-reaching goals. It has never been possible to capture the inventiveness of the human spirit on paper!

There are many factors other than difficulties with intellectual functioning that can lead to low IQ scores. Factors such as cultural or linguistic differences, distractibility or anxiety, refusal to cooperate, and disabling conditions such as autism and deafness can all limit a person's ability to perform the tasks on an IQ test. Research has shown that the norms for intelligence tests become dated over time and that IQ scores gradually drift upward. When current norms are used, a child's score may be slightly lower [12].

Intelligence tests give a wide range of information about children's abilities in several areas of functioning. Wechsler considered intelligence a combination of abilities reflecting an overall level of intellectual capability. The newly revised Wechsler Intelligence Scale for Children-Fourth Edition (WISC-IV) provides subtest and composite scores in specific areas as well as an overall cognitive score representing general intellectual ability (i.e., Full Scale IQ) [12]. This revised edition has updated norms, new subtests, and greater emphasis on discrete domains of cognitive functioning. It is easier to administer and score. The revisions were based on research findings on cognitive development and intellectual assessment. Ten subtests have been retained from the WISC-III, and there are five new subtests (Picture Concepts, Letter-Number Sequencing, Matrix Reasoning, Cancellation, and Word Reasoning). The subtests of the WISC-IV cover a wide variety of abilities that can contribute to successful performance in school (Table 2.1).

For a 16-year-old whose ability is above average, the Wechsler Intelligence Scale-III test for adults may be most appropriate.

The Wechsler Preschool and Primary Scale of Intelligence-III (WPPSI-III), available since 2002, offers an assessment of the intelligence of children ages two years, six months through seven years, three months [13]. Like the other Wechsler tests, it provides an overall cognitive score as well as scores for verbal and performance abilities. A major advantage of the WPPSI-III is that it follows the same structural format and philosophy as the WISC-IV. The seven Core subtests are: Block Design; Information; Matrix Reasoning; Vocabulary; Picture Concepts; Word Reasoning;

Table 2.1 The WISC-III subtests grouped according to scale.

Verbal	Performance
2. Information	1. Picture Completion
4. Similarities	3. Coding
6. Arithmetic	5. Picture Arrangement
8. Vocabulary	7. Block Design
10. Comprehension	9. Object Assembly
12. Digit Span†	11. Symbol Search*
	13. Mazes†

* Supplementary subtest that can substitute only for Coding.
† Supplementary subtest.
From Wechsler D: *Wechsler Intelligence Scale for Children – Third Edition: Manual.* New York: Harcourt Brace Jovanovich; 1991:5.

and Coding. There are seven Supplemental subtests: (Symbol Search); (Comprehension); (Picture Completion); (Similarities); (Receptive Vocabulary); (Object Assembly); and (Picture Naming). For a six-year-old child whose ability is below average, the best choice for intelligence testing may be the Wechsler Preschool and Primary Scale of Intelligence-III (WPPSI-III).

One of the advantages of ability testing is that it provides us with information on the pattern of strengths and weaknesses that can affect the student's ability to function in the classroom (Table 2.2). It gives information to the educator about the special needs and learning style of the student. In clinical practice, several findings can be significant. When there is a low score on the Coding subtest relative to the other scores, for example, the child often has difficulty with handwriting and motor performance in the classroom. Some children may exhibit only this single deficit. These children struggle greatly to perform written work in the classroom, particularly in the primary grades, and are often labeled as 'lazy,' when in fact their neurologic processing proceeds at a different rate than that of other children in the classroom. The Similarities subtest scores can be quite important, since they relate specifically to abstract reasoning and what we commonly consider overall intelligence. All of the areas assessed on the WISC-IV, however, are relevant for understanding the child's functioning in the classroom.

Children who have marked discrepancies between the Verbal Comprehension Index (VCI) and Perceptual Reasoning Index (PRI) can experience difficulty functioning in the classroom (Table 2.3, Table 2.4). Any child who has a severe deficit may be affected severely, even if many other subtest scores are average

Table 2.2 Scales derived from factor analyses of the WISC-III subtests.

Factor I Verbal Comprehension	Factor II Perceptual Organization	Factor III Freedom from Distractibility	Factor IV Processing Speed
Information	Picture Completion	Arithmetic	Coding
Similarities	Picture Arrangement	Digit Span	Symbol Search
Vocabulary	Block Design		
Comprehension	Object Assembly		

From Wechsler D: *Wechsler Intelligence Scale for Children – Fourth Edition: Manual.* New York: Harcourt Brace Jovanovich; 1991:7.

Table 2.3 Abbreviations of composite scores.

Composite Score	Abbreviation
Verbal Comprehension Index	VCI
Perceptual Reasoning Index	PRI
Working Memory Index	WMI
Processing Speed Index	PSI
Full Scale IQ	FSIQ

or above average. Children with high verbal scores but low performance scores struggle with the production of work in the classroom. Children with high performance scores and low verbal scores are often impulsive, action-oriented individuals who have difficulty reflecting or using language to process their experience. The psychologist should look for unique patterns of strengths and weaknesses and attempt to understand them in relation to the overall functioning and personality of the child.

Some children, such as the learning disabled (LD)/gifted child, have complex combinations of cognitive abilities. There appear to be multiple patterns of scores for LD/gifted students. One pattern involves high reasoning/verbal abilities with deficiencies in performance abilities or slow fine-motor coordination (shown by a low Coding score); there may also be difficulties with attention span and focusing. Another pattern is high performance abilities combined with a low verbal score; this pattern may be particularly difficult to identify, because we usually rely on children's verbal functioning as an overall indication of high intelligence. Another pattern is characterized by a relatively high overall IQ but a high degree of distractibility. In the classroom, several areas of special needs should be addressed, including distractibility, slowness in handling written work, difficulty with organization, emotional lability, and negative self-concept [14].

How does ADHD affect intelligence test results? No conclusive battery of tests exists for this disorder. ADHD children often score low on one or more subtests of the WISC-III, including Arithmetic, Coding, Information, and Digit Span. The Freedom from Distractibility factor is not a pathognomonic indicator of ADHD, however. There is tremendous variability in the relative abilities of children with ADHD, and ADHD thus negatively affects performance on structured tests in varied ways. Further, ADHD symptoms present in several childhood disorders. Suggestions for diagnosis include using a variety of assessment instruments to improve convergent validity as well as taking a thorough history from multiple sources if possible. Believe your data. Carefully review intratest and intertest scatter, behavioral observations as the child approaches tasks, and unusual errors; work hard to communicate to others the importance of your assessment data for intervention and treatment planning.

The Stanford–Binet Intelligence Scale – fourth Edition yields scores for Verbal Reasoning, Abstract/Visual Reasoning, Quantitative Reasoning, and Short-Term Memory [15]. The current edition includes many performance items and so has addressed earlier criticism of the Binet that it was too verbally oriented. Using either the WISC-IV or the Binet to ascertain strengths can provide useful information for guiding an individual in school and in making later career choices. Our schools tend to be highly verbally and language oriented. Not all careers require such a strong emphasis in this area; some use performance abilities, for example. It is often difficult for the classroom teacher to realize the ability areas of children who exhibit low verbal and language abilities but stronger performance abilities.

The Leiter International Performance Scale-Revised has the strong advantage of being a nonverbal test of intelligence [16]. It can be used to evaluate children with sensory or motor deficits or language problems,

Table 2.4 Comparison chart.

	Leiter-R	WISC-IV	WPPSI-III	SB-4	WJ-R
Completely nonverbal	Yes	No	No	No	No
Domains measured					
Visualization	Yes	Yes[1]	Yes[1]	Yes	Yes[1]
Reasoning	Yes	Yes[1]	Yes[1]	Yes	Yes[1]
Memory	Yes	Yes[1]	No	Yes	Yes
Attention	Yes	No	No	No	Yes[1,4]
'Growth' scores	Yes	No	No	No	Yes[6]
Age range	2–21	6–16	3–7	2–90	2–90
Appropriate for					
Cognitive delay	Yes	Yes[3]	Yes[3]	Yes[3]	Yes
ESL	Yes	No	No	No	No
Limited English	Yes	No	No	No	No
Learning disabilities	Yes	Yes	Yes	Yes	Yes
ADHD	Yes	Yes	No	Yes	Yes
Deafness	Yes	No[5]	No[5]	No[5]	No[5]
TBI	Yes	No[5]	No	Yes[4,5]	Yes[4,5]
Communication disorders	Yes	Yes[5]	No	No[5]	No[5]
Diverse cultures	Yes	No[5]	No[5]	No[5]	No[5]
Motor impaired	Yes	Yes[2,5]	Yes[2,5]	Yes[2,5]	Yes[2,5]
Fast screening	Yes	No	No	No	No

1. Some subtests measure related areas, but require hearing, language, reading or motor skills.
2. Verbal skills only.
3. Restricted lower bound of IQ ranges.
4. Some areas, but not the complete spectrum provided in Leiter-R.
5. Adjusted administration required.
6. Uses Rasch modeling to derive other special scores.
ADHD = Attention deficit hyperactivity disorder; ESL = English as a second language; Leiter-R = Leiter – Revised; SB-4 = Stanford–Binet – 4th Edition; TBI = traumatic brain injury; WISC-III = Wechsler Intelligence Scale for Children – 3rd Edition; WJ-R = Woodcock–Johnson – Revised; WPPSI-R = Wechsler Preschool and Primary Scale of Intelligence – Revised.
From Leiter RG: *Leiter International Performance Scale – Revised*. Wood Dale, IL: Stoelting; 1997.

or those who speak a different language from the examiner. It contains 54 tests from levels II to XIV and takes 30–45 minutes to complete. The tests involve arranging a series of blocks initially from pairings of colors, shapes, and objects to analogies, perceptual patterns, and concepts at later levels. Instructions are given in pantomime. The Leiter has recently been revised and may thus address uneven item difficulty at various levels. This test is certainly less culturally loaded than other IQ tests, but there is no evidence on whether it is 'free' of cultural bias (Table 2.4).

A quick assessment of intelligence is provided by the Kaufman Brief Intelligence Test (K-BIT) [17]. This can be used for children, adolescents, and adults from the ages of 4 to 90 years. The test has the advantage of taking between 15 and 30 minutes to administer with only two subtests including Vocabulary and Matrices. It appears to be useful for establishing a baseline of intelligence but does not provide in-depth information on strengths and weaknesses. Specifically, the many difficulties with cognitive functioning that a child or adult may show may not be revealed. The use of the K-BIT, therefore, is limited from a clinical perspective.

Another relatively brief assessment of capability is found in the Peabody Picture Vocabulary Test-Third Edition (PPVT-III) [18]. This test is designed to measure receptive vocabulary over a wide range using a friendly approach. The subject is shown four pictures and given a single word. The child then indicates either verbally or nonverbally which picture best represents that word. The simplicity of the test is useful in some situations when a more comprehensive assessment might not be possible, and it may enhance the likelihood of cooperation as well.

The Woodcock–Johnson-III Tests of Achievement (WJ-III) [19] and the Wechsler Individual Achievement Test-Second Edition [20] provide information on basic academic skills. Learning disabilities are defined as major discrepancies between IQ level and tested academic skills. Some children, however, experience significant learning problems in the classroom but do not show such severe discrepancies. The field of education is moving toward a team-based method of assessing learning problems and special educational needs, but individual psychoeducational testing should remain an integral part of this assessment process.

IQ scores should never stand alone in patients being diagnosed for developmental disabilities or mental retardation. Rather, clinicians should consider the pattern of strengths and weaknesses on IQ tests, assess adaptive and other behaviors, and use common sense.

When assessing a child, it is important to seek multiple sources of data, including information on the child's personal and social sufficiency at home, at school, and in the community. The Vineland Adaptive Behavior Scales can be used to measure communication, daily living skills, socialization, and motor skills in children from birth to 18 years and 11 months of age or in low-functioning adults [21]. The scales can be used for handicapped individuals as well. The Vineland requires a respondent who is familiar with the individual's behavior. The survey form contains 297 items, although only those items necessary to establish basal and ceiling levels are used. The test takes 20–30 minutes to administer and yields useful information on strengths and weaknesses in adaptive behavior.

Two additional tools may be helpful. First, the Achievement Identification Measure by S. Rimm can be used to assess underachievement [22]. It identifies students who are performing in school below their ability level. Some may be sliding through on the basis of 'brains,' not effort, whereas others may be in the early stages of underachievement before it has been noted on their report card. The scale measures six dimensions of adaptive attitudes toward academic competition, responsibility, control, achievement, communication, and respect—as well as a total score that reflects a child's overall potential for success in school. Second, Light's Retention Scale can assist in objectifying the issues involved in retaining a child

below his or her grade level [23]. This can be a difficult, emotional process of decision making, so it helps to have a systematic method of weighing the facts. In addition, the book *Summer Children: Ready or Not for School* can be reviewed [24].

Drawings

DiLeo acknowledged that interpreting children's drawings requires more than one approach to understanding [25]. In the correlational approach, data are collected and statistically analyzed to determine any correlation between a characteristic in the drawing and the significance that the clinician attaches to it. In the longitudinal approach, the clinician performs an in-depth study of the patient and examines the relationship between characteristics shown in the patient's drawings and the patient's behavior and overall development.

Clinicians use subjectivity as well as a backlog of clinical experience in interpretating children's drawings. This process involves generating hypotheses to be tested with the use of other data and behavioral observations. Drawings should never be used by themselves to establish clinical 'facts.'

The age and developmental level of the child need to be considered in the interpretation of drawings, and the clinician should be familiar with what is normative for specific developmental levels. Preschool children, for example, often fail to integrate parts into a whole, but this failure is abnormal in an older child. Developmental milestones and stage-dependent theories have been presented by Freud, Erickson, Piaget, and Gesell.

Drawing characteristics that have interpretive significance include the use of space; the quality of line; orientation; shading (as an indicator of anxiety); integration of the human figure drawings, symmetry, and balance; and style. Drawings are also reflective of cognitive development. The drawing of a person 'yields an overview of intellectual maturity' [25]. House drawings give information about the change from an egocentric to an objective view (Table 2.5 and Appendix 2.2).

DiLeo discussed several pitfalls in the analysis of drawings, including inconsistency in drawing performance [25]. When features appear consistently in several drawings, there is a great likelihood that they have been integrated into the child's concept. Particularly when working with young children, therefore, the clinician should obtain several drawing specimens. Another pitfall is to assign excessive weight to specific details. It is important to use a holistic approach and examine the overall impression of the drawing and to appreci-

Table 2.5 Development of drawing related to Piaget's stages of cognitive development – A synoptic view.

Approximate age (yr)	Drawing	Cognition
0–1	*Reflex response* to visual stimuli. Crayon is brought to mouth; the infant does not draw.	*Sensorimotor stage* Infant acts reflexively, thinks motorically.
1–2	At 13 months, the first scribble appears: a zig-zag. Infant watches movement leaving its marks on a surface. Kinesthetic drawing.	Movement gradually becomes goal-directed as cortical control is gradually established.
2–4	Circles appear and gradually predominate. Circles then become discrete. In a casually drawn circle, the child envisages an object. A first graphic symbol has been made, usually between three and four years.	The child begins to function symbolically. Language and other forms of symbolic communication play a major role. The child's view is highly egocentric. Make-believe play.
4–7	*Intellectual realism* Draws an internal model, not what is actually seen. Draws what is known to be there. Shows people through walls and through hulls of ships. Transparencies. Expressionistic. Subjective.	*Preoperational stage* (intuitive phase) Egocentric. Views the world subjectively. Vivid imagination. Fantasy. Curiosity. Creativity. Focuses on only one trait at a time. Functions intuitively, not logically.
7–12	*Visual realism* Subjectivity diminishes. Draws what is actually visible. No more X-ray technique (transparencies). Human figures are more realistic, proportioned. Colors are more conventional. Distinguishes right from left side of the figure drawn.	*Concrete operations stage* Thinks logically about things. No longer dominated by immediate perceptions. Concept of reversibility: things that were the same remain the same though their appearance may have changed.
12+	With the development of the critical faculty, most lose interest in drawing. The gifted tend to persevere.	*Formal operations stage* Views his/her products critically. Able to consider hypotheses. Can think about ideas, not only about concrete aspects of a situation.

From DiLeo JH: *Interpreting Children's Drawings*. New York: Brunner/Mazel; 1983:38.

ate that environmental factors, such as the season of the year or specific holidays, influence the content of children's drawings. DiLeo cautions against overinterpreting ambiguous sexual symbols in the drawings of young children or using a mechanistic, point-by-point analysis [16]. It should be recognized that drawings can be misleading.

For the Kinetic Family Drawing (KFD), the child is asked to 'draw a picture of everyone in your family, including you, doing something. Try to draw whole people, not cartoons or stick people. Remember to make everyone doing something – some kind of activity' [26]. The child is given a plain white 8½″ × 11″ piece of paper with a No.2 pencil placed in the center of the paper and is seated individually in a chair at a table of appropriate height. The examiner leaves the room and checks back periodically. Noncompliance is extremely rare. If children say 'I can't,' they are encouraged periodically and left in the room until they complete the KFD.

Characteristics of individual figures that are analyzed in the KFD include arm extensions, elevated figures, erasures, figures on the back of the page, hanging, omission of body parts, omission of figures, eyes, and rotated figures. The action depicted is also analyzed in terms of intensity, symbolism, fixation, conflict, internalization, avoidance, and harmony. The mean age for both boys and girls performing the KFD is about 10 years, and ages range from 5 to 20 years, skewed toward the '10 and below' age group. Data are also available elsewhere on the actions of individual KFD figures and the frequency of actions for various family members, including father, mother, and self [26]. One should also consider the type of action between KFD figures, such as throwing balls, and the existence of barriers, dangerous objects, or heat, light, and warmth. Drawing styles can be categorized as compartmentalization, encapsulation, lining at the bottom, underlying individual figures, edging, lining at the top, folding compartmentalization, and evasions.

In addition to the Draw-A-Person test (DAP) and the KFD, the House–Tree Person test (HTP) developed by J. Buck in 1948 can also be revealing [27]. In this approach, the house is viewed primarily as a reflection of the home environment and family functioning, the tree is viewed as a reflection of psychosexual-psychosocial history, and the person is viewed as a reflection of interpersonal functioning and relationships with others. The HTP can be used for children five or six years of age, although some children of this age may not be mature enough in terms of their drawings skills. One major advantage of this test is that it uses a projective technique that taps into unconscious behavior and cannot be faked, except possibly to 'fake bad.' (It is considered unlikely that individuals can 'fake good.')

Drawings are useful for children to express their feelings regarding their parents' divorce. Cordell and Berman-Meador suggested that having children 'draw a picture of [their] family divorcing' can help them express underlying attitudes regarding the divorce as well as their attitudes or misconceptions about the process [28]. The four rating scales are denial/acknowledgment, emotionality, aggression, and the use of people. Children's divorce drawings can be rated '0' or 'I' for the absence or presence of each of these four items (Figures 2.2 and 2.3).

Characteristics of children's drawings can point to underlying fears and concerns that may be related to coping styles such as repression or sensitization. This technique can be used in initial assessments for treatment during the therapy process or for court-ordered evaluations regarding custody or visitation.

Projective Testing

Projective tests have received extensive criticism, because they are based on theories of unconscious internal processes and are therefore difficult to establish in terms of reliability and validity. According to Klein, the most commonly used projective tests are the following [29]: Rorschach; Thematic Apperception Test (TAT) Children's Apperception Test (CAT); Blackey Pictures Drawings; Bender Gestalt Test.

Klein discussed the origin of projective tests from psychoanalytic theory, which interprets all human experiences as colored by unconscious repressed mental content [29]. More intrapsychic material can be expected during ambiguous tasks. Projective techniques provide the individual with an ambiguous stimulus, and the individual's response is thought to reflect underlying conflicts, needs, and features of personality. Klein argued that projective testing cannot pinpoint types of personality organization, specific personality characteristics, or the diagnosis of mental disorders [29]. Further, the TAT has failed to show satisfactory validity, and in Klein's view too little work has been done with the Rorschach to assess its validity with children. Given our state of knowledge, it is certainly unjustified to rely on projective test results to rule out the presence of disorders when symptoms are evident, or to assume from the tests that personality deviance is present when it is not shown in the child's behavior. For diagnosis, Klein maintained that projective tests are not useful except in instances of mental retardation and specific developmental disorders. She maintained that when test results can be used accurately to diagnose, the deviance may already be obvious [29]. Similarly, it is unreliable to reconstruct the child's early developmental psychologic history based on projective tests or to use projective tests to predict what is likely to happen to a child.

Despite the strength of the previous criticism, projective tests are used extensively. So what is the usefulness of these procedures? Projective tests can first and foremost provide a structured format for assessing a child's reactions and observing his or her behavior. It takes the focus off the child and the need for verbal response and instead allows the child to engage in action-oriented activity. Thus, the child can be more comfortable and spontaneous. Second, projective tests allow the psychologist to understand more about the individual child's worldview. The Rorschach provides information on processing, and the TAT provides information on interpersonal relationships. Third, the structural approach, as exemplified by Exner, fulfills criteria of the scientific method [30]. Projective

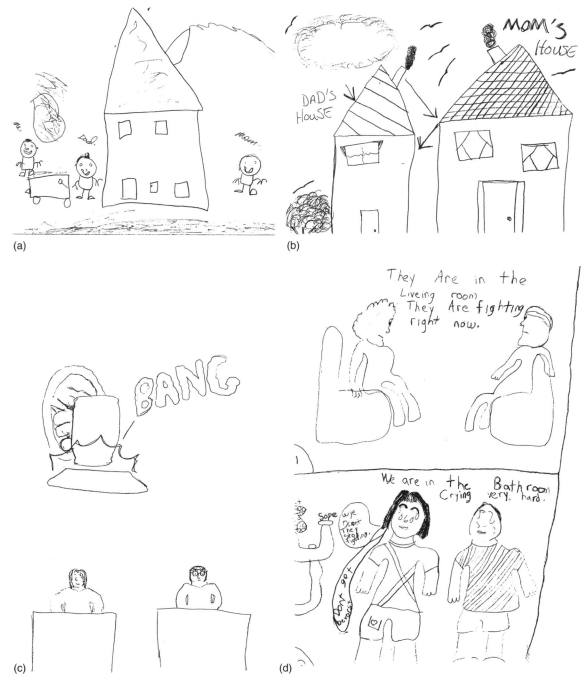

Figure 2.2 (a), seven-year-old boy, Scale I – acknowledgment, 0 = no direct reference to divorce; (b), 13-year-old girl, Scale I – acknowledgment, 1 = divorce clearly acknowledged; (c), 12-year-old boy, Scale II – emotionality, 0 = no emotion directly depicted; (d), seven-year-old girl, Scale II – emotionality, 1 = emotion shown.

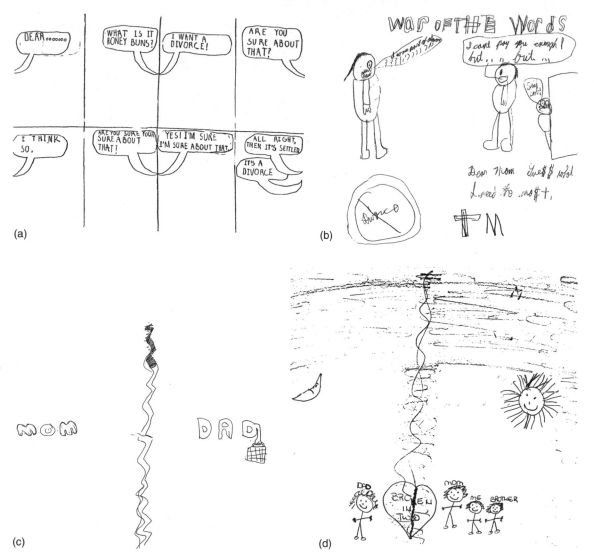

Figure 2.3 (a), nine-year-old boy, Scale III – aggression, 0 = no idication of aggression, conflict, or fighting; (b), 11-year-old boy, Scale III – aggression, 1 = aggression, conflict, or fighting depicted; (c), 12-year-old girl, Scale IV – use of people, 0 = no people pictured; (d), teenage girl, Scale IV – use of people, 1 = people pictured.

information can be useful in planning the treatment process and in identifying important goals and effective strategies.

Projective tests appear to be particularly useful for children who are anxious or depressed or who have a history of abuse and neglect. One area in which projective tests can be quite misleading, however, is in the assessment of children with conduct disorders. From a clinical perspective, these children often have projective test responses that reflect a wide range of feelings and

reactions and do not seem substantially different from those of children with other diagnoses. Their responses may not necessarily reveal the characteristics that could be considered indicators of conduct disorder. In fact, 'projective techniques do not enjoy widespread use for conduct disorders' (p. 301 [31]). This may be unfortunate, because the child's worldview can still significantly affect the treatment process.

Exner and Weiner discussed the nature of the Rorschach test and on what basis Rorschach interpretations can be justified [32]. The Rorschach was developed as a psychodynamic reflection of personality. It is now viewed as a 'perceptual–cognitive task,' however, and we can be more certain in our interpretation of the Rorschach results. When the Rorschach is viewed as a perceptual–cognitive task, the ink blots are considered an ambiguous source of stimulation in which the client imposes structure and organization; interpretations are based on the structure of how individuals process stimuli. Rorschach scoring allows us to derive data on how individuals perceive and respond to their environment. We can then draw inferences about personality functioning, including traits, dispositions, coping styles, and sources of concern that lend consistency to individual behavior.

When interpreting the Rorschach, clinicians need to be aware of situational and developmental factors that influence the stability of the Rorschach indices. Rorschach results generally give a picture of stable personality characteristics. The results are also representative of behavior; the task presented on the test is a sample of behavior, and behavior is the best predictor of future behavior. Interpretations on the Rorschach are reasonably certain and require 'very few levels of inference' [32].

When the Rorschach is viewed as a stimulus to fantasy, different guidelines are applied in the analysis, and interpretations may be based on Rorschach content. What individuals say as they respond with images is particularly revealing. Content interpretations come from the language or words that the individuals use and can be used to address personality dynamics; in this sense, Rorschach responses can also be viewed as symbolic of behavior. Interpretations should be relatively speculative and phrased only as hypotheses. Interpreters should remember that the two forms of interpretation have differing levels of certainty.

Special consideration should be used to guide the evaluation of Rorschach records obtained from younger clients. Knowledge of the normative data is critical. The proper procedures must be used in collecting the data, and the interpreters working with children should have a solid understanding of developmental psychology and developmental psychopathology. (Exner and Weiner argued, however, that 'Rorschach behavior means what it means regardless of the age of the subject' [32]).

The TAT requires patients to examine picture cards and then devise stories inspired by the cards. Henry's book *The Analysis of Fantasy* described how stories reflect thought processes as well as emotional functioning [33]. The interpretation of thematic appercep-

tion uses the overlapping frameworks of private, or less conscious, motives and the public, more conscious approach to social interactions. Thus, the stories are derived from personal experiences as translated into our social world [33].

Individuals learn societal expectations through a series of daily interactions in which skills and feelings are required. As individuals learn to conform to these expectations, they develop and organize their own personality. Their personality receives and processes the demands of social interaction and is also projected outward onto behavior, including responding to the TAT cards, for example. Telling stories is similar to the tasks involved in typical social interactions; in other words, the individual responds to the pictures in terms of both personal significance and 'cultural training.' People respond to the TAT pictures according to their own techniques of adapting to emotions and social demands as well as the manifest content and latent content of the pictures. For some people, the form and content of the picture draw emotional reactions that are termed the latent stimulus of the picture. Thus, the TAT is able to produce material that reflects the deeper emotional issues of the individual as stories are told.

Henry discussed analyzing TAT stories in terms of form, content, and dynamic structure, including the interpretation of symbolic content [33]. In the conceptual framework for individual case analysis, Henry considered several areas: mental approach, imaginative processes, family dynamics, inner adjustment, emotional reactivity, sexual adjustment, behavioral approach, and descriptive interpretive summary [33].

Children generally enjoy the TAT, because they find it relatively undemanding and nonthreatening. Some five- and six-year-olds can handle the TAT cards, as opposed to the CAT. Stories are often a transparent reflection of a child's point of view. Occasionally, a child will exclaim, 'This is just like me!' In these instances, children typically proceed comfortably with their storytelling. The TAT is a popular technique clinically. It may bias toward stimulating negatively toned stories, however, and the cards themselves are somewhat dated.

The Roberts Apperception Test for Children (RATC) is also a popular projective test to aid in assessing the psychological development of children [34]. The RATC was specifically designed for children age 6 through 15 years and depicts children in all 16 of the cards. The current set of stimulus cards was drawn up in 1968 and later compared by Roberts to the Children's Apperception Test and the Thematic Apperception Test. The cards are realistic drawings of children and adults engaged in everyday interpersonal events. The RATC is easily scored with objective measures and a high degree of agreement between raters. Its goal is to assess children's perceptions of interpersonal situations. The scoring system assesses both adaptive and maladaptive traits. There is both qualitative and quantitative interpretation, so structural analysis is possible. There is normative data for a sample of 200 well-adjustment children ages 6 through 15 years. The categories depicted on the cards include: Family Confrontation; Maternal Support; School Attitude; Support/Aggressions; Parental Affection; Peer/Racial Interaction; Dependency/Anxiety; Family Conferences; Physical Aggression Toward Peer; Sibling Rivalry; Fear; Parental Conflict/Depression; Aggression Release; Maternal Limit-Setting; Nudity/Sexuality; and Paternal Support.

The CAT was designed for children aged 3–10 years and was inspired by the TAT [35]. It was hypothesized that children would identify easily with animal figures. A set of 10 pictures of animals in a variety of situations is used with an apperception method that studies personality by examining individual differences in response to standard stimuli and the dynamic significance of these differences. The CAT provides data on how children relate to the key individuals in their life and to their own needs. The cards stimulate issues related to eating, sibling rivalry, relationships to parents as individuals and as a couple, aggression, acceptance of the adult world, loneliness at night, and toileting.

Like the TAT, the CAT is concerned with content and what children see and think. The developers of the CAT acknowledge that it may not facilitate formal diagnosis like the Rorschach, but it is 'better able to reveal the dynamics of interpersonal relationships, of drive constellation, and the nature of defenses against them' (p. 2 [35]). The animal pictures are equally applicable for all groups of children, so the CAT is 'relatively culture free' [35]. The examiner tells the child, 'We are going to engage in a game in which [you have] to tell a story about pictures; [you] should tell what is going on, what the animals are doing now.' At suitable points, the child may be asked what went on in the story before and what will happen later (p. 2 [35]).

More recently, cards with human figures have been provided [36]. Some preliminary studies have indicated that human figures may have greater stimulus value than drawings of animals. Some children may do better with the animal cards and some with the human ones; the regular CAT is recommended for use first. The CAT-Human Figures, however, might be considered for children 7–10 years of age or those who are particularly bright; it is available when the CAT has not yielded satisfactory results or vice versa. The Children's Apperception Test, Supplemental (CAT-S) is also available for exploring special circumstances such as physical disability, psychosomatic disorder, or the mother's pregnancy [37].

The Projective Storytelling Cards are useful in depicting a wide array of situations [38]. The 25 cards represent a variety of themes dealing with problems that children and teens face, with a focus on traumatic events, conflict in the family or social arena, and possible physical and sexual abuse. These cards can be used at any time during treatment, but they are especially useful for diagnosis and for establishing rapport. They have the goal of inspiring children to express their feelings, attitudes, and experiences in thematic form. The cards are particularly useful in helping children set goals to cope with physically or sexually abusive situations.

The Adoption Story Cards developed by R. Gardner can be used diagnostically as well as therapeutically to evoke issues relating to adoption [39]. This is a particularly difficult area to assess, since denial is often very strong. The cards were designed to provide the therapist with some access to information that children may otherwise be resistant to reveal.

Child Questionnaires

The Incomplete Sentences Blank forms are useful for young people in high school or college [40]. The Sentence Completion Test for Children has been used in this practice for the past 25 years (Appendix 2.3). It is a simple, two-page sentence completion form with 25 items. It is useful for children ages 5 through 12 years. For some children, it may help for clinicians to read the questions out loud and write down the child's responses. Other children, particularly older children or those who seem very private, might respond more openly by doing it themselves in their own handwriting. In one evaluation, an 11-year-old girl gave as little response as possible on all other assessment tools, including an interview. The sentence completions, however, were extremely revealing about the depth of feeling and dissatisfaction toward her parents and family. It was the only time in the entire evaluation process during which she shared these feelings.

The Child Anxiety Scale (CAS) can be useful in some instances for children 5 through 12 years of age [41]. It involves 20 straightforward questions in which a child marks on either a red circle or a blue circle. It can be administered through a tape or by the clinician. Children who are very anxious, however, may base their responses on denial. CAS users need to note extremely high or extremely low scores: high scores consistently reflect a high level of anxiety; and low scores could indicate a high anxiety level that is being systematically denied. Further, studies have shown that children may often resist reporting negative experiences and instead present a favorable view that may underestimate their actual anxiety levels.

The Children's Depression Inventory (CDI) is the most popular child questionnaire for assessing depression in children [42]. It was developed by Kovacs based on the Beck Depression Inventory for adults [43]. The long form has 27 items, and a short form (CDI-S) has 10 items. It is suitable for children 7–17 years of age and requires only a third-grade reading level, the lowest of any childhood depression measure. For each item, children choose one of three statements reflecting minimal, moderate, or severe depression in the past two weeks. The items pertain to depressive symptoms such as a negative mood, a lack of pleasure, sleeping or eating disturbances, their self-image, and behavior with peers or at school. There are high positive correlations of test scores with self-reported anxiety and negative correlations of test scores with self-esteem. Self-esteem, defined as the 'extent to which the individual believes himself to be capable, significant, successful, and worthy' (p. 5 [44]) is measured by items such as 'I'm doing the best work that I can,' 'I'm pretty sure of myself,' 'I wish I were someone else,' and 'I often get discouraged in school.' Self-esteem involves a personal assessment of worthiness and capability that is apparent in the beliefs and attitudes that children maintain toward themselves. Although the CDI has been shown to be a reliable measure of distress and depressive symptoms, it should not be used alone to diagnose depression.

Following a social learning analysis, Harter discussed how competence motivation leads children toward independent attempts at mastery [45]. They may receive positive or negative feedback from several sources, including their own assessment of the outcome as well as the reactions of others. Positive feedback leads to feelings of success, renewed efforts, an inner sense of capability, and worthiness or high self-esteem. Overly negative feedback can lead to a sense of failure and lower competence motivation. It can contribute to a tendency to avoid challenges, to depend on others to solve problems, and ultimately, to fail more often – low self-esteem.

Among the self-esteem inventories, the Culture-Free Self-Esteem Inventory can be useful in assessment and preassessment for both individual and group treatment [46]. The Piers–Harris Self-Concept Inventory is also available. With self-esteem measures, however, there is a strong tendency for children to report what they think the adult wants to hear or they themselves want to believe [47]. Such inventories may be less revealing of deeper feelings than many other assessment tools.

Seligman and colleagues emphasized success at performance and accomplishment as a pivotal component of self-esteem [48]. They did not support the theory that we can 'give' our children self-esteem by seeking only to help them 'feel good' and instead designed a program for children to learn the skills of optimism. Their Children's Attributional Style Questionnaire measures aspects of self-esteem based on performance capability rather than the 'feel good' school of thought. Attitudes toward self and events contribute to the experience of success.

Kurdek and Berg developed a helpful assessment tool for children of divorce who are 5–18 years of age [49]. The Children's Beliefs About Parental Divorce Scale has six scales that reflect peer avoidance, paternal blame, fear of abandonment, maternal blame, hopes of reunification, self-blame, as well as a total score for maladaptive attitudes. The questionnaire allows questions to be structured around divorce and is therefore more revealing than generic questions that do not relate to divorce specifically, or questions that make children feel put on the spot or require them to 'criticize' their parents. This scale has been used in our office since it was developed and has been found useful even when the divorce occurred at some considerable time in the past.

Behavioral Assessment

The behavioral assessment of children follows a problem-solving strategy. It is an empirical approach to clinical child assessment, utilizing what we know of child development and developmental psychopathology. Behavioral assessment allows for the evaluation of treatment outcome and can improve the effectiveness of services for children. Certain concepts are pivotal, such as the importance of situational influences, direct observation of behavior, and treatment evaluation. This is a rapidly emerging field that is still refining techniques for clinical practice. Accurate observations and objectivity in reporting are guiding principles. Behavioral assessment does not rely on inferences or underlying personality constructs but is instead concerned with the child's actual behavior in certain situations.

For example, in the behavioral assessment of enuresis, it is helpful to inquire whether children sleep in their own room or with siblings, where they sleep relative to their parents' bedrooms, and the time at which the children and their parents go to bed. Further, it is important to assess what children know about the problem and the treatment. They may feel that the bedwetting is their fault. Do they realize that it is a common problem among other children? Projective assessment can be used to determine how concerned children are about bedwetting and how much they want to be cured. Sometimes embarrassment or denial can lead parents to feel that their children are indifferent to the symptoms. Also, when children are dry sleeping away from home, the parents might think that they are bedwetting on purpose at home. Usually, however, children simply sleep less soundly in an effort to prevent the bedwetting away from home.

When treating encopresis, the clinician should assess the frequency of the problem, when it occurs during the day or night, how much occurs, and variations in the pattern. The clinician should also ask who has the responsibility for the clean-up. Further, the clinician should inquire of the parents the exact words used in talking to the child as well as what the child actually does in response. The parents can keep a behavioral record for a week to answer some of these questions. Since this is an extremely frustrating symptom for parents, their tolerance level has usually been exceeded, and they may be extremely angry and frustrated. It is important for the clinician to be able to get past the emotional reactions into a more objective evaluation of what is actually occurring. In addition, it is important to assess how emotions are handled generally within the family. A merely mechanistic record of behavior cannot by itself be definitive.

Another symptom that can be usefully evaluated from a behavioral perspective is children's fears. One useful method with school-age children six years and older as well as teenagers is to use systematic desensitization, beginning with constructing a rank ordering of fears. For older children, a 10-point scale can be used, with '10' indicating the situation in which they would feel the most fear and '1' the situation in which they would feel the most relaxed and comfortable. As children are selecting situations to put on their scale, their reactions and feelings in many situations can be effectively diagnosed. This simple assessment can then be used in a systematic desensitization routine in which the child is taught a method of relaxation and then imagines a situation on the scale and practices relaxing. This is an instance in which assessment and treatment are closely combined. Given the aversiveness of

anxious reaction, this approach is often used immediately in treating an anxious child.

There are refined behavioral techniques for assessing obsessive–compulsive disorder (OCD) in childhood [50]. The Leyton Obsessional Inventory-Child Version and the 20-item Leyton Obsessional Inventory are extremely helpful in assessment and treatment planning [50]. In addition, the Yale–Brown Obsessive–Compulsive Scale has specific instructions for children [50]. There is also a National Institute of Mental Health (NIMH) Teacher Rating of OCD [50].

Behavioral assessment of conduct disorders in children has expanded rapidly in recent years (Table 2.6). Atkeson and Forehand discussed characteristics of conduct-disordered children, which include a high rate of negative commands, disapproval, humiliation, noncompliance, negativism, teasing, physically negative acts, and yelling, as well as high-intensity deviant behavior such as destructiveness [51].

These children also exhibit a low frequency of positive behavior, such as approval expressed to others, positive attention, independent activity, laughing, and talking. Further, 'in the negative reinforcement model, coercive behavior on the part of one family member is reinforced when it results in the removal of an aversive event being applied to another family member'(p. 188 [51]). Three strategies have been employed in the assessment process; behavioral interviews, behavioral questionnaires, and behavioral observations; see Holland's Interview Guide (p. 1951 [51]). Behavioral questionnaires have included the Becker Bipolar Adjective Checklist [51], Parent Attitude Test [51], Walker Problem Behavior Identification Checklist [51], and Behavior Problem Checklist [51]. Direct observations of parent–child interactions are considered the most valid source of data.

Researchers have developed elaborate coding systems for research in the home environment, such as the Family Interaction Coding System by Patterson and colleagues [52]. Since few clinical settings have the resources for this, structured clinical observations of parent–child interactions are instead recommended. One simple technique that can be used is the Behavior Management Questionnaire, completed by parents, which covers the activities and interests of the child and disciplinary practices of the parents. This was developed for use with autistic children [53].

Barkley presented an extensive training program for parents of children who have behavior problems, including ADHD and conduct disorders [54,55]. Decreasing noncompliance, decreasing disruptiveness, and increasing independent play are major components of the program. Children are also taught a 'think

Table 2.6 Selected measures of antisocial behaviors for children and adolescents.

Measure	Response format	Age range*	Special features
Children's Hostility Inventory†	38 true–false statements assessing different facets of aggression and hostility.	6–13 yr	Derived from Buss-Durke Hostility Guilt Inventory. A priori subscales from that scale comprise factors that relate to overt acts (aggression) and aggressive thoughts and feelings (hostility).
REPORTS OF OTHERS			
Eyberg Child Behavior Inventory	36 items rated on 1 to 7 points scale for frequency and whether the behavior is a problem.	2–17 yr	Designed to measure wide range of conduct problems in the home.
Sutter-Eyberg Student Behavior Inventory	36 items identical in format but not content to the Eyberg Child Behavior Inventory.	2–17 yr	Measures a range of conduct problem behaviors at school.
Peer Nomination of Aggression	Items that ask children to nominate others who show the characteristics (e.g., 'Who starts a fight over nothing'?).	3rd through 13th grade	Items reflect the child's reputation among peers regarding overall aggression. Different versions of peer nominations have been used.
DIRECT OBSERVATIONS			
Adolescent Antisocial Behavior Checklist	57 items to measure antisocial behavior during hospitalization. Behaviors are rated as having occurred or not based on staff observations.	Adolescence	The items can be scored using different sets of subscales; one set focuses on the form of the problems (e.g., physical vs. verbal harm); another set focuses on the objects of aggression (e.g., toward self, others, property). Different versions are available and differ in scoring.
Family Interaction Coding System (FICS)	Direct observational system to measure occurrence or nonoccurrence of 29 specific parent–child behaviors in the home. Each behavior is scored within small	3–12 yr	Individual behaviors are observed but usually summarized with a total aversive behavior score. The general procedure can be adopted using some or all of the behaviors of the FICS.

Table 2.6 *Continued*

Measure	Response format	Age range*	Special features
	intervals for an hour each day for a period of several days.		
Parent Daily Report	Parents identify symptoms of antisocial behavior. After symptoms are identified, the parent is called daily for several days. Each day the parent is asked if each behavior has or has not occurred in previous 24-hr period.	3–12 yr	Measure does not reflect a standardized set of items but rather refers more to an assessment approach for collecting date on behaviors at home.
SELF-REPORT			
Children's Action Tendency Scale	30 items in forced-choice format, child selects what he or she would do in interpersonal situations.	6–15 yr	Scores for response dimensions: aggressiveness, assertiveness, and submissiveness.
Adolescent Antisocial Self-Report Behavior Checklist	52 items, each of which is rated by the child on a 5-point scale (from never to very often).	Adolescence	The measure samples a broad range of behaviors from mild misbehavior to serious antisocial acts. The items load four factors: delinquency, drug usage, parental defiance, and assaultiveness.
Self-Report Delinquency Scale	47 items that measure frequency with which individual has performed offenses included in the Uniform Crime Reports. Responses provide frequency with which behavior was performed over the last year.	11–21 yr	Measure has been developed as part of the National Youth Survey, an extensive longitudinal study of delinquent behavior, alcohol and drug use, and related problems in American youths.
Minnesota Multiphasic Personality Inventory Scales	True–false items derived from Scales F (test-taking attitude), 4 (psychopathic deviate) and 9 (hypomania) are summed to yield an aggression/ delinquency score.	Adolescence	Part of more general measure that assesses multiple areas of psychopathology.

Table 2.6 *Continued*

Measure	Response format	Age range*	Special features
Interview for Aggression†	Semistructured interview, 30 items pertaining to aggression such as getting into fights, starting arguments. Each item rated on a 5-point scale for severity and 3-point scale for duration.	6–13 yr	Yields scores for severity, duration, and total (serverity + duration) aggression. Separate factors assess overt and covert behaviors.

* The age ranges are tentative and derived from the ages of cases reported rather than inherent restrictions of the measure.
† This measure has separate versions: (1) a self-report measure for children, and (2) a parent-report measure to evaluate children's behavior.
From Kazdin AE: Conduct disorder. In: Ollendick TH, Herson M, eds. *Handbook of Child and Adolescent Assessment*. Boston: Allyn & Bacon; 1993:295. Copyright ® 1993 by Allyn & Bacon. Reprinted by permission.

aloud-think ahead' self-control technique. Parents may be trained in the office, but in-home practice methods are also an integral part of the program.

Useful assessment tools of Barkley's program include the Parent–Child Interaction Interview Form, Home Situations Questionnaire, Parent's and Teacher's Questionnaire, and School Situations Questionnaire [55]. In addition, there are behavioral sheets for observing the parents and child together, which include Recording Observations of Parent–Child Interactions and Coding Form for Recoding Parent–Child Interactions. Barkley also assists parents in understanding their problems through the Profile of Child and Parent Characteristics and the Family Problems Inventory [55].

Kazdin stresses that the assessment of conduct disorders should be multimodal [31]. The process should include different methods (interviews and direct observations), perspectives (child, parent, and teacher) domains (affect, cognition, and behavior), and settings (home, school, and community). Further, prosocial behavior and adaptive skills should be assessed as well as the theory that 'antisocial behavior is not merely the opposite of prosocial behavior' (p. 392 [31]).

Play Observations

The importance of play and the use of imagination in child development cannot be overstated. The use of fantasy enables children to delay gratification and to deal more effectively with frustration, which in turn has implications for their success in the classroom [56]. By studying preschool children, Parten identified five ways that children play: (1) in solitary play, children are unaware of others and play alone; (2) in onlooker play, children watch others play; (3) in parallel play, children play side by side with little interaction; (4) in associative play, children interact and share; and (5) in cooperative play, they relate to each other, helping and taking turns [57]. Piaget described three types of play – practice games, symbolic games, and games with rules – through which children learn the rules of social exchange and enhance their sense of competence and self-esteem [58].

It has long been recognized that children use play as their natural medium of self-expression and as an avenue for cognitive development. It can therefore be useful to incorporate some opportunity to observe unstructured play in child assessment procedures. Typically, a doll house, large blocks, and trucks can be used. Children's personalities are revealed in the way that they approach these materials. Straightforward observation of their behavior can indicate how they typically behave in similar situations. Some children are quiet and resilient, seeking permission before beginning play, whereas others race rambunctiously into the thick of it, with nary a thought to protocol or manners. Some children play quietly without verbalization, whereas others talk constantly.

Clinicians can use some of their own feelings and reactions to the child to diagnose potential problem areas, as demonstrated by the following case study.

CASE STUDY

A six-year-old girl was demanding and bossy with her therapist; she would sweetly ask the therapist to play with her and seemed dependent in this respect. Every time the therapist picked up a toy to begin to play or make some independent gesture, however, the girl would give orders for it to be done differently. The therapist, being very accommodating, tried to comply, only to find herself feeling irritated. Finally, the therapist identified that this little girl was likely to be bossy and demanding in a sweet way in her interactions with both peers and adults. This became a major focus of the treatment plan.

The themes of play can also be meaningful, although the style of approaching the play materials should be observed as well.

Many youngsters who come for assessment and treatment have difficulties engaging in pretend play. Their play doesn't hang together; it may seem disconnected, a fragmented puzzle, hardly a way for them to learn about themselves and the world around them (p. 153 [59]). Different ways of using play in diagnosis and treatment have been presented that offer observation of the child's verbal and nonverbal reactions, thought process and decision making, style in using materials, nature and content of play, and interaction with the clinician. Children reveal individualized aspects of personality in their responses as well as in their interests and preferences.

Behar and Rapoport discussed the usefulness of summarizing play behavior of young children as a general clinical screening tool: 'The diagnostic play interview seems particularly important for children before they have found more adult, or structured, outlets' (p. 193 [60]). These authors recommended play assessment when: (1) parents and teachers offer conflicting reports; (2) reports and clinical observation differ; (3) verbal communication is inadequate or the child is too young; or (4) when there is shyness or withdrawal in the child's behavior. Children's play can reveal: (1) the style of interaction with a parent; (2) the style of separation from parent; (3) the style of relating to the examiner; (4) the use of toys in play; (5) spontaneous behavior; and (6) play behaviors relevant to the diagnosis [51]. Play may be particularly useful in diagnosing young or nonverbal children.

In an extensive manual, Schaefer and colleagues presented a variety of uses for the assessment of play [61].

There are articles on scales for developmental play, diagnostic play, parent–child interaction, peer interaction, projective play assessment, and play therapy. As noted by Westby, the 'evaluation of children's play skills permits assessment not only of the knowledge children have, but also of how they use this knowledge in a real-world context' (p. 133 [62]). The Westby Symbolic Play Scale presents developmental levels for play shown by children from eight months to five years of age [62].)

Family Interaction

Family interaction should be considered in any assessment of children. Family sessions can be used for diagnostic purposes and are also particularly useful when working with children and their parents to teach child management techniques for externalizing disorders such as ADHD and oppositional defiant disorder (ODD). In all families, however, the child's role within the family strongly affects his or her feelings, attitudes, and behaviors, and clinicians should assess these characteristics when planning for treatment. Baumrind demonstrated that a child's characteristics are closely related to the structure of that child's family [63], and Hetherington and Parke compared parenting styles with children's behavior and self-esteem [64]. Clinicians often assess the child individually, although others advocate 'incorporating family assessment into comprehensive child assessment' (p. 136 [65]). The latter approach may make it more difficult to develop a rapport with the child or teenager, however. Both approaches have their advantages and disadvantages. In general, it is important for the individual conducting the assessment to be aware of certain common family patterns that can influence a child's behavior.

It is important for clinicians to assess parental warmth, a factor important to the child in terms of seeking approval. Parents showing this warmth may be more likely to provide information about alternative social responses available to the child. 'Warm' parents also frequently use reasoning and explanations that permit children to internalize social rules and to identify and discriminate situations in which a given behavior is appropriate. Warmth is likely to be associated with responsiveness to the child's needs. Warm parents do not have to resort to methods that are frustrating to the child, and children are less likely to avoid contact with the parents; this facilitates the socialization process.

Clinicians should also evaluate parental control. Parental restrictiveness or permissiveness can lead to problems in child functioning. A permissive family can cause problems of neglect and may also damage a child's adaptive ability. Authoritarian family approaches may have the advantage of preparing children to deal with rules and limits but the disadvantage of limiting overall competence.

In families of neglect, the mother often exhibits depression and detachment. Depressed mothers have difficulty finding the energy to take care of their children. Parental detachment may be encouraged by our narcissistic culture that gives permission for seeking personal gratification before the needs of others. Divorce also contributes to parental neediness.

Beavers and Hampson presented a paradigm for analyzing family interaction in terms of overall competence and family style [66]. Family style relates to the positioning of the family in the community: centripetal families bind their members to the family, making any absence difficult; and centrifugal families expel the child from the family before individuation is complete. Family style and level of competence are used to classify families into types that may be relevant to the problems shown by offspring. For example, it is hypothesized that severely centrifugal families often have sociopathic offspring.

Beavers and Hampson developed a comprehensive scale to rate the nature of family interaction, termed the Beavers Interactional Scale: Family Competence and Family Style [66]. This scale is used by clinicians and allows ratings on the following dimensions: (1) structure of the family (specifically overt power, parental coalitions, and closeness); (2) mythology; (3) goal-directed negotiation; (4) autonomy, including clarity of expression, responsibility, and permeability; and (5) family affect, assessed through range of feelings, mood and tone, unresolvable conflict, and empathy. In addition, the Global Health-Pathology Scale includes a Self-Report Family Inventory and an Individual Family Style Scale for family members to fill out, which can be useful in the assessment process [66]. The Self-Report Family Inventory (SFI) includes a scoring system for health/competence, conflict, cohesion, leadership, and expressiveness [66]. A similar test that can be used in family sessions, called FACES II, was developed by Olson and colleagues at the Department of Family Social Science at the University of Minnesota [67]. It yields information on family cohesion and adaptability, indicating family type.

A discussion of family interaction would not be complete without considering the profound effect of extended family interaction, both for children who have an intact nuclear family and for those who are being raised by other family members including grandparents. Further, extended family members may share in the upbringing of children significantly. These trends appear to be increasingly prominent. As clinicians, we see many children who are being raised by their grandparents. We also see many situations that are essentially shared parenting between parents and grandparents or other family members.

Grandparents may be raising children when they have little access to resources outside of their own family. In addition, in many states there is no legal provision for grandparents to have parental rights or legal rights to parenting time. In some situations, it even makes sense for a parent and grandparents to have shared parenting with each other. This can be a useful arrangement, but Courts may be reluctant to encourage these arrangements without legal procedure that require cooperation between family members.

Special Issues

Social Skills and ADHD

It has recently been estimated that there are over two million school-age children in the United States alone with ADHD [68].) These are children who show significant behavioral problems that are very stressful for family life. There is often conflict over chores, homework, and getting along with siblings, with the ADHD child showing antagonistic behavior at school and in the neighborhood. Further, ADHD children typically have difficulties modulating their own emotional reactions. Such intense reactions create difficulties in social relationships. Children with ADHD tend not to see the connection between their behavior and the outcome, whereas other children learn this automatically. Low self-esteem results from the negative reactions of others, and specific social skills are lacking in children with ADHD.

There is a wide variety of social skills, including communication skills, sharing, social initiation, joining strategies, determining appropriate behavior for a given situation, listening and asking questions about ambiguous messages, smiling, sharing, positive physical contact, verbal complimenting, using instructions, modeling, praise, labeling emotions and facial expressions, referential communication accuracy, taking perspective, listening, making friends (including greeting), asking for information, including extension, giving information, giving help, and being observant of appropriate classroom behavior. Children with ADHD may be deficient in any number of these skills. Sometimes they have acquired certain steps but not the entire sequence of behaviors necessary for positive social exchange.

Fortunately, there has been great interest in developing procedures for enhancing children's interpersonal relationships with peers, since having well-developed social skills corresponds to fewer mental health problems. Popular children behave in specific ways, initiate interactions, smile, and make positive comments. The fact that children can be taught social skills has been applied to a wide variety of problems and disorders, including ADHD.

A variety of intervention strategies have been used to effectively teach social skills. These include contingent positive reinforcement, modeling, coaching and behavioral rehearsal, and peer initiation. The first step is to evaluate the strengths and weaknesses of each child individually, as there is a wide variety of specific deficits.

Social skills can be evaluated using the Social Skills Rating System for parents, teachers, and children [(69]. Behaviors that influence a child's social capability and adaptive skills at home and school can be assessed systematically, which can help in further assessment and treatment planning as well as the outcome evaluation of individual or group intervention. Teacher and parent forms are available for preschool, kindergarten through grade 6, and grades 7 through 12. Separate self-rating forms are available for students in grades 3 through 6 and in grades 7 through 12. Prosocial behaviors that are assessed include cooperation, assertion, responsibility, empathy, and self-control.

Goldstein and colleagues' skillstreaming material allows for the assessment of a wide variety of specific social skills [70]. There are 50 social skills that can be taught, and the curriculum even includes listening! The Structured Learning Skill Checklist is used in the assessment process.

Adolescents

Teens may be reluctant to sit and talk about their feelings and experiences with a grown-up, particularly a professional. They generally respond well to structured assessment procedures, however, including drawings, projective tests, and sentence completions. Establishing rapport is possible by allowing teens 'space' to express themselves in their own way.

The Millon Adolescent Clinical Inventory (MACI) for teens 13–19 years is both useful and relatively short, consisting of only 160 items [71]. The recent revision gives information on borderline tendencies and abuse experiences. The four new personality scales for the MACI measure self-demeaning, forceful, doleful, and borderline tendencies. The majority of teens complete the MACI easily. Occasionally, a younger teenager makes a comment implying that they do not know how to answer the items relating to sex, such as 'I enjoy thinking about sex,' or 'Sex is enjoyable.' It is helpful to review the form carefully before sending it in for computer analysis, because some teenagers leave too many items blank. It is important for the teens to have a sense about why they are going through the assessment process. There will occasionally be difficulty with compliance, in which case it is best to move on to other assessment methods. We have found the narrative description of personality provided by the MACI to be accurate and useful in treatment planning. It includes a section on pointers for psychotherapy as well.

There is a new Millon assessment tool available January, 2005, for younger preteens ages 9–12 years called the Millon Pre-Adolescent Clinical Inventory (M-PACI) [72].) It contains fewer than 100 questions and takes only 15–20 minutes for youngsters to finish. It has been validated and there are up-to-date national norms with a detailed interpretative report for the clinician. The M-PACI focuses on clinical problems comprehensively, not just a single issue, and identifies emerging personality styles that will aid the clinician in planning intervention and pinpointing effective methods.

Teens can be engaged in assessment and treatment if the goals are defined on their terms. Many teens like the idea of 'learning more' about themselves. Psychoeducational assessment can also be interesting to them as a way of developing strategies for success in school and planning for college (viewed as a chance to be away from home!).

Of particular interest to teens are the personality styles of the Myers-Briggs Type Indicator [73].) This is a 'nonpathologizing' measure of personality. Its analysis of personality types provides a comprehensive theory of personality functioning by describing four types of mental processes: sensing (S), intuition (N), thinking (T), and feeling (F). Sensing is the ability to understand through observation and the senses; intuition is the conceptualization of possibilities; thinking is the process of linking ideas together in a logical way; and feeling is a more subjective process based on values. There are four basic personality types and the possibility of 16 subtypes when two additional dimensions are added (extrovert–introvert and judgment–perception). The four basic types of individuals are as follows: ST, sensing and thinking; SF, sensing and feeling; NF, intuition and feeling; NT, intuition and thinking. STs focus on facts and the use of interpersonal analysis. They tend to be practical and matter-of-fact and to develop technical skills with facts and objects. SFs focus on facts and the use of personal warmth. They tend to be sympathetic and friendly and emphasize practical help and services for people. NFs focus attention on possibilities and the use of personal warmth. They are enthusiastic and insightful and have strengths in understanding and communicating with people. NTs focus on possibilities by using impersonal analysis. They are logical and ingenious and emphasize theoretical and technical developments. Teens can be intrigued with learning more about themselves and, without realizing it, may apply this information to help them cope with their own lives.

Although teens may be anxious and avoid responsibility for planning for the future, they also typically lack skills for systematically addressing these issues. They often respond favorably to discussions on this topic as well as to specific assessment procedures such as the Harrington-O'Shea Career Decision-Making System-Revised [74]. In their responses to the Survey Booklet, teens express their likes and dislikes for many activities, and Career Clusters that match their interests are then suggested to the teens. Their interests only suggest jobs that they might like, however. Teens also need to consider ability, values, training, and employment outlook to make career decisions.

Such nonpathologizing ways of working with teens can be surprisingly effective. They learn problem-solving skills that can help them overcome their difficulties. The process also emphasizes teens' independence from their family and their own responsibility for their futures.

It is easy for mental health clinicians to sidestep the issues of substance abuse as they are facing a young and seemingly healthy individual who does not as yet typically show the long-term effects of substance use. To aid in assessing teens for substance abuse issues, the adolescent form of the Substance Abuse Subtle Screening Inventory (SASSI) is available for ages 12 through 18 year [75]. Many teenagers will give significant information regarding substance abuse habits on a questionnaire when they may volunteer no information in an interview. Teenagers may not spontaneously provide information but may provide information on their use if asked specific questions. However, the clinician may worry that it is easy to produce false positives by asking leading questions. Further, it is difficult to distinguish between the acting-out adolescent who is chemically dependent and the acting-out adolescent who is not.

Sexual Abuse

Evaluation for child sexual abuse should be comprehensive and cover all aspects of personality function-

ing. Such evaluations are extremely complex. Some of the following questionnaires may be useful as part of a comprehensive assessment.

Petty developed a Checklist for Child Abuse Evaluation [76]. This is an expensive questionnaire that covers all aspects of child abuse cases, including the following: the accuracy of validations by the reporter; interview with the child – physical or behavioral observations; interview with child – disclosure; child psychologic status; history and observed or reported characteristics of the accused; and credibility of the child – observed or reported. Conclusions cover the competence of the child as a witness, the level of stress on the child, and the protection of the child. Treatment recommendations are also included.

The Sex Abuse Legitimacy (SAL) Scale developed by Gardner attempts to differentiate between legitimate and fabricated child sexual abuse allegations [77]. It is most effective when the child, accuser, and accused all are interviewed. The scale is less valuable but may still be used, however, when the alleged perpetrator is unavailable. The SAL Scale was developed from studies conducted between 1982 and 1987 of children who made allegations of sexual abuse. It helps to organize data but does not produce a definitive conclusion and therefore should not be used as a questionnaire or a standardized psychological test. It can only be used as a guideline and should not be used as evidence in court proceedings.

Peterson [78] proposed a child dissociation problem checklist to be used in diagnosing the dissociation identity disorder now included in the *Diagnostic and Statistical Manual for Mental Disorders-Fourth Edition Text Revision* (DSM-IV-TR) [79]. The clinician may not be diagnosing this disorder in early childhood, because it is extremely rare and in fact may not exist in childhood. It may be misdiagnosed, exist along with another disorder, or have an atypical presentation in childhood (i.e., with fewer elaborate complex personalities and their alters). In addition, clinicians may not ask the appropriate questions to make an accurate diagnosis. For example, they should ask about missing blocks of time or other aspects of dissociation, and should also note if the child appears to be in a trance at any point. These experiences may not be discussed by children, owing to a fear of not being believed or being punished. There may be less differentiation between personality aberration and the age appropriate behaviors of a child.

The presentation of multiple personality disorder (MPD) in childhood may be different than in adulthood, since the common characteristics of MPD in adults are not present in children. These characteristics in adults include persecutor personalities, inner self-helper personalities, and special-purpose fragments and systems of personalities. There may also be somatic complaints and severe headaches. Putnam and colleagues developed a child dissociation scale to be completed by the parents [80].

Conclusion

Psychological testing allows the clinician to collect a wide range of information about the child both effi- ciently and in a standardized way. The data that are generated have specific applications and usefulness for diagnosis and treatment planning. A broad approach that includes multiple sources of data and allows us to understand children in the context of their lives is recommended. Since children do not have the facility or experience to fully express themselves verbally, we as clinicians are interested in their worldview and how it can be revealed to us.

Appendix 2.1 Assessment Protocol

PSYCHOEDUCATIONAL TESTING

Cognitive Tests

Stanford–Binet – 4th Edition
Wechsler Preschool and Primary Scale of Intelligence
Wechsler Intelligence Scale for Children – 3rd Edition Leiter – Revised
Peabody Picture Vocabulary Test
Bender Gestalt Test
Achievement Tests
Woodcock–Johnson – Revised
Wechsler Individual Achievement Test

Note: The average psychoeducational assessment can be completed in two sessions. Exceptions include teenagers, very bright 10–12-year-olds, and children experiencing unusual emotional reactions to testing. Be sure to prepare the parents that a third session for psychoeducational testing may be necessary.

PRESCHOOL (INFANCY TO FIVE YEARS)

First Session

Background information from parents or guardian
Questionnaires
Eyberg Child Behavior Inventory
Parenting Stress Index
Vineland Social Maturity Scale
Orientation

Second Session

Developmental measures
Bayley Scales of Infant Development
Stanford–Binet
Wechsler Preschool and Primary Scale of Intelligence
Kaufman

Third Session

Personality assessment
Drawing
Rorschach (use modified method with no inquiry)
Children's Apperception Test
Observation
Consider parent–child interaction

Fourth Session

Consultation with parents
Note: Assessment should be collapsed to three sessions when feasible.

SCHOOL-AGE (6–12 YEARS)

First Session

Background information from parents or guardian
Questionnaires
Eyberg Child Behavior Inventory
Parenting Stress Index
Achenbach
Attention–Deficit Disorders Evaluation Scale
Orientation with child
Testing with child
Draw-a-Person
Kinetic Family Drawing
Sentence Completion Test for Children

Second Session

Personality testing
Rorschach
Thematic Apperception Test
Interviewing

Third Session

Interviewing
Exploring treatment goals and possible intervention strategies and enlisting child's cooperation

Fourth Session

Consultation with parents and treatment planning

Note: Additional sessions are required for psychoeducational testing, but in this instance, another option is to collapse the second and third sessions into a one-hour session to reduce the number of sessions. Family interaction session frequently follows the consultation session with parents.

TEENS

First Session

Background information from parents
Achenbach (if needed)
Orientation with teen
Millon (some teens may not be ready)
Draw-A-Person
Kinetic Family Drawing
Rotter Sentence Completions

SECOND SESSION

Personality testing
Rorschach
Thematic Apperception Test
Interviewing

Third Session

Interviewing
Exploring treatment goals and possible intervention strategies (assess teen's preferences)
Fourth session
Consultation with parents and treatment planning (teen can be invited to participate in part of session)

Note: Modifying the protocol may be needed in crisis situations or with teens who are seriously uncomfortable. A family interaction session frequently follows the consultation session with parents.

Appendix 2.2 Interpretation of Drawings: Suggested Procedure

I. GLOBAL IMPRESSIONS (HOLISTIC VIEW)

Spontaneous selection of subject
Assigned topic

Pleasant effect of the whole
Unpleasant effect

Drawn from memory
Copied or imitating comic-strip character

Freely drawn and bold
Tiny and at bottom or well away from center

Elaborate
Limited

Vivid fantasy
Poor in content

Own sex drawn first in Draw-A-Person test
Other sex drawn first

Omission of self or other in family group
Inclusion of all members

Excessive shading
'Artistic' shading for modeling of figure

Static figures
Movement indicated

Full-face
Profile

Well-coordinated figure
Disjointed figure

Symmetry
    Preoccupation with perfect symmetry
    Excessive disregard

Quality of line
    Broken
    Continuous

Pressure
    Barely visible figure
    Well defined
    Heavy, may punch holes through paper

Velocity
    Speedy and careless
    Exasperatingly slow

Mood
    Peaceful
    Turbulent

Organization
    Orderly
    Chaotic

Composition
    Simple
    Complex

II. CONTENT (ITEM ANALYSIS OF HUMAN FIGURE)

Head
    Huge
    Disproportionately small

Eyes
    Large
    Small
    Empty
    With pupils

Ears
    Prominent
    Absent

Hair
    Abundant, coiffured
    Scribbled
    Scant, absent

Fingers
    Five, supernumerary or absent stick- or clawlike

Mouth
    Absent or emphasized
    Cosmetic or minimally represented

Arms
    Large, muscular
    Absent or sticklike

Legs
    Two or more
    Wide apart or close together

Crotch
    Excessive attention, erasures
    Shading, covered by hands

Trunk
    Absent or tiny, smaller than head
    Emphasized, organs or navel visible

Nose
    Absent or tiny
    Large, nostrils shown

Breasts
    Emphasized, firm or drooping
    Absent

Genitalia
    Suggested
    Explicitly shown, exaggerated
    Apparently ignored
    Concealed

Teeth
    Large, pointed
    Not visible

Clothing
    Appropriate
    Incongruous
    Profession or occupation shown
    Scant or absent
    Jewelry, ornaments

From DiLeo JH: *Interpreting Children's Drawings.* New York: Brunner/Mazel, 1983:217–220.

Appendix 2.3

SENTENCE COMPLETION TEST FOR CHILDREN

Name:

Date of Test:
  1. At times I feel . . .
  2. At home . . .
  3. Other kids . . .
  4. My mother . . .
  5. My biggest worry . . .
  6. I feel happy when . . .
  7. My dad . . .
  8. What I like best is . . .
  9. I cry . . .
  10. I get mad when . . .
  11. When I get mad, I . . .
  12. If I could do anything, I would . . .
  13. Boys . . .
  14. Daddy gets mad when . . .
  15. People are . . .
  16. I feel sad when . . .
  17. Girls . . .
  18. What bothers me is . . .
  19. Mommy gets mad when . . .
  20. When I get nervous, I . . .
  21. People think that I . . .
  22. I cannot . . .
  23. When I grow up . . .
  24. In school I . . .
  25. When I was little . . .

References

1. Mooney KC, Harrison AJ: A content of analysis of child psychological evaluations. *J Child Adolesc Psychother* 1987; **4**(4):275–282.
2. Eyberg SM, Ross AW: Assessment of child behavior problems: The validation of a new inventory. *J Clin Child Psychol* 1978; **7**:113–116.
3. Abidin RR: *Parenting Stress Index: Professional Manual.* 3rd ed. Odessa, FL: Psychological Assessment Resources, 1995.
4. Sheras PL, Abinin, RR, Konold, TR: *Stress Index for Parents of Adolescents: Professional Manual.* Odessa, FL: Psychological Assessment Resources, 1998.
5. Achenbach TM: *Manual for the Child Behavior Checklist/4–18 and 1991 Profile.* Burlington, VT: University of Vermont, 1991.
6. Achenbach, TM: *Manual for the Teacher's Report Form and Profile.* Burlington, VT: University of Vermont, 1991.
7. Achenbach, TM, Rescorla, LA: *Manual for ASEBA Preschool Forms & Profiles.* Burlington, VT: University of Vermont, 2000.
8. Conners CK: *Conners' Rating Scales-Revised.* North Tonawanda, NY: MHS, 1997.
9. McCarney SB: *ADDES.* 2nd ed. Columbus, MO: Hawthorne Educational Services, 1995.
10. Randolph EM: *Attachment Disorder Questionnaire.* 1993. Call 910/674–8045 for information.
11. Kaufman AS, Ishikuma T: Intellectual and achievement testing. In: Ollendick H, Hersen M, eds. *Handbook of Child and Adolescent Assessment.* Boston, MA: Allyn and Bacon, 1993:192–207.
12. Wechsler D: *Wechsler Intelligence Scale for Children-Fourth Edition: Manual.* New York: Harcourt Brace Jovanovich, 2003.
13. Wechsler, D: *Wechsler Preschool and Primary Scale of Intelligence-Third Edition: Manual.* San Antonio, TX: Harcourt Assessment, 2002.
14. Cordell AS, Cannon T: Gifted kids can't always spell. *Acad Ther* 1985; **21**(2):143–152.
15. Thorndike RL, Hagen EP, Sattler JM: *Stanford-Binet Intelligence Scale-Fourth Edition: Manual.* Chicago, IL: Riverside Publishing, 1986.
16. Leiter RG: *Leiter International Performance Scale-Revised.* Wood Dale, IL: Stoelting, 1997.
17. Kaufman AS, Kaufman NL: *Kaufman Brief Intelligence Test: Manual.* Circles Pines, MN: American Guidance Service, 1990.
18. Williams KT, Wang JJ: *Peabody Picture Vocabulary Test-Third Edition: Manual.* Circle Pines, MN: American Guidance Service, 1997.
19. Woodcock RW, McGrew KS, Mather N: *Woodcock-Johnson-III (WJ-III) Tests of Achievement.* Allen, TX: DLM Teaching Resources, 1989.
20. The Psychological Corporation: *Wechsler Individual Achievement Test-Second Edition: Examiner's Manual.* New York: Harcourt Assessment, 2002.
21. Sparrow SS, Balla DA, Chicchetti DV: *Vineland Adaptive Behavior Scales.* Circle Pines, MN: American Guidance Service, 1984.
22. Rimm S: *Achievement Identification Measure,* Watertown, WI: Educational Assessment Service, 1985.
23. Light W: *Light's Retention Scale,* Novato, CA: Academic Therapy Publications, 1981.
24. Uphoff JK, Gilmore JE, Huber R: *Summer Children: Ready or Not for School.* Middletown, OH: J&J Publishers, 1986.
25. DiLeo JA: *Interpreting Children's Drawings.* New York: Brunner/Mazel, 1983.
26. Burns RC, Kaufman SH: Actions, Styles, and Symbols in Kinetic Family Drawings (KFD), New York: Brunner/Mazel, 1972.
27. Buck IN: *The House-Tree-Person Technique: Revised Manual.* Los Angeles: Western Psychological Services, 1970.
28. Cordell AS, Berman-Meador B: The use of drawings. *J Div Remarr* 1991; **17**(1–2).
29. Klein RG: Questioning the clinical usefulness of projective psychological tests for children. *Dev Behav Pediatr* 1986; **7**(6):378–398.
30. Finch AJ, Belter RW: Projective techniques. In: Ollendick TH, Hersen M, eds. *Handbook of Child and Adolescent Assessment.* Boston, MA: Allyn and Bacon, 1993: 224–236.
31. Kazdin AE: Conduct disorder. In: Ollendick TH, Hersen M, eds. *Handbook of Child and Adolescent Assessment.* Boston, MA: Allyn and Bacon, 1993: 292–310.

32. Exner JE, Weiner IG: *The Rorschach: A Comprehensive System, vol.* 3. *Assessment of Children and Adolescents.* New York: John Wiley and Sons, 1982.

33. Henry W: *The Analysis of Fantasy.* New York: John Wiley and Sons, 1956.

34. McArthur D, Roberts G: *Roberts Apperception Test for Children: Manual.* Los Angeles: Western Psychological Services, 1982.

35. Bellak L, Bellak SS: *The Children's Apperception Test* (CAT). Larchmont, NY: C.P.S., 1976.

36. Bellak L, Hurvich MS: *Manual for the CAT-H.* Larchmont, NY: C.P.S., 1984.

37. Bellak L, Bellak SS: *Manual for Supplement to the Children's Apperception Test (CAT-S).* Larchmont, NY: C.P.S., 1978.

38. Caruso KR: *Basic Manual to Accompany Projective Storytelling Cards.* Redding, CA: Northwest Psychological Publishers, 1987.

39. Gardner RA: *The Adoption Story Cards.* Cresskill, NJ: Creative Therapeutics, 1978.

40. Rotter J: *Incomplete Sentences Blank.* New York: Harcourt Brace Jovanovich, 1977.

41. Gillis JS: *Child Anxiety Scale Manual.* Champaign, IL: Institute for Personality and Ability Testing, 1980.

42. Ollendick TH, Hersen M, eds: *Handbook of Child and Adolescent Assessment.* Boston, MA: Allyn and Bacon, 1993.

43. Kovacs M: *Children's Depression Inventory (CDI).* New York: Multi-Health Systems, 1992.

44. Coopersmith S: *The Antecedents of Self-Esteem.* San Francisco: Freeman, 1967.

45. Harter S: Competence as a dimension of self-evaluation. Toward a comprehensive model of selfworth. In: Leahy R, ed. *The Development of Self.* New York: Academic Press, 1983:51–121.

46. Battle J: *Culture-Free SEI: Self-Esteem Inventories for Children and Adults.* Seattle, WA: Special Child Publications, 1981.

47. Piers EV, Harris DB: *The Piers-Harris Children's Self-Concept Scale.* Los Angeles: Western Psychological Services, 1969.

48. Seligman ME, Reivich K, Jaycox L, Gillham J: *The Optimistic Child: A Revolutionary Program that Safeguards Children Against Depression and Builds Lifelong Resilience.* New York: Houghton Mifflin, 1995.

49. Kurdek LA, Berg B: The Children's Beliefs About Parental Divorce Scale: Psychometric characteristics and concurrent validity. *J Consul Clin Psychol* 1987; **55**:712–718.

50. Berg CZ: Behavioral assessment techniques for childhood obsessive-compulsive disorder. In: Rapoport JL, ed. *Obsessive-Compulsive Disorder in Children and Adolescents.* Washington, DC: American Psychiatric Press, 1989:41–70.

51. Atkeson BM, Forehand R: Conduct disorders. In: Mash El, Terdal LG, eds. *Behavioral Assessment of Childhood Disorders.* New York: Guilford Press, 1981:185–219.

52. Patterson GR, Reid JB, Jones RR, Conger RW: *A Social Learning Approach to Family Intervention.* Eugene, OR: Castalia, 1975.

53. Newsom C, Rincover A: Autism. In: Mash EL, Terdal LG, eds. *Behavioral Assessment of Childhood Disorders.* New York: Guilford Press, 1981:414–415.

54. Barkley RA: *Defiant Children: A Clinician's Manual for Parent Training.* New York: Guilford Press, 1987.

55. Barkley RA: *Defiant Children: Parent-Teacher Assignments.* New York: Guilford Press, 1987.

56. Singer JL: *The Child's World of Make-Believe: Experimental Studies of Imaginative Play.* New York: Academic Press, 1973.

57. Parten MB: Social participation among pre-school children. *J Abnorm Soc Psychol* 1932; **27**:243–260.

58. Pulaski MA: Play symbolism in cognitive development. In: Schaefer C, ed. *Therapeutic Use of Child's Play.* New York: Jason Aronson, 1976:27–41.

59. Irwin EC: The diagnostic and therapeutic use of pretend play. In: Schaefer CE, O'Connor KL, eds. *Handbook of Play Therapy.* New York: John Wiley and Sons, 1983:148–173.

60. Behar D, Rapoport JL: Play observation and psychiatric diagnosis. In: Schaefer CE, O'Connor KL, eds. *Handbook of Play Therapy.* New York: John Wiley and Sons, 1983:193–199.

61. Schaefer CE, Gitlin K, Sandgrund A, eds: *Play Diagnosis and Assessment.* New York: John Wiley and Sons, 1991.

62. Westby CE: A scale for assessing children's pretend play. In: Schaefer CE, Gitlin K, Sandgrund A, eds. *Play Diagnosis and Assessment.* New York: John Wiley and Sons, 1991:131–161.

63. Baumrind D: Effective parenting during the early adolescent transition. In: Cowan PA, Hetherington EM, eds. *Family Transitions.* Hillsdale, NJ: Erlbaum, 1991:111–164.

64. Hetherington EM, Parke RD: *Child Psychology: A Contemporary Viewpoint,* 4th ed. New York: McGraw-Hill, 1986.

65. Hughes IN, Baker DB: *The Clinical Child Interview.* New York: Guilford Press, 1990.

66. Beavers WR, Hampson RB: *Successful Families: Assessment and Intervention.* New York: W.W. Norton, 1990.

67. Olson DH, Portner J, Bell R: *FACES II.* St. Paul, MN: Family Social Science, University of Minnesota, 1982.

68. Barkley RA: *Attention-Deficit Hyperactivity Disorder.* New York: Guilford Press, 1990.

69. Gresham FM, Elliott SN: *Social Skills Rating System.* Circle Pines, MN: American Guidance Service, 1990.

70. Goldstein AP, Sprafkin RP, Gershaw NJ: *Skillstreaming the Adolescent: A Structured Learning Approach to Teaching Prosocial Skills.* Champaign, IL: Research Press, 1980.

71. Millon T, Millon C, Davis R: *The Millon Adolescent Clinical Inventory.* Minneapolis, MN: Pearson Assessments, 2004.

72. Millon T, Tringoner, Millon C, Grossman S: *Millon Pre-Adolescent Clinical Inventory.* Minneapolis, MN: Pearson Assessments, 2004.

73. Myers IB, McCaulley MJ: *Manual: A Guide to the Development and Use of the Myers-Briggs Type Indicator.* Palo Alto, CA: Consulting Psychologists Press, 1992.

74. Harrington TF, O'Shea A1: *The Harrington-O'Shea Career Decision-Making System Revised.* Circle Pines, MN: American Guidance Service, 1992.

75. Miller: *The Substance Abuse Subtle Screening Inventory (SASSI) Manual: Chapter 8, The SASSI Adolescent Manual.* Addiction Research & Consultation: Call 1–800–726–0526 for more information.

76. Petty J: *Checklist for Child Abuse Evaluation.* Odessa, FL: Psychological Assessment Resources, 1990.

77. Gardner RA: *The Sex Abuse Legitimacy Scale*, Cresskill, NJ: Creative Therapeutics, 1987.

78. Peterson G: *Diagnosis and Child and Adolescent Multiple Personality*, Chapel Hill, NC: Southeast Institute for Group and Family Therapy; 1989.

79. American Psychiatric Association: *Diagnostic and Statistical Manual of Mental Disorder*, 4th ed. Text revision. Washington, DC: American Psychiatric Association; 2000.

80. Putnam FW, Helmers K, Trickett PK: Development, reliability, and validity of a child dissociation scale. *Child Abuse Negl* 1993; **17**:731–741.

3

Neurobiological Assessment

George Realmuto

Introduction

Neurobiological assessment for psychiatric disorders can't come along too quickly. Child mental health has several needs for such technology. The field needs to rapidly and easily measure the various capacities of the central nervous system (CNS) so that we can accurately evaluate cognitive, emotional and behavioral variation. We need to go further and measure the genetic variation of these domains to understand risk and vulnerability prior to their developmental manifestations. The discovery, testing, validation and dissemination of technological procedures to fill gaps in our assessment protocols could reshape our practice of patient care, standards of treatment, the scope of our intervention goals and the direction that resources are expended on mental health care. There are many problems that we face with assessment that are now answered in ways that are not different from an approach that is decades old. What tools do we need, for example, that would allow us to know if a child with poor academic progress and identified dyslexia also had attentional problems that were consistent with attention deficit hyperactivity disorder (ADHD) inattentive type? Or if an adolescent presented as withdrawn, isolated and self-destructive, what neurobiological assessment would allow us to easily tell whether this was an acute reaction to significant loss, a major depressive disorder or bipolar disorder? Could we use neuroimaging to separate very early prodroms of schizophrenia from Asperger syndrome? Could we curtail the time burden of developmental, family and medical history taking by simply applying a piece of modern day miracle technology? Do we have the neurobiological tools to refine diagnosis and treatment planning? At this point we do not. If we could, our entire nomenclature might need changing. For example, if neuroimaging provided enough informa-

tion about brain–behavior relationships we might decide that disorders of the frontal cortex should be a major DSMx category. Limbic system disorders might encompass depression, anxiety and adjustment disorders if assessment techniques could discriminate among them. New categories would group global brain problems such as mental retardation and autism together. Specific brain region disorders would be a collection of problems such as simple motor tic disorder, habit disorders and blephrospasm. Rapid neurobiological assessment using one of the many forms of imaging such as positron emission tomography (PET), single-photon emission computed tomography (SPECT), and the various forms of magnetic resonance imaging (MRI) would improve identification and move treatment to early onset or even prodromal stages. We now have these technologies but they have not revolutionized the way we work with patients and it may be time to hope the next generation of technologies will create these opportunities. An alternative is to start to look elsewhere for technologies that are waiting to be brought to clinical practice.

Pharmacogenomics

Pharmacogenomics may be a new place to start. It is a field that is as new as the effort to completely sequence the human genome. Only in 2001 was a first draft sequence of the entire human genome made available to the public by Lander and Venter. The human genome includes 22 pairs of autosomal chromosomes and an additional pair of sex chromosomes. The entire cellular DNA consists of approximately three billion base pairs that may encode 30 000–70 000 genes. One way of inquiring into this massive storehouse of our potential is the field of pharmacogenomics. What is pharmacogenomics not? It is not

Clinical Child Psychiatry, Second Edition. Edited by W.M. Klykylo and J.L. Kay
© 2005 John Wiley & Sons Ltd.

pharmacogenetics. Pharmacogenetics is the study of inheritance (a gene) and its interactions with medications. Pharmacogenomics is the convergence of advances in pharmacology and genomics. Pharmacogenomics is a scientific body of knowledge and procedures that allows for genotypic screening to arrive at an informed clinical choice for psychotropic medication. Genomics is the study of whole sets of genes, gene products and their interactions. Genomics is the study of groups of related function genes as compared to genetics that is limited to the study of single genes. Pharmacogenomics then asks questions about medications as it relates to an array of genes that influence these medications. In some sense pharmacogenomics is a study of the heritability of the variance that exists in drug effect. The implications of utilization of this expertise are enormous as it applies to medicine. One example is the choice of a chemotherapeutic agent for the treatment of cancer. One treatment may be intolerable for one cancer patient because drug metabolic processes cause intolerable side effects and the full dosage cannot be applied. Another example is the widespread use of an effective analgesic medication. While safe and effective in most patients in some cases, popular accounts suggest that a very small group had very serious and life-threatening adverse effects. The pharmaceutical company established that this group had a variant of a metabolic pathway that caused large accumulations of the drug leading to near fatal consequences. A simple test was devised to identify patients belonging to this group. Physicians were warned of this potential hazard, educated about identification procedures and screening, and at-risk patients were excluded from treatment with it. As compelling as these scenarios may seem in general medicine, in order for mental health to adopt pharmacogenomics a clear application needs to be found. Then why should pharmacogenomic technology become part of a practical and effective neurobiological assessment?

There is significant variation among individuals in the way they metabolize medications. For example among individuals of European origin, one in ten metabolize certain antidepressants poorly. A much smaller group metabolizes the same drug rapidly. If the clinician knew the status of a particular patient would that clinician make a more informed choice and reduce the risk of adverse side effects, i.e., slow metabolism and adverse effects, i.e., quick metabolism and poor response?

Fluorescence *In Situ* Hybridization

Genetic testing is not new to psychiatry. We may not think too much about the procedure that we choose when a genetic disorder with significant behavioral and cognitive features is suspected. Fluorescence *in situ* hybridization (FISH) is a method of creating a sequence of DNA, attaching an identification tag on it called a fluorophore and incubating it with the genetic material in question. If the complementary sequence of genetic material to be tested is present, the probe will stick and the fluorophore will mark its presence through a light-emitting signal. FISH was developed in 1986 by Pinkel *et al.* His group found a method to visualize chromosomes using fluorescent-labeled probes. The procedure involves the annealing of the FISH probe DNA with complementary DNA sequences in the chromosomes. The presence or absence of the signal is observed with a fluorescence microscope. FISH probes have been developed for many disorders of interest to psychiatry. These include Fragile X, Velocardiofacial syndrome, Smith–Magenis syndrome, Prader–Willi and Angelman syndrome and Williams syndrome. New tests could be developed at any time. A psychiatric researcher who had reason to believe that a specific sequence of DNA was responsible for a product that affected CNS functioning could develope a systematic test for that DNA sequence. FISH is less useful when variation in gene sequence is the question, but it is very suitable for an application in which the presence or absence of a known DNA base pair sequence is the question to be answered.

Polymerase Chain Reaction

An important procedure that underlies the incredible advances that have taken place in DNA sequencing is the polymerase chain reaction (PCR). It is the most widely used molecular procedure and it underlies most genetic testing strategies. PCR permits copying pieces of DNA multiple times to produce exact replicas of the original. The procedure begins with the identification of the double stranded DNA template to be copied. The double stranded DNA is heated to break the hydrogen bonds between the base pairs and separate the DNA into two complementary single strands. Other ingredients required include a synthetic or laboratory constructed version of DNA sequences called oligonucleotide primers. These primers are complementary to a short segment of DNA sequence at either end of the template to be replicated. They serve as starting points for the replication to take place. In addition the building blocks – nucleotide triphiophates – for DNA construction must be present. There are four types of nucleic acid: adenine, guanine, thymine and cytosine that are subsequently attached to a sugar–phosphate backbone. Finally the enzyme that catalyzes the reaction is the DNA polymerase. This is an enzyme that synthesizes DNA by successively adding nucleotides to the free 3′ hydroxyl group of the growing strand. This enzyme is heat stable allowing for cooling and heating cycles. Each cycle involves binding of the primer to the DNA sequence that is immediately adjacent to the target sequence to be replicated, which sets into play the extension of the bound oligonucliotide primer which can then add free nucleotides. Each cycle results in doubling of the number of target DNA regions with a final target amplification of approximately more than a million copies.

Microarray Analysis

Microarray technology is a novel tool to evaluate many genes and gene products en masse with high efficiency. Microarray analysis, as its name suggests, is possible with the availability of miniaturized, computer assisted imaging systems. If an investigator thought that a disease state was caused by or associated with a particular gene polymorphism or cluster of genes, multiple patients with this disorder could have this combination of genes evaluated and commonalties of specific polymorphisms could be determined. For the clinician, once this grouping is identified treatments could be devised to alter gene expression. The possible applications of DNA microarray analysis include identification of a specific gene of interest, screening for mutations or polymorphisms, and comparative genomic hybridization.

The physical features of a microarray chip might be consistent with a view of computers in general. The chip is made of chemically coated glass to which a nylon membrane is attached. A coating of polylysine or silane allows for the adhesion of the test probes. The cells are small, less that 250 µm in diameter (Figure 3.1(a)), and are topographically organized into columns and rows capable of being assessed by computer-directed robotic readers with the input being systematically recorded. A place on the microarray – cell – the intersection of a column and a row, designates the location for the quantification of the expression of a gene for a particular subject or patient. The microarray chip containing these cells is embedded with a small fragment of DNA (Figure 3.1(b)). The DNA molecule that is attached to each cell on the chip is referred to as a probe. Probes are used to detect targets. The target is usually complementary DNA, made by synthesis using an RNA sequence as the template. The advantages of complementary DNA is that it is devoid of introns, sequences that are not represented in the product sequence of a gene. Introns are removed by a process known as intron splicing. Probes are looking for targets and the interaction between probes and target is simply the processes of hybridizing or alignment and attachment of base pairing. However some experimental tasks require the use of genomic DNA. If a single DNA base pair distinguishes the subject from the norm, genomic DNA rather than expressed DNA or DNA made from RNA would be the target of choice. These are searches for single nucleotide polymorphism or SNP. A particular gene's activity or efficiency, or developmental time sequence to come on line may be influenced by a SNP. A SNP requires very fine scale detection procedures, and preparation of the probes needs to be carefully thought through. As mentioned above PCR techniques can produce large quantities of DNA products or probes. Where should one choose to obtain these probes? When looking for the variant it may be best to have probes of the wild type or most common genetic variation. The absence then of a match between probe and target says that a difference has been detected. Databases exist currently that detail extensive information about each probe at each cell location.

How are Matches and Nonmatches Detected?

First, complementary DNA is deposited on the microarray cells by a computer assisted high-speed robot. The number of cells on a chip depends on the private company who supplies the chip. Some chips carry as many as 65 000 cells. The probes are then processed with florochrome dye that is applied to the probes so that they can report the presence or absence of a target match. When a laser is focused onto a cell, a light is emitted and each lit cell is detected and computer coded. The laser beam excites the fluorescent dye linked to the probe that has been hybridized with the target DNA (Figure 3.2(a)). A scanner can monitor fluorescence from each cell. The degree of fluorescence correlates with the abundance of target molecules at a specific cell (Figure 3.2(b)).

While the technology and processes are very sophisticated, the advantage for clinical practice can be exciting and practical. One application already past the pilot stage is the identification of differences in enzyme systems that influence psychoactive drug metabolism. Of special interest to child and adolescent psychiatry is the P450 group of enzymes expressed in the liver. This family of enzymes is responsible for all of currently available selective serotonin reuptake inhibitors, tricyclic and some antipsychotic metabolism. There are 10 enzyme systems in this family and each of the genes has an array of alleles that confer variability of meta-

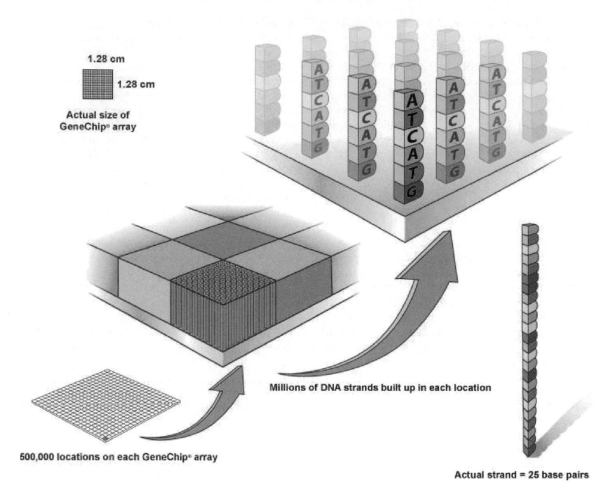

1.28 cm

1.28 cm

Actual size of GeneChip® array

ATCATG

ATCATG

ATCATG

ATCATG

ATCATG

Millions of DNA strands built up in each location

500,000 locations on each GeneChip® array

Actual strand = 25 base pairs

Figure 3.1(a) GeneChip™; Single feature cartoon depicting a single feature on an Affymetrix GeneChip™; microarray. Image courtesy of Affymetrix.

bolic rate. Within different ethnic groups there may be less heterogeneity. One of these is the CYP2D6 allele. Humans have two copies of this allele. Since this enzyme is responsible for the metabolism of some antidepressants, the activity of a particular inherited variant may play a part in effectiveness of treatment. The version of the gene inherited will be demonstrated by a specific expression of metabolic activity. The kinds of gene differences that might lead to different outcomes could include a deletion of the allele, a redundant version due to duplication of the gene or one-nucleotide differences or SNPs that have a spectrum of effects. CYP2D4 has as many as 12 known variants. The variations are produced by a different kinds of base pair alterations including shifts, addi-

tions, deletions or single nucleotide substitutions. The consequences for metabolic activity span slow to ultrarapid. The slowest activity may be due to deletion or inactivation of both copies of the gene. Another version is the heterozygous variant with one inactive gene resulting in an intermediate level of metabolism. The most common variant metabolizes some drugs in this class fairly extensively, and finally there is a very rapid metabolic type that is due to multiple duplications of the gene. It is not uncommon for individuals with the highest level of metabolism to be unresponsive to treatment.

To know how to proceed clinically, a sample of the patient's blood sample is required, and DNA extracted. Multiple copies of cDNA that is represen-

RNA fragments with fluorescent tags from sample to be tested

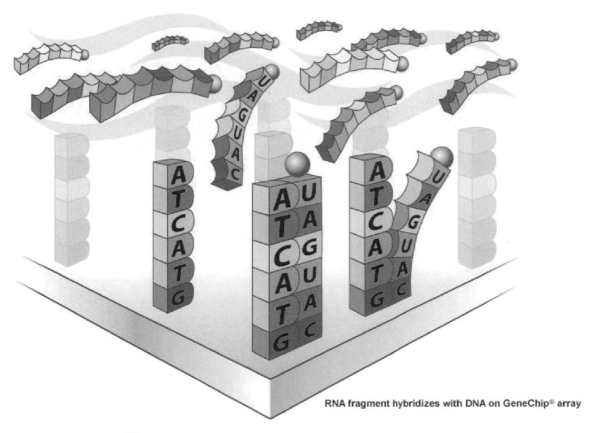

RNA fragment hybridizes with DNA on GeneChip® array

Figure 3.1(b) GeneChip™; Hybridization cartoon depicting hybridization of tagged probes to Affymetrix GeneChip™; microarray. Image courtesy of Affymetrix.

tative of this allelic site can be produced by PCR. A specific chip with probes for each variant can be prepared and depending on the hybridization that occurs on the chip and the detection of target/probe matching through fluorescent emission, information about that individual's genetic variant can be determined. This may be very useful for clinical decision-making. Since different SSRI antidepressants have a different profile of P450 enzyme metabolism, a specific choice of SSRI might be made on grounds other than 'best guess.' Paroxitine and fluoxitine are metabolized by the CYP2D6 enzyme system. This family is even more genetically diverse than the CYP2D4. It has been shown to have more than 50 allelic polymorphisms. As noted above, different ethnic groups have different profiles of polymorphisms that in some cases can increase the accuracy of clinical guessing about the possible

success of an antidepressant in a member of that group. However, we now have the laboratory capacity to determine in an individual the specific polymorphism of each of the P450 enzyme families. Therefore with a high degree of certainty, a laboratory test can determine rate of metabolism and clearly indicate which antidepressant is likely to be effective or produce side effects, according to the rate of metabolism predicted from the presence of particular polymorphisms. There are several implications of these procedures. Genetic profiling may identify patterns of gene variants that at some point in time may be linked to risk for disease. Informing a patient about their genotype for clinical decisions about medication choice today may expose them to knowledge about risk for disease in the near future: a decision to know that was not included in the informed consent that accompanied

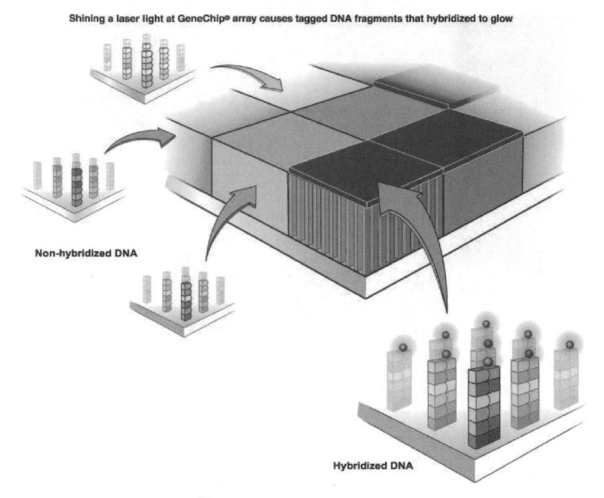

Figure 3.2(a) Hybridized GeneChip™; Microarray cartoon depicting scanning of tagged and un-tagged probes on an Affymetrix GeneChip™; microarray. Image courtesy of Affymetrix.

their decision to obtain information for medication decision-making. Therefore additional consent about the possible use of genetic testing would need to include a discussion about how the information would be documented and to whom the information would be or would not be transferred now and in the future. Another implication is the role of pharmacogenomic testing for practice standards. If there is a way to choose a medication that will have fewer side effects and better efficacy should we not adopt such a test?

These tests are really here now. A well-known medical clinic in the Midwest is already making this test available for a small sum of about $300 (personal communication Dr. David Mrazek). The test will provide a clinician with a profile of a patient's cytochrome P450 2D6 genotype with information about the activity of each of the identified variants. The laboratory can be reached at 800 533 1710. Matching these genetic determinates with a drugs preferred metabolic pathway can be lifesaving: for example a patient is admitted to an inpatient unit for continued suicidal ideation and attempt, and it is determined that the current SSRI is ineffective; making a wrong therapy choice could lead to a lengthy hospitalization whereas cytochrome P450 information could lead to an informed choice. The costs of the tests would quickly be recouped through shorter length of stay. We have been disappointed by the promises that imaging and other technology were expected to bring to child and

Figure 3.2(b) GeneChip™; Array output data from an experiment showing the thousands of genes detected by a single GeneChip™; probe array. Image courtesy of Affymetrix.

adolescent psychiatry. Although new, we seem to have a need for a test for and a rationale for pharmacogenomic testing. Will we adopt it?

Promising Technologies for Neurobiological Assessments

Many tools currently used for research show promise of making their way into clinical practice. These technologies are dependant upon sophisticated computer hardware and software. In some cases, scientists with special expertise are needed beyond the highly trained technicians who prepare the patient and operate the equipment. However, the costs of individual examinations have been decreased, bringing such methods of examination closer to clinical practice than ever before.

What follows is a brief description of the methods and principles of experimental neurobiologic assessment techniques (Table 3.1).

Single-Photon Emission Computed Tomography

The technique of single-photon emission computed tomography (SPECT) detects and images gamma rays produced by radioactive isotopes. These gamma-emitting radiolabeled substances produce a single photon of energy that is detected by single-crystal scintillation instruments external to the subject. The radioactive distribution is analyzed by a computer and displayed as an image based on the energy produced and the position of the source of the energy (Figure 3.3). The procedure has gone through several refinements, including an improved detection of photon emissions of new radiopharmaceuticals.

There are several important differences between SPECT and PET. SPECT radioscopes produce lower-energy gamma rays than the photons produced by the radionuclides used in PET. As a result, the former are more easily absorbed by the body and therefore require longer scanning sessions for adequate resolution. In addition, lower-energy isotopes result in deeper structures of the brain absorbing or attenuating emitted radiation, which requires some adjustment of the signal to decrease artifact.

SPECT has been successfully used in the study of patients with ADHD. In a series of studies in which children and adolescents with ADHD inhaled radio-labled xenon, results were consistent with other evidence for hypofrontality as well as hypoperfusion of the caudate nuclei. Administration of methylphenidate to a subgroup of these patients had a normalizing effect on brain activity as shown after rescanning [6]. Another center studied a larger and better-described group of children and adolescents with ADHD under resting and stress conditions. Again, prefrontal problems were noted [2].

There have been advances in the radiolabeling of a variety of pharmaceutical antagonists whose application is important to psychiatry, such as radio-labeled probes for D1 and D2 dopamine receptors [14,15]. Poor morphologic resolution and the use of radioactive substances that convey some small risk in developing children may limit the overall potential for child psychiatry. However, improved detection enhanced through computer software and other technical improvements as well as targeted probes identifying neurotransmitters and receptors may improve to the point that SPECT closely rivals PET.

Positron Emission Tomography

PET permits measurements of the rate of radioactive substrate consumption. If the radioactive substrate collects at points of increased neural activity, the decay of the substrate at that locale will identify such processes. If the substrate binds to a particular receptor, then the receptor will be localized during the degradation of the radioactive substrate.

Table 3.1. Potential neurobiologic techniques.

Technique	Description	Potential application	References
Event-related potentials	Summed electrical activity form groups of neurons responding to a time-locked stimulus	Neurodevelopmental disorder, early identification, and qualification of impairment	[1–3]
Magnetic resonance imaging	Detection of radio waves from atomic particles and translation into computerized images	Brain behavior correlations, identification of structures abnormal for volume and blood flow	[4,5]
Single-photon emission computed tomography	Radioactive substance produces an emission that can be detected and visualized	Identification of subgroups within diagnostic groups that may have different pathophysiologic processes requiring different interventions	[6,7]
Positron emission tomography	Radioactive substance emits protons that produce photons that are detected and imaged, creating maps of activity or localization	Anatomic localization of important brain events of locales that underlie disorders or responses to treatments	[8–12]
Functional magnetic resonance imaging	T2*, the modified time constant for transverse relaxation, is measured in various tissues whose differences emerge as a result of the imposition of a field magnet	Structure/function relationships of the central nervous system	[13]

The physics of PET scanning are founded on principles governing the emission of protons from radioactive nuclei as the radioactive substance decays. The emitted proton inevitably collides with an electron, resulting in two photons traveling in almost opposite directions. The PET scanner can record these photons with scintillation detectors using sodium iodide or bismuth germanate crystals. The scintillation detectors convert the photon energy into visible light that can be recorded on film. Only those photons traveling in linear but opposite directions are saved as data points through the encircling array of scintillation detectors. The activity produced by the radioactive nuclei can be pinpointed in two-dimensional space and reorganized spatially to produce a graphic representation of the photons.

The advantages of PET over SPECT include higher-energy reactions and thus the emission of higher-energy protons with smaller attenuation from surrounding tissue that produces cleaner images. Also, PET does not use collimators or parallel filters to focus photons that may compromise the resolution of SPECT technologies.

There are limitations of PET, however. First, the energy of the radioactive substance used to generate protons is considered more hazardous to the host than that of the lower-energy chemicals in SPECT and this is an important factor in limiting the recruitment of children for PET studies. Second, the collision of proton and electron does not always produce photons traveling in exactly opposite directions, thus adding some blur to the image. Third, the scintillation detectors themselves bear physical limits that affect clarity. What begins as a single point of activity in the brain may ultimately emerge as a 10 cm image. Fourth, the mathematical modeling methods used to extract absolute measurements are highly controversial. Because of differences between imaging centers'

Right **Anterior** **Left**

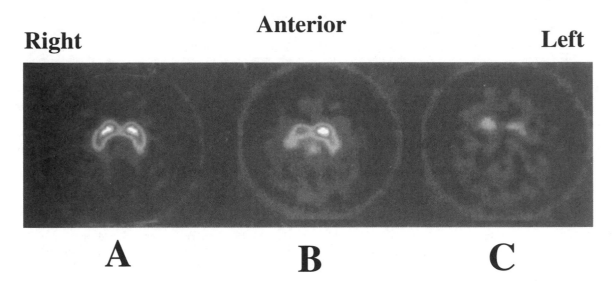

A **B** **C**

Figure 3.3 Transaxial single-photon emission computed tomography (SPECT) images at the level of the striatum in a healthy subject (A) and two patients with Parkinson disease (B, early stage; C, late stage). The ^{123}I-labeled radiopharmaceutical β-CIT binds to dopamine transporters on the presynaptic terminals of dopamine neurons. The SPECT images demonstrate that patients with Parkinson disease have fewer striatal uptake sites than healthy subjects, with greater loss in the putamen (posterior) region than in the head of the caudate. (Courtesy of John Seibyl, MD, Ken Marek, MD, and Robert Innis, MD, New Haven, CT).

methods and equipment and mathematical algorithms, results might best be considered relative rather than absolute quantities. Finally, a unique requirement for PET scanning is the production of a radioactive tracer. High-energy radiolabeled pharmaceuticals with definable parameters of energy, proton emissions, and other physical characteristics must be created in a cyclotron. The substrates are bombarded with protons in the cyclotron to produce the desired probe. Since the probe decays rapidly, this technique requires on-site facilities to create tracer substances along with the personnel and capacity to deal with the spent low-level radioactive waste [16].

PET scan studies of interest to child and adolescent psychiatry were begun in 1990 by Zametkin and colleagues, using a sample of adults with ADHD [8]. In 1993, 10 adolescents with ADHD were studied, and six brain regions showed differences in activity when compared to controls. These included frontal, thalamic, hippocampal, and temporal areas with findings distributed by both hemisphere and rate (increase or decrease in brain metabolic activity) [9].

Further extension of these studies was pursued to evaluate the metabolic activation of brain areas stim-

ulated by dextroamphetamine and methylphenidate [11,17]. Unfortunately, the findings about the action sites of drugs did not give clear inferences about brain response to medication in regions specific to ADHD. A more promising study recently published by Matlay and colleagues used PET to view the action of medication in adults [12]. In this study, cognitive tasks of executive brain function were administered to subjects to stimulate metabolism in brain regions subserving those functions. Differential oxygen uptake enhancement by stimulant drug was observed in the prefrontal cortex and hippocampus.

In summary, although PET methodology was applied in a research setting to differentiate ADHD subjects from controls and to evaluate drug treatment effects, the results were disappointing. Few adolescents and no children participated in the studies because of concerns about the protection of human subjects, thus significantly limiting application to the patients of prime interest. Also, the results were neither anatomically specific nor, for the most part, consistent with hypothesized defects derived from other sources. The long-term prospective of PET scanning for the child and adolescent population may not be bright, since other technologies subserve similar goals. Functional MRI (fMRI) has several advantages over PET and obtains similar information (see next section). Competition among technologies is good for the field, improving the time, convenience, cost, and information delivered.

Magnetic Resonance Imagining

The technologic procedure that appears to have the easiest entry into child and adolescent mental health is MRI. The equipment required includes a high-powered magnet, which lines up protons according to the direction of the magnetic field, and coils conducting radio waves. Radio waves alter the alignment of the protons, and the resulting signal produced from this realignment can be detected and fashioned into images using computer software. Stronger magnets, better software, and more experience with the location and pulse frequency of coils have improved the quality of the images (Figure 3.4).

Interesting work with MRI has elucidated the size of important brain structures and allowed for clearer correlations between structure and function. For example, a recent report contributed to a better understanding of the basal ganglia in patients with obsessive–compulsive disorder (OCD). Basal ganglia volumes measured with MRI were compared with symptom severity at different times, and as treatment removed antistreptolysin O antigens, caudate size diminished and symptoms decreased [4]. In the future, an evaluation of structures such as caudate size may be useful in differential diagnosis and the evaluation of treatment response. Defining caudate volume may be useful in differentiating habit disorders from adjustment disorders, and neurobiologic phenomena such as Tourette syndrome and OCD, and may also give specific direction to treatment interventions and permit clearer measures of treatment response.

Limitations to this procedure are minimal. Contraindications include mainly the presence of ferrous metals in the body, although this is probably not a significant problem in the child and adolescent population. Multiple exposures were originally a concern, but these are now being permitted when clinically indicated, with few adverse experiences. Rapidly changing the direction of the magnetic field potentially produces electric shock and tissue damage, and alternations that are too rapid in magnetic polarity may induce electric currents within the body and may thus produce an activation of peripheral nerves that the patient may feel. In addition, tissues that have few ways to dissipate heat can be exposed to the hazard of energy produced by a rapidly changing magnetic field. The Food and Drug Administration has set limits on these parameters, and most MRI scanners have these upper limits built

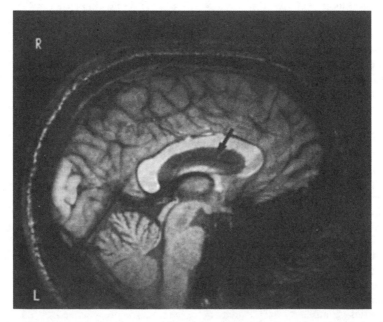

Figure 3.4 Sagittal view of the human brain at 4.1 Tesla demonstrating exquisite neuroanatomic resolution. (Courtesy of Dr. Jullie W. Pan and Hoby Hetherington, PhD, Birmingham, AL).

into the system software to prevent untoward events. Another limitation of use has been cost, particularly in setting up such equipment, but competition and the portability of the equipment have made MRI virtually universally available.

Given the opportunities for better definition of CNS substrates of psychopathology, it behooves the profession to develop medical necessity guidelines and criteria so that this and other technologic procedures will be approved for use in children and adolescents as a standard of care.

Functional Magnetic Resonance Imaging

Mapping of physiologic activity is a capacity of MRI technology shared with PET, SPECT, and evoked potentials. However, high temporal and spatial resolution and the ability to repeatedly scan subjects give fMRI an advantage over other imaging techniques. Although this technique may circumvent many of the hazards that have precluded children from entering research protocols, fMRI has arrived only recently, and there is little in the literature to demonstrate its superiority over other methods [18].

As described for MRI (see previous section), the physical basis of fMRI is the systematic manipulation of changes to the precession of atomic nuclei around its axis. The activity of spinning atomic nuclei results in minute magnetic fields, and anatomic structures differ in their chemical composition and thus magnetic characteristics. Differences in the magnetic susceptibility of these anatomic structures make it possible for these magnetic dipoles to be manipulated to produce radio frequencies that can be detected by specialized receiver coils. Using sophisticated computer technology, these differences are then spatially arranged into images. The largest magnetic fields are produced at the boundaries of volumes with the largest differences in magnetic susceptibility.

Magnetic susceptibility is caused by the propensity of a material to develop an internal magnetic field in response to one applied from the outside. In the case of the fMRI, the field that is applied is the large magnetic field applied to the body [23]. Of particular importance in fMRI are the physiologic changes that occur in the blood as it perfuses neural tissue. Activated tissue deoxygenates blood, and thus maps can be produced of localities in the brain where oxygen is being consumed at rates statistically different from baseline. Oxygen changes the magnetic properties of hemoglobin, and deoxygenated blood has very different magnetic properties from surrounding brain parenchyma, which can be detected as differences in magnetic field frequencies.

The specific type of MRI frequency that is measured in fMRI is the T2*. When a static magnetic field is applied to a volume of tissue, atomic nuclei can respond by developing a magnetic field and thus magnetic susceptibility. However, the random directions of the magnetic fields of surrounding nuclei result in the neutralization of any particular summed field strength. These events are generated in the direction transverse to the static magnetic field. This equilibration of the magnetic field is called relaxation and it occurs over a specific time course. T2* therefore represents the modified time constant for transverse relaxation (Figure 3.5).

Little work has been done with fMRI in any population. Teicher and colleagues reported the effects of methylphenidate on ADHD symptoms and fMRI in children and showed a strong correlation between the number of child movements on placebo and T2* relaxation times of the right caudate [13]. The optimal dose of methylphenidate exerted significant effects on frontal and caudate T2*, which affected the right hemisphere more than the left. Another recent publication investigating the neuroanatomy of OCD symptoms in adults showed the activation of specific brain regions, including limbic structures that had been identified previously for subjects but not controls [19].

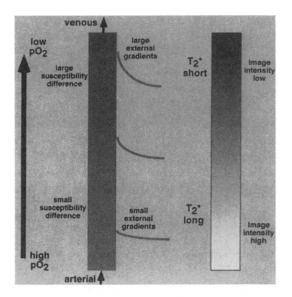

Figure 3.5 The physical basis of fMRI signal changes. From left to right, decreasing blood oxygenation increases field gradients surrounding vessels, which in turn decreases T2* and image intensity. Neuronal activity increases capillary level oxygenation, which is detected as an increase in T2*-weighted image intensity. (From [16]).

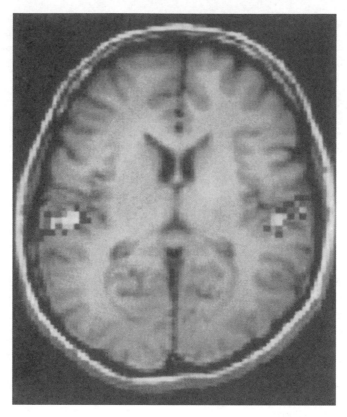

Figure 3.6 Functional magnetic resonance (MR) map of the primary auditory cortex. Pixels with significant signal changes associated with the presentation of sounds are shown in color (greater significance in lighter shades), superimposed on a conventional MR scan of the same slice through the brain (Courtesy of Rene Marois, Yale University, New Haven, CT).

Conceptually, fMRI is more complicated than other imaging systems. The master of fMRI requires skills in many technical and clinical areas. The first wave of studies to be published will likely be a replication of studies that have previously used other imaging procedures. These replication studies may allow fMRI to quickly emerge as the imaging standard, and studies of all ages and conditions will likely follow (Figure 3.6).

Magnetic Resonance Spectroscopy

Preceding the more widely used imaging techniques of MRI was magnetic resonance spectroscopy (MRS), a novel investigative tool developed to understand the functional basis of disease [20]. MRS is capable of identifying important events in cell metabolism such as energy production and dissipation through the identification of chemicals that are produced or consumed by these processes.

The basic principles of MRS and MRI are identical. MRS, however, records differences in activity based on the detection of chemical shift. As described previously, atomic nuclei possessing magnetic properties rotate around an axis based on the strength of the magnetic field applied. For MRS, however, detection of the differences in chemicals is based on the magnetic properties of atomic nuclei as they are influenced by the quantity of electrons possessed by a given chemical. This is the key point of the technique. Hydrogen protons may precess at a certain frequency, but differences exist if the hydrogen atom is part of water, with an electric cloud produced by two oxygen atoms, or if it is a hydrogen atom that is part of a methane moiety of a large organic molecule. Since each hydrogen atom experiences a slightly different local magnetic field owing to shielding by different clouds of electrons, each chemical shift is the difference in resonance frequency caused by the characteristics inherent in a particular nucleus. Detection of these differences is similar to procedures described for MRI and includes tipping the axis of the spinning atomic nuclei with a specific radio frequency and recording changes in magnetic field. Relaxation time as nuclei reequilibrate is transformed into frequency values and displayed as unique frequency spectra [21].

MRS can detect cellular activity involving phosphorylated compounds including adenosine triphosphate and its phosphorylated intermediates. Chemical products available for measurement with this technique include choline and lactate. Further extension of this technology includes quantitative measurement of neurotransmitter and neurochemical levels. Limitations that are generic to magnetic resonance technologies are also present with spectroscopy, including slow acquisition time, artifact created by patient movement, and relatively poor spatial resolution. However, more powerful computer software, higher field strengths of the magnet, and creative ways of improving patient cooperation may allow the detection of chemical events related to specific psychopathologic processes [21].

Electrophysiologic Procedures: Event-Related Potentials

The event-related potential is a neural phenomenon captured with a relatively noninvasive procedure, and some applications are not particularly demanding of a child's attention or self-discipline. Brain electrical activity can be recorded through the placement of electrodes on the skull in a system similar to that of electroencephalogram electrode placement. The brain produces a sequence of positive and negative deflections that are consistently observed as a consequence of auditory, visual, or somatosensory stimuli. These waves are generated by groups of aligned cells that together reach a state of depolarization or hyperpolarization that is detected by electrodes—much the same way the center of an earthquake is detected by seismologic instruments distributed across the Earth's crust. Courchesne and colleagues have done considerable work using this technique to further our understanding of autistic disorder [2]. It is with such neuropsychiatric conditions that organ level measurements become most useful, because of the significant communicative disability that makes direct inquiry difficult, if not impossible. One of the many findings contributed by a series of studies with autistic subjects was the reduction of amplitude of the P300 waveform. The P300 waveform is a characteristic positive deflection occurring approximately 300 milliseconds after the onset of a stimulus. The P300 response is generally invoked by target- or task-related events and may be influenced be the relevance of the stimuli, the motivation of the subjects, and other subject and stimuli variables. This late-appearing wave may therefore have something to do with cognitive processing as compared to earlier-appearing waves that may measure the 'hard wiring' of the CNS. The subject is asked to complete a cognitive task that is reflected in the P300. The finding that nonretarded adolescent autistic subjects demonstrate smaller P300 amplitudes as well as other parameters suggests that autism is a disorder of focused attention in which novel and common stimuli are perceived with equal relevance [2]. Evoked potential procedures have been applied to infants and very young children who have experienced prenatal or perinatal insults [22], and in a growing body of work, the examination of risk for chemical dependency has been quite fruitful [1].

Current limitations of this procedure include costs for computer hardware and software and ongoing technical support as well as the time and energy consumed by technical and computer glitches that appear to be a by-product of cutting-edge technology.

Electroencephalography

Old technology namely the electroencephalogram (EEG) continues to have a place in the neurobiological assessment of children and adolescents. The earliest work on EEG dates to the German psychiatrist Hans Berger who published the EEG of his son in 1929. He showed that changes occurred in his son's alpha rhythm due to mental activity. EEG instrumentation identifies changes in direction of the flow of electrons from electrodes placed on the patient's scalp. As groups of neurons depolarize an electrical field is developed the direction of which can be noted by the electrode. Fluctuations in field strength for each electrode are recorded on paper and more recently captured by sophisticated computer software.

Among the disorders relevant for EEG assessment is autism. Differentiation of a disorder such as Landau–Kleffner syndrome, which has a specific treatment, from autism is very important. Also since autism has an incidence of seizures of about 20–30% with a peak risk for onset in early adolescence, the clinician should consider ordering an EEG as part of a workup for any unusual change in the adolescent's clinical condition. EEG differences from normal have been noted for ADHD, conduct disorder, and learning disorders but the findings are nonspecific and may not be helpful for guiding treatment. Medication monitoring for drug treatments that lower seizure threshold may continue to define a use for EEG testing.

Conclusion

Neurobiologic assessment has a bright future in identifying clinically significant differences in activation levels of specific brain regions, in measuring neurohumoral proclivities associated with fundamental biologic activities, and in parceling out genetic and environmental endowment associated with diagnostic entities and behavioral, emotional, and ideational symptoms. Further, the wedding of information generated by these laboratory procedures to biologic responses from the next generation of psychopharmacologic agents may detail new insights into neurochemical brain–behavior relationships. This may provide the child and adolescent psychiatrist a powerful technology to explore symptoms as well as comprehensive and integrative techniques that allow for predictive statements about disease progression and outcome. How this is to evolve is unclear. As with many challenges, the conquerors may already be staging an assault. It was premature a decade ago to assume that the dexamethasone suppression test would provide diagnostically useful information. We now know much more about cortisol and its relationship to acute and chronic stress and psychiatric disorders. That experience should have taught us that we cannot clearly predict the utility of our enhanced neurobiologic assessment tools. We must also be concerned that, at this point in the evolution of managed care, investment in these approaches may be minimal. As with all leaps forward, all the right ingredients need to come together. Economic advantage, charismatic spokespersons, and a critical event are at least three of the requisite pieces to fuel this leap.

Glossary

Allelic polymorphisms
One of a pair or series of genes that occupy a specific position on a specific chromosome [24].

Angelman syndrome
A genetic disorder with developmental and neurologial symptoms including severe mental retardation, seizures, ataxic gait, jerky movements, lack of speech, microencephaly, and frequent smiling and laughter [25].

Complementary DNA
cDNA is complementary to RNA. The RNA serves as a template for synthesis of the complimentary DNA in the presence of the enzyme reverse transcriptase [25].

DNA polymerase
Any of various enzymes that function in the replication and repair of DNA by catalyzing the linking of dATP, dCTP, dGTP, and dTTP in a specific order, using single-stranded DNA as a template [24].

Fluorescence *in situ* hybridization (FISH)
A process which vividly paints chromosomes or portions of chromosomes with fluorescent molecules [26].

Fluorophore
An atomic group with one excited molecule that emits photons and is fluorescent; also written fluorophor [28].

Fragile X
Fragile X syndrome is a hereditary condition that causes a wide range of mental impairment, from mild learning disabilities to severe mental retardation. It is the most common cause of genetically-inherited mental impairment and is associated with a number of physical and behavioral characteristics [30].

Genome
All the DNA contained in an organism or a cell, which includes both the chromosomes within the nucleus and the DNA in mitochondria [26].

[comparative] Genomic hybridization
Comparative genomic hybridization (CGH) is a powerful molecular and cytogenetic technique that provides an overview of genetic imbalance within the entire genome [29].

Genomics
The study of all of the nucleotide sequences, including structural genes, regulatory sequences, and noncoding DNA segments, in the chromosomes of an organism [24].

Genotype
(i) The genetic makeup, as distinguished from the physical appearance, of an organism or a group of organisms. (ii) The combination of alleles located on homologous chromosomes that determines a specific characteristic or trait [24].

Microarray analysis
A new way of studying how large numbers of genes interact with each other and how a cell's regulatory networks control vast batteries of genes simultaneously [26].

Oligonucleotide primers
Short sequence of single-stranded DNA or RNA. Oligonucleotides are often used as probes for detecting complementary DNA or RNA because they bind readily to their complements [26].

Pharmacogenetics

The study of genetic factors that influence an organism's reaction to a drug [24].

Pharmacogenomics

A biotechnological science that combines the techniques of medicine, pharmacology, and genomics and is concerned with developing drug therapies to compensate for genetic differences in patients which cause varied responses to a single therapeutic regimen [25].

Polymerase chain reaction

A fast, inexpensive technique for making an unlimited number of copies of any piece of DNA [26].

Polymorphisms

The regular occurrence of two or more alleles of a gene [25].

Prader–Willi syndrome

Prader–Willi syndrome is characterized by severe hypotonia and feeding difficulties in early infancy, followed in later infancy or early childhood by excessive eating and gradual development of morbid obesity, unless externally controlled. All patients have some degree of cognitive impairment; a distinctive behavioral phenotype is common. Hypogonadism is present in both males and females. Short stature is common. Accurate consensus clinical diagnostic criteria exist, but the mainstay of diagnosis is DNA-based methylation testing to detect the absence of the paternally contributed Prader–Willi syndrome/Angelman syndrome (PWS/AS) region on chromosome 15q11.2–q13. Such testing detects over 99% of patients. Methylation-specific testing is important to confirm the diagnosis of PWS in all individuals, but especially those who are too young to manifest sufficient features to make the diagnosis on clinical grounds or in those individuals who have atypical findings [31].

Single nucleotide polymorphism

Common, but minute, single base pair variations that occur in human DNA at a frequency of one every 1000 bases. These variations can be used to track inheritance in families [26].

Smith–Magenis syndrome

Smith–Magenis syndrome (SMS) is characterized by distinctive facial features, developmental delay, cognitive impairment, and behavioral abnormalities. The facial appearance is characterized by a broad square-shaped face, brachycephaly, prominent forehead, synophrys, upslanting palpebral fissures, deep-set eyes, broad nasal bridge, marked mid-facial hypoplasia, short, full-tipped nose with reduced nasal height, micrognathia in infancy changing to relative prognathia with age, and a distinct appearance of the mouth, with fleshy everted upper lip with a 'tented' appearance. Individuals with SMS function in the mild to moderate range of mental retardation. The behavioral phenotype includes significant sleep disturbance, stereotypies, and maladaptive and self-injurious behaviors. Childhood and adulthood are characterized by inattention, hyperactivity, maladaptive behaviors including frequent outbursts/temper tantrums, attention seeking, impulsivity, distractibility, disobedience, aggression, toileting difficulties, and self-injurious behaviors (SIB) including self-hitting, self-biting, and/or skin picking, inserting foreign objects into body orifices (polyemoilokomania), and yanking finger nails and/or toenails (onchyotillomania). Two stereotypic behaviors, spasmodic upper-body squeeze or 'self hug' and hand licking and page flipping ('lick and flip'), seem to be specific to SMS.

Diagnosis/testing. The diagnosis of SMS is confirmed either by detection of an interstitial deletion of the short arm of chromosome 17 band p11.2 (del17p11.2) by G-banded cytogenetic analysis and/or by fluorescence in situ hydridization (FISH) [32].

Velocardiofacial syndrome

The most common features are cleft palate, heart defects, characteristic facial appearance, minor learning problems and speech and feeding problems. The gene or genes that cause VCFS have not been identified; most children who have been diagnosed with this syndrome are missing region 22q11 of the genome. VCFS is an autosomal dominant disorder; in most cases neither parent has the syndrome or carries the defective gene. The cause of the deletion is unknown [27].

Williams' syndrome

A rare genetic disorder characterized especially by hypercalcemia of infants, heart defects (as supravalvular aortic stenosis), characteristic facial features (as an upturned nose, long philtrum, wide mouth, full lips, and pointed chin), a sociable personality, and a high verbal aptitude, but with mild to moderate mental retardation [29].

References

1. Begleiter H, Porjesz B, Bihari B, Kissan B: Event-related potential in boys at risk for alcoholism. *Science* 1984; **225**:1493–1496.

2. Courchesne E, Lincoln AJ, Yeung-Courchesne R, *et al.*: Pathophysiologic findings in nonretarded autism and receptive developmental language disorder. *J Autism Dev Disord* 1989; **19**:1–17.

3. de Regnier RA, Georgieff MK, Nelson CA: Visual event-related brain potentials in 4-month-old infants at risk for neurodevelopmental impairments. *Dev Psychobiol* 1997 30(1):11–28.

4. Giedd JN, Rapport JL, Leonard H, *et al.*: Case study: Acute basal ganglia enlargement and obsessive-compulsive symptoms in an adolescent boy. *J Am Acad Child Adolesc Psychiatry* 1996; **35**:913–915.

5. Piven J, Arndt S, Bailey J, Andresen N: Regional brain enlargement in autism: A magnetic resonance imaging study. *J Am Acad Child Adolesc Psychiatry* 1996; **35**:530–536.

6. Lou HC, Henricksen L, Bruhn P: Focal cerebral hypoprofusion in children with dysphasia and/or attention-deficit disorder. *Arch Neurol* 1984; **41**:825–829.

7. Amen DG, Paldi JH, Thisted RA: Brain SPECT imaging. *J Am Acad Child Adolesc Psychiatry* 1993; **32**:1080–1081.

8. Zametkin AJ, Nordahl TE, Gross M, *et al.*: Cerebral glucose metabolism in adults with hyperactivity of childhood onset. *N Engl J Med* 1990; **323**:1361–1366.

9. Zametkin AJ, Liebenauer LL, Fitzgerald GA, *et al.*: Brain metabolism in teenagers with attention-deficit hyperactivity disorder. *Arch Gen Psychiatry* 1993; **50**:333–340.

10. Matochik JA, Nordahl TE, Gross M, *et al.*: Effects of acute stimulant medication on cerebral metabolism in adults with hyperactivity. *Neuropsychopharmacology* 1993; **8**:377–386.

11. Matochik JA, Liebenauer LL, King AC, *et al.*: Cerebral metabolism in adults with attention-deficit hyperactivity disorder after chronic stimulant treatment. *Am J Psychiatry* 1994; **151**:658–664.

12. Matlay VS, Berman KF, Ostrem JL, *et al.*: Dextroamphetamine enhances "neural network-specific" physiological signals: A positron-emission tomography rCBF study. *J Neurosci* 1996; **16**:4816–4822.

13. Teicher M, Polcare A, Anderson C, *et al.*: Methylphenidate effects on hyperactivity and fMRI in children with ADHD. *Sci Proc Am Acad Child Adolesc Psychiatry* 1996; **12**:120.

14. Mozley PD, Zhu X, Kung HF: The dosimetry of iodine-123 labeled TISCH: A SPECT imaging agent for the D1 dopamine receptor. *J Nucl Med* 1993; **34**:208–213.

15. Seibyl JP, Woods SW, Zoghbi SS, *et al.*: Dynamic SPECT imaging of dopamine D2 receptors in human subjects with iodine-123-IBZM. *J Nucl Med* 1992; **33**:1964–1971.

16. Anderson AW, Gore JC: Neuroimaging. *Child Adolesc Psychiatr Clin North Am* 1997; **6**(2):213–264.

17. Ernst M, Zametkin AJ, Matochik JA, *et al.*: Effects of intravenous dextroamphetamine on brain metabolism in adults with attention-deficit hyperactivity disorder: Preliminary findings. *Psychopharmacol Bull* 1994; **30**:219–225.

18. Belliveau JW, Kennedy DN, McKinstry RC, *et al.*: Functional mapping of the human visual cortex by magnetic resonance imagining. *Science* 1991; **254**:716–719.

19. Breiter H, Rauch S, Kwong K, *et al.*: Functional magnetic resonance imaging of symptom provocation in obsessive-compulsive disorder. *Arch Gen Psychiatry* 1996; **53**:595–606.

20. Lauterbur PC: Image formation by induced local interactions: Examples employing nuclear magnetic resonance. *Nature* 1973; **242**:190–191.

21. Dager RS, Steen G: Applications of magnetic resonance spectroscopy to the investigation of neuropsychiatric disorders. *Neuropsychopharmacology* 1992; **6**:249–266.

22. DeRegnier RAO, Georgieff MK, Nelson CA: Visual event-related brain potentials in four-month-old infants at risk for neurodevelopmental impairments. *Dev Psychobiol* 1997; **30**:11–28.

23 Lim KO, Tew W, Kushner M, *et al.*: Cortical gray matter volume deficit in patients with first-episode schizophrenia. *Am J Psychiatry* 1996; **12**:1548–1553.

24. *The American Heritage Dictionary of the English Language*, 4th ed. Boston, MA: Houghton Mifflin Company, 2000.

25. *Merriam-Webster Medical Dictionary.* Springfield, MA: Merriam-Webster Inc., 2002.

26. National Human Genome Research Institute. [n.d/2005]. Talking Glossary. [WWWdocument]. URL http://www.genome.gov/10002096

27. National Institute on Deafness and Other Communication Disorders. 2005. Health Information: Voice, Speech, and Language. [WWWdocument]. URL http://www.nidcd.nih.gov/health/voice/velocario.asp

28. *Webster's New Millennium Dictionary of English*, Preview Edition (v 0.9.5). 2003, 2004 Lexico Publishing Group, LLC.

29. Corso C, Parry EM: The application of comparative genomic hybridization and fluorescence in situ hybridization to the characterization of genotoxicity screening tester strains AHH-1 and MCL-5. *Mutagenesis* 1999; **14**:417–426.

30. Fast D: The National Fragile X Foundation: What is Fragile X Syndrome? [WWWdocument] URL http://www.fragilex.org/html/what.htm. 2003.

31. Cassidy SB, Schwartz S: Prader-Willi Syndrome. [WWWdocument] URL http://www.geneclinics.org/profiles/pws/. 1998–2004

32. Smith ACM, Allanson JE, Allen AJ, *et al.* Smith-Magenis Syndrome. [WWWdocument] URL http://www.geneclinics.org/profiles/sms&id=8888888&key=r5uHMS56EheaU. 2001–2004

4

Educational Assessment and School Consultation

Dorothyann Feldis

Introduction

School is an environment in which children are asked to learn certain basic academic and social skills and in which their performance is judged and compared with that of other children. If children perform well, they learn that success provides opportunities and social status. If, on the other hand, they perform poorly for whatever reasons, they learn about failure and restricted opportunities. It is demoralizing to try to maintain a sense of self-worth and enthusiasm for learning within the confines of educational expectations that are impossible to achieve. Very early in their school careers, children essentially learn whether they are to be a success or a failure. The dilemma of failure is exacerbated by the fact that children are powerless to change their environment; they need adult support to identify learning problems and effective solutions to these problems. Child and adolescent psychiatrists and other professionals involved with children who are experiencing difficulty in school must understand the devastating impact that school failure has on a child's life and act swiftly to resolve the situation.

The first step in understanding a child's learning problems in school is devising some method of gathering information to help us understand the factors influencing the student's performance for the purpose of generating a solution. Historically, assessment has been used as a method of sorting students to be channeled into 'various segments of our social and economic system' rather than a method of 'tracking and enhancing growth toward standards' as well as a method of motivating students 'to strive for academic excellence' (p. 15 [1]). Classroom teachers are quick to state that assessment is effective only if used as a problem-solving mechanism; data not directly related

to improving school performance have little value to the classroom teacher. Lerner (2003) defines assessment as 'the process of collecting information about a student that will be used to form judgments and make decisions concerning that student' (p. 62 [2]). She also states that the 'closer the connection between education assessment and instruction the more effective the assessment–teaching process will be' (p. 62 [2]).

The educational assessment of children is a specialized process that directly addresses overall achievement in school. Generally, success in school is based on academic performance. Students who achieve well academically are usually considered successful and those who perform poorly are targets for academic assistance and adjustments. However, variables considering student's dispositions 'motivations, feelings and desires' must be included in that they 'directly influence academic achievement' (p. 199 [1]). This , of course, implies that the assessment process must have a collaborative approach: one that includes not only teachers, parents, diagnosticians but also the child. The child must be more than the object of the process but a part of the process. Stiggins (2005) asks us to consider the child as a 'consumer of assessment results' (p. 19 [1]). Positive, constructive results of continuous assessment builds self-esteem along with feelings of 'hopefulness' and the 'expectation of more success in the future' (p. 19 [1]). The outcome of any assessment process should provide information that allows teachers, parents and others to better create effective positive learning environments: environments that allow students to assume control of their own destiny in school. The performance of the child is not viewed in isolation but as part of a large ecosystem containing numerous interdependent variables. This approach acknowledges that factors other than ability affect learning and therefore

Clinical Child Psychiatry, Second Edition. Edited by W.M. Klykylo and J.L. Kay
© 2005 John Wiley & Sons Ltd.

requires that the environment adjust to support the special learning needs of the child.

Who is Qualified to Conduct an Educational Evaluation?

Individuals who conduct educational evaluations are usually called diagnostic educators; they must be able to collect the data necessary to identify a learner problem and then use those data to devise educational intervention strategies. Their academic training should consist of at least a master's degree in education combined with clinical testing and teaching experience, and knowledge of reading disorders. This diagnostic role is relatively new for educators, however, and it is therefore important to understand and distinguish the skills of the diagnostic educator from those of other professionals. The diagnostic educator must be able to identify and analyze the child's learning patterns and assist the classroom teacher in implementing instructional methods that can accommodate learning differences. To help accomplish this, he or she must understand the cause and nature of learning disabilities as well as methods of accommodating learning differences in the classroom. The diagnostic educator must understand the purpose of a school-based problem-solving team and be able to use this team to help facilitate change in both attitudes and approaches to learning and assessment of outcomes. Because the role of the educational diagnostician involves interpreting performance in the classroom, teaching experience often validates these individuals' credentials.

When Should A Referral be Made?

The psychiatrist may have to request an educational evaluation when there is a question about school performance or the need to adjust a child's educational program. The problem may be a new development or a chronic or crisis situation. A new problem is a recent situation without an identified history, for example, a child in kindergarten or first grade for whom the teacher has expressed concerns about progress. Problems such as these might be considered 'developmental,' and teachers and other professionals might choose to take the 'wait and see' approach. Many of these issues, however, often materialize into significant learning problems in the second or third grade, when the child actually begins to fail. Serious consideration should therefore be given to early concerns about a child's progress, before school expectations begin to appear insurmountable to the child and his or her family. Other new problems might be caused by illness or other family trauma that has affected school performance for a child who historically has been considered a typical learner.

In some chronic situations children may have received some form of assessment or intervention, and in other cases they may not have received any consideration. An example of the former would be a sixth-grade child with a history of reading problems who has received some individual tutoring but whose report cards continue to indicate little or no improvement. An example of the latter would be a ninth-grader with a history of learning problems who has managed to perform adequately through elementary and junior high school, but who has significant difficulty adjusting to the expectations of the secondary school environment.

A crisis situation needs immediate action and has the potential for seriously compromising the future academic progress of the child. There are various circumstances that might generate a crisis, but two situations should be addressed without hesitation: grade retention and school suspension or explusion. In the case of grade retention, one ground rule exists: no decision should be made until the child receives an interdisciplinary evaluation that includes an educational, psychological, psychiatric, and speech and language assessment. The reason for failure must be specifically identified and a plan for intervention designed; the child deserves every resource available to resolve the problem. In the case of school suspension or explusion, the child also needs an interdisciplinary evaluation to determine the variables affecting behavioral issues, and to rule out other contributing factors such as learning disorders and psychiatric illness. If the child has been assessed in the past, these reports need to be reviewed and updated. If the child has been suspended, the present education program is not helping him or her adjust to the expectations of the learning environment, and the child's situation needs to be reconsidered.

The cause of problematic behavior must be identified and an intervention plan developed, if reentry is to be successful. In these cases the psychiatrist needs the educator to assess academic performance and identify the necessary accommodations required for successful progress to occur. Whatever the problem, it is important to remember that children cannot usually develop coping mechanisms on their own or adjust their school environment to help them better meet expectations. If professionals hesitate in obtaining an assessment there can be misdirected, inefficient, and often disappointing results for all.

Legislation and Rights

Historically, classroom teachers have assessed children by trying to discover what they do or do not know and why they have learned some things and not others. If a teacher is skilled and the system supportive, this method can be effective. The individual skill of the teacher and the random sensitivity of the system, however, do not ensure that all children experiencing problems in school will be appropriately identified and provided with the adaptations necessary for learning to occur. The enactment of Public Law (PL) 94–142, the Education of Handicapped Children Act (1975), changed this process. Instead of depending on good teachers and interventions, the law mandated that all children aged 5–21 years with an identified handicap will have a free and appropriate education. It also provided procedures to determine eligibility for special education services and appropriate programming. This legislation was revised in 1990 (PL 101–476) and renamed Individual with Disabilities Education Act (IDEA) recognizing the concept of considering individuals first, then identifying their characteristics and extended the mandate to serve children aged 3–21 years. The most recent revision of the Individuals with Disabilities of 1997 includes raising expectations for children with disabilities, ensuring that children with disabilities have increased access to the general education curriculum and strengthening the role of parents.

This legislation emphasizes educating children in the least restrictive learning environment possible, one that can provide inclusion in the general curriculum. Good program decisions usually consider the child's educational needs, the support services needed to accommodate those needs, and methods of imbedding supports into the general curriculum.

The Ohio Department of Education suggests that 'a child's placement is presumed first to be the general education environment' (p. 14 [3]). If the child is not participating with nondisabled children, the IEP team must provide an explanation.

The legislation also provides a specific set of procedures for identifying a child's disability and determining an appropriate educational program (Table 4.1). These procedures ensure the right of all children to receive services for which they are eligible. Any child suspected of a disability must have a multifactored evaluation (MFE), which assesses all areas related to the suspected disability, and an individualized education program (IEP) conference to review the MFE data, determine eligibility for special services, and define the least restrictive learning environment to be used. Because of the school's obligation to determine an IEP for each identified child and to define general educational goals and teaching strategies, educators have begun to perfect the educational assessment as a means of providing data pertinent to classroom learning and curricula.

Table 4.1 Identifying a child's disability: procedural safeguards.

Stage	Components
Preferral	Parents discuss program with teacher and request intervention, or school requests referral for evaluation in writing.
Referral	School explains referral process to parent. Parents receive copy of parent's rights. Parents give permission for testing.
Evaluation	Parents participate in and contribute to team evaluation activities. School completes evaluation and team determines eligibility for special education services.
IEP meeting	Parents participate in IEP activities. Evaluation team jointly develops IEP. Parent gives consent for placement to receive special education services which will enable child to participate in general education curriculum.
Annual review	School and parents review child's progress and current IEP.
Reevaluation	School initiates reevaluation every three years. Parents initiate sooner needs of child change.
Independent educational evaluation	Parent has a right to an independent evaluation if there is a disagreement over the evaluation. School may initiate due process if evaluation team believes the evaluation is fair and accurate.

IEP, Individual education program. Adapted from Ohio Department of Education Office for Exceptional Children: *Whose Idea Is This? A Resource Guide for Parents*. Columbus, OH: Ohio Department of Education, 2004.

Schools must by law provide an MFE for any child suspected of having a disability. The referral may be made by the parents, school personnel, or community agency personnel. If parents are making the referral, they should do so in writing, indicating that they suspect that their child has a disability and requires an MFE. If the school district refers the child, the parents must be contacted by the school and asked for their consent to evaluate [3]. Prior to referral parents should expect the school to contact them to discuss the problem and obtain additional information. The school is also required to organize a team of professionals consisting of the parents, teachers, principal and other school personnel such as the school psychologist or speech and language therapist, who might help generate interventions strategies. If these strategies are not effective within a designated period, this team, often called an intervention-based assistance team, then refers the child for an MFE. Schools sometimes ask professionals not part of the school's team, including child psychiatrists or pediatricians, to assist in the problem-solving and evaluation process. If the school requests this assistance, it is obliged to pay for the service. If there is a disagreement over the evaluation, the parent has the right to an independent evaluation at the school's expense. Sometimes parents decide to pursue an independent MFE rather than using services provided by the school. This is a legitimate choice for parents, and the results must be considered by the school, as long as the professionals have the appropriate certification or license in their specific discipline. In this situation, however, the parents are obliged to cover the cost.

The school is required to hold an IEP conference to review the results of the MFE, determine eligibility for services, and plan an appropriate education program. This meeting must include parents as joint decision makers. Parents may request other individuals to attend this meeting. These individuals may include professionals from outside the school who conducted all or part of the MFE or who were involved in implementing treatment programs – namely tutors, child and adolescent psychiatrists, occupational or physical therapists, and speech and language therapists. Parents may also invite an advocate or mentor to help them deal with the educational system on behalf of their child. Advocates or mentors are available through parent or child advocacy programs in the community. Many school districts are instituting parent mentor programs to help parents understand and effectively access the IEP process. Special education regional resource centers exist in some areas and may also provide advocates.

Once a child is enrolled in special education, the school district is obliged to conduct an annual review of the child's progress and notify parents of current IEP goals. A reevaluation by the school district is required every three years. Parents should be notified of and informed about this process.

In summary, children with disabilities have a legal right to a free and appropriate education, and schools are legally obligated to meet these needs. Parents often require the support of mentors and professionals to ensure that their children's needs are in fact met.

The Evaluation

The purpose of the education evaluation is to collect the data necessary for determining eligibility for special education services and to identify specific learning needs and intervention strategies. Eligibility is ultimately a procedural and legal decision that depends on present levels of performance and standardized data; the identification of specific learning needs requires additional data emphasizing an analysis of the student's learning patterns, the school environment and other social and cultural influences. Each component of an educational evaluation should contain information necessary to help to determine eligibility but also to identify specific learning strategies. These components usually include background information, descriptive data, test data, and the educational plan (Figure 4.1).

Background Information

The background information in an evaluation includes school history, relevant medical history, the presenting problem, the duration of the problem, and the effect the problem has had on the child's development at home and in school. This information may be collected from parents, teachers, and other professionals and individuals involved in the care of the child. At this point in the process, the educational diagnostician determines how parents, teachers, and the student each perceive the problem. Do teachers perceive parents as helpful and supportive to the child and his or her learning process? Do parents view the teachers and other school personnel as willing to adjust teaching strategies to accommodate the child?

How does the child perceive his/her performance? Can the student identify problems and possible solutions? How have teachers and parents responded to the students school failure? Does the student view himself to be in a hopeless situation? Differences in these per-

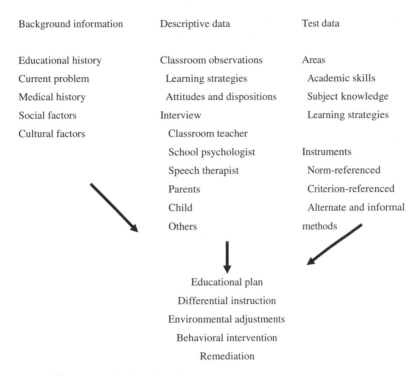

Figure 4.1 Components of an educational evaluation.

ceptions may have a significant impact on the resolution of the problem.

Test Data

An educational assessment usually includes both norm- and criterion-referenced testing of academic achievement, general knowledge, and specific skill mastery. Most tests divide the academic areas of reading, mathematics, and written language into different components to allow a more thorough analysis of the child's abilities.

In addition to providing information about what the child knows the educational assessment also needs to focus on how the child learns. This requires a careful analysis of the results including the child's responses to content as well as different test requirements. For example, some students do better on items that require a verbal response rather than timed, written responses. If these types of responses are a theme throughout the assessment process, and also evident in the classroom, the educator can begin to identify effective learning strategies. Lerner (2003) states that when teachers 'help students acquire learning strategies, students learn how to learn' [2]. This, of course, is the ultimate goal of the educational evaluation.

Depending on the presenting problem, information required for eligibility for special education services emphasizes test performance in specific areas of academic, cognitive, language, and behavioral development. This information compares the child with others and is called norm-referenced. Information generated from norm-referenced tests compares the child's performance to a group of children similar in age, grade and sometimes other characteristics. Criterion-referenced tests, also standardized, identify a student's mastery of specific skills based on an established criterion usually aligned with classroom curriculum. Criterion-referenced tests do not compare the child to a group of peers.

Because criterion-referenced tests tend to be more closely aligned with classroom curricula they allow for a more detailed interpretation of the child's performance than do norm-referenced tests. A norm-referenced test in reading and written language, for example, may indicate that a child's performance in reading comprehension and written language is within two standard deviations below the mean. This information probably confirms the teacher's concerns that the child can read but is not comprehending or expressing thoughts well; it does not, however; identify learning processes that might help the child or teacher to better understand their performance. More specific analysis of reading comprehension and written language is necessary. In this instance, criterion-referenced tests can help the educator to better analyze the child's ability to manage specific aspects of the learning process required in the classroom.

Although criterion-referenced tests do allow a more specific analysis of a child's performance, they may also suggest solutions based on isolated skill deficits, thus neglecting the effect of other variables within the learning environment. Additional data are required to adequately characterize a student's learning and to provide a more detailed analysis of the learning process.

Descriptive Data

Descriptive data help to identify the environmental variables, teaching approaches, and other factors that might be affecting a child's progress in school. The data are usually collected via classroom observation and interviews with teachers, parents, and other specialists involved in the child's educational program. The child should also be included in this process and provided the opportunity to contribute their perception about the problem, its cause, and even possible solutions.

Classroom observation can provide information about a child's behavior, attention, and general ability to adapt to school expectations. The educational diagnostician is interested in the child's ability to learn in the classroom. Understanding how material is presented to the child, how the child is requested to respond, how the child responds, and the attitudes attached to the child's performance are all indicators of overall performance. For example, a child with a written language problem might be required to answer essay questions to pass tests in social studies. As a result of this testing procedure, the child will probably fail. To generate effective intervention strategies, the educator must not only identify the child's ability in social studies and written language but also understand the relationship between the two within the structure of the classroom. All this may become apparent only after classroom observation and discussion with the teacher, the child and the parents. Descriptive data help to answer the following questions:

Is the child motivated and interested in school?
Is the child attentive in the classroom?
Is homework and/or organization a problem?
What is the child's attitude about school?
How does the child respond to discipline?

What are peer interactions like in the school environment?
How do other students and the teacher respond to the child's performance?
How is the child recognized in the classroom?
Is the child regarded as is a successful or unsuccessful learner?
How frequently does the child receive positive feedback in the classroom?

Each source of information provides a different perception of the problem, and information from all these sources needs to be analyzed to identify the child's learning problems, teaching approaches that might enhance or obstruct learning and possible solutions. The expectations and responses of all people involved must be understood if adjustments in the educational program are to be successful.

Educational Plan

The final component of an educational evaluation is the educational plan, which provides a framework for generating solutions. In the case of a child with written language problems, for example, the educational diagnostician and the teacher must generate two solutions: (1) a way to evaluate the child's knowledge of content that does not employ a weak skill as the vehicle for testing, and (2) a plan to improve knowledge and, where possible, deficient skills. In the past, solutions have focused on requiring the child to improve performance through remediation and, of course, 'try harder' without any significant environmental adjustments. Creating a more accessible learning environment that emphasizes strengths and decreases negative outcomes is crucial, however, if children with learning problems are to succeed. Even with the appropriate intervention, some children will never totally correct these weaknesses and must instead learn how to compensate. Although children may have some ability to identify stumbling blocks in their learning environment, they are almost always powerless to change them. Adults must ensure that the necessary adjustments occur.

When a child is referred for educational testing, the problem has already been identified. Assessment should do more than confirm the referral question; it should identify skills or learning behaviors that are interfering with learning, as well as a set of effective learning strategies. The educational plan should identify ways to adjust negative variables, introduce remediation, and emphasize possible variables to enhance learning. This purpose implies that intervention will focus on implementing changes in the environment and in instruction. The most difficult aspect of this approach is that persons other than the child may be expected to change and, consequently, that the child's progress may be dependent on changes in the environment.

Consultation, Collaboration, and Educational Planning

Historically, the medical literature has described consultation as a process by which one physician requests expert advice from another, usually pertaining to the condition or situation of a patient [4]. In these situations the consultant providing the advice has assumed no responsibility for the outcome but has merely shared knowledge. Although this is an accepted practice in medicine, educators are attempting to approach consultation as a process wherein teachers, parents, and others involved with a child work jointly to solve a problem. This usually involves adapting the learning environment to better meet the specific needs of the child. It also emphasizes the need for professionals to collaborate as a team to generate workable solutions that might involve joint responsibility for implementation and outcome – a process called collaborative consultation.

School Dynamics and Collaborative Consultation

The IDEA requires that a 'multifactored team' assess the child's learning problems and develop intervention plans. Successful intervention, particularly in inclusive learning environments, requires that parents, administrators, support services, and teachers work together with the student to create a more effective learning environment All professionals involved in the care of children, then, must understand the process of educational consultation and school dynamics.

West and Idol defined consultation as 'a term used across various disciplines to refer to some type of triadic relationship among consultants, consultees, and clients or problems' (p. 395 [5]). The expert consultation model may be distinguished from the collaborative consultation model: the former refers to a type of consultation in which an 'expert,' usually a school support professional such as a school psychologist, analyzes the problem, evaluates options, and prescribes interventions for the teacher to implement [6]. His is the model that many teachers have experienced, one in which they are given little input but all the responsibility for change. Idol and colleagues defined collaborative consultation as 'a process that enables people

with diverse expertise to generate creative solutions to mutually defined problems' (p. 1 [7]). Such a model allows teachers equal participation in a process that will generate solutions for them to implement. Friend and Cook (2000) further describe school consultation as a 'voluntary process' where 'one professional assists another' to help a third (p. 73 [8]).

Historically, teachers have voluntarily sought information from colleagues. The process of collaboration is complicated, however, when professionals from outside the school become involved in the process and in fact might initiate the process. Although these individuals may have crucial information that needs to be incorporated into the educational plan, effective results are dubious unless professionals understand teachers' expectations and roles within the configuration of the school. In the hierarchy of professional competence, physicians have historically been rated higher and teachers lower than most other professionals. Teachers, of course, have resented interference by physicians, who are viewed as more knowledgeable than themselves yet are deficient in knowing how to teach children. Many teachers return to their classrooms after planning meetings mumbling 'I'd like to see them manage a class like this alone for just one day.' The lack of support and professional respect has promoted in teachers an attitude of suspicion of 'outsiders.' The psychiatrist must understand the process of collaboration in schools as well as the various levels of competence that exist. Some schools have established effective collaborative intervention models, some are in the process of developing these models, and some have not yet begun. Whatever the status of a school, the model of consultation used must be collaborative. IDEA, as well as good educational practice, expects team collaboration.

To begin the process of collaboration, schools are required by law to hold an IEP meeting to review the results of a multifactored assessment. Many schools also establish teams to address the needs of a child who may not have been referred for a multifactored assessment but who is experiencing learning or behavioral problems. These teams provide a mechanism for teachers to discuss these problems with support personnel, parents and other teachers, and to collaboratively plan intervention strategies. It is fair to expect the child's psychiatrist to also become a part of this problem-solving team. Although this meeting involves energy as well as time, the therapeutic process is augmented by securing teacher cooperation and a formal method for problem solving in the school.

Psychiatry, particularly child and adolescent psychiatry, is mysterious to the general public. Unless faced with a child who requires the services of a child and adolescent psychiatrist, most people are unfamiliar with the psychiatrist's role in the care of children. As psychiatrists begin to interact with schools, they may need to explain to school personnel their goals for the child and his or her family and intervention strategies such as therapy and medication. If medication is being considered for treatment, psychiatrists should explain the medication and the expected outcome as they relate to the overall treatment goals. They should emphasize the need for teachers to report behavioral changes in order to help determine the effectiveness of the medication. It may help to provide teachers with a specific format or behavior checklist for collecting this information and to periodically contact them by phone. Establishing clear avenues of communication is crucial; whatever method is chosen, psychiatrists should be proactive in establishing communication with teachers and other school personnel. Often, the most efficient way of achieving these goals and providing the family with the appropriate support is to attend the IEP meeting.

The family as well as the child should play an equal part to that of the psychiatrist and the teacher in the collaboration process. The IDEA actually requires that parents and the child become involved in the IEP assessment and planning process. This process is effective only if all members of the team appreciate the contribution of the family members and are skillful in including their participation. Many parents are proactive and aggressively solicit intervention for their child; others, however, are timid and unfamiliar with their rights as parents and the capacity of their influence. Whatever the circumstances, the psychiatrist should facilitate the process of collaboration by helping parents understand their child's needs, as well as the roles of parents and the process of collaboration in the problem-solving process.

Whereas parents, teachers, and other professionals join together to plan educational programs for children, the child is often absent from the discussions. Young children, of course, are usually not able to contribute directly to this process and depend on the parents and others involved to represent their best interests. As Friend (2000) explains, the child, ' not a direct participant in the interaction' is the beneficiary of the process (p. 73 [8]). This is an interesting situation, since most professionals and parents believe that they are acting on behalf of the child but may in fact have other agendas. Schools are affected by financial boundaries and legislative mandates as well as their responsibility to accommodate the needs of an individual child. Accommodations to the learning environment may require financial commitment and a change in the school's perception of its responsibilities. Parents make requests influenced by their perception of the child's problem in school, the school's legal responsibilities to assist the child, the developmental issues affecting the child's performance, and their ultimate goals for the child. Conflict arises when perceptions of the school and the family differ; resolution, then, can occur only if both sides are able to jointly address the child's learning needs and adjust environmental variables accordingly.

The planning process can sometimes be augmented by inviting children to participate. Their interpretation of the situation should be considered, even if they are not present at the meeting, and their capacity to state their own educational needs should not automatically be dismissed. Children can often be helped in focusing on their school problems and beginning to identify intervention strategies that will help them succeed. If the child does not wish to be present or is too young to understand the purpose of the meeting, the child psychiatrist can be helpful in articulating the child's perceptions of the problem and possible ideas about the solution. Adolescents should definitely be given the option to contribute to the planning process and, if comfortable, to be present at planning meetings. If the adolescent is embarrassed to go to the office to be given medication, or if the adolescent is teased about leaving class for tutoring, there is a good chance that he or she will not cooperate and the plan will fail. These procedures should be adjusted whenever possible to preserve the child's dignity among his or her peers, because the success of any intervention program depends on the cooperation of the child or adolescent.

Techniques of School Collaboration

Successful communication with schools depends on understanding the general administrative structure of schools as well as the function of individuals in the schools. Different problems require different administrative authority, and knowledge about these lines of authority can be important (Table 4.2). Issues that focus on curriculum and adjustment in the classroom or school are generally managed by the teacher and the principal. If a teacher is resistant to adjusting classroom procedures or using a curriculum agreed on by the planning team, this problem becomes the principal's responsibility. Issues involving finances or the implementation of legislative mandates, including referral, evaluation, and eligibility for services, are responsibilities of the director of special education and the superintendent. Principals control building issues

Table 4.2 The function of school personnel in resolving school issues.

School personnel	Issue(s)
Principal	School entry
Principal and teacher	Classroom issues
	Curriculum
	Instruction
	Environmental
	variables
Support services	School adjustment
School psychologists	Referral and
Speech/language	assessment
therapist	Behavior management
Reading specialist	Individualized
OT/PT	intervention
Administration personnel	Procedural issues
Principal	Eligibility for special
Pupil personnel director	services
Superintendent	Due process
	procedures
	School safety
	Quality control
	Curriculum guidelines

be knowledgeable about special education procedures and services, including the referral process and legislative mandates, the director of special education may need to be contacted directly. The superintendent is, of course, responsible for all activities in the school district and should be contacted if other administrators are unresponsive to the educational needs of a child. In practice, collaboration with a school is seldom successful without the wholehearted support of the principal.

For child psychiatrists, the most important part of collaboration with schools is to participate as much as possible. Whatever the situation, open communication with the school is important. Schools should be aware of the psychiatrist's involvement with the child, and the psychiatrist should be aware of the child's performance and adjustment to the school environment. The psychiatrist must willingly share information with the school but at the same time help the child and his or her family separate those issues that should be discussed with the school and those that should remain confidential. Children often have a clear perception of the things they would like teachers to know or not know about them. The psychiatrist can become an important conduit between the child, family members, and the school. This role, if supportive to all people involved, can have a positive effect on the problem-solving process.

The child psychiatrist should remember the following rules when collaborating with schools.

Always:

- initiate contact with the school
- share information
- explain your role
- represent the child's perspectives
- request school evaluation data
- expect team effort in problem solving
- expect parents to collaborate as team members
- be a team member

and the functions of the school intervention or child study team; the director of special education, however, becomes involved when a child is suspected of having a developmental disability that would qualify him or her for special education services.

Contact with the school should generally begin with the school principal. The principal should introduce professionals from outside the school to the teacher, clarify the role of these professionals, and ensure that communication with the teacher has been authorized by the parents or guardian. It is important for 'outsiders' to understand that the principal establishes the culture of the school building. This does not mean that the principal obstructs contact between teachers and outside professionals, rather that he or she is aware of individuals contacting teachers and monitors these contacts, particularly if he or she is concerned about the ability of a teacher to interact appropriately. Thus failure to contact the principal before communicating with a teacher can be an irreparable mistake. The principal also arranges for the involvement of the director of special education and other school support personnel (e.g., the school psychologist or a speech and language pathologist). If a principal does not appear to

References

1. Stiggins R: *Student-Involved Assessment For Learning.* Upper SaddleRiver, New Jersey: Pearson Merrill Prentice Hall, 2005.
2. Lerner J: *Learning Disabilities – Theories, Diagnosis, and Teaching Strategies.* Boston, MA: Houghton Mifflin Company, 2003.
3. Ohio Department of Education: *Whose Idea Is This? A Resource Guide for Parents.* Columbus, OH: Ohio Department of Education, 2004.
4. Caplan G: *The Theory and Practice of Mental Health Consultation.* New York: Basic Books, 1970.

5. West FJ, Idol L: School consultation. Part 1: An inter-disciplinary perspective on theory, models, and research. *J Learn Disab* 1987; **20**(7):388–408.

6. Reeve PT, Hallan DP: Practical questions about collaboration between general and special educators. *Focus Except Child* 1994; **26**(7):1–11.

7. Idol L, Paolucci-Whitcomb P, Nevin A: *Collaborative Consultation*. Rockville, MD: Aspen Publishers, 1986.

8. Friend M, Cook L: *Interactions-Collaboration Skills for School Professionals, 3rd ed*. New York: Longman, 2000.

5

Psychiatric Assessment in Medically Ill Children, Including Children with HIV

David M. Rube, G. Oana Costea

Introduction

The majority of children with chronic medical problems do not have a psychiatric illness. However, the risk for psychological and social adjustment problems in those children is approximately twice the risk of healthy children. Additionally, comorbid psychiatric and pediatric medical problems contribute to increased health care costs, less satisfactory outcomes, and increased diagnostic uncertainty. The consultation-liaison child psychiatrist's role is to help educate the pediatric colleagues about the comorbidity of medical and psychiatric disorders, the importance of psychiatric consultation and to work as part of the multidisciplinary team in order to provide comprehensive care for these children. This chapter examines the: (1) epidemiology and characteristics of psychiatric disorders in medically ill children; (2) reasons for psychiatric consultation; (3) psychiatric assessment; (4) psychiatric sequelae of chronic medical problems; and (5) pediatric HIV infection including epidemiology, neuro-developmental and psychological manifestations, psychiatric assessment and treatment considerations. Illustrative clinical cases are included.

refusing visitors. He was belligerent throughout the day and consistently removed IVs. The consultation was held to evaluate Stephen's behavior. On examination, Stephen met criteria for a depressive disorder with associated anxiety symptoms. Individual psychotherapy and a trial of fluoxetine were initiated. Psychotherapy entailed play, drawing, story-telling and also distraction and relaxation techniques to help him cope with the procedures. Areas of focus included: education about his illness, the effects of his cancer and its treatment on body image, issues of life, death and grief, at a developmentally appropriate level. Gradually, Stephen was noted to be more upbeat, cooperative, pleasant, more open to procedures, and more emotionally open to discuss his medical condition. He started to interact more appropriately with physicians and staff and was more able to talk about death and dying to his parents and family.

CASE ONE

A psychiatric consultation was received for Stephen, a nine-year-old boy with stomach cancer. The hematology/oncology team and the nursing staff found Stephen to be belligerent and aggressive during medical procedures. During 'off hours' he would be found in his room in the dark with the shades pulled,

CASE TWO

During her second hospital admission for an evaluation of abnormal wheezing, Sarah, a 12-year-old girl, underwent a psychiatric consult. An extensive workup for wheezing, including X-rays, sweat tests, and a computed tomography (CT) scan, all proved negative. The only procedure that helped Sarah not wheeze was

Clinical Child Psychiatry, Second Edition. Edited by W.M. Klykylo and J.L. Kay
© 2005 John Wiley & Sons Ltd.

lying recumbent. A psychiatric consultation was requested to elucidate any psychiatric factors that might be contributing to Sarah's medical condition. After interviews with Sarah and her parents, the physician found no evidence of depression, hypochondriasis, or any reported anxiety symptoms. During the interview, Sarah described an adult supervisor at recess who had been harassing her on the playground. This harassment consisted of teasing as well as telling other girls not to play with Sarah. The parents had brought this issue to the local school board but had received little assistance. Sarah had made a presentation and written a letter to the school board herself describing this harassment. It was about that time that Sarah's wheezing began. A school consultation was initiated by Sarah's psychiatric consultant. The harassment ended and so did Sarah's wheezing.

These two cases illustrate the necessity and importance of the appropriate use of psychiatric consultation in the pediatric population. One- to two-thirds of in-patient pediatric patients have to cope with psychological issues [1,2] and could potentially benefit from psychiatric consultation. Chronic physical illness appears to be a significant risk factor for emotional and behavioral difficulties, while emotional, behavioral and family difficulties can negatively affect the course of physical disease [3]. In addition, comorbid psychiatric and pediatric medical problems contribute to increased health care costs, less satisfactory outcomes, and increased diagnostic uncertainty [4]. In this day of children who survive severe medical illnesses such as leukemia, who undergo transplantation (e.g., cardiac, liver, lung, bone marrow), and who live with chronic illnesses for much longer than previously (e.g., cystic fibrosis, diabetes mellitus, infection with the human immunodeficiency virus HIV), psychiatric sequelae are common. It is incumbent on child and adolescent psychiatrists to work in collaboration with pediatricians in an effort to provide comprehensive care for these children.

Traditionally, consultation-liaison child psychiatry has taken place on pediatric wards and in hospital units. The influence of managed care, however, has shortened hospital stays, and more care is now being provided in the outpatient setting as well as in the home or day hospital. This implies that consultation-liaison must adapt to the outpatient and homecare setting. In this chapter, we discuss the epidemiology and characteristics of psychiatric disorders and diagnostic dilemmas in the medically ill child. We follow this with discussions of the consultation and assessment process and the psychiatric sequelae of chronic medical problems. We conclude with pediatric HIV infection including epidemiology, neurodevelopmental and psychological manifestations along with the psychiatric assessment and treatment considerations in this patient population.

Epidemiology

Consultation-liaison child psychiatrists work with their pediatric colleagues to convey to them the importance of psychiatric consultation. When we assume the role of a consultant, we should help our pediatric colleagues by informing them of the data that exist regarding the comorbidity of medical and psychiatric disorders. The majority of children with chronic medical problems do not have a psychiatric illness. Reports indicate, however, that the risk for psychological and social adjustment problems in children with chronic medical problems is about twofold compared with the risk of healthy children [5–7]. Emotional and behavioral problems have been found to affect 18–20% of children in pediatric primary care practice [8] while estimates of psychological morbidity associated with chronic illness in childhood range from 10 to 30% [1]. Ten to 15% of the population under 18 years of age has chronic medical problems. A Swedish primary care district, however, estimated the prevalence of chronic illness in childhood to be 6% [9]. In the Isle of Wight Survey, 6% of the population had chronic physical illnesses [10]. In the latter study, Rutter and colleagues found that the prevalence of child psychiatric disorders in the general population was 7% and that the prevalence of psychiatric conditions in children with chronic physical illnesses was 12% (illnesses without brain lesions) and 34% (illnesses with brain lesions).

The National Survey of Health Development in England, Wales, and Scotland and the Rochester Child Health Survey showed that the prevalence of chronic medical problems ranges from 10 to 20% [11]. The former survey observed that 25% of physically ill children younger than 15 years of age had two or more symptoms of behavior disorder, compared to 17% of the healthy population [11]. Similarly, the Rochester survey showed that the rates of behavior problems in the chronically ill children were consistently higher than in healthy children and were reflected in behaviors such as a poor attitude toward school and truancy [12,13]. Additionally, studies showed higher frequency of oppositional disorder and conduct disorder in children with cystic fibrosis compared with children with sickle cell disease. The treatment regimen for cystic fibrosis being highly demanding and involving daily numerous medications and chest physical therapy may contribute to this difference [14].

Different theories attempt to explain this comorbidity and to identify factors that account for the variability in the psychological adjustment of children with chronic illness. Reports have described risk factors at multiple levels that can impede the psychological adjustment to chronic illness (Table 5.1). In this regard, studies suggest that severe asthma, inflammatory bowel disease (Crohn disease or ulcerative colitis) and diabetes may have specifically elevated rates of depression

Table 5.1 Risk factors affecting psychological adjustment in medically ill children.

Illness related factors [1,8,14,19,20]
  1. Frequent or chronic pain (e.g., sickle cell disease)
  2. Brain dysfunction as a result of illness or treatment
  3. Physical disability (e.g., decreased exercise endurance in advancing cystic fibrosis)
  4. Invisible condition
  5. Uncertain prognosis
  6. Multiple hospitalizations
  7. Intrusive care routines (e.g., numerous medication and chest physical therapy in cystic fibrosis)
  8. Dietary restrictions (e.g., diabetes)

Patient related factors [8,18,19,20]
  1. Young age
  2. Male gender (immunoreactive theory)
  3. Genetic loading
  4. History of psychiatric illness
  5. Insecure attachments
  6. Difficult temperament
  7. Low self-esteem
  8. Coping style with depressive behavior in reaction to daily problems

Family related factors [1,8,20]
  1. Single parent
  2. Low family income
  3. Parental anxiety, anger, sadness, guilt, blame
  4. History of psychiatric illness
  5. Poor family support
  6. Inadequate parenting

[15]. Additionally, a meta-analysis of depression in children with chronic medical conditions showed higher rates of depression in children with asthma and sickle cell anemia as compare with children with cancer. The unpredictable and long-term course of those illnesses may potentially explain the difference [16].

Adolescent females with chronic medical conditions were found to have greater emotional problems, depression, sadness, anhedonia, and suicidal thoughts than were adolescent males with chronic medical conditions [17]. However, male gender may potentially pose a higher risk of emotional problems as suggested by the immunoreactive theory [8]. It is hypothesized that males are selectively afflicted with neurodevelopmental and psychiatric disorders of childhood and this may relate to the relative antigenicity of the male fetus which may induce a state of maternal immunoreactivity leading to fetal damage [57]. There are protective factors as well. Children's personal strengths, whether in academia, sports, music or interpersonal skills could help maintain self-esteem and build important relationships [1]. The coping style confrontation characterized by active and purposeful problem solving along with seeking social support were found to be related to positive psychosocial functioning [18]. Additionally, family flexibility, positive meanings ascribe to the condition, social integration, good communication, clear boundaries, support network in the community appear to be also protective [19].

The epidemiologic evidence indicates a role for liaison to medical subspecialties to educate other physicians about psychiatric disturbances that may become evident in their patients. Since not all children develop psychiatric symptoms, baseline evaluations or screening devices are needed to clarify which children and families are at risk. The Pediatric Symptom Checklist developed by Jellinek and Murphy has been shown to be a helpful, user-friendly screening device for pediatricians and pediatric residents [21]. Jones and colleagues recommend the Pediatric Symptom Checklist to routinely screen all pediatric patients and, for those patients who meet the cut-off criteria, then using the Child Behavior Checklist [22]. This approach therefore provides an efficient means of screening for and then identifying child psychosocial problems in general pediatric populations.

The Consultative Process and Assessment

Reasons for Consultation

Consultation-liaison child psychiatrists, like other pediatric subspecialists, are called to consult on challenging or difficult cases. The most common reasons for psychiatric consultation encountered in major academic centers and tertiary care hospitals are presented in Table 5.2.

Five Fundamental Questions

Question 1

Is this patient safe to himself or herself or others in the current treatment setting?

The issues that may drive this question arise from individuals who attempt suicide and who may then need to be hospitalized for medical treatment in the intensive care unit (ICU) or on the general pediatric unit and may also require one-on-one intensive supervision. Other examples of this question may be the child who develops delirium and has visual or auditory hallucinations.

CASE THREE

Nancy is a 12-year-old girl with a previous medical history of Burkitts' lymphoma, which was treated approximately three years prior to the consultation and was currently in remission. She came to the children's hospital emergency department (ED) after having a seizure. She was loaded with phenytoin in the ED and became highly agitated and needed restraints. She professed to see airplanes going through her room and stated that she had to follow them, even if it meant jumping out the window to get them. A psychiatric consultation was called to best evaluate where in the hospital this patient should be placed and to help manage her delirium.

Another example in which this question is pertinent is with a child who in the hospital manifests severe behavioral dyscontrol that interferes with his or her treatment. This often takes the form of hyperactivity and aggressive behavior to the staff and other patients. A corollary to this question is, 'What is the next treatment setting for this patient?' This latter question is particularly important for individuals who have attempted suicide. Referral to an inpatient psychiatric setting, an outpatient mental health agency, or private psychiatric practice depends on the nature and the

Table 5.2 Common reasons for child and adolescent psychiatric consultation [23,24].

1. Emergencies (e.g., suicide attempts, mental status changes)
2. Differential diagnosis of somatoform symptoms
3. Collaborative care of children with stress-sensitive illnesses
4. Diagnosis and care of children with psychiatric symptoms following a somatic illness
5. Chronic illness (e.g., major depression in a patient with cystic fibrosis)
6. Reactions to major pediatric treatment techniques (e.g., post-traumatic stress disorder following stem cell transplantation)
7. Reactions to pediatric illnesses
8. The child's reaction to his or her illness and hospitalization
9. Nonadherence to medical plan
10. Family assessments
11. Pretransplant (e.g., cardiac, liver, bone marrow) psychiatric evaluation

assessment of the child's suicide attempt, as well as the presence of a major psychiatric disorder.

Question 2

Why is our patient not cooperating with treatment?

This consultative question is seen in numerous areas, e.g., the cancer patient who is extremely anxious and fearful around medical procedures, the diabetic child who is noncompliant, and the depressed mother who has trouble following directions from the nursing staff. The differential diagnosis of noncompliance with treatment is broad and includes the following behaviors or characteristics:

- inability to understand directions
- lack of education
- opposition and defiance
- developmental issues (IQ, PDD, etc.)
- a passive wish to die
- anxiety
- depression
- denial of illness
- passive vs. active coping style [1]
- embarrassment vs. pride with respect to self-care [1]
- limited family or peer support [1]
- relationship with medical providers [1]

All of the above phenomena confront general pediatricians in their practice on a daily basis. Our liaison work, therefore, must focus increasingly, in view of the shorter hospital stays, on teaching our pediatric colleagues to ask the appropriate questions to achieve the right answers.

CASE FOUR

Amber was a 16-year-old girl who was admitted to the diabetic service in a coma caused by diabetic ketoacidosis. Five days prior to admission she had refused all laboratory tests during a clinic visit when she stated, 'I'm fine and I don't care.' The patient had a long history of noncompliance with her diabetic regimen. A psychiatric consultation was requested to evaluate Amber's noncompliance. During the assessment Amber admitted to being embarrassed by her illness and avoiding social contact. She stated that she slept most of the day, was truant from school, couldn't concentrate, had little energy, and was anhedonic. Although she was not actively suicidal, she was aware that noncompliance could lead to death. A diagnosis of major depression was made, with a recommendation for antidepressant medication and a trial of brief psychotherapy. The patient was agreeable to this plan. Psychotherapy sessions focused on psychoeducation regarding diabetes and its treatment and the impact of illness on her social, academic and family functioning. Cognitive behavioral interventions were employed to address her depressogenic cognitions and promote behavioral activation. Her mood symptoms gradually improved and there was subsequent improvement in her diabetic symptoms.

Question 3

This patient has had an extensive and expensive medical workup that has yielded no findings. Is there a psychological or psychiatric reason for the patient's medical symptoms?

Studies of somatization in children showed that medically unexplained physical symptoms are common in childhood and include in descending order of frequency:

- headaches
- recurrent abdominal pain
- limb pain
- chest pain
- fatigue [8]

Additionally, patients could present with complex syndromes involving both medical or neurological and somatoform symptoms (e.g., a patient with both seizures and pseudoseizures). Many parents with children present with these medical complaints are fearful of possible psychiatric consultation. As a result, there can be a relentless and aggressive medical workup. The primary fear of the child or family is that they are not being taken seriously or that nobody believes them. The fear of calling a psychiatric consultation is that the physician might think, 'It is all in your head' or, 'I think you're crazy.' The primary care physician fears losing the alliance developed with the family.

CASE FIVE

A seven-year-old hyperactive child had a joint in his toe removed due to osteomyelitis and appeared despondent. The mother refused a psychiatric consultation but agreed to let a third-year medical student pediatric clerk work with the boy. The clerk was supervised on various techniques to engage the child and establish rapport with the mother. On discharge, the mother arranged an appointment with a child psychiatrist.

The consultant's goal is twofold: to consult with the primary care physician on how to best approach the patient, and to be empathic with the patient and his or her family in their frustration with not getting answers. A common approach is to present the psychiatric consultant's role as an adjunct to ongoing medical care, to help the child cope with the chronic symptoms interfering with his functioning, the stress of being in the hospital or the frustration of 'not finding the answer.' Interaction with families should be supportive and nonconfrontational, hopefully to begin the process of forming a therapeutic alliance that will allow the consultant to make recommendations to the family and primary care physician. It is essential in the assessment of such cases to view the physical symptoms as real even if they seem to be occurring in the context of stress or psychiatric illness. These children are generally not faking or malingering and the symptoms are as real to them as the physical symptoms from a medical illness [25].

CASE SIX

Jane is a 15-year-old girl diagnosed as idiopathic pain syndrome fibromyalgia at age 11, re-admitted to the pediatric ward for further assessment and recommendations. The presentation at age 11 included abdominal and joint pain, migraines and fever followed thereafter by multiple episodes of joint pain of increasing severity and duration. The current episode of one year includes right leg pain and shakiness, only present upon weight bearing and absent when lying down, leading to a significant walking impairment and a subsequent need to use a walker for assistance. For the last year she has been home schooled. There is a history of multiple failed treatment interventions including medication trials (e.g., analgesics, antidepressants), inpatient and outpatient rehabilitation, homeopathic treatment with acupuncture. A psychiatric consultation was requested to evaluate the underlying psychosocial factors for Jane's presentation and rule out the presence of a depressive condition.

The above question is also relevant to cases in which both psychiatric treatment and medical treatment are necessary, as in diseases such as anorexia nervosa or bulimia nervosa. With the number of eating disorder units decreasing, hospitals are administering more medical and psychiatric care for anorexia and bulimia nervosa on the general pediatric unit. Medical hospitalization is usually prompted by a rapid or profound weight loss, cardiovascular abnormalities, electrolyte imbalance, hypothermia and may represent a failure of outpatient psychotherapy [1]. The psychiatric consultant's role is to 'jump start' the psychiatric treatment for these patients and make recommendations regarding the level of psychiatric intervention after medical stabilization.

Question 4

I think my child is having a hard time since her diagnosis. Can you please send someone to talk with her?

This question is generally posed by parents to their primary care physicians, especially in the face of chronic illness. At times, parents will state that they are concerned that their child is having difficulty adjusting to a new diagnosis or may be suffering from depression as a result of treatment or the news of the diagnosis of a chronic illness. Or it may be a subtle request for the parents or other family members themselves, who may be experiencing difficulty adjusting to their child's chronic illness. Often, parents request that the patient's siblings or other family members be informed about their loved one's medical problems. As previously noted, disturbances requiring psychiatric attention are manifest in a greater proportion of chronically medically ill patients and their families than in healthy children. This is extremely important in the context of managed care, in which sicker and more unstable patients are at times the only patients on a hospital unit or ICU.

Parents sometimes request a psychiatric consultation to discuss how to tell their child bad news, or to prepare the child for medical procedures. The child psychiatric consultant is uniquely qualified to give the parents developmental guidelines with which to discuss these issues with their children.

Question 5

This patient has an end-stage organ disease and would require a pre-transplant psychiatric evaluation as part of the multidisciplinary transplantation assessment.

Solid organ transplantation has become recognized as a legitimate treatment for many types of end-stage organ failures. Hence, this question is frequently encountered by the psychiatric consultant in major academic centers where he or she is a member of the multidisciplinary transplantation team. The consultant's role is to conduct a thorough evaluation of the child and family with an emphasis on identifying psychopathology, potential risk factors for adjustment reactions or nonadherence to treatment and the adequacy of social supports [26].

Assessment

1   Consultative Question

A significant challenge for the consultant is determining and often narrowing the question raised by the primary care team – framing the consultative question. When training for this specific task, the students and residents can be given clinical vignettes and asked to arrive at the consultative question. Training our future colleagues to ask appropriate consultative questions will help teach them how to best work with their consultants, and it will help us as psychiatric consultants to best fulfill our responsibilities to the treatment team and to the patient and family. An important component of an appropriate consultative request is to ascertain who is asking the question. This helps focus the intervention and recommendations of the consultant. The following case illustrates this point.

CASE SEVEN

Mark was a six-year-old boy who was admitted to the burn unit after spilling hot water on most of his body. Prior to this hospitalization, Mark was completely toilet trained and was progressing in his development. During his hospitalization on the burn unit, he received numerous procedures and operations, including skin grafts. He became enuretic and encopretic in his bed. A psychiatric consultation was ordered when the patient became encopretic in the middle of the hospital unit. It became clear throughout the consultative process that the consult was requested by the charge nurse and the nursing staff, for they had to clean up after the child. The consultant worked with the staff to institute a behavioral program to help the child regain control and limit his regression.

In addition, it is helpful to clarify who the 'identified patient' and who the 'real patient' are. For example, this question is critical when diagnoses such as a failure to thrive or Munchausen syndrome by proxy are being considered in the differential diagnosis of the consultative request.

2 Consent of the Parent and 'Assent' of the Child

It is imperative that the team requesting the consult notify the family (in the form of a request) of the need for psychiatric consultation and also inform the child that someone will be coming to talk with him or her. This is an area in which residents and medical students are fearful of patient reactions and need help in being able to discuss the potential for psychiatric problems with the parents of their patients. An appointment is scheduled with the parents so that the consultation can be completed, as quickly as possible. At this stage of clinical practice, the primary care team's responsibility is to inform the patient and help the family obtain authorization for a mental health consultation through third-party carriers.

3 Medical Record Review

It is imperative that the consultant be thoroughly informed about the child's medical condition, the treatment of this condition, and the related side effects of treatment. The patient's laboratory values, electrocardiograms, and medications, etc., need to be reviewed thoroughly. A major component often lacking in psychiatric–pediatric collaboration has been communication. Stereotypes of psychiatrists depict them as impractical, unavailable, and not knowledgeable about medical illnesses and their treatment [27]. As psychiatrists, we can debate whether this is appropriate or not; however, these are the impressions that consultation-liaison psychiatrists face every day. Being aware of all the medical issues ensures that the pediatrician and the consulting psychiatrist speak the same language and thus provide the patient with the best service. In addition, the best way to collaborate is to be familiar with each other's work. An important finding is that child psychiatrists and pediatricians are better able to collaborate when they have been trained in a setting in which they worked together [28]. Working together is illustrated by the next case.

CASE EIGHT

A psychiatric resident was called to the ICU to evaluate a schizophrenic teenager who was still psychotic, despite what appeared to be adequate antipsychotic treatment. The patient was being treated for multiple infections and was intermittently in septic shock. On review of the patient's chart, the consultant noticed that the patient's blood cultures revealed that her current antibiotic therapy was inadequate. A recommendation was made that the antibiotics be changed and psychiatric follow-up conducted as needed.

---

4 Psychiatric interview

In Chapter 2, the details of the psychological assessment are discussed; however, the special considerations needed to evaluate a child with a medical condition are highlighted here. First, the psychiatrist should directly observe the patient and conduct an initial observation of the patient's status, regardless of whether his or her family members are staying overnight or are available for the appointment or where the patient is located (such as the day hospital, inpatient unit, ICU step-down unit, and burn unit). This provides a rapid assessment of the patient's medical needs at the time of consultation. Is the patient in bed, awake, alert, interacting with staff, watching television, playing games, or engaging in childlike activities? Is the child demonstrating that he or she is in pain? In general, for school-age children up to age 11 years, the consultant should meet with the parents first. The parents should be asked if their physician or treatment team requested this consultation and whether they were aware of it, or whether they requested the consultation themselves. It is important to ascertain the goals of the evaluation early in the process. A full history of the medical episode as well as a psychiatric review of systems, family history, social developmental history, current living situation, and school performance is obtained from the parents.

Based on the information gathered from the treatment team and the parents, the next step in the consultation is interviewing the child. The interview is generally briefer as the child could be too weak, irritable due to being ill and to tolerate a lengthy examination [29]. In addition to conducting the general child psychiatric evaluation and mental status examination, the physician should direct special attention to the feelings and reactions toward the child by the family (such as overprotective, distant, or fearful) and the child's understanding of his or her own illness; the identification of any fantasy about the cause of illness is critical. It is important to know what the child experiences and their perceptions of their medical condition. The child may have fantasies of what caused their illness i.e., punishment, etc., which would be important in assessing the patient. Assessing how well family members are coping with the child's illness is also significant. Studies have measured the child's ability to cope and assessed what type of coping strategies children use to deal with their illnesses [30,31]. This coping ability is especially important for children with chronic illness and their families. A thorough understanding of the patient's and family's coping strategies and defense mechanisms yields important information on how they cope with ongoing treatment and improvement or worsening of the medical condition.

5 Discussion of the Findings with the Referring Team

Once the assessment is completed it is helpful for the consultant to discuss the findings directly with the team or physician calling the consultation. This allows the consultant to fill in the gaps between the parental and the child interview. This will also allow the consultant to tailor psychiatric interventions that may be necessary and that are practical for this particular patient, family, and treatment team and the medical setting in which the patient is found.

Report and Recommendations

Our general medical and pediatric colleagues have reported over time that, although they appreciate detailed psychological and psychiatric reports, they find practical and concrete suggestions and recommendations for their patients to be the most helpful. It is not helpful, then, to submit a long report with only short, possibly unclear, recommendations. With those considerations in mind, a consultation report could be designed as follows:

(1) Reason for consultation
(2) Patient's identifying data (age, gender, race, level of education, living arrangements, household and family structure)
(3) Sources of information (e.g., patient, family members, friends, medical records).
(4) History of present illness:
   • brief summary of the current medical condition and treatment
   • psychiatric review of systems with pertinent positives and negatives; onset, duration and course of the psychiatric symptoms relative to the course of the medical condition
   • recent psychosocial stressors
(5) Past psychiatric history
(6) Family history
(7) Social/developmental history
(8) Medical/surgical history
(9) Current medication, laboratory data, vital signs
(10) Mental status examination including the assessment of cognitive function
(11) Assessment and diagnosis
(12) Plan and recommendations: will address the specifics of the consultation request and will include specific, concrete recommendations in nonpsychiatric jargon and follow up, presented in list form and in decreasing order of importance; patient's safety must be addressed first.

Table 5.3 Characteristics of an effective consultant and consultation.

1. Available
2. Knowledgeable regarding medical issues
3. Communicative
4. Gives practical recommendations in non psychiatric jargon
5. Provides or arranges outpatient or ongoing follow up

The psychiatric consultant must remain involved with the patient's care throughout both hospitalization and follow-up to the outpatient setting, if indicated. The psychiatric consultant should keep the patient's primary care physician informed of the type of treatment and its specific mode and goals. In our experience, pediatricians rarely receive these types of calls. The parents of the children appreciate that their child's psychiatric care is being discussed with their primary care physician. Table 5.3 summarizes the characteristics of an effective consultant and consultation.

Psychiatric Aspects of Chronic Medical Illness

The psychiatric aspects of chronic medical illnesses are well documented [20,32–34]. A few additional points need to be made, especially for the child psychiatry/psychology trainee that must be assessed. (1) Does the illness or its treatment, such as brain tumor, diabetic ketoacidosis, or steroids, affect the brain? (2) What is the patient's knowledge and information regarding his or her illness?

CASE NINE

Anna was an 18-year-old female who had had diabetes mellitus since the age of eight years. She had been repeatedly hospitalized for non-compliance. During the evaluation, the psychiatry resident discovered that the patient had little knowledge and understanding of her illness. During the consultation and therapy sessions, the resident explained in detail about diabetes, insulin, the pancreas, hormones, and other aspects of the illness. The patient began to show more interest in caring for herself after these sessions. She actively sought out the diabetic educator as well as other patients who had diabetes and began to take an active interest in diabetic control.

The consultation-liaison psychiatrist may help the treatment team explain and educate about a newly diagnosed illness. A psychiatric consultation may be called to evaluate the educational level or developmental level of a family, patient, or child and to assist the treatment team in explaining the child's illness in a way that can be more easily understood.

(3) Developmental sequelae of chronic medical illness. Children need to be children. The goal of treating pediatric illnesses is to keep or return a particular child and family to their normal developmental trajectory. Having an illness that results in multiple hospitalizations, clinic visits, injections, breathing treatments, physical changes such as hair loss, and other effects of medical problems or their treatments can change the way a child views his or her body and his/her self-esteem. It can also alter academic potential because of absence from school or cognitive changes. Sometimes these children have difficulty with peers who lack understanding about them and their medical problem.

CASE TEN

Billy was an eight-year-old boy diagnosed with rhabdomyosarcoma of his finger, which required amputation. He did not want to leave the hospital on discharge, and a psychiatric consultant was called. During the evaluation, it became clear that the patient was fearful of leaving the hospital because he did not know how to hold a baseball bat after his surgery. He was afraid that other kids would make fun of him. The consultant worked with the child and his father, as did physical and occupational therapists, to show Billy how to hold a baseball bat.

(4) Family dynamics. As is true with all child psychiatric assessments, careful attention must be directed to the family, both immediate and extended, of a child with a chronic medical illness. Illness can change the family milieu, due to parents staying with the child, possibly taking, time off from work, and losing income. Family sessions may be needed to help a family adjust. Marital issues may arise owing to the extra strain of caring for a medically ill child. At times it is up to the psychiatric consultant to remind these parents to spend time together to keep the marriage and family functioning. Siblings also need attention

from the treatment team and the psychiatric consultant to discuss issues about their ill brother or sister and their feelings regarding family changes.

(5) Education of allied professionals. In these days of managed care and short hospital stays, it is imperative that treatment teams have in-services regarding 'the psychiatric review of systems.' As previously mentioned, medically ill children report more psychiatric symptoms than do well children [10–12]. It is important to have refresher courses in psychiatric signs and symptoms to enable the staff to identify children who may have developed new psychiatric symptoms.

Medical illnesses may present as psychiatric illnesses. Children with brain disorders report psychiatric symptoms four to five times more than do well children [10]. At times, a change in mental status may be the first sign of a medication side effect, a recurrence of cancer, connective tissue diseases, or HIV. It is incumbent on consultation-liaison psychiatrists to work closely with residents and the nursing staff to observe and identify subtle mental status changes.

Psychiatric conditions may present as medical illnesses. In one study, psychosomatic disorders accounted for 28% of all child psychiatric consultations [24]. The Ontario Child Health Study estimated a prevalence rate of somatization syndromes of 4.5% for boys and 10.7% for girls aged 12–16 years [8]. These children had medical workups that were negative, and the presenting problems included failure to thrive, abdominal pain, headache pain, and eating disorders. In our hospital, gastrointestinal complaints by far constitute the majority of consultation requests in this area. As mentioned previously, one of the difficulties the house staff tends to have with these patients is telling a parent that a psychiatric consultation is needed; they are fearful of parental reaction. We suggest the following approaches for house staff to deal with these issues:

(1) Emphasize the need for multiple team members on the treatment team, including mental health professionals.
(2) Do not imply that you are giving up on the patient and his or, her problem.
(3) Feel free to express frustration at not being able to arrive at a medical diagnosis.
(4) At times, request a consultation for the purpose of offering support to the patient and family in dealing with medical complaints.

These suggestions may help patients accommodate to the possibility that a psychiatric component may have initiated or maintained their ongoing medical problem.

Pediatric HIV Infection

Epidemiology

Worldwide 38 million people were living with HIV/AIDS in 2003 and almost five million people acquired the virus, a rate that is higher than any year before [35]. The new infections emerged particularly in women and children. By the end of 1999, 1.2 million children under the age of 15 years were living with HIV/AIDS while 470 000 children died from AIDS [36].

In the USA one million people were living with HIV/AIDS in 2003. In the year 2002, there were 877 275 adult and adolescent AIDS cases and 9300 AIDS cases in children under the age of 13 years [37]. In the 15–24-years old age group AIDS is the sixth leading cause of death [38].

Worldwide, over five million infants have been infected with HIV since the beginning of the pandemic, 90% of whom were or are in Africa [39]. Other areas of increased incidence rate include Central and South-East Asia, Eastern Europe, and India [39].

Children at risk for HIV infection include infants of intravenous (IV) drug abusers, sexually abused children, children who have received blood products between 1982 and 1985, adolescent IV drug abusers, gay adolescents, and those who are sexually promiscuous with multiple partners [40]. In the USA, pediatric AIDS is over-represented among ethnic minorities (62% African–American, 25% Hispanic) [36,38], socioeconomically disadvantaged [36], in large metropolitan areas (New York City, Miami, Newark) [36], and among the offspring of IV drug users [36].

Child and adolescent psychiatrists are likely to encounter HIV-positive children and adolescents in the course of their clinical work, 'unless their practice excludes contact with minorities, chronically ill children, sexually active adolescents, gay youth, and abused or molested children' [41]. Advances in HIV treatment have led to survival past five years of age in more than 65% of children with HIV and many of those children will be encountered by mental health professionals [38]. Child psychiatry liaison service is used by multiple medical services to assist in the psychosocial aspect of treating families with infected children. The entire range of child psychiatric expertise, such as family therapy, psychotherapy, crisis intervention, and knowledge of neuropsychology and psychopharmacology, is required to help these families receive services [42]. Even if a vaccine or cure is found, psychiatrists will be called on to respond to the psychiatric sequelae of the AIDS epidemic for the next generation.

Sources of Infection in Children

Vertical transmission

Perinatal transmission accounts for more than 90% of pediatric HIV infection and could occur during pregnancy, labor, delivery or breastfeeding [39]. The rates of mother-to-child transmission range from 15–25% in industrialized countries to 25–35% in developing countries [39]. Maternal transmission could be influenced by factors such as age of the child, severity of maternal HIV, amniocentesis, specific blood type or vitamin deficiency (e.g., vitamin A) [38]. Vertical transmission of HIV infection has been substantially reduced by the pre- and perinatal use of zidovudine (AZT) [36,38]. It is not usually possible to determine whether a child is infected at the time of delivery due to the maternal HIV antibodies that cross the placenta. For the majority of children, it is not known with certainty if the child is free from infection until maternal antibodies disappear and the HIV antibody test becomes negative, a process that occurs most commonly between 9 and 15 months of age. This unknown period will likely be a particularly difficult time for parents and other caregivers [43]. Additionally, infected infants not identified in the nursery may be diagnosed later by monitoring their serostatus or by observing when they develop failure to thrive and frequent infections.

Infection by Blood Products

The majority of cases of infection via blood products are in patients with hemophilia who received nonheat-treated quality concentrates prior to 1983. Since 1985, blood banks have been effectively monitored for heat-treated factor VIII concentrates. Prior to the use of this precaution, the risk of infection depended on the severity of hemophilia: about 75% of patients in the severe group were infected, 45% in the moderate group, and 25% in the mild group [44].

Sexually Transmitted Disease

Child sexual abuse is another cause of childhood HIV infection [38,39], therefore HIV testing is clinically indicated in assessing children who have been abused or molested. Additionally, a random sampling of youths in public health clinics showed that having a history of physical abuse, sexual abuse, or rape is related to practicing high-level HIV-risk behaviors [45]. Of note, female adolescents are at the highest risk for completed rape and other forms of sexual assaults [46].

Adolescent Risk Factors

Adolescents constitute one of the fastest growing risk groups [36] and sexual intercourse accounts for the majority of new AIDS cases [38]. National data on adolescents with AIDS indicate that 73% were infected by intravenous drug use or sexual activity, and 22% through exposure to infected blood products [47]. Additionally, children who are runaways are at risk for having multiple sexual partners and engaging in prostitution, hence are at great risk for infection.

With these risk factors in mind during a thorough psychiatric assessment, psychiatrists should assess these issues in all of their patients. Risk factors for HIV should be noted and a test performed when indicated.

Neurodevelopmental Aspects of Pediatric HIV Infection

Many children with HIV are considered to be asymptomatic, one study showing only 10% of children being symptomatic before the onset of an AIDS-defining illness [48]. However, numerous studies document at least some cognitive and language delays that could be quite subtle [38,48]. Additionally, the severity of the neurological and the neuropsychological compromise positively correlate with the severity of HIV related-illness [36].

Two relatively distinct neurodevelopmental patterns have been described: static encephalopathy and progressive encephalopathy [36]. Static encephalopathy is characterized by non-progressive neurologic and neurodevelopmental deficits and is likely etiologically related to non-HIV risk factors such as prematurity, low birth weight, prenatal toxins or infectious agents exposure, and or genetic factors [36,49].

Progressive encephalopathy, which corresponds with the AIDS dementia complex in adults, can be the initial presenting problem of acquired immunodeficiency syndrome (AIDS) in up to 18% and eventually up to 30–60% of affected children in adolescence [50–52]. In a series that included both asymptomatic children and children with advanced disease, a 19.6% prevalence rate of progressive encephalopathy was reported [49]. The progressive encephalopathy is felt to result from both direct and indirect effects of HIV-1 infection on the central nervous system and eventually results in an insidious and severe clinical neurological deterioration [52,53]. Progressive encephalopathy is observed when immunosuppression is present, however there is no correlation between the immunologic status (e.g., CD4 cell count) and the degree of neurocognitive impairment [38]. HIV-associated progressive encephalopathy in children is characterized by a triad of symptoms:

(1) impaired brain growth, with either a decrease or plateau of head growth velocity or a progressive loss of brain parenchymal volume, as seen on neuroimaging studies;

(2) progressive motor dysfunction;

(3) loss or plateau of the acquisition of age-appropriate neurodevelopmental milestones [51–54].

Additionally, encephalopathic children manifest apathy, decreased social interaction and symptoms of depression and irritability as compare with non-encephalopathic children [36]. Developmental problems are often multifactorial, and environmental, psychosocial and nutritional factors may have an important influence on neurodevelopmental outcome and testing [52]. Formal developmental testing of HIV-1-infected infants has yielded conflicting results, with abnormalities in age-appropriate testing of motor skills or prelinguistic abilities predominating [49,52]. The school-age child is at risk for impaired cognitive functioning including declining IQ scores, increasing difficulties with language, and attention and memory.

Neurodevelopmental testing should be an integral part of the assessment of HIV-1-infected pediatric patients, especially those with known neurologic abnormalities or receiving antiretroviral therapy. Additionally, one study found that the overall CT brain scan severity rating to be highly predictive of the level of cognitive functioning [38]. In a sample of HIV-infected children under the age of 10 years, CT scan abnormalities were significantly correlated with poorer receptive and expressive language functioning, the latter being more severely impaired among encephalopathic children [38]. A review of neuroimaging studies found that 79% of the patients studied had at least one abnormality on CT brain scan [55]. Most frequently, cortical atrophy was found with ventricular dilatation and/or sulcal enlargement, both of which were associated with white matter abnormalities. These lesions were equally common in vertically transmitted and other infected patients. Intracerebral calcifications were only seen in vertically infected children. The lesions tended to be bilateral and symmetrical, occurring in basal ganglia and spreading to the periventricular frontal white matter [55]. Current antiretroviral treatments have the potential to improve the cognitive deficits in children with AIDS and the improvement is independent of the immune status or the presence of encephalopathy at baseline [38]. However the effect is not sustained in many children beyond six months of treatment [38].

Emotional and Behavioral Manifestations in HIV-Infected Children

Pediatric HIV patients are at risk for psychological disturbance due to both the direct effects of HIV infection on brain structures and indirect effects related to coping with the range of medical, psychological and social stressors associated with HIV disease [56]. Such stressors include the repeated hospitalizations, fears of death, disclosure of HIV infection, social ostracism, and family conflict [38]. Additionally, HIV is associated with other high-risk factors such as poverty, prenatal drug exposure, birth complications, and heritable parental psychopathology that may be more potent mediators of mental health problems in HIV infected children than HIV itself [36].

Developmental disabilities, learning disorders, behavior syndromes, anxiety, bereavement reactions and depression have been reported in HIV-infected children [36,38,52]. Additionally, attention deficit hyperactivity disorder-like symptoms were reported to be highly prevalent among school-age children [36,38,52]. Learning disabilities are prevalent in HIV-infected children, and these children often require special education services [52].

Psychiatric Assessment and Interventions

A multidisciplinary team including professionals in general pediatrics, infectious diseases, child neurology, child and adolescent psychiatry, nursing, social work, and special education is needed to treat these children and their families. Table 5.4 [54] provides an outline

Table 5.4 Psychosocial assessment in HIV-infected patients and families.

Family	History of illness Child
Constellation	Pre-illness
Reaction to diagnosis	School performance
Support system	Relationships with peers
Health status	Development
Previous losses and coping skills	Current reaction to diagnosis
	Behavioral changes
	Cognitive development
	Coping skills

Adapted from Weiner L, Septimus A: Psychosocial support for child and family. In: Pizzo PA, Wilfert CM, eds. *Pediatric AIDS: The Challenge of HIV Infection in Infants, Children, and Adolescents,* 2nd ed. Baltimore, MD: Williams & Wilkins; 1994: 809–828.

geared toward evaluating children and families with HIV.

In addition to performing a thorough psychiatric assessment of the child and his or her family, it is critical that the child and adolescent psychiatrist works on behalf of the family with other practitioners and with schools. These children are at risk for learning disabilities, cognitive impairment, and behavior problems. Psychiatrists can ease the transition to school by working with school officials to educate them about HIV and discuss their worries about dealing with an HIV infected child.

Little data are available on the pharmacological treatment of psychiatric disorders in HIV-infected children, however treatment approaches similar with those used for noninfected patients are likely employed [38]. Specific considerations include:

(1) Behavioral syndromes first require a thorough neurological assessment to rule out any organic causes.
(2) A review of the antiretroviral, antimicrobial and antifungal agents due to their potential neuropsychiatric side effects [36,38].
(3) The patients require lower start dose, slower titration and close monitoring of the medications.
(4) The patients are more sensitive to drug side effects.
(5) Many antiretroviral (especially protease inhibitors) and psychotropic medications are metabolized by the cytochrome P450 system and they are also inducers or inhibitors of the different P450 isoenzymes. Therefore, it is important to review the potential drug–drug interactions between antiretroviral and psychotropic medications before initiating any psychoactive medications.

Conclusion

The role of the child and adolescent consultation in liaison psychiatry is currently in a state of flux, as both the mode of health care delivery and the patterns of reimbursement for consultation are changing. When evaluating many perplexing and difficult patients, liaison psychiatrists find themselves needing to adapt to various settings and lengths of time given for assessments. The opportunity to interact with our colleagues is also lessened because, to keep up with demand, primary care physicians and pediatric specialists are seeing four to eight patients per hour. Nevertheless, the need for child and adolescent psychiatrists for consultation continues to be high.

In this context, the consultation-liaison child psychiatrist's task is to help educate the pediatric colleagues about the comorbidity of medical and

psychiatric disorders, the importance of psychiatric consultation and to work as part of the multidisciplinary team in order to provide comprehensive care for these children. Additionally, due to the advances in HIV treatment with HIV infection becoming a subacute, chronic disease, the child psychiatrist is being called upon to help address the newly posed challenges to the neurocognitive and psychosocial development of children and families [38].

The liaison child psychiatrist has the additional important task of educating the patients and their families, in a developmentally appropriate way, about medical procedures, medical illness and its potential psychological consequences. Additionally, in working with adolescent patients, the educative role with focus on the risks for HIV infection is essential, given their especially increased risk.

Using the clinical skills and research in our field, child and adolescent psychiatrists are well prepared to deal with the complex psychological and social consequences of chronic medical illness.

While there is a growing body of literature on the psychosocial adjustment in children with chronic medical illness and specifically in children with HIV infection, more work would be needed especially in the area of treatment interventions both nonpharmacological and psychopharmacological. Additionally, the collaboration between the child psychiatrists, primary care physicians and pediatric specialists will require ongoing attention and research in order to optimize the multidisciplinary approach to the chronically ill pediatric patients.

References

1. Rauch P: Paediatric consultation. In: Rutter M, Taylor E, eds. *Child and Adolescent Psychiatry* 4th ed. Oxford: Blackwell Science Publishing, 2002:1051–1066.
2. Shugart MA: Child psychiatry consultations to pediatric inpatients: A literature review. *Gen Hosp Psychiatry* 1991; **13**:325–336.
3. Campo JV, Kingsley RS, Bridge J., Mrazek D: Child and adolescent psychiatry in general children's hospitals. A survey of chairs of psychiatry. *Psychosomatics* 2000; **41**(2):128–133.
4. Steiner H, Fritz GK, Mrazek D, *et al.*: Pediatric and psychiatric comorbidity. Part I: The future of consultation-liaison psychiatry. *Psychosomatics* 1993; **34**(2):107–111.
5. Pless IB, Roghmann KJ: Chronic illness and its consequences: Observations based on three epidemiologic surveys. *J Pediatr* 1971; **79**:351–359.
6. Cadman D, Boyle M, Szatmari P, *et al.*: Chronic illness disability and mental and social well-being. *Pediatrics* 1987; **79**:805–813.
7. Gortmaker SL, Walker DK, Weitzman M, *et al.*: Chronic conditions, socioeconomic risks, and behavioral

problems in children and adolescents. *Pediatrics* 1990; **85**:267–276.

8. Knapp PK, Harris ES: Consultation-liaison in child psychiatry: A review of the past 10 years. Part I: Clinical findings. *J Am Acad Child Adolesc Psychiatry* 1998; **37**(1):17–25.

9. Westborn L: Well-being of children with chronic illness: A population-based study in a Swedish primary care district. *Acta Paediatr* 1992; **81**:625.

10. Rutter M, Tizard J, Whitmore K: *Education, Health and Behavior*. New York: Wiley, 1970.

11. Douglas JWB, Blomfield JM: *Children Under 5*. London: Allen and Unwin, 1958.

12. Haggerty RJ, Roghmann KJ, Pless IB: *Child Health and the Community*. New York: Wiley Interscience, 1975.

13. Pless IB, Douglas JWB: Chronic illness in childhood. Part I: Epidemiological and clinical characteristics. *Pediatrics* 1971; **47**:405–414.

14. Thompson RJ, Gustafson KE, Gil KM, Godfrey J, Murphy LM: Illness specific patterns of psychological adjustment and cognitive adaptational processes in children with cystic fibrosis and sickle cell disease. *J Clin Psychology* 1998; **54**(1):121–128.

15. Burke P, Elliott M: Depression in pediatric chronic illness. A diathesis-stress model. *Psychosomatics* 1999; **40**(1):5–17.

16. Drell MJ, Hanson White TJ: Children's reaction to illness and hospitalization. In: Sadock B, Sadock V, eds. *Kaplan & Sadock's Comprehensive Textbook of Psychiatry*. 7th edition. Philadelphia: Lippincott Williams & Wilkins, 2000:2889–2897.

17. Suris JC, Parera N, Puig C: Chronic illness and emotional distress in adolescence. *J Adolesc Health* 1996; **19**: 153–156.

18. Meijer SA, Sinnema G, Bijstra JO, Mellenbergh GJ, Wolters WHG: Coping styles and locus of control as predictors for psychological adjustment of adolescents with a chronic illness. *Soc Sci Med* 2002; **54**:1453–1461.

19. Huurre TM, Aro HM: Long-term psychosocial effects of persistent chronic illness. A follow-up study of Finnish adolescents aged 16 to 32 years. *Eur Child Adolesc Psychiatry* 2002; **11**:85–91.

20. Mrazek DA: Psychiatric aspects of somatic disease and disorders. In: Rutter M, Taylor E, Hersov L, eds. *Child and Adolescent Psychiatry: Modern Approaches*. London: Blackwell Scientific Publications, 1994:697–710.

21. Jellinek MS, Murphy M: Use of the Pediatric Symptom Checklist in outpatient practice. In: Jellinek MS, ed. *Current Problems in Pediatrics: Psychosocial Aspects of Ambulatory Pediatrics*. Littleton, MA: Mosby-Year Book, 1990:602–609.

22. Jones RN, Latkowski ME, Green DM, *et al.*: Psychosocial assessment in the general pediatric population: A multiple-gated screening and identification procedure. *J Pediatr Health Care* 1996; **10**(1):10–16.

23. Lewis M: The consultation process in child and adolescent psychiatric consultation-liaison in pediatrics. In: Lewis M, ed. *Child and Adolescent Psychiatry: A Comprehensive Textbook* Baltimore, MD: Williams & Wilkins, 1996, 935–939.

24. Jellinek MS, Herzog DB, Selter LF: A psychiatric consultation service for hospitalized children. *Psychosomatics* 1987; **22**:29–33.

25. Slater JA: Deciphering emotional aches and physical pains in children. *Pediatrics Annals* 2003; **32**(6):402–407.

26. Slater JA: Psychiatric issues in pediatric bone marrow, stem cell, and solid organ transplantation. In: Lewis M, ed. *Child and Adolescent Psychiatry: A Comprehensive Textbook*. Baltimore, MD: Williams & Wilkins, 1996: 1147–1175.

27. Granger RH, Stone EL: Collaboration between child psychiatrists and pediatricians in practice. In: Lewis M, ed. *Child and Adolescent Psychiatry: A Comprehensive Textbook*. Baltimore, MD: Williams & Wilkins, 1996: 940–943.

28. Fritz GK, Bergman AS: Child psychiatrists seen through pediatricians' eyes: Results of a national survey. *J Am Acad Child Adolesc Psychiatry* 1985; **24**:81.

29. Slater JA: The medically ill child or adolescent. In: Scahill L, Martin A, eds. *Textbook of Pediatric Psychopharmacology*. New York: Oxford University Press, 2003:631–641.

30. Milousheva J, Kobayashi N, Matsui I: Psychosocial problems of children and adolescents with a chronic disease: Coping strategies. *Acta Paediatr* 1996; **38**:41–45.

31. Ryan-Wenger NA: Children, coping, and the stress of illness: A synthesis of the research. *J Soc Pediatr Nurs* 1996; **1**:126–138.

32. Krener PKG, Wasserman AL: Diagnostic dilemmas in pediatric consultation. *Child Adolesc Psychiatr Clin North Am* 1994; **3**:485–512.

33. Stuber ML: Psychiatric sequelae in seriously ill children and their families. *Psychiatric Clin North Am* 1996; **19**: 481–493.

34. Rubinstein B: Psychological factors influencing medical conditions. In: Kestenbaum CJ, Williams DT, eds. *Handbook of Clinical Assessment of Children and Adolescents*. New York: New York University Press, 1988:771–799.

35. UNAIDS AIDS Epidemic Update, July 2004. World Health Organization, Joint United Nations Program on HIV/AIDS.

36. Havens J, Mellins CA, Hunter JS: Psychiatric aspects of HIV/AIDS in childhood and adolescents. In: Rutter M, Taylor E, eds. *Child and Adolescent Psychiatry* 4th ed. Oxford: Blackwell Publishing, 2002:828–841.

37. UNAIDS/WHO Epidemiological Fact Sheet, 2004.

38. Brown LK, Lourie KJ, Pao M: Children and adolescents living with HIV and AIDS: A review. *J Child Psychol Psychiat* 2000; **41**(1):81–96.

39. Paediatric HIV/AIDS: UNAIDS Point of view, September 2002.

40. Krener P: Neurobiological and psychological aspects of HIV infection in children and adolescents. In: Lewis M, ed. *Child and Adolescent Psychiatry: A Comprehensive Textbook*. Baltimore, MD: Williams & Wilkins, 1996, 1006–1015.

41. Krener P, Miller FB: Psychiatric response to HIV spectrum disease in children and adolescents. *J Am Acad Child Adolesc Psychiatry* 1989; **28**:596–605.

42. Stuber ML: Psychiatric consultation issues in pediatric HIV and AIDS. *J Am Acad Child Adolesc Psychiatry* 1990; **29**:463–467.

43. Adnopoz JA, Forsyth BWC, Nagler SF: Psychiatric aspects of HIV infection and AIDS on the family. *Child Adolesc Psychiatr Clin North Am* 1994; **3**:543–555.

44. Eyster ME: Transfusion and coagulation factor acquired disease. In: Pizzo PA, Wilfert CM, eds. *Pediatric AIDS: The Challenge of HIV Infection in Infants, Children, and*

Adolescents, 2nd ed. Baltimore, MD: Williams & Wilkins, 1994:22–37.

45. Cunningham RM, Stiffman AR, Dore P, *et al.:* The association of physical and sexual abuse with HIV risk behaviors in adolescence and young adulthood: Implications for public health. *Child Abuse Negl* 1994; **198**(3): 233–248.

46. Prothrow-Smith O: Drug treatment planning, sexuality and privacy, management of fertility. *J Adolesc Health Care* 1989; **10**:5–8.

47. Braverman PK, Strasburger VC: Adolescent sexuality. Part 3: Sexually transmitted diseases. *Clin Pediatr (Philadelphia)* 1994; **33**:26–37.

48. American Psychiatric Association: Practice guidelines for the treatment of patients with HIV/AIDS, November 2000.

49. Brouwers P, Belman AL, Epstein L: Central nervous system involvement: Manifestations, evaluation and pathogenesis. In: Pizzo PA, Wilfert CM, eds. *Pediatric AIDS: The Challenge of HIV Infection in Infants, Children, and Adolescents.* 2nd ed. Baltimore, MD: Williams & Wilkins: 1994:433–455.

50. Belman AL, Ultmann MLT, Horoupian D, *et al.*: Neurologic complications in infants and children with

acquired immune deficiency syndrome. *Ann Neurol* 1985; **18**:560–566.

51. Epstein LG, Sharer LR, Oleske JM, *et al.*: Neurologic manifestations of human immunodeficiency virus infection in children. *Pediatrics* 1986; **78**:678–687.

52. Mintz M: Neurological and developmental problems in pediatric HIV infection. *J Nutr* 1996; **126**:2663S–2673S.

53. Mintz M: Clinical comparison of adult and pediatric NeuroAIDS. *Adv Neuroimmunol* 1994; **4**:207–221.

54. Weiner L, Septimus A: Psychosocial support for child and family. In: Pizzo PA, Wilfert CM, eds. *Pediatric AIDS: The Challenge of HIV Infection in Infants, Children, and Adolescents.* 2nd ed. Baltimore, MD: Williams & Wilkins, 1994:809–828.

55. Brouwers P, Decarli C, Heyes MP, *et al.:* Neurobehavioral manifestations of symptomatic HIV -1 disease in children: Can nutritional factors play a role? *J Nutr* 1996; **126**:2651S–2662S.

56. Bachanas PJ, Kullgren KA, Schwartz KS, Lanier B, McDaniel JS, Smith J, Nesheim S: Predictors of psychological adjustment in school-age children infected with HIV. *J Pediatric Psychology* 2001; **26**(6): 343–352.

6

How to Plan and Tailor Treatment: An Overview of Diagnosis and Treatment Planning

Brian J. McConville, Sergio V. Delgado

Introduction

The purpose of this chapter is to address the increasing imperative in child and adolescent psychiatry to form a coherent diagnostic and initial treatment plan for a child, adolescent, or family, and to do so in such a way that this plan will be logical and agreed upon by the consumers of mental healthcare – including the patients themselves, their families, employers and insurers. It is also important to be flexible, so as to alter treatment approaches with evolving clinical realities.

Contemporary medicine, including psychiatry, is subject to specific treatment guidelines, such as the well-known Milliman and Robertson standards [1]. The argument that this is unfeasible because of the imprecise nature of psychiatric diagnosis is invalid, since the precision of psychiatric assessment measures is comparable to that of physical diagnoses, and the overall results of treatment in child and adolescent psychiatry, especially for the Axis I diagnoses, are comparable to those in adult psychiatry [2]. As have other specialty organizations, the American Academy of Child and Adolescent Psychiatry has developed practice parameters [3]. In pediatric pharmacotherapy, the results for treatment of attention-deficit hyperactivity disorder (ADHD), obsessive–compulsive disorder (OCD), bipolar disorder, depressive disorder, and other conditions have been empirically validated and are extremely promising [4–8]. A perception of uncertainty still exists for the results of child and adolescent psychotherapy and other psychosocial interventions. Currently, insurance companies award a limited number of sessions annually and require the designa-tion of goals both initially and during the period of therapy. Such goals are usually imprecise, partly because of the paucity of outcome data in psychotherapy research [9].

Earlier models of a more reflective form of psychotherapy, with indefinite goals and time periods, are still necessary to obtain knowledge of certain aspects of the psychotherapeutic process, especially during the training of child psychiatrists. These patterns remain present especially in psychoanalytic psychotherapy [10]. But there is also a need for formal training in more directive types of therapy, especially those directed toward specific diagnoses (such as affective disorders or OCD), or specific family and social situations and modes of community intervention. Psychopharmacologic and psychotherapeutic approaches are often used together, and need to be so, since pharmacotherapy essentially aims to reduce or suppress problematic symptoms, and does not directly lead to new behavior. The usefulness of such combination approaches has been recently demonstrated in the MTA study of the combination of behavior therapy and psychostimulants [11]. In the TADS study for cognitive behavior therapy (CBT) and antidepressants for child and adolescent depression, the combination showed clear improvement over the use of either medication or CBT alone [12]. However, the lack of clear separation between those treated with antidepressant medication and those on placebo, as well as the inadequate capture of initial and/or emerging suicidality during these studies, has lead in part to recent concerns about the use of antidepressants and suicidality in children and adolescents [13]. There is an emerging consensus about

Clinical Child Psychiatry, Second Edition. Edited by W.M. Klykylo and J.L. Kay
© 2005 John Wiley & Sons Ltd.

the necessity of combining pharmacotherapy and psychotherapy, with a need for collaboration between the pharmacotherapist and the psychotherapist, who need to work closely together. We believe that ideally these roles should be fulfilled by the same person, since otherwise it is problematic for either therapist to know what the other is doing. However, this belief awaits substantiation.

A General Framework for Diagnosis and Treatment Planning

In the next two sections, general principles of diagnosis and modes of therapy will be summarized, as to how to select and alter modes of therapy as needed. Following this, brief descriptions of the different therapies will be given. Finally, combinations of therapies will be discussed, and clinical vignettes will be given.

Models of Diagnostic Classification

There are three general models for classifying disorders: categorical, dimensional, and ideographic [14]. This distinction is important because it is tempting to believe that the ordinary method of classification used, the clinical–categorical approach, is the only feasible one.

The categorical approach, which is similar to the general medical model of classification, is dichotomous in that it views disorders as either present or absent. This approach implies that cases of a particular disorder show certain characteristic symptoms, which in turn suggests an underlying pathophysiology, or cause of disorder and treatment. But even in such systems as the *Diagnostic and Statistical Manual of Mental Disorders, Fourth Edition, Text Revision (DSM-IV-TR)* [15] or the still-evolving (in the US) International Classification of Diseases (ICD-10) [16], this approach is not always followed. Some disorders, such as depressive disorders, require cardinal features such as anhedonia, dysphoria, or irritability as cardinal symptoms, as well as a number of other symptoms for full diagnosis. In other disorders, such as ADHD, six of nine symptoms of inattention or hyperactivity/impulsivity or a combination of both allow for the diagnosis. Hence, disorders support the 'Chinese menu' style of diagnosis, rather than with a strictly convergent system where a given number of symptoms always indicates a particular diagnosis [17].

The most commonly used pattern of categorical diagnosis in child psychiatry in North America is the DSM-IV-TR [15]. This consists of a number of axes:

- Axis I: Major clinical diagnoses
- Axis II: Developmental disorders and personality disorders
- Axis III: Physical disorders
- Axis IV: Psychosocial stressors
- Axis V: Global assessment of functioning

In contrast, the dimensional or multivariate statistical system, such as that used in the Child Behavior Checklist of Achenbach and colleagues [18], uses the convention that symptom groups indicate the universe of behaviors in a given population. These symptom groups are selected from a fixed group of behavioral symptoms derived from factor analysis and varying with age and sex. Those cases that occur above a given cutoff point (usually the 98th percentile) are abnormal. Individual symptoms and particular 'narrow band' syndromes (those defined by scores in a narrow range) may therefore occur or disappear at different ages and also differ between sexes. Comorbidity frequently occurs, and rarer disorders such as autism do not emerge in the usual analyses of normative or clinical populations. In addition, using the list of symptoms found at the predetermined cutoff point for abnormality may affect the frequency of the disorder [19]. This system has been widely used in epidemiologic studies, including international studies in which the general nature of the questions tends to minimize cultural differences in syndrome expressivity [20–22].

The third system, ideographic diagnosis, uses an approach that focuses on the totality of the individual child's life and circumstances and avoids simple descriptive labels. Despite the seeming inherent validity of this approach, the lack of labels makes it difficult for clinicians to communicate with each other regarding such studies of unique individuals. Moreover, proponents of this approach usually operate from some strict theoretical framework that slants their clinical approach, as in psychoanalytic, behavioral, family, sociologic, or psychopharmacologic viewpoints.

Other diagnostic systems can be used, including psychodynamic diagnosis, which has been proposed in the past for inclusion in the DSM system of classification, and family diagnosis [23]. The psychodynamic diagnosis approach has been implicit in a number of systems, such as that espoused by Freud [24] and later by Nagera [25].

More recently, diagnostic systems have attempted to avoid theoretical or etiologic considerations [26] and instead have widely used the phenomenological approach that operated in the original definition of

Research Diagnostic Criteria [27]. Even under these conventions, however, disorders such as post-traumatic stress disorder or reactive attachment disorder of childhood clearly imply etiology.

It does not necessarily follow that the disease concept is the most useful one to employ. An approach favoring an extension of the DSM-IV TR Axis V, and stressing functional impairment may be more generally useful [28], as in patients with mental retardation or autism. A number of recent rating systems use this concept, as in the Children's Yale-Brown Obsessive–Compulsive Scale (C-YBOCS) [7], which measures the number and nature of symptoms, but then uses the degree of functional impairment as the most important component.

Other Considerations in Child Psychiatric Diagnosis

A further aspect is to consider the question of what is being classified. Cantwell noted that diagnoses classified disorders, but not individual children [29]. Diagnosis refers to a process of assigning a label to a particular problem or a group of problems to allow for greater precision about treatment, prognosis, and possible etiology. But the diagnosis given to a child may vary from time to time, or be relatively fixed, depending on whether the disorder is an adjustment to some external stressor or a more internalized disorder following prolongation of a particular stressor, or the emergence of other internal and probably neuropathologic factors, as in schizophrenia.

In contrast to adult psychiatry, where the opinions of various informants about a person's degree of impairment are often overlooked, child and adolescent diagnosis implies the gathering of information not only from the child but also from parents, teachers, and others. One of the earliest studies in this area, Rutter's Isle of Wight Epidemiologic Study [30], focused on the number of behavior problems shown in children in a particular village, as determined by different informants. When a group of village members was asked to name those children who had the most problems, the group of children selected showed a high degree of reliability among informants. Similarly, when the children's teachers were asked to name their problematic children, they replied with a high degree of inter-rater reliability about their chosen group. All the children came from the same pool of children in the village; however, there was little overlap between the two groups selected by village members and teachers, respectively. There was not only a difference in perceived behavior between informants, but also a difference in particular situations (as in school and home).

This implies that different patterns of pathology may appear among the same children in different settings.

There are also times when the existence of problems relates more to 'goodness of fit' between parents and the infant rather than to a uniformly recognized disorder in the child [31]. The child's and the parents' temperamental characteristics may interact negatively. In 1960, Kanner commented that behaviors thought of as disturbing by one set of parents were not necessarily thought of similarly by other parents; he made a distinction between the 'disturbing' and the 'disturbed' child [32]. The work of Werner and Smith showed that the prognosis of children with behavior disorders was dependent both on parenting techniques and social support [33]. LaRoche indicated that children of parents who were depressed were particularly at risk of perceiving their children as having behavioral problems, and that those parents who had violent and abusive parents were in turn likely to be abusive [34]. The work of David Reiss and his associates has demonstrated effects of differential parenting and the interplay of environmental and genetic factors upon the outcome of adolescents [35,36].

Diagnosis in children, therefore, relates largely to the issue of social context and also to factors of tolerance, parenting skills, temperament, and economic disadvantage [37]. There are also reasons to believe that cultural factors may determine what is seen as problematic in children.

Therapeutic Interventions: Models for Selection and Utilization of Different Forms of Child and Adolescent Psychotherapy

A General Model for Sequential Strategies in Child and Adolescent Psychotherapy

To simplify the complex array of possible psychotherapies, a general model will first be presented, focusing particularly on the strategies used or required to establish particular goals. In turn, the type of therapy used will be selected for its utility for stipulated goals at particular times during the course of the therapy. To this extent, the idea of adhering only to a particular form of psychotherapy – especially one with dedicated disciples – for all cases is nonsensical. It attempts to fit the patient into a Procrustean bed in conformity to the therapist's particular enthusiasms or limitations of training, rather than being responsive to the patient's needs. Good therapists can alter their approaches flexibly as need be, ideally with the knowledge and assent of the patient and/or parents, while still largely remaining within their preferred or initial psychotherapeutic

Table 6.1 Patterns in sequential child psychotherapy.

Therapy spectrum	Directive ←————————————————— Nondirective —————————————————→			
Therapy type	Custodial-supportive	Part-relationship	Complex relationship	Analytic relationship
	'Do therapy to the patient'	'Do therapy to or with the patient'	'Do therapy with the patient'	'Be with the patient while he or she re-experiences or works through past issues'
Associated strategies	Supportive	Concrete reward systems	Negotiated behavioral rehearsals	Verbal or play therapy; re-experiencing
	Suppressive	Induced partial modeling	Induced full modeling	Corrective experience with new skills; tension relief

métier. Implicit in this approach is that the therapist must be broadly and flexibly trained. This is why general strategies rather than labeled therapies are stressed in this section.

Psychotherapies with their attendant strategies can be conceptualized as existing in a spectrum between more goal-directed, behaviorally oriented modes and more nondirective analytic therapies [38]. Intermediate are those directed relationship therapies that use the therapist as a partial model for limited patterns of social interaction, as in assertiveness training techniques [39], or as a total model of an adult or parent figure (Table 6.1).

In addition, the concept of 'patient unit' is introduced here to stipulate whether the therapy is with the individual child, the parent(s), the parents plus child, the family, the group, the immediate society in general, or other units, for example, residential groups. Again, the 'unit' may vary from time to time, but always within the context of clinical evolving realities. Put another way, the therapist should be able to define at any time why he or she is following a certain pattern of therapeutic intervention in a case.

The various psychotherapeutic strategies, viewed as a continuum or spectrum, can be classified from directive to nondirective, and also as suppressive to expressive. There is a general parallel between these two dimensions, although they are not necessarily synonymous. The model to be presented will describe how a variety of therapies may be selected depending on the diagnosis of the child, family or group, and also point out how the style of therapy may evolve over time, related in part to what occurs in therapy and to other events or clinical considerations. The model also indicates how both the therapeutic relationship and the therapy style are also dependent on diagnosis. Therapy often evolves from simpler to more complex phases – or sometimes vice versa – using a sequential approach that allows for interphase negotiations with the child and family about how to proceed throughout therapy. Such an approach is particularly suited to episodic and planned therapies with associated specified outcome goals; both apply to the realities of practice in the current clinical environment.

The strategies associated with this sequence of directive to nondirective child therapies frequently evolve from behavioral methods to more dynamic approaches, especially with action-oriented and mistrustful children, as suggested by the left–right sequence in Table 6.1. Such an evolving sequence of strategies, however, has also been found useful in more internalizing children with subjective inner distress. After a full initial clinical diagnosis, there follows in sequential psychotherapy a first stage of initial contract negotiation with different styles as required by the type of case (as described below), followed by a second stage of rehearsal of more simple interactional and affectual behaviors, and a possible third stage of exploration of more complex intrapsychic, intercommunicational, and intrafamilial issues. To illustrate these points, examples follow of the three-stage, sequential psychotherapy approaches to children with different diagnoses. However, this sequence is not invariant, and may vary with different children.

Stage I: Initial Contract Negotiation and Formation, with Different Styles of Therapist–Patient Relationship

Several clinical variants of stage 1 occur, requiring different styles of approach by the therapist. Examples of three common styles follow. These are defined by the context of the relationship.

Style A: Therapist as 'Manipulated' Helper: 'What's In It For You to be in Therapy?'

In children with disruptive behavior disorders, interactions with authority figures are usually both unsatisfactory and punitive. Such children are often mistrustful, action-oriented, and desirous of escaping from the therapeutic situation. Therapists must formulate the initial contract in terms of 'what's in it for you?' They stress the therapist's role as a helpful adult, pointing out how the child might, for example, be able to remain in school or avoid further punishment by the law if he or she conforms to certain rules. Therapists are not the law but merely members of that particular society. As 'manipulated' helpers rather than prime authority figures, they act in response to the communication of the patient. Out of respect for the patient's needs they are able to avoid moralizing – but they do indicate the logical consequences involved in the child's antisocial actions.

Therapists should refrain from imposing their own values. Novice clinicians may be at special risk to manifest their own values of permissiveness or punishment. For most children, a decision to avoid misbehavior to avert the response that will follow from school or other authorities is sufficient motivation for therapy to proceed. Once this understanding has been reached, the child and therapist can move on to specific behavioral rehearsals in the second stage of sequential psychotherapy.

Style B: Therapist as Nonmanipulated Helper: 'How Can I Help – or Take Good Enough Care of You?'

In a more trusting child the therapeutic relationship can become more personalized. In a suicidal child, for example, formation of the initial contract stressed that the child should be cared for in a structured and protective setting. This fulfilled the child's need for nurturance and protection. This general point of 'good enough' care is similar to Winnicott's concepts [40]. In another child with asthma and associated depression, the initial contract for 'good enough' care involved assurance of adequate pediatric help while avoiding the overprotection and subsequent shame–rage reactions that had plagued the child in relationships with his own family.

The therapist in this situation is cast into a nurturing role with a child who can accept the usefulness of helping adults and has therefore achieved a degree of trust, or at least a suspension of mistrust. If this is not initially possible for the child, a brief period of more neutral contractual maneuvering in the 'what's in it for you?' style may be required. In reality, very few therapeutic interactions are exclusively or perpetually Style A or Style B.

Style C: Therapist as Empathic Participant: 'What's It Like Being You?'

The two former patterns in contract formation have stressed doing things with or for the child. In contrast, questions asked about 'What's it like being you?' relate to the therapist's wish to understand the child and also achieve some notion of the child's own perceptions.

In all three styles the therapist's total understanding of the child must of necessity be limited; the child is still guarded, and the time available for obtaining information is short. But the therapist does signal his or her basic interest in the child as a person, and the contractual position of usefulness, helpfulness, and empathy reflects an honest transaction between one person and another.

During this initial contract formation, there may have been an unfolding elaboration of roles, from the therapist as a nonpersonalizing informer of consequences or routes of legal or social redress, to that of parenting caretaker in the second style, to that of an interested and empathic person in the third style. Many children and adolescents may progress through all three styles in contract formulation, but such a sequence is not invariable or even necessary for successful therapy. Such contractual groundwork provides a basis for the second stage in sequential psychotherapy.

Stage 2: From Instrumental to Interactional Patterns: 'Doing Therapy To or With the Patient'

This stage initially employs an elaboration of simple to more complex behavior modification methods. Therapists may initially use concrete reward systems and behavioral rehearsals, but then develop more complex interactional patterns by using themselves as models of interactions, while augmenting the child's capacity to observe himself or herself interacting more successfully. Similarly, children progress in their perception of the therapist. Whereas initially they may regard the therapist as somebody to be manipulated for gain, they are secondarily involved with the therapist as a model towards whom they have ambivalent liking. Finally, they understand being with the therapist and share their excitement about increasing capacities. Following the formation of the initial contract, a number of possible therapies may therefore occur.

The next case examples illustrate this approach with children with different diagnoses and attitudes towards the therapist.

The Children with Externalizing Disruptive Behavior Disorders

These children are best approached by directive therapies for agreed-on target behaviors such as high intensity aggression or other maladaptive social behaviors. Often such target behaviors are best approached by using rewards and time-outs for positive and negative behavior. This therapeutic interchange in the 'what's in it for you' relationship spells out to children the consequences of their actions, but also avoids the intense and often exhortative personalizing that has often taken place with other adult figures.

In group interactions dominance–submission maneuvers with other children usually predominate, since such children have frequently not managed to achieve sharing or a capacity to delay gratification. As a result, social skills training with peers and adults can sometimes be employed. Often group approaches are used: group peer interactions may be broken down into such simple behavioral objectives as 'spending more time with the group by avoiding fights and tantrums,' with later sequential elaboration into more complex patterns of 'doing something that somebody would like,' and then into 'doing something so that someone will try to please a third person' [41].

In later individual or group therapy, techniques to limit or redirect excessive and ineffective verbal expression may be used once a child has experience with more concrete reward systems. The primary therapist can also use direct modeling to channel the child into more effective modes of affectual assertion. Role-playing techniques of possible aggressive techniques may be employed, along with role reversals; here, the child can try out different patterns of verbal and physical behav-

ior and demonstrate in a concrete way that such interactions are possible.

The Children with Internalizing and/or Psychophysiologic Disorders

The sequential psychotherapy model is also relevant for children and adolescents with internalizing or psychophysiologic disorders. In the suicidal child mentioned previously in the vignette in Style B, one of the key conflicts addressed in therapy related to his ineffective aggressive assertion. This in turn followed from his unmastered and murderous rages toward his mother, arising from a recently threatened separation from his father. Such murderous rages were immediately internalized because of the family's structure of strict and punitive values, leading to internalizing aggression and a resultant suicidal attempt. The key strategy area (after basic nurturance was achieved) was to encourage effective aggression. Accordingly, aggressive–assertive role playing was used, with role reversal to decrease the child's anxiety when necessary. With coaxing and support, he managed to express his anger first at the therapist in a role, and then in a real fashion-playing the person who would not allow him to return home for the weekend. He initially became more comfortable in therapy sessions, but as he expressed conscious anger during later sessions, he suddenly became aware of murderous rage impulses, followed immediately by a wish to kill himself and an absolute conviction of his own wickedness.

These emotions were dalt with directly by telling him about the nature of such early and primitive feelings, and by demonstrating that the therapist did not 'drop dead' or attack him for his anger – even when the child said he 'really meant it.' The child then relaxed, although further working through was required as part of a continuing process of interpretation and identification of affects.

In another example, an asthmatic child also had his aggression toward his mother identified, but initial attempts to have this well-socialized, charming child express and channel his anger were unsuccessful. In one session, however, a childcare worker to whom the patient related warmly as a mothering person role – played his attacking and rejecting mother. The patient immediately became suffused with rage and attempted to attack her physically. Afterward, when this event was examined, the therapist was able to help the patient recognize the presence of his emotions and explore their source. Subsequently, they were able to rehearse this sequence with good results.

In summary, the second stage of behavioral rehearsals focuses on a series of simple to more complex behavioral, interactional, and affective rehearsal systems. Such intervention increases children's learned ability to perform social maneuvers, as well as their internalization and comfort in their own abilities, which is often associated with more positive self-esteem.

Renegotiation at the End of the Second Stage: 'Do You Want To Go On, or Stop at this Stage?'

In sequential psychotherapy it is frequently possible to stop at the end of the second stage. In the case of the disruptive behavior-disordered child, the acquisition of more appropriate social behaviors usually leads to better acceptance by the family and society, although there may be technical difficulties. For example, counter-reactions by the family may follow the use of reward systems; parents may feel that a child should not be rewarded for fulfilling only normal expectations. Alternatively, guilty, self-punitive behaviors may emerge from the behavior-disordered child once more effective social maneuvers have been learned; this may arise from an internalizing of the anger that had previously been contained by the aggressive acting out. Again, the emphasis on behavioral reinforcers throughout the second stage might result in the parents and child still dealing with each other at the end of this stage of therapy as 'good' or 'bad,' rather than as loving or loved persons. Hence the very use of social learning techniques might lead to the child's using adults in a more facile nature, but still with problems in affectual expression.

Many behavior-disordered children who have been brought up in a fashion that values objects and concrete transactions over affective interactions may experience considerable difficulty with affect verbalization [42]. But both they and their parents are often capable of a general but strong warmth, which is released once more effective modes of expression and interaction are demonstrated. Once satisfactory behavioral interchanges have been elaborated, increased comfort between child and parent is often sufficient to allow the termination of therapy. Malone made this point in his analysis of the role of family therapy in different social classes, noting that families from different backgrounds may manifest very different patterns of communication that are nonetheless still imbued with positive affective content [43].

Many children and parents will accept the symptom change in social and affectual behavior accomplished during this second stage, and in the renegotiation phase will tell the therapist of their wish to stop therapy at this point. In other cases, the child or family will wish to explore more complex issues.

Stage 3: 'Let's Go On': Exploration of More Complex Intrapsychic, Intercommunicational, and Intrafamilial Issues

In more verbal and subjectively oriented children, the behaviorally oriented techniques used in the second phase facilitate exploration during the third stage into more complex individual and familial psychodynamic material.

In the depressed suicidal child described earlier, the rehearsal of more effective aggressive–assertive patterns was initially paralleled by an increase in rage toward his mother. Further exploration in therapy revealed that he had always been angry at his mother for her threats of deserting the family. He also felt that his death by strangulation might cause his mother to feel guilty in this life, and also to be punished in the next life for her lack of attention to him. This led to an associated fantasy of their being linked together in life and death, since he would also be punished in Hell because of his suicide.

The ambivalent association between the child and his mother was also sustained by the family structure. The mother had formed a close alliance with the child, using him as a shield against the aggressive and sexual advances of her husband. Moreover, her basic ambivalence toward the boy was heightened because she became pregnant with him soon after she had adopted her first daughter, at a time when she felt – or had convinced her husband – that it was not possible for her to have a child. The child's perception of himself as unloved and unwanted was at the heart of his depression.

An interesting question asked by behavior therapy colleagues is whether knowledge of such dynamic material alters subsequent therapeutic strategies. In practice, such knowledge does seem to be useful. In the above case, knowledge of the use of the patient and his sister as defenses against sexuality was addressed directly in family therapy, as was the unsuccessful attempt at dominance of the father. Behavioral and insight approaches often coexist; the prime symptom of aggression in this patient was treated concomitantly by rehearsal of increasingly modulated aggressive behaviors. The child later observed that he was more comfortable in expressing anger toward his peers and his parents; as he did this, his suicidal wishes decreased and he was able to cry. His extremes of murderous rage had been modulated into more useful affects, which resulted in his being more spontaneously cheerful and less depressed. Therapeutic strategies therefore continued to come directly from previous stages of behavioral rehearsal, even though new treatment dealing with family relationships, sexual impulses, and other aspects of his life then entered into therapy.

In the case of the child with asthma described above, the demonstration of increased ability to cope added to his general self-esteem and capacity to envision himself as exploring the world. Although he had previously avoided school, the child now planned successful reentry. He began learning again and also started to play with other children; this replaced his previous behavior of sitting sadly with adults, endlessly reciting tales of the sports heroes he had observed in hours of passively looking at television.

The model of sequential psychotherapy presented therefore indicates a reasonable and rational approach for planning the initial moves and subsequent strategies to be used in therapy with many different types of children. The different stages are as follows: (1) an initial diagnostic evaluation; (2) a period of contractual negotiation; (3) a stage of behavioral, interactional, and affectual rehearsal; and (4) a possible stage of further exploration into more involved intrapsychic, environmental, and intrafamilial issues. Although the complexities of the case often suggest many complicated possibilities, initial therapeutic strategies are often couched in rather simple behavioral terms. Similarly, even though strategies become more complex as therapy progresses, they still maintain their inner consistency. As children achieve greater skills, they internalize increasing self-esteem and are therefore able to attack the more internalized and often frightening material that emerges in therapy. Even when such material emerges, behaviorally based approaches often provide the best inroads to these complex interactional and intrapsychic problems.

One final caveat regarding either simple or complex accounts of the mechanisms of therapy remains. Whatever elegant hypotheses might be made by the therapist, the focus or impetus for change might follow from basic and simple perceptions of the patient. The noted Canadian psychoanalyst analyst Stanley Greben wrote a book about a particular analysis, which contained complex descriptions of the analytic process. In contrast, the patient's remark at the end of the analysis was: 'He was always there!' [44].

Commonly Described Forms of Psychotherapy

The following sections refer to the most commonly described forms of psychotherapy and pharmacotherapy. Basic underlying concepts in each form of therapy will be outlined; and it will be noted that there are frequently a number of different strategies and even schools of thought in each general form of therapy. Usually, these concepts and strategies overlap with those described above under the general model, although the jargon associated may be different.

Child and Adolescent Psychopharmacotherapy

Recently, there has been a rapid evolution in the psychopharmacotherapy of children and adolescents [5]. Given the recent changing patterns of psychiatric practice, there is now great emphasis on this mode of therapy.

The ordinary purpose of pharmacotherapy is to reduce the severity of selected target symptoms. Maturational and developmental issues may influence physiologic, cognitive, psychological, and experiential factors. The provision of pharmacotherapy is part of an overall treatment plan that includes comprehensive diagnostic formulations as well as the involvement of the family. Compliance with medication is an issue of particular importance. It is a reflection of the doctor–patient relationship and of family experience and expectation, and a powerful determinant of outcome.

Each medication and its effects need to be explained fully to the child and adolescent. Medico-legal and ethical concerns require that the parent or guardian also understand the medication and its effects. In addition, several issues concerning informed consent will require discussion. There may be unknown risks when taking medication, especially when novel psychopharmacologic treatments are used or when the risks versus benefits are uncertain. Since many medications are not specifically designated by the Food and Drug Administration (FDA) as being safe or effective for children, many are used in an off-label (non-FDA-approved) fashion. In all cases, however, the use of such medication should be consistent with ordinary clinical practice, and there should be some notation in the chart that the available literature has been studied.

Medication should continue to be monitored using the appropriate physical examination and laboratory tests and procedures such as complete blood count with differential, urinalysis, liver, renal and thyroid profiles, and electrocardiograms (ECGs) and electroencephalograms (EEGs) as required. Baseline clinical observations may include standard rating scales such as the Conners Parent/Teacher Scale and the Abnormal Involuntary Movement Scale. And because of recent concerns about antipsychotic weight gain, leading to predictable increases in insulin resistance, and risk for hyperglycemia, hypertension, dyslipidemias and cardiovascular disease, monitoring guidelines have recently been issued. These include personal/family history, weight, waist circumference, blood pressure, and fasting glucose and lipid profiles during antipsychotic therapy [45].

In this age of cost-consciousness, the clinician will often be required to distinguish between generic and brand-name preparations. In general, it is probably wise to start off with the brand name and then see whether the patient can be switched to a generic preparation without loss of effect or the development of unknown side effects due to the congeners found in some generic preparations.

Since some children may require more than one drug, they may experience significant drug interactions, particularly interactions involving the cytochrome P450 isoenzyme systems. The drug dosage varies with age, with younger children often requiring larger doses proportional to age. Pharmacokinetics and pharmacodynamics (the interactions of one drug with another) are seldom fully studied in children, and much additional research is needed in this area. Some drugs and/or their metabolites require monitoring of blood levels, particularly those drugs used for bipolar disorders, such as lithium, valproic acid, and carbamazepine. For most other medications, including methylphenidate, levels are not usually obtained nor are they clearly related to clinical response.

Other than for finite problems, it is customary to continue psychotropic medication for a considerable time, often for many years. Periodic withdrawal and tapering of medications may be undertaken, if the patient's clinical state allows, to determine if it is possible to discontinue such medications. In the case of methylphenidate or other psychostimulants, medications may be withheld during the weekends or summer because of possible adverse effects on growth and height, or because the patient can function adequately without them. In disorders such as bipolar disorder and schizophrenia, however, it may be difficult to reduce the dosage of medication, especially in those medications that require an adequate blood level. When drugs are withdrawn or tapered, relapse or withdrawal effects may occur.

In summary, pharmacotherapeutic agents are essentially suppressive, in that they reduce unwarranted symptoms or behaviors. They may also in some cases be neuroprotective, as current studies of antidepressants suggest [46]. However, by themselves they rarely allow for the development of new behavior.

The Verbal/Behavioral Psychotherapies

Psychotherapy, in contrast to pharmacotherapy, usually aims to change behavioral maladaptive patterns and may allow for longer-term remissions [47] than pharmacotherapy, in which stopping medication usually results in the return of symptoms. This section outlines the more common child and adolescent psychotherapies.

Psychodynamic Psychotherapy

Historically, child and adolescent psychotherapy has tended to focus on intensive individual psychodynamic psychotherapy [48]. The approach is to form a trusting relationship between the therapist and the patient and to allow the verbal expression of feelings with increasing self-knowledge and self-mastery [49]. While these elements exist in all psychotherapies, in psychodynamic models they are considered to be primary to the therapeutic process. Formation of the therapeutic alliance is fundamental, especially in the initial phase when children are told that they will have a series of times set aside to begin to understand the their problems. Children may indicate particular problems through play and with defensive structures. Following the initial phase, the therapist moves into the middle phase of psychotherapy, whose goals are to work through problems and also interpret the transference by which conflicts and associated symptoms experienced by the child are passed on to the therapist. As Lewis pointed out, the normal dependent development of the child throughout therapy may modify the transference [48].

For example, a very young child would be expected to establish a transference with infantile aspects, which might become less regressive and more assertive as the child grows older.

Linking the child's behaviors with fantasies may be helpful, especially in the context of a personal myth held by the child. This myth may be used to link current and earlier behavior and to help explicate defenses. During the interpretative process, the therapist may place observations in the context of what has previously taken place or what is happening during the relationship between the child and the therapist. This process models that of the observing ego initially in the adult therapist, and then in the child. In the case of child therapy, this needs to be spelled out in a concrete way, given the child's relative inability to abstract [50]. The process of working through requires a sustained therapeutic effect, since repetitive defensive conflicts will remain relatively unchanged unless the affects contained by such conflicts are able to be expressed. Often a process of mourning occurs, as children let go of worked-through material, and also during the subsequent formation of alternate modes of coping. For example, in a session a child may set aside a favorite toy or game, but do so with reluctance or sadness. The process of gaining insight gradually leads to change of thought and behavior.

As in most models, during the termination phase, the goals of therapy are to reduce anxiety, increase frustration tolerance, and improve relationships and the capacity for pleasure. The termination phase often brings up issues of separation and loss, relating both to previous experiences and the loss of the therapist. These issues may relate to more global concerns regarding the acceptance of limitations in life.

Play is a frequent feature of psychodynamic psychotherapy [51]. Anna Freud and Melanie Klein [52,53] initially provided principles for the use of play in child therapy as well as the understanding that play had unconscious meaning. Winnicott [54] expanded these concepts, using play as an intermediate or transitional object between fantasy and reality. Currently the techniques in psychodynamic psychotherapy are modified to meet the developmental needs of the child and there is active involvement of the parents in the process. Other aspects of play therapy include the mastery of conflictual situations, with the therapist suggesting alterations in repetitive or nonproductive play sequences, even in children with ADHD [55]. Alternatively, the therapist may remain an observer, while the child seeks his or her own solutions. Coppolillo indicated the powerful effects of play therapy, including the child's immersion into play and how possible affects are offset by the reality of the therapist's presence and his or her capacity to tolerate the child's impulses [51].

The effectiveness of psychodynamic therapy is unclear, since most therapies are used by individual clinicians. Weisz and Weiss [56] and Weisz et al. [57] reported that psychodynamic therapies had less measured therapeutic effect than behavioral treatments. On the other hand Fonagy and Target found that children with disruptive behavior who remained in psychodynamic psychotherapy for more than a year '69% were no longer diagnosable on termination' [58]. In any case psychodynamic therapies have been less rigorously tested than behavioral treatments.

Behavior Therapy

As described by Vitulano and Tebes [59] behavior therapy originated from the well-known experiments of Pavlov, who found that when an unconditioned stimulus appeared repeatedly with a previously neutral stimulus, this neutral stimulus would eventually elicit a conditioned response that resembled the unconditioned reflex [60]. For example, Pavlov's dogs, who initially salivated at the presentation of food, eventually salivated at the sound of a bell. Similarly in humans, a young boy named Albert heard a loud noise when he began to play with a rat and subsequently became fearful of the rat and other 'furry animals,' illustrating stimulus generalization [61]. A more flexible pattern of conditioning identified by Skinner as operant conditioning involved behaviors that could be modified or maintained by their consequences [62]. Behavior followed by pleasant consequences was likely to increase in frequency, whereas that followed by unpleasant consequences was likely to decrease.

A third development was cognitive behavior therapy, which has been widely used in both adult and child psychiatry [63,64]. The basic assumption is that cognitive processes, including expectations, beliefs, or attributions, influence behavior and affect. Irrational and faulty cognitive processes foster maladaptive behaviors, which can be reversed by modification of this cognition. The cognitive behavioral approach is therefore less concerned with the influence of affect. This approach recognizes the field-dependence of children, and emphasizes that other individuals in the child's environment should be enlisted in the treatment of the child. The cognitive behavioral model requires that the success of therapy should be determined from observed behaviors rather than reported subjective experiences, and that all treatment techniques should be based on empirically derived clinical techniques.

In contrast to cognitive behavioral models, social learning theory, developed by Bandura, includes observational learning, in which behaviors change as a result of observing a model [65]. A child who views another child being rewarded for a particular behavior is more likely to perform similar behavior. Hence, the child is able to effect change by himself or herself.

Behavior Therapy Techniques Particularly Used for Disruptive Behavior Disorders

Several terms are frequently used in the behavioral literature, many of which refer to the treatment of disruptive behavior disorders. General techniques of behavior therapy include reinforcement, in which behavior is strengthened by its consequences, as in operant conditioning. In positive reinforcement the reward is presented after the occurrence of a desired behavior, and in negative reinforcement the reward involves the removal of an aversive stimulus after the desired behavior happens. Continuous reinforcements are administered each time a response occurs. In contrast to intermittent reinforcement, in a fixed, interval schedule a child is reinforced after a specific time period regardless of the response, and in a variable interval schedule, the rate of reinforcement varies randomly. A fixed ratio technique administers reinforcement after a specific number of the child's responses, whereas a variable ratio technique reinforces randomly around a specific average of desired responses by the child. Intermittent reinforcement responses may be difficult to change; compulsive gambling, for example, demonstrates how intermittent reinforcement can lead to high rates of response. Parents who are inconsistent and variable in their responses to a child may reinforce the behaviors they wish to extinguish.

Other techniques include reinforcing a particular response in the presence of one stimulus but not in the presence of another. Common examples include shaping, in which closer and closer approximations of behavior produce a final desired behavior. In this approach, rewarding and reinforcing initially occur for small changes of behavior, and as the behavior becomes closer to the goal, the rewards continue but the tasks and standards of behavior become more stringent. In contrast, fading involves changing a stimulus so that a new stimulus eventually produces the same response. Chaining involves reinforcing more and more links to produce a complex chain of behavior, as in teaching an autistic child the sequence of dressing. Contracting is primarily used to increase specific behaviors or eliminate unwanted behavior. Contracts for particular patterns of performance commonly involve sequences about what the child and the parents should do. They are used especially with adolescents and have the advantage of distancing: the contract involves a relatively neutral, agreed-on interchange that is distinct from high-level arguing. Finally, modeling is frequently used in modifying parent–child or other adult–child interactions at home or at school.

Several suppressive techniques in behavior therapy are used to reduce or eliminate behavior; some of these techniques have achieved a degree of notoriety [66]. For example, the use of massive negative stimuli such as cattle prods to change the behavior of autistic children gave rise to justifiable concern. More generally, extinction occurs when reinforcement is withheld after an offered response in order to reduce the frequency of this response. For example, parents may be taught to respond to a child's crying at night by not going into the room immediately and to progressively increase the length of time before they go in. A similar response is that of differential reinforcement, in which reinforcement is given for nonoccurrence or low rates of occurrence of a problem behavior, such as hitting teachers or other children.

Punishment such as scolding, spanking, or removing privileges is used to reduce undesirable behavior through the introduction of an aversive stimulus or the removal of a positive stimulus. Punishment is able to elicit a rapid decrease in problem behaviors and may be useful for some self-injurious or aggressive behaviors. The behaviors usually change only temporarily, however, and may be associated with fear or escape responses, or even by reinforcement due to the negative attention the child receives during punishment (as distinct from the lack of attention otherwise received from the parent). The behavior may simply be displaced. Parental commands such as 'Don't let me see you hit your sister' may lead to the child hitting his or her sister somewhere else; the parent who punishes may in turn model aggressive, physical, or verbal behavior as well as a lack of respect for the rights of others. Children who are physically aggressive have often seen such behavior modeled by others; similarly, those who have been severely beaten will frequently continue this behavior as they grow older.

Punishment procedures that appear to be effective include time-out, in which the child is removed from the setting where the behavior occurred and is placed in a restrictive environment such as his or her room for a brief period, and response cost, in which a reinforcer is removed because of misbehavior. In the latter case, a child may have privileges such as the use of a television or telephone temporarily removed, with the opportunity to earn back these privileges. In overcorrection, the child may be required to negate the effects of his or her actions, for example in cleaning crayon off the walls or contributing toward the cost of repairing damage in the house. Alternatively, the child may be required to practice positive behavior incompatible with misbehavior; for example, a child who leaves his or her books around in a messy fashion may be required to line up the books in a particularly neat fashion.

The treatment of conduct disorder and antisocial behavior may consist of problem-solving skills training (PSST) or behavioral parent training [67,68]. Kazdin and colleagues [69] and Barkley et al. [70] showed that a combined approach of PSST and parent training is effective in treating antisocial behavior in children. As in all therapies, those children who respond best, may have more internal motivation and more motivated parents.

Behavior therapy for ADHD has been shown to enhance learning and improve academic performance, although the usefulness of such techniques in the absence of psychostimulant medication is still a matter of discussion [71]. This issue has been clarified by results of the National Institute of Mental Health multimodality treatment study of children with ADHD [11,72]. In this large study, subjects were randomly assigned to one of three manually based protocols –

medication only, psychosocial therapy only, or combined medication and psychosocial therapy – versus a community standard treatment (assessment and referral).

Other areas for behavioral techniques include pervasive developmental disorders, autism, and mental retardation, all of which focus on suppressing unwanted behaviors and teaching new skills [73,74]. Behavioral approaches have also been used for enuresis and encopresis. The 'bell and pad treatment' for enuresis has been in use since its description in 1938 by Mowrer and Mowrer [75]. This technique is effective in 75–80% of cases but also has a relapse rate of about 40%. The dry-bed training technique of Azrin and colleagues incorporates several behavioral techniques, including positive practice, reinforcement, punishment, and the urine alarm and thus may be more effective than the urine alarm only [76]. Behavior therapy for functional encopresis uses positive conditioned reinforcement and/or regular checks toward full cleanliness. Laxatives or suppositories are often used as adjuncts.

Behavior Therapy Techniques Particularly Used for Internalizing Disorders

Desensitization has been widely used to reduce children's fears, as in the gradual exposure of a child to a conditioned stimulus such as separation, test taking, or frightening animals [77]. An extension of this technique is participant modeling, in which a parent models a lack of fear of a particular animal, for example, and the child is then able to follow this behavior. In systematic desensitization, the child works with the therapist to establish a hierarchy of fears about anxiety-provoking stimuli; these stimuli are then provided during therapy from the least to the most anxiety producing. This may be done either in imagination or in vivo, as in taking a child to school who has school phobia. Flooding or implosion therapy involves having the child come into contact with the most feared item in the hierarchy. It has been found useful for children not responding favorably to gradual desensitization, but its general use is discouraged because it is often anxiety producing and may be used as a punishment technique.

Other behavioral therapies for anxiety or depression that stress a more cognitive approach include cognitive behavioral therapy (CBT) and interpersonal therapy. As Petti has noted [77], in the former therapy, cognitive distortions or errors in reasoning (such as those noted by Beck and colleagues [78], and Kovacs and Beck [79]) include arbitrary inferences, selective abstraction (details taken out of context), personaliza-tion (being blamed for particular events), and dichotomous thinking (which does not allow for intermediate positions).

Therapists may use such cognitive techniques to explore the bases of faulty assumptions and to teach alternate coping skills such as assigning measures of probability and reassigning attribution. In contrast, more formal cognitive behavioral techniques help patients test their dysfunctional cognitions and change their behavior by using homework assignments or time structuring, increasing specific activities, or carrying out exercises related to specific situations. Some studies have described the successful use of cognitive therapy in adolescents with issues such as depression and distorted perceptions regarding appearance, sexuality, and competency [79]. Leahy has suggested using a representation of dichotomy, with figures such as 'the bad thoughts monster' and 'the smart thoughts man' [80], but challenging assumptions may be difficult with children [81,82].

A variant of the cognitive approach, which has been particularly used for depression among adolescents, is interpersonal therapy, as described by Moreau and colleagues [83]. In contrast to formal cognitive behavioral therapy with its emphasis on internal cognitions and relatively less emphasis on affect, interpersonal psychotherapy emphasizes particular emotional and cognitive situations that exist between the patient and stressful circumstances or persons. By going through these areas, it is possible for the patient not only to recognize how certain situations may provoke depression or other affects but also to work on alternate strategies.

Behavior therapy has been used for child and adolescent depression dealing with poor self-esteem, social isolation, and hopelessness, and self-control training has demonstrated efficacy in treating depression in children and adolescents. As noted, it has also been shown to be effective in a recent study of depression the combination of fluoxetine and CBT by March and colleagues, where again the combination was more effective than either individually, but the CBT had a more robust effect [12]. Previously, Brent and colleagues found that individual cognitive behavior therapy was superior to systemic behavior family therapy and individual nondirective supportive therapy in the treatment of adolescents with major depressive disorders [84]. OCD has been shown by March and colleagues [85] to be responsive to exposure and response prevention techniques, where patients are asked to expose themselves to real or imagined distressing thoughts or experiences until the distress caused by these agents has abated. This technique, combined with medication to offset the more severe forms of OCD, has been shown to be particularly effective and often utilizes manuals that lead to a more rational cognitive behavioral therapy approach.

In contrast to the above cognitive approaches, rational emotive therapy emphasizes an active dispute with the patient concerning fundamental dysfunctional thoughts and teaches the evaluation of actions [86]. Waters used rational emotive therapy for disturbed youth and focused on cognitions and the identification of sources causing specific problems [87]. Goals for young children are to identify emotions, distinguish thoughts from feelings, be alert to self-talk (private speech about oneself), connect self-talk and feelings, and develop rational coping statements. There is a possibility of confrontation in this technique, which may cause concern to some patients and families, and which must be handled in a tactful fashion.

Interpersonal cognitive problem solving, which Shure and Spivack found effective with pupils in poor urban preschools, is conducted by teachers and stresses alternative solution thinking as well as means-end thinking, which in turn leads to better interpersonal adjustment and less psychopathology [88]. Self-management skills in cognitive therapy include self-regulation for some phobias and self-instructional training. The latter may be particularly useful for children with concrete thinking or learning problems and either low to average intelligence or retardation [89,90].

In summary, the various behavior therapies presented have been found to be particularly useful for treating internalizing disorders.

Adlerian Psychotherapy

Although not generally described in many compendia of therapy, the Adlerian or NeoAdlerian approach described by Dinkmeyer and McKay is often extremely useful, especially with intelligent verbal children with oppositional defiant disorder whose parents are also intelligent and verbal [91]. The 'goals of misbehavior' as defined in this form of therapy include: (1) requiring attention in which children only feel they belong when they are being noticed or served; (2) power, in which children feel that they belong only when in control; and (3) revenge, in which children feel that hurting others is necessary because they cannot be loved. Displays of inadequacy also convince others not to expect anything from the child. In contrast, the goals of positive behavior include involvement and contribution, feelings of power and autonomy, feelings of justice and fairness, and feeling the opportunity to withdraw from conflict. (It is not necessary to fight all battles!)

These points are described in the manual on systematic training for effective parenting [91]. In contrast to behavior therapy, which emphasizes doing things to or with the child, Adlerian therapy aims to give the child as much power as possible, including allowing the child to make choices. These choices are often demarcated by the parent, as in 'You have a choice – to stop hitting your brother or to go to your room,' but are nonetheless choices. If the child cannot make a decision, then the parent has the option of taking over and making the decision for the child. The child is told, however, that the parent is willing to hand back the decision to the child as soon as the child is capable of doing this. The general phraseology is, 'I see that you are unable to choose how to sort out your problem. I will take care of your problem, but then I will solve it my way. You may have your problem back at any time when you are able to solve it.'

It is important for the parents to give directions as neutrally as possible, and for the therapist to reinforce this. Usually a prior group program of parent training is useful. A somewhat counter-intuitive approach is that when a child is being aggressive or oppositional, parents should be free to remove themselves from the scene, on the basis that quarreling cannot occur in the absence of one of the two parties.

Family and Group Therapies

There are many models of family therapy with different theoretical bases. They have in common a focus on treating the family as the defined unit for therapy: problems evolve from the family structure and history, and although the child or adolescent may be the 'identified patient,' the basic problems rest within the family. These approaches therefore address interactional components, although Ravenscroft has noted that earlier patterns of family therapy stressed psychoanalytic principles [92]. Satir and colleagues at the Mental Health Institute in 1958 focused on a communications family therapy model, which later led into Haley's concepts of strategic family therapy [92]. Minuchin developed structural family therapy based on working with multiproblem families from low socioeconomic groups [93]. Earlier systemic approaches to family therapy were based on general systems theory, including the concept of cybernetics, which held that families tend to maintain equilibrium: a tension always exists between homeostasis and change, balancing stability and self-preservation with change and adaptation. Strategic and structural family therapy arose from this theory and focused on observable as well as reported family behavior. Structural family therapy requires that dysfunctional family structures are observed when the family is in action and allows for active suggestions for change. Strategic family therapy primarily emphasizes deciphering the family communication rules that underlie problems, leading to planned strategies for change and greater emphasis on cognition (Table 6.2).

Other schools of family therapy include behavioral approaches such as the parent behavioral training model for family therapy described by Griest and Wells [94]. Another behavioral approach is functional family therapy, in which maladaptive behavior evolving from the family context becomes more interpersonally adaptive [95]. This active approach has been widely used in intervention and prevention programs for children with substance abuse and antisocial problems, and

Table 6.2 Varieties of Family Therapy.

Strategic (Haley, Madanes)
The pattern of symptomatic behavior is the best solution to conflicts that the family has developed
The therapist disrupts negative patterns of interaction by prescribing tasks that the family as a whole needs to contribute

Structural (Minuchin)
The therapist recognizes dysfunctional patterns within the family that leads to children to exhibit behavioral problems. Frequent dysfunctional patterns are enmeshment (ineffective closeness), disengagement (excessive distance) and scapegoating

Systemic (Bowen)
The therapist promotes differentiation and may use triangulation (therapist may pair with family member to understand other member) to elicit help within the family to reflect and work through intergenerational conflicts. Genograms are used to help explore the way the family system has created rules, and hierarchy

Behavioral (Patterson)
The therapist identifies problematic behavior in children and helps parents reinforces positive behavior. This form of therapy focuses on the here and now conflicts

Psychodynamic/object relations (Ackerman, Framo)
The therapist helps members of the family recognize that their needs in the family are based on their own early parent–child experiences. The insight gained helps members appreciate their limitations and understand the distortions they have of others intentions

---

stresses phases of engagement and motivation, behavioral change, and generalizations which are linked to specific goals for each family. Further forms of family therapy include extended family therapy and object relations family therapy; the former obviously relates to extended family and social networks, and the latter returns to the psychoanalytic roots of family therapy, in which internal psychologic development occurs in relation to significant caretakers.

There are a number of schools of family therapy, whose basic components are often associated with particular therapists who in turn tend to have their own disciples. The style of family therapy used is frequently overly dependent on the practitioner's schooling. Alternatively, family therapists may eschew labels for an 'eclectic' approach; frequently, however, the therapist functions flexibly with patients but then has difficulty defining what he or she is doing.

Family diagnosis as such is not a major feature of family therapy, although a number of clinicians, including Epstein and colleagues [23] and more recently the Family Therapy Committee of the Group for the Advancement of Psychiatry, have advanced concepts for family therapy diagnosis. Other 'diagnostic' models and typologies include the Beavers systems model of family competence and adaptability versus family interaction styles versus the Olson circumplex model, which measures dimensions of family behavior such as cohesion, adaptability, and communication [96]. Combrinck-Graham described families in a more developmental fashion, with the introduction of the family life cycle [97]. The multiplicity of models allows family therapies to evolve from more behavioral to intercommunicational and intrapsychic functioning, in line with the general sequential model of psychotherapy.

Group Therapy for Children and Adolescents
As described by Cramer-Azima [98] group therapy started with group analytic models, as with that of Anthony [99] and then evolved to activity group therapy, focusing on observation of the child's behavioral and motoric communications in a particular group action. Most group therapists now use a mixture of developmental and group assignment frameworks, either with parents in parallel treatment with younger children or with groups of children who have common or at least interconnected problems. One of the technical difficulties is to focus on what represents a group. The group allows for a commonality in approach, but it may lead to a number of children or adolescents held to be similar for therapy purposes, but actually very

different individually and clinically. The observation that other children have similar problems is nonetheless useful in reducing a child's anxiety and may lead to the evolution of shared coping skills.

A number of groups for special populations therefore exist, including those for social skills, underachievement in school, divorce, abused children, and drug-using children, as well as parent/family groups stressing family evolution and parent training [100]. Groups for older children and adolescents using interpersonal and cognitive behavioral models have been established [100–102].

Groups can be used in an evolutionary fashion, changing over time from behavioral to more communicational emphases. Group therapies are often attractive to a number of insurance companies, because they give the impression that more can be achieved for a greater number of children with less cost; the hard evidence for this is unclear, however. In one analysis, group therapy treatment was found to be more effective than individual treatment in 31% of the cases. Some studies have discussed the effects of group therapy for particular diagnoses. Fine and colleagues, for example, found that depressed adolescents in a therapeutic support group showed a greater decrease in depressive symptoms and increased self-support than those not receiving group therapy [103].

In summary, group therapy is an important but somewhat understudied mode of therapy for children and adolescents. It is already undertaken with great enthusiasm in several settings but will benefit from more rigorous research.

Special Population Therapies

Because of the high prevalence of children and adolescents with problems not easily amenable to therapy, as in conduct disorders, there has been an increased interest in using multiple arenas for intervention. Some of the more dramatic forms, such as the use of 'Boot Camps' have not been proven effective [104], but others such as the Multi-Systemic Therapy (MST) of Bourdin and colleagues have been tested satisfactorily, and show considerable promise [105]. This is an intensive family and community-based treatment that address the multiple determinants of serious antisocial behavior in juvenile offenders. It views individuals as being nested within a complex network of interconnected peer, family, and neighborhood systems, and targets necessary interventions in one or more of these systems. It has produced very favorable outcome data compared to previously studied interventions.

Summary

In this chapter, the processes of diagnosis and psychopharmacologic and other psychotherapeutic treatments in children and adolescents has been outlined. A sequential model was described that allows for a rational selection of therapies for the complex problems met by child and adolescent psychiatrists. Such an approach, which leads to the sequential descriptions of defined goals and objectives, is increasingly important in an era marked by increasing impetus for accountability. Finally, the complex and rapidly adumbrating areas of 'specific' forms of psychotherapy have been briefly discussed. Child psychiatrists and others training in this area need to have a broad training, probably with an emphasis in a particular area. But they should also be able to tailor their approaches to the varying clinical needs of the child, parent or society. It is hoped that this brief summary will help child psychiatrists choose competently and selectively from among the often-bewildering mosaic of available therapies.

References

1. Doyle RL, Feren AP, Jacobs RJ: *Ambulatory Care Guidelines: Health Care Management Guidelines Manual.* Vol. 3. New York: Milliman and Robertson Inc., 1996.
2. Somoza E, Soutullo-Esperon L, Mossman D: Evaluation and optimization of diagnostic tests using receiver-operating characteristic analysis and information theory. *Int J Biomed Comput* 1989; **24**:153–189.
3. Bernet W: Introduction: Tenth Anniversary of AACAP Practice Parameters. *J Am Acad Child Adolesc Psychiatry* 2002; **41**:S001–S003.
4. Flament MF, Rapoport JL, Berg CJ, *et al.*: Clomipramine treatment of childhood obsessive compulsive disorder: A double-blind controlled study. *Arch Gen Psychiatry* 1985; **42**:977–983.
5. Green WH: *Child and Adolescent Clinical Psychopharmacology.* 2nd ed. Baltimore: Williams & Wilkins, 1995.
6. DeLong GR, Aldershof AL: Long-term experience with lithium treatment in childhood: Correlation with clinical diagnosis. *J Am Acad Child Adolesc Psychiatry* 1987; **26**:389–394.
7. Riddle MA, Scahill L, King RA, *et al.*: Double-blind, crossover trial of fluoxetine and placebo in children and adolescents with obsessive-compulsive disorder. *J Am Acad Child Adolesc Psychiatry* 1992; **31**:1062–1069.
8. Ryan ND, Puig-Antich J, Cooper T, *et al.*: Imipramine in adolescent major depression: Plasma level and clinical response. *Acta Psychiatr Scand* 1986; **73**:275–288.
9. Kazdin AE: Psychotherapy for children and adolescents: Current progress and future research directions. *Am Psychol* 1993; **48**(6):644–657.

10. Shapiro T: The psychodynamic formulation in child and adolescent psychiatry. *J Am Acad Child Adolesc Psychiatry* 1989; **28**:681–684.

11. MTA Co-operative Group 1999. A 14-month randomized clinical trial of treatment strategies for attention-deficit/hyperactivity disorder. *Arch Gen Psychiatry* 1999; **56**:1073–1086.

12. March J, Silva S, Petrycki S, Curry J, *et al.*: Fluoxetine, cognitive-behavioral therapy, and their combination for adolescents with depression: Treatment for Adolescents With Depression Study (TADS) randomized controlled trial. *JAMA* 2004; **292**:861–863.

13. U.S. Food and Drug Administration: FDA Public Health Advisory; Suicidality in Children and Adolescents Being Treated With Antidepressant Medications. October 15, 2004.

14. Werry JS: ICD-9 and DSM-III classification for the clinician. *J Child Psychol Psychiatry* 1985; **26**:1–6.

15. American Psychiatric Association: *Diagnostic and Statistical Manual of Mental Disorders*, 4th ed. *Text Revision. DSM-IV-TR*. Washington, DC: American Psychiatric Association, 2000.

16. Bramer G: Tenth revision of the International Classification of Diseases (in progress). *Br J Psychiatry* 1988; **152**(suppl):29–32.

17. Spitzer R, Williams JBW: Classification in psychiatry. In: Kaplan H, Freedman A, Sadock B, eds. *The Comprehensive Textbook of Psychiatry,* 3rd ed. Baltimore: Williams & Wilkins, 1980.

18. Achenbach TM, Edelbrock CS: The classification of child psychopathology: A review and analysis of empirical efforts. *Psychol Bull* 1978; **85**:1275–1301.

19. Anderson J: Personal communication; 1995.

20. Verhulst FC, Berden GFG, Sanders-Woudstra JAR: Mental health in Dutch children: (II). The prevalence of psychiatric disorder and relationship between measures. *Acta Psychiatr Scand* 1985; **72**:1.

21. Vikan A: Psychiatric epidemiology in a sample of 1510 ten-year-old children. I Prevalence. *J Child Psychol Psychiatry* 1985; **26**:55.

22. Xin RE, Chen SK, Tang HQ, *et al.*: Behavioral problems in preschool-age children in Shanghai: Analysis of 3000 cases. *Can J Psychiatry* 1992; **37**:254–258.

23. Epstein NB, Bishop DS, Baldwin LM: McMaster model of family functioning: A view of the normal family. In: Walsh F, ed. *Normal Family Processes.* New York: Guilford Press, 1982:115–141.

24. Freud A: *Normality and Pathology in Childhood.* New York: International University Press, 1965.

25. Nagera H: *The Developmental Approach in Childhood Psychopathology.* New York: Aronson, 1981.

26. Stengel E: Classification of mental disorders. *Bull World Health Org* 1959; **21**:601–663.

27. Feighner J, Robbins ED, Guze DB, *et al.*: Diagnostic criteria for use in psychiatric research. *Arch Gen Psychiatry* 1972; **26**:57–63.

28. Volkmar FR: Classification in child and adolescent psychiatry: Principles and issues. In: Lewis M, ed. *Child and Adolescent Psychiatry: A Comprehensive Textbook.* 2nd ed. Baltimore: Williams & Wilkins, 1996: 418–422.

29. Cantwell DP: DSM-111 studies. In: Rutter M, Tuma H, Lann IS, eds. *Assessment and Diagnosis in Child Psychopathology.* New York: Guilford Press, 1985:3–36.

30. Rutter M: Isle of Wight revisited: Twenty-five years of child psychiatric epidemiology. *J Am Acad Child Adolesc Psychiatry* 1989; **28**:633–653.

31. Chess S, Thomas A: *Temperament in Clinical Practice.* New York: Guilford Press, 1986.

32. Kanner L: Do behavior symptoms always indicate psychopathology? *J Child Psychol Psychiatry* 1960; **1**:17–25.

33. Werner EE, Smith RS: Overcoming the odds: High-risk children from birth to adulthood. Ithaca, NY: Cornell University Press, 1992.

34. LaRoche C: Children of parents with major affective disorders: A review of the past 5 years. *Psychiatr Clin North Am* 1989; **12**:919–932.

35. Kim JM, Hetherington, EM, Reiss, D: Family, school, and community associations among family relationships, antisocial peers, and adolescents' externalizing behaviors: gender and family type differences. *Child Dev* 1999; **70**(5):1209–1230.

36. McGuire S, Manke B, Sandino KJ, Reiss D, Hetherington EM, Plomin R: Perceived competence and self-worth during adolescence: A longitudinal behavioral genetic study. *Child Dev* 1999; **70**(6):1283–1296.

37. Farrington DP, West DJ: The Cambridge study in delinquent development. In: Mednick SA, Baert AE, eds. *Prospective Longitudinal Research: An Empirical Basis for the Primary Prevention of Psychological Disorders.* New York: Oxford University Press; 1981:137–145.

38. McConville BJ: Opening moves and sequential strategies in child psychiatry. *Can Psychiatric Assoc J* 1976; **21**:295–301.

39. Bandura A, Walters RH: *Social Learning and Personality Development.* New York: Holt, Rinehart & Winston, 1963.

40. Winnicott DW: *The Maturational Processes and the Facilitating Environment.* New York: International Universities Press, 1965:145–146.

41. Elkin AE: Behavioral strategies in group psychotherapy. Paper presented to the Ontario Group Psychotherapy Association, Opinicon; 1973.

42. Singer RD, Singer A: *Psychological Development in Children.* Toronto: WB Saunders Co., 1969:274–297.

43. Malone CA: Observations on the role of family therapy in child psychiatry training. *Am J Psychiatry* 1974; **13**:437–458.

44. Greben SE: *Love's Labor: Twenty-Five Years of Experience in the Practice of Psychotherapy.* New York: Schocken Books, 1984.

45. American Diabetes Association; American Psychiatric Association; American Association of Clinical Endocrinologists; North American Association for the Study of Obesity: Consensus development conference on antipsychotic drugs and obesity and diabetes. *Diabetes Care* 2004; **27**:596–601.

46. Thomas M, Peterson DA: A neurogenic theory of depression gains momentum. *Mol Interv* 2003; **3**(8):441 444.

47. Franklin M, Foa E, March JS: The pediatric obsessive-compulsive disorder treatment study: Rationale, design, and methods [review]. *J Child and Adolescent Pharmacol* 2003; **13**(Suppl 1):S39–S51.

48. Lewis M: Intensive individual psychodynamic psychotherapy: The therapeutic relationship and the

technique of interpretation. In: Lewis M, ed. *Child and Adolescent Psychiatry: A Comprehensive Textbook,* 2nd ed. Baltimore: Williams & Wilkins, 1996:802–809.

49. Karasu TB: Psychotherapies: An overview. *Am J Psychiatry* 1977; **134**:851–863.

50. Piaget J: *The Child's Conception of the World.* New York: Harcourt Brace, 1929.

51. Coppolillo HP: Use of play in psychodynamic psychotherapy. In: Lewis M, ed. *Child and Adolescent Psychiatry: A Comprehensive Textbook,* 2nd ed. Baltimore: Williams & Wilkins, 1996:809–815.

52. Freud A: *The Psycho-Analytical Treatment of Children.* London: Imago, 1946.

53. Klein M. *The Psycho-Analysis of Children.* London: Hogarth, 1932.

54. Winnicott DW: *Therapeutic Consultations in Child Psychiatry.* New York: Basic Books, 1971.

55. O'Brien NJ: The psychotherapy of children with attention-deficit hyperactivity disorder and their parents. In: O'Brien, Pilowsky D, Lewis O, eds. *Psychotherapies with Children and Adolescents.* Washington DC,: American Psychiatric Press, 1992:109–124.

56. Weisz B, Weiss JR: Conceptualization, assessment, and treatment of depression in children. The impact of methodological factors on child therapy effectiveness. *J Am Acad Child Adolesc Psychiatry* 1990; **31**:703–709.

57. Weisz JR, Weiss B, Donnenberg GR: The lab versus the clinic: Effects of child and adolescent psychotherapy. *Am Psychol* 1992; **47**:1578–1588.

58. Fonagy P, Target M: The psychoanalysis for children with disruptive disorders *J Am Acad Child Adolesc Psychiatry* 1994; **33**:45–55.

59. Vitulano LA, Tebes JK: Child and adolescent behavior therapy. In: Lewis M, ed. *Child and Adolescent Psychiatry: A Comprehensive Textbook,* 2nd ed. Baltimore: Williams & Wilkins, 1996:815–831.

60. Pavlov IP: *Conditioned Reflexes: An Investigation of the Physiological Activity of the Cerebral Cortex.* London: Oxford University Press, 1927.

61. Watson JB, Ryanor R: Conditioned emotional reactions. *J Exp Psychol* 1920; **3**:1–14.

62. Skinner BF: *Science and Human Behavior.* New York: Free Press, 1953.

63. Beck AT: *Cognitive Therapy and the Emotional Disorders.* New York: International Universities Press, 1976.

64. Meichenbaum DH: *Cognitive Behavior Modification.* New York: Plenum Publishing Corp., 1977.

65. Bandura A: *Social Learning Theory.* Englewood Cliffs, NJ: Prentice-Hall, 1986.

66. Lovaas I, Koegel RL, Simmons JW, *et al.*: Some generalization and follow-up measures on autistic children in behavior therapy. *J Appl Behav Anal* 1973; **6**:131–166.

67. Kazdin AE: *Conduct Disorders in Childhood and Adolescence.* Newbury Park, CA: Sage, 1987.

68. Patterson GR: *Families: Applications of Social Learning to Family Life.* Champaign, IL: Research Press, 1975.

69. Kazdin AE, Siegel T, Bass D: Cognitive problem-solving skills training and parent management training in the treatment of antisocial behavior in children. *J Consult Clin Psychol* 1992; **60**:733–747.

70. Barkley RA, Shelton L, Crosswait C, Moorehouse M, Fletcher K, Barrett S, Jenkins L, Metevia L: Multi-method psycho-educational intervention for preschool children with disruptive behavior: Preliminary results at post-treatment. *Br J Child Psychol Psychiatry* 2000; **41**(3):319–332.

71. Barkley RA: Attention deficit disorders. In: Bornstein PH, Kazdin AE, eds. *Handbook of Clinical Behavior Therapy with Children.* Homewood, IL: Dorsey Press, 1985:158–217.

72. Richters JG, Arnold LE, Jensen PS, *et al.*: NIMH collaborative multisite multimodal treatment study of children with ADHD: Background and rationale. *J Am Acad Child Adolesc Psychiatry* 1995; **34**:987–1000.

73. Eason LJ, White MJ, Newsom C: Generalized reduction of self-stimulatory behavior: An effect of teaching appropriate play to autistic children. *Ann Intervent Dev Disabil* 1982; **2**:157–169.

74. Foxx RM, Azrin N: The elimination of autistic self-stimulatory behavior by overcorrection. *J Appl Behav Anal* 1973; **6**:1–14.

75. Mowrer OH, Mowrer WM: Enuresis: A method for its study and treatment. *Am J Orthopsychiatry* 1938; **8**:436–459.

76. Azrin NH, Sneed TJ, Foxx RM: Dry-bed training: Rapid elimination of childhood enuresis. *Behav Res Ther* 1974; **12**:147–156.

77. Petti TA: Cognitive therapies. In: Lewis M, ed. *Child and Adolescent Psychiatry: A Comprehensive Textbook,* 2nd ed. Baltimore: Williams & Wilkins, 1996:832–840.

78. Beck AT, Rush AJ, Shaw BF, *et al.*: *Cognitive Therapy of Depression.* New York: Guilford Press, 1979.

79. Kovacs M, Beck AT: An empirical-clinical approach towards a definition of childhood depression. In: Schulterbrandt JG, Raskin A, eds. *Depression in Children: Diagnosis, Treatment and Conceptual Models.* New York: Raven Press, 1977:1–25.

80. Leahy RL: Cognitive therapy of childhood depression: Developmental considerations. In: Shirk SR, ed. *Cognitive Development and Child Psychotherapy.* New York: Plenum Publishing Corp., 1988:187–204.

81. Wilkes TCR, Rush AJ: Adaptations of cognitive therapy for depressed adolescents. *J Am Acad Child Adolesc Psychiatry* 1988; **27**:381–386.

82. Kaslow NJ, Rehm LP: Conceptualization, assessment, and treatment of depression in children. In: Bornstein PH, Kazdin AE, eds. *Handbook of Clinical Behavior Therapy with Children.* Homewood, IL: Dorsey Press, 1985:599–657.

83. Moreau D, Mufson L, Weissman MM, Klerman GL: Interpersonal psychotherapy for adolescent depression: Description of modification and preliminary application. *J Am Acad Child Adolesc Psychiatry* 1991; **30**:642–651.

84. Brent DA, Holder D, Kolko D, *et al.*: A clinical psychotherapy trial for adolescent depression comparing cognitive, family and supportive therapy. *Arch Gen Psychiatry* 1997; **54**:877–885.

85. March JS, Mulle K, Herbel B: Behavioral psychotherapy for children and adolescents with obsessive-compulsive disorder: An open trial of a new protocol-driven treatment package. *J Am Acad Child Adolesc Psychiatry* 1994; **33**:333–341.

86. Ellis A, Bernard ME: An overview of rational-emotive approaches to the problems of childhood. In: Ellis A,

Bernard ME, eds. *Rational-Emotive Approaches to the Problems of Childhood.* New York: Plenum Publishing Corp., 1983:3–37.

87. Waters V: Rational emotive therapy. In: Reynolds CR, Gurkin TB, eds. *The Handbook of School Psychology.* New York: John Wiley & Sons, 1982:570–579.

88. Shure MB, Spivack G: Interpersonal cognitive problem solving. In: Price RH, Cowen EL, Lotion RP, *et al.*, eds. *Fourteen Ounces of Prevention: A Casebook for Practitioners.* Washington, DC: American Psychological Association, 1988:69–82.

89. Whitman T, Burgio L, Johnson MB: Cognitive behavioral interventions with mentally retarded children. In: Meyers AW, Craighead WE, eds. *Cognitive Behavior Therapy with Children.* New York: Plenum Publishing Corp., 1984:193–228.

90. Ollendick TN, Mayer JA: School phobia. In: Turner SM, ed. *Behavioral Theories and Treatment of Anxiety.* New York: Plenum Publishing Corp., 1984.

91. Dinkmeyer D, McKay GD: *Parents' Handbook: Systematic Training for Effective Training for Effective Parenting.* Circle Pines, MN: American Guidance Service, Inc., 1976.

92. Ravenscroft K: Family therapy. In: Lewis M, ed. *Child and Adolescent Psychiatry: A Comprehensive Textbook.* 2nd ed. Baltimore: Williams & Wilkins, 1996:848–862.

93. Minuchin S: *Families and Family Therapy.* Cambridge, MA: Harvard University Press, 1974.

94. Griest DL, Wells KC: Behavioral family therapy for conduct disorders in children. *Behav Ther* 1983; **14**:37–53.

95. Barton CV, Alexander JF: Functional family therapy. In: Garman AS, Kniskern DP, eds. *Handbook of Family Therapy.* New York: Brunner/Mazel, 1981:403–443.

96. Beavers WR, Voeller MN: Family models: Comparing and contrasting the Olson circumplex model with the Beavers systems model. *Fam Process* 1983; **22**:85–98.

97. Combrinck-Graham L: A model of family development. *Fam Process* 1985; **24**:139–150.

98. Cramer-Azima FJ: Group psychotherapy for children and adolescents. In: Lewis M, ed. *Child and Adolescent Psychiatry: A Comprehensive Textbook*, 2nd ed. Baltimore: Williams & Wilkins, 1996:840–846.

99. Anthony EJ: Group-analytic psychotherapy with children and adolescents. In: Foulkes SH, Anthony EJ, eds. *Group Psychotherapy.* Baltimore: Penguin Books, 1965:186–232.

100. Toseland RW, Siporin M: When to recommend group treatment: A review of the clinical and the research literature. *Int J Group Psychother* 1986; **36**: 171–201.

101. Hayward C, Varady S, Albano AM, Theimann M, Henderson L, Schatzberg AF: Cognitive-behavioral therapy for social phobia in female adolescents: results of a pilot study. *J Am Acad Child Adolesc Psychiatry* 2000; **39**(6):721–726.

102. Wilfley DE, Agras WS, Telch CF, Rossiter EM, Schneider JA, Cole AG, Sifford LA, Raeburn SD: Group cognitive-behavioral therapy and group interpersonal psychotherapy for the nonpurging bulimic individual: a controlled comparison. *J Consult Clin Psychol* 1993; **61**(2):296–305.

103. Fine S, Forth A, Gilbert M, *et al.*: Group therapy for adolescent depressive disorder: A comparison of social skills and therapeutic support. *J Am Acad Child Adolesc Psychiatry* 1991; **30**:79–85.

104. Group for the Advancement of Psychiatry; Committee on Preventive Psychiatry: Violent behavior in children and youth; preventive intervention from a psychiatric perspective. *J Am Acad Child Adolesc Psychiatry* 1999; **38**:235–241.

105. Bourdin CM: Multisystemic treatment of criminality and violence in adolescents. *J Am Acad Child Adolesc Psychiatry* 1999; **38**:242–249.

7

Assessment of Infants and Toddlers

Martin J. Drell

Introduction

In this chapter, I explain the basics of conducting an infant assessment. I do so by answering three questions:

(1) What are the fundamental aspects of an infant assessment?
(2) What models does one use to conceptualize infant assessments?
(3) How does one actually conduct an infant assessment?

As I address each of these questions, I suggest general modifications and accommodations to make when assessing very young children. Other articles address the specific content of infant assessments in more detail [1–4].

Fundamental Aspects of an Infant Assessment

The purpose of the assessment is to define the problem and elucidate its cause. An assessment is triggered by the perception that there is a problem. In the case of very young children, the perception is usually voiced by a parent or caregiver. The problems generally center on aspects of normal daily activities such as eating, sleeping, bathroom functions, motor activities, and interactions. Based on their own experiences including those with other very young children, what they read, and what they are told by others, the parents have a general idea of what their child should be doing. When their child does not meet these expectations, they become concerned and try to figure out whether there is a problem and, if so, what to do about it. In the vast number of instances, this perception of something being wrong is not enough to lead to a formal assessment. Parents assume that the problem is transient, that it is within the range of normal behavior, or they deny that there is a problem. And indeed, due to the dynamic nature of very young children, their relationships, and the unending march of development, the problems noted often change with time or even disappear. It is only when caregivers perceive that there is a significant problem and the problem endures despite their best efforts to solve or deny it that they seek an assessment.

The overall goal of an infant assessment is to collaborate with the caregivers to identify the problem, mutually agree on the factors that contribute to the problem, and design an appropriate treatment strategy. If any members of this 'team' of caregivers and professionals disagree, this constitutes a separate therapeutic problem. Often, important clinical information can be ascertained while working from disagreement toward mutual agreement. Like any diagnostic assessment, such a process provides an absolutely unique entree into how the caregivers see the world, get along with people in this world, and solve problems.

CASE ONE

A couple brought in their 24-month-old son for an evaluation. The mother was upset that her child was hyperactive and unmanageable. The father felt that there was no problem, stating that 'boys are just that way.' He went on to denigrate his wife's parenting skills. The evaluation showed a child who was caught in the middle of his parents' marital problems. The child's behavior was a response to these difficulties. The behaviors ceased immediately after the parents were counseled on the impact of their difficulties on the child and sought marital therapy. They were astounded that a two-year-old could pay attention to these issues. This is an example of how disagreements about what the problem is can be used in the treatment effort.

Clinical Child Psychiatry, Second Edition. Edited by W.M. Klykylo and J.L. Kay
© 2005 John Wiley & Sons Ltd.

Most experts agree that it is helpful to gather data from many sources. As in the first case study, differences in perception often occur between the various persons involved. It is also vital to observe the infant and to judge the infant's interactions with the key persons in the infant's life, as well as with the assessor. The importance of these interactions is a key focus in infant work. Finally, most experts admit that no one specialty or person has a mastery of all the knowledge needed to assess infants and their caregivers. As a result, infant assessments often involve the expertise of numerous disciplines, including, but not limited to, child and adolescent psychiatry, pediatrics, clinical psychology, developmental psychology, speech and hearing, physical therapy, genetics, and social work. Each of these disciplines has its own approaches, knowledge base, and formal assessment tools. When integrated, the information provided by these disciplines can be invaluable in defining problems and formulating what needs to be done to help moderate the problem.

Models of Infant Assessment

I use a systems oriented developmental, biopsychosocial model. The term 'systems' refers to the belief that people are best understood when they are viewed as important interacting parts of a larger family system that is in turn part of still larger social systems such as peer groups, religious groups, organizations, and cultures. This emphasizes the importance of the continuous interaction of all these systems and it assumes the continual evolution of problems and people. A systems approach also implies interest in the antecedents of the problem as well as its consequences.

A developmental perspective implies that children develop over time. It stresses the need to examine the child against established norms for other children his or her age. This perspective recognizes that development occurs in numerous areas of the child's life. The Denver Developmental Screening Test, a long standing and popular screening instrument for very young children, categorizes the areas of development in the following way [5].

- Personal–social. Does the child smile? Does the child respond to his or her caregivers in ways that indicate that they are special? Does the child respond differentially to strangers? Does the child indicate his or her needs? Does the child imitate other people?
- Fine motor-adaptive. Does the child grasp a rattle? Does the child sit? Does the child have the ability to transfer an object from one hand to the other?

- Language. Does the child laugh? Does the child turn in response to another's voice? Does the child imitate speech sounds? Does the child speak? How complex is his or her speech?
- Gross motor. Can the child roll over? Can the child sit? Can the child stand? Can the child walk? Can the child walk backward? Can the child walk upstairs? Can the child kick and throw a ball? Can the child balance on one foot?

All these skills have been tested on thousands of children to determine what are the normal ranges of behaviors in each of these categories. A failure to develop appropriately in any of these areas may indicate a deviation. Certain types of developmental failure are indicative of specific types of problems and disorders. For example, children with early autistic disorder show a cluster of abnormalities in their ability to interact with people, in their ability to play, and perhaps in some of their motor skills. A fundamental component of assessing young children is appreciating what is normal and abnormal development for a particular age group. This is learned over time by seeing many young children.

A biopsychosocial approach implies that problems (and their solutions) evolve from the interaction of biologic, psychologic, and social phenomena. These phenomena should not be considered all negative and include protective factors and individual resiliences. During assessments, one must attend to these strengths and weaknesses and the possibility of problems in all these overarching categories. Unfortunately, when dealing with infants or toddlers and their caregivers, there has been a tendency to accept the first reasonable theory. For example, in the 1950s it was thought that autistic disorder was caused by faulty parenting. The experts who believed this at the time were correct that the parents of autistic children acted differently than the parents of other children. They were incorrect, however, in attributing the cause of the disorder to the parenting. Subsequent research has shown that the abnormalities in parenting noted are within the norm of expectable responses of parents faced with a young child who is different and who therefore poses unique parenting challenges. The cause of early infant autism is now believed to be neurodevelopmental (i.e., a disruption in early brain development). Numerous prenatal, perinatal, and postnatal biologic events are also known to cause the types of behaviors that lead to the diagnosis of autistic disorder. A short list of these includes maternal rubella, untreated phenylketonuria, tuberous sclerosis, anoxia during birth, encephalitis, infantile spasms, and fragile X syndrome.

Neurodevelopmental problems also affect a young child's social skills, which in turn have consequences for the caretakers. A systemics oriented developmental, biopsychosocial approach assumes that the behaviors of the parents reciprocally affect the social skills of the child, which may in turn affect the biology and brain development of the child.

Development is a dynamic process that affects and is changed by interacting biologic, psychologic, and social events. Thankfully, for the assessor, these interactions usually have a predictable quality that facilitates diagnosis. As with the psychiatric disorders of older children and adults, there are key behaviors and interactions that differentiate the infant disorders from one another.

In 1989, Stern-Bruschweiler and Stern proposed a systems model for conceptualizing the role of the mother or primary caregiver in mother–infant therapies [6]. I find this model helpful in my approach to infant and toddler assessments. The model consists of four interdependent elements in constant dynamic equilibrium (Figure 7.1). These elements are the following:

(1) the infant's overt interactive behavior;
(2) the mother's overt interactive behavior (items 1 and 2 together constitute 'the interaction');
(3) the infant's representation of the interaction (i.e., how the infant understands what is happening in the situation, including what's happening to him or her and others in the interactions);
(4) the mother's representation of the interaction.

All four elements together constitute 'the relationship.' In the assessment, this translates into the need to evaluate three major categories of information:

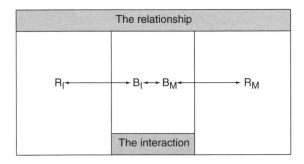

Figure 7.1 The Stern-Bruschweiler and Stern model. Reproduced from Plotkin J: The at-risk infant. In: Parmelee DX, ed. Child and Adolescent Psychiatry. New York: Mosby, 1994:194. With kind permission of Dean Parmelee, M. D.

(1) What the mother (and other key persons involved in the infant's caregiving system, including pediatricians) thinks is happening. This constitutes the R_M (mother's representation) part of the model.
(2) How the mother and the other involved caregivers behave and interact with the infant (and each other) as well as how the infant behaves and interacts with the mother and other caregivers. This constitutes the B_M (behaviors of the mother)/B_I (behaviors of the infant) part of the model, which defines 'the interaction.'
(3) What the infant thinks is happening. This coincides with the R_I (infant's representation) part of the model. Knowledge concerning the representations of infants is sparse and remains speculative, since it is difficult for researchers to ascertain with certainty what goes on in an infant's mind [7].

An infant assessment, then, involves asking questions about what may have occurred to get things to their present state and then developing a coherent story concerning the relationship of these four elements.

Conducting an Infant Assessment

There are varying ways to accumulate the essential data for a comprehensive assessment. All the techniques are directed at clarifying the nature of the problem and constructing a formulation that will serve as the basis for a treatment plan. This section is organized around the three major categories of information set forth in the Stern-Bruschweiler and Stern model.

Assessing the Perceptions of the Mother and Other Caretakers

The first step of any evaluation is to identify the people who are involved with the infant. One then asks each of these individuals to define the problem. Consider speaking to the person who made the initial contact with you, since this person has probably been chosen as the spokesperson for the family. It is often best to start with the family's perception and move from there. Often this means dealing with the fears, misperceptions, misunderstandings, and defenses of the family, all of which can interfere with an accurate accounting of what is happening. The same processes are critical to each step of the treatment.

People to be interviewed are those who can provide information on problem definition, who might have been involved in the creation of the problem, and who might be involved in solving the problem. This almost always includes the parents, and it can also include grandparents, siblings, and other caregivers such as foster parents, community agencies involved in the care of young children, pediatricians, professionals from other medical disciplines, and daycare providers.

Having identified these key people, the clinician must investigate their unique stories concerning the infant under assessment. One should cover the five Ws: when, where, why, what, and who. Make sure everyone is asked about their impression of the problem. It is important to collect data on antecedents, behaviors, and consequences (the 'ABCs' in behavior terminology). Thus, the assessment will investigate events before the problem started, while the problem occurs, and what happens as a result of the problem. Are there times and situations when the problem doesn't occur or things that make the problem better or worse? It is important to determine with whom the problem occurs, since the infant's behavior can be person specific. The clinician should understand that at this stage in the assessment, the perceptions of key people vary. Problems are, of course, in the eye of the beholder. Often one parent may feel that there is no problem (e.g., 'He's just a spirited boy,' or 'My parents told me I was just like that when I was that age, and I turned out OK'). When faced with differing perceptions, the assessor should ask questions about these differences. This line of questioning elicits people's differing perceptions of what is normal or not normal. It also allows the assessor to identify misconceptions or knowledge deficits about infants that can be remedied through education. Such differences of perception are often the first sign the assessor receives of problems between the parents that may be contributing to the infant's or toddler's behavior.

It is wise to ask questions about how and why the parent has arrived at his or her perception. 'How did you come to that idea?'; 'What does the infant do that leads you to believe that?'; 'Who told you that?' If these initial questions are not productive, the answer needs to be pursued in the past history of the parent. This approach is reflective of the early infant work of Selma Fraiberg on what she called 'ghosts in the nursery' [8]. In this pioneering work, Fraiberg hypothesized that many infant and toddler problems stem from unresolved parental conflicts that distort their interactions and behaviors with their children in the 'here and now.' To emphasize this point, I often tell parents: 'You raise your kids exactly as you were raised or exactly the opposite, and both are wrong because you aren't your parents and your child isn't you!' This starts parents thinking about their pasts.

A more formal technique for getting at the ghosts in the nursery uses family of origin work, wherein specific, detailed information is gathered about the parents' families [9]. In some cases this is done in separate sessions (one with each parent) that discuss how each parent's family functioned as they grew up. Parents are told that such information is valuable in learning about the forces that molded them into the people and the parents they are. Ghosts from the past can lead to inconsistent or nonexistent disciplinary habits and confusing interactions for infants and their parents. Frequently family of origin issues arise naturally during the assessment as parents associate to events, often stressful, in their past lives.

CASE TWO

A mother brought her two-year-old in for an evaluation to see if he was hyperactive. The child was indeed more hyperactive than most children his age. In the interview, I was puzzled that the mother put extraordinary emphasis on the fact that she had read that hyperactive children had something wrong with their brains. After a successful behavioral intervention and parenting work, the child's behavior moderated. Rather than being pleased, the mother continued to worry about her son and the possibility of brain damage. She especially wanted to know if he would 'get better.' More careful family of origin work on my part unearthed a brother with profound mental retardation that had been sent to live in an institution at an early age. A discussion of the impact of this brother on the mother's family when she was growing up provided clues about the mother's concern over 'damaged brains' that do not get better.

The assessor should gather information concerning the infant's development and maturation, including gestation, birth, perinatal events, and developmental milestones. The assessor should also ask about medical problems, medical procedures, current medications, allergies, and hospitalizations. Information should be received from the pediatrician when indicated, especially if there is suspicion of a biologic disorder. In cases in which the infant has not had routine pediatric care, this should be suggested as a means of providing preventive care.

CASE THREE

A mother was very concerned about her 12-month-old daughter who was not responding to her. She worried that her daughter might have autistic disorder. The assessment showed that the child was hearing impaired. Referral to speech and hearing specialists led to a dramatic improvement in the responses of her child.

The assessment should seek to elicit key events in the past history of the infant and his or her family that might perturb or influence the families' interactions. These events include deaths in the family, the subsequent reactions to these deaths by family members, separations, medical or emotional problems in other family members that might change the parent–infant interaction (e.g., postpartum depression or medical illness of a parent), accidents, fires, or persons being laid off from work.

CASE FOUR

The 22-month-old daughter of a single father whose wife had recently died in an auto accident was having temper tantrums daily and was kicking, refusing to go to sleep at the proper time, and incredibly oppositional. The father was overwhelmed both with his grief and with his new duties as a single parent. The father was helped to appreciate that his daughter had equally strong feelings concerning the death of her mother. He was instructed to talk to his daughter about the death and to 'open this area' for discussion. He was counseled on what to expect from his daughter and how to deal with her emotions. He was further supported in the process by the therapist, who helped the father with his own grief. As part of the process, the father and daughter put together a scrapbook of mementos and pictures of the mother. The oppositional symptoms lessened over several weeks.

In cases in which the assessor has specific questions concerning the child's development or lacks the knowledge base or expertise to properly assess his or her development, referral to a developmentally trained psychologist is suggested. These psychologists have access to and knowledge of specific developmental tests and instruments that usually yield a clear profile of the infant's strengths and weaknesses (Table 7.1).

As the assessor gathers the history, usually a story or major themes emerge that create a clearer sense of the problem. In a few cases, the caregiver's information is sufficient to determine the problem and suggest a solution. In most cases, however, the clinician assesses the behaviors and interactions of the infant and the caregivers through interactional sessions.

Assessing the Interaction

The interactional approach may include sessions with the evaluator and the infant as well as with the infant and family members. Sessions with the infant help the assessor better understand the infant outside the context of his or her caretaking environment. Sleep disorders, attention deficit hyperactivity disorder, developmental disabilities, and anxiety disorders can prove important in the genesis of interactional problems. In short, if the evaluator is overwhelmed by the child, uncomfortable with the child, or cannot get the child to interact normally, then this is important information. Likewise, it is equally important if the evaluator has no difficulty interacting with a child who appears normally behaved. It may indicate that the problem stems from something the parents are doing or not doing to which the infant is reacting with relationship or situation-specific problematic behaviors.

CASE FIVE

A two-year-old with severe temper tantrums played beautifully with the evaluator. The same two-year-old was then observed while she played with her mother. This play session was punctuated by numerous temper tantrums. The evaluator noted that these occurred when the mother intervened to finish play sequences that the two-year-old wanted to do herself. The mother would repeatedly tell her child that she was 'doing it wrong' and, in frustration, would take over the play. At this point, the child would complain. If the mother did not turn the play back over to the child, then she would begin to tantrum.

Table 7.1 Infant development screening tests.

Screening test	Age range	Time to administer (min)
Batelle Developmental Inventory	0–8 yr	30
Bayley Scales of Infant Development	1–30 mo	45–90
Clinical Adaptive Test/Clinical Linguistic Auditory	1–36 mo	15–20
Denver Developmental Screening Test II	0–6 yr	30
Developmental Screening Inventory – Revised	1–18 mo	20–30
Early Language Milestone Scale	0–36 mo	5
Gesell Preschool Test	2.5–6 yr	40
Infant Monitoring Questionnaire	4–36 mo	15–20
Miller Assessment for Preschoolers	8 mo–5 yr	20–30
Minnesota Child Development Inventory	1–6 yr	10–15
Peabody Picture Vocabulary Test	2.5–4 yr	10–20
Vineland Adaptive Behavior Scales	0–19 yr	20–60

From Plotkin J: The at-risk infant. In: Parmelee DX, ed. *Child and Adolescent Psychiatry*. New York: Mosby; 1994:194.

Interactive sessions can provide information that cannot be gathered by parental interviews alone, as some problems are outside the awareness of the parents. Calling such patterns to the attention of the parents during the assessment can allow the parents to see their child's problems in a new light. Parents can be quite resistant to such insights, however. Because of this, the material elicited by the assessor must be handled with great therapeutic sensitivity. The evaluator must be empathic to the fear and guilt in many parents that they are responsible for their child's problems. In cases in which the interactions are too subtle, too complex, or too confusing to keep track of in real time, videotaping the sessions can be useful. Be sure to obtain appropriate consent for these procedures.

CASE SIX

A mother was concerned that her three-month-old son was not breast feeding properly. The history proved noncontributory, so the breast feeding was videotaped. This showed that the son would interrupt his feeding at regular intervals to make eye contact with his mother. Whenever the mother did not reciprocate the eye contact, the baby would become upset and interrupt the feeding until eye contact was made. Once this pattern was identified, the mother was able to adjust her responsiveness, which caused the feedings to improve.

CASE SEVEN

A father complained that his 21-month-old was not obedient. In a videotaped play sequence, it was noted that the father would ask his young son to do something but would not give his son adequate time to respond. The fact that the son did not respond immediately frustrated the father, who would then re-ask his son in a louder voice. The son who wanted to respond but didn't have time also became frustrated and began to say 'No.' At this point, the father became angry and began to yell at his child, who he felt was being disrespectful. The evaluator showed the videotape sequence to the father, who was able to see how his son was really trying to please him. The father was given some developmental guidance on what a 21-month-old is capable of and was told to wait at least three seconds for a response. This allowed the son to respond to his father's requests. The father–son relationship improved measurably after this session.

It is not uncommon for infant experts to videotape interactions (usually between the expert and the infant or between the infant and his or her caregiver) and to repeatedly replay the tape to catch all of these nuances. Often combinations of unstructured time (free play in which you ask the parent to be with the child as they normally would be at home) and structured time (in which you ask the parent to perform a specific inter-active task such as feeding or playing a simple game with the infant) are more helpful and time conserving than videotaping a regular session. To facilitate inter-actions, the assessor is advised to equip his or her office with toys, games, furniture, and equipment developmentally suitable for very young children. Any combination of age-appropriate toys will do (Table 7.2). If the evaluator does not have toys, he or she can ask the parents to bring favored examples of the child's play equipment from home. This, however, does not allow the evaluator to see what play is like with new toys (a crude test of curiosity) or toys that might be too difficult for the child's developmental level (a crude test of frustration tolerance).

CASE EIGHT

A mother complained that her six-month-old infant cried incessantly and seemed to not like her. The history proved unhelpful. During a subsequent observation session, the evaluator noted that the mother was grossly overstimulating the child with her constant and intrusive rocking and bouncing of the infant. It was further noted that the mother would become increasingly frustrated and increase her intrusive behaviors the more the child cried, thus further exacerbating the situation. The evaluator then videotaped the interaction and showed it to the mother, who was able to moderate her responses. Her infant's crying subsequently decreased. The mother was quite pleased by the change in her infant and admitted that she had been told that rocking and forceful bouncing were what one should do when babies begin to cry.

In several cases, I have suggested that the parents set up a video camera at home to record problematic behavior. This is especially helpful in those instances in which the infant, for whatever reason, does not display the problem behaviors during the assessment. Home videos can provide wonderful additional material and often can be a vindication for parents who can be quite embarrassed and angry when their infant fails to 'show' the problem to the evaluator.

Some clinicians have a routine for their evaluative sessions. Some have very structured assessments that include specific questions, tests, and tasks based on the

Table 7.2 Typical set of toys.

1. Doll house and family figures
2. Tea set
3. Trucks
4. Nesting cups
5. Pop-it beads
6. Playpath, with small balls in large ball
7. Wooden blocks
8. Pounding bench and hammer
9. Dolls
10. Book
11. Play telephones (2)
12. Stuffed bear
13. Fisher-Price hourglass
14. Playskool school bus and seven passengers
15. Playskool teddy bear shape sorter
16. Fisher-Price stacking rings
17. Fisher-Price ring stand
18. Plastic bowl and lid
19. Pie plate
20. Wooden spoon
21. Gabriel busy driver
22. Fisher-Price musical roller (push toy)

From Harmon R: How to do an infant psychiatry assessment: Fundamental knowledge for clinical work with infants and toddlers. Paper presented to the premeeting institute, American Academy of Child and Adolescent Psychiatry, Los Angeles; 1986.

type of problem noted, such as eating disorders, temper tantrums, and sleep disorders. The latter approach is especially useful for research and for gathering a personal database on the range of interactions noted in infant work.

While interacting with the infant, the assessor should conduct a mental status evaluation to provide a baseline snapshot of how the child looks, acts, and responds. Such baselines are extremely valuable to monitor subsequent behavioral changes. Assessors new to this population could profitably use the five developmental areas in the Denver Developmental Screening Test to organize their remarks [5]. Researchers of infants and toddlers are currently trying to formally define an appropriate mental status examination for this population [10]. Their initial attempts include the following categories:

- physical appearance, including dysmorphic features;
- motor functioning, tone, coordination, gross and fine tics, abnormal movements, seizure activity;

- reaction to new settings and people, adaptation during evaluation;
- self-regulation: state regulation, sensory regulation, activity level, attention span, frustration tolerance, unusual behaviors;
- speech and language, expressive and receptive language, speech production;
- thought: hallucinations, dissociative states, nightmares, fears;
- affect and mood: behavioral, nonverbal cues to affect, intensity, range, modes of expression;
- play: structure, content, symbolic functioning, expressions of and control of aggression;
- intellectual functioning;
- relatedness: to parent figures, other caregivers, examiner.

Assessing the Perceptions of the Infant

The third category of information in the Stern-Bruschweiler and Stern model is assessing the subjective experience of the infant. This often proves difficult because of the lack of knowledge about the mental processes of infants. The younger the child is, the greater the challenge. We cannot easily ask infants to tell us their opinions of their problems. We can, however, make assumptions based on how infants interact with their parents and the evaluator. These assumptions are based on response patterns such as smiles, reaching for objects, putting objects in their mouth, periods of rapt attention, noting what is attended to, crying, pouting, insistent grunts, falling asleep, crawling away, and avoiding certain people or objects.

As infants grow older, they develop an increased ability to share their experiences. The most significant of these advances is the addition of babbling at 4–5 months, words at 12 months, and the ability to think symbolically at 16–18 months. The latter two abilities allow skilled assessors to engage the infant in play therapy-type assessments. The developmental achievements that occur at around 18 months, which include the ability to truly pretend play, to pretend with other people, to use one object to represent another, to use personal pronouns, and to realize the difference between self and others, distinguish infancy from toddlerhood. Just as an assessor uses different strategies for children in middle childhood versus adolescence because of their different developmental levels, an infant assessor needs different strategies for toddlers versus infants. Strategies for working with toddlers include spending more individual time with the toddler than with an infant, with a corresponding emphasis on relationship building. Within this relationship, there is

an increased use of words and play. Toddler assessments also take into consideration the fact that toddlers increasingly spend time with people other than their parents. Thus, toddler assessments more often include information about daycare and peer interactions.

Having conducted a thorough assessment in which you have assessed the perceptions of the key players involved in the presenting problem, viewed their interactions, assessed the infant's and parents' interactions with you, taken a past history and a developmental history, performed a mental status examination, and tried to assess what is going on in the child's mind, a reasonable formulation of the problem should be made. The assessor should be able to view the problem from a systems' perspective and determine its developmentally influenced biopsychosocial causes. At this point, the assessor should share this formulation with the parents and gather their feedback concerning their reactions. Any discrepancies between the assessor's perception of the problem and those of the parents should be clearly addressed. These discrepancies can be due to simple straightforward misinterpretations and misunderstandings of the facts, but they may also be due to resistances. When resistances arise, the assessor should interrupt the process and try to empathically understand their causes. Such processing of resistances ensures that the therapeutic relationship is maintained and that treatment can continue.

No effective treatment can occur unless the parents 'buy into' the formulation. This is not the same, however, as saying that the formulation cannot change over time as new information is gained. My particular style is to share my formulations with the parents as the assessment unfolds. I talk out loud and share my best guess of what is occurring at the moment and challenge the parents to tell me what is right or wrong with my guesses. This technique involves the parents and gives them a feel for the way I think, prioritize, and solve problems. It also allows for modeling and numerous mid-course corrections as the evaluation proceeds.

If the assessor has gathered the appropriate data and is unable to arrive at a formulation, some key element or point has probably been missed. Such a situation should prompt the evaluator to reanalyze the questions asked and the data gathered. If this reanalysis fails to clarify the situation, then a consultation is probably needed. A consultant can bring additional expertise and more objective 'fresh eyes' to the situation. In some cases, however, the family and assessor need to take a 'wait and see' approach, in which time either clarifies the missing element or solves the problem, or the problem evolves into another form.

Table 7.3 Diagnostic Classification: Zero to Three.

The diagnostic framework is multiaxial. It consists of five axes:

AXIS I: PRIMARY CLASSIFICATION
Traumatic stress disorder
Disorders of affect
  Anxiety disorders of infancy and early childhood
  Mood disorder: Prolonged bereavement or grief reaction
  Mood disorder: Depression of infancy and early childhood
  Mixed disorder of emotional expressiveness
  Childhood gender identity disorder
  Reactive attachment deprivation or maltreatment disorder of infancy
Adjustment disorder
Regulatory disorders
  Type I – Hypersensitive
  Type II – Underreactive
  Type III – Motorically disorganized, impulsive
  Type IV – Other
Sleep behavior disorder
Eating behavior disorder
Disorders of relating and communicating
  Multisystemic developmental disorder

AXIS II: RELATIONSHIP CLASSIFICATION
Overinvolved relationship
Underinvolved relationship
Anxious or tense relationship
Angry or hostile relationship
Mixed relationship
Abusive relationship
  Verbally abusive
  Physically abusive
  Sexually abusive

AXIS III: MEDICAL AND DEVELOPMENTAL DIAGNOSES

AXIS IV: PSYCHOSOCIAL STRESSORS
Mild effects
Moderate effects
Severe effects

AXIS V: FUNCTIONAL EMOTIONAL DEVELOPMENTAL LEVEL

From *Diagnostic Classification: Zero to Three. Diagnostic Classification of Mental Health and Developmental Disorders of Infancy and Early Childhood.* Arlington, VA: Zero to Three; 1994.

Should the assessor wish to make a diagnosis, he or she can do so using the *Diagnostic and Statistical Manual of Mental Disorders, Fourth Edition (DSM-IV-TR)*, which includes the standard diagnostic nomenclature for the field [11]. Unfortunately, the DSM-IV was not developed with very young children as its main priority. It contains only a few infant and toddler diagnoses (e.g., separation anxiety disorder, reactive attachment disorder, early infant autism, and pica) and does not capture the interactive realities of most infant and toddler problems [12]. A group of infant experts have attempted to address the weaknesses of the DSM-IV-TR by designing a diagnostic classification especially for children younger than four years of age. It is entitled Diagnostic Classification: Zero to Three (Table 7.3) [13]. Like the DSM-IV, the classification system consists of five axes, each of which focuses on varying factors thought to be important to an infant's or a toddler's problems. Owing to the differing developmental realities of this population, the axes are not all similar to those of the DSM-IV-TR. The Diagnostic Classification: Zero to Three has allowed a new generation of infant/toddlers diagnosis and research to occur [14–19].

Conclusion

Although performing a psychiatric assessment on a very young child can be intimidating, it can be successfully achieved by keeping track of the fundamental aspects of any assessment and modifying them to the needs of infants and toddlers. The assessor must have a solid understanding of development in this age range, as in all other ages of children and adults.

References

1. Greenspan S, Wieder S: The assessment and diagnosis of infant disorders: Developmental level, individual differences, and relationship-based interactions. In: Osofsky J, Fitzgerald H, eds. *Early Intervention, Evaluation, and Assessment I*, Vol II. New York: John Wiley & Sons, 2000:207–237.
2. Meisels S, Atkins-Burnett S: The elements of early childhood assessment. In: Shonkoff J, Meisels S. eds. *Handbook of Early Childhood Intervention*, 2nd ed. Cambridge, UK: Cambridge University Press, 2000:231–257.
3. Seligman S: Clinical interviews with families of infants. In: Zeanah C, ed. *Handbook of Infant Mental Health*, 2nd ed. New York: Guilford Press, 2000:211–221.
4. Gilliam W, Mayes L: Development assessment of infants and toddlers. In: Zeanah, C. ed. *Handbook of Infant Mental Health*, 2nd ed. New York: Guilford Press, 2000:236–248.
5. Frankenburg W, Dobbs J, Fandal A, *et al.*: *Denver Developmental Screening Test.* Revised ed. Denver: Denver Developmental Materials, 1975.

6. Stern-Bruschweiler N, Stern D: A model for conceptualizing the role of the mother's representational world in various mother-infant therapies. *Infant Ment Health J* 1989; **10**:142–156.

7. Stern D: *Diary of Baby.* New York: Basic Books, 1990.

8. Fraiberg S, Adelson E, Shapiro V: Ghosts in the nursery: A psychoanalytic approach to the problems of impaired infant-mother relationship. In: Fraiberg S, ed. *Clinical Studies in Infant Mental Health: The First Year of Life.* New York: Basic Books, 1980:164–166.

9. Bowen M: *Family Therapy in Clinical Practice.* New York: Jason Aronson, 1978.

10. Benham A: The observation and assessment of young children including the Infant Toddler Mental Status Exam. In: Zeanah C, ed. *Handbook of Infant Mental Health,* 2nd ed. New York: Guilford Press, 2000:249–265.

11. American Psychiatric Association: *Diagnostic and Statistical Manual of Mental Disorders,* 4th ed., text revision. Washington, DC: American Psychiatric Association, 2000.

12. Gadow K, Sprafkin J, Nolan E: DSM-IV symptoms in community and clinic preschool children. *J Am Acad Child Adolesc Psychiatry* 2001; **40**:1383–1392.

13. *Diagnostic Classification: Zero to Three. Diagnostic Classification of Mental Health and Developmental Disorders of Infancy and Early Childhood.* Arlington, VA: Zero to Three; 1994.

14. Lieberman A, Wieder S, Fenichel E: *DC: 0-3 Casebook.* Washington, DC: Zero to Three: National Center for Infants, Toddlers and Families, 1997.

15. Wright C, Northcutt C: Brief clinical report: Schematic decision trees for DC: 0-3. *Infant Mental Health J* 2004; **25**(3):171–174.

16. Scheeringa M, Zeanah C, Myers L, Putnam F: New findings on alternative criteria for PTSD in preschool children. *J Am Acad Child Adolesc Psychiatry* 2003; **42**:561–570.

17. Luby J, Heffelfinger A, Mrakotsky C, Brown K, Hessler M, Wallis J, Spitznagel E: The clinical picture of depression in preschool children. *J Am Acad Child Adolesc Psychiatry* 2003; **42**:340–348.

18. Luby J, Heffelfinger A, Koenig-McNaught A, Brown K, Spitznagel E: The preschool feelings checklist: a brief and sensitive screening measure for depression in young children. *J Am Acad Child Adolesc Psychiatry* 2004; **43**:708–117.

19. Thomas J, Guskin K: Disruptive behavior in young children: what does it mean? *J Am Acad Child Adolesc Psychiatry* 2001; **40**:44–51.

8

Play Therapy

Susan Mumford

Introduction

'Childhood ain't what it used to be,' so say professionals and parents alike. The whirlwind of activities in which children have become involved often leave families overscheduled, with woefully little time for spontaneous interactions. Concern about the accelerated pace of children's lives emerged in the mid-1980s. The 'hurried child' was now reported to be missing crucial elements of childhood as he rushed from one activity to another. However, despite this call for simplification, there has been little change in the complexity of life for many children [1]. The dramatic surge in the identification of childhood mental health disorders in part reflects the mounting pressures on today's children yet there has not been a comparable increase in treatment methods or opportunities. The onset of managed care has reduced care options for patients and treatment restrictions have discouraged some mental health experts from participating in modalities such as individual therapy or groups. For the child patient in particular, receiving appropriate treatment has become especially challenging as the treatment balance tilts toward pharmacology rather than psychotherapy or a mixture of the two. Despite this trend, play therapy, the traditional therapeutic approach with children, remains a viable treatment option. The purpose of this chapter is to familiarize the reader with the basic principles of play therapy including its history, definition and technique.

History

As early as 1905, Sigmund Freud's writings contained references to play [2]. Freud maintained that play facilitates instinctual discharge as well as mastery of traumatic or unpleasant events. It provides a safe medium through which the repetition compulsion functions to help the child patient gain control over otherwise unmanageable feelings or situations. Play allows for the process of catharsis and reflects both the child's wishes and wish fulfillment. Fantasy, and the break it offers from reality, facilitates the growth of the ego in children. In the fluid atmosphere of fantasy, the ego can reckon with both id and superego demands, enabling the child to experiment with novel solutions to conflict. Freud followed up these early discussions of play with the publication of 'Little Hans,' one of the first pieces about psychotherapy with a child. Melanie Klein and Anna Freud subsequently emerged as the major theorists of child development and one of its natural subsets – play. Both offered significant but different ways of treating the conflicts of children. Klein's theory of object relations, which placed great importance on the preoepidal period of human development, distinguished her from classical psychoanalysts. Her revolutionary work posited that children have a rich and complicated internal life that can be shown to the therapist through the use of toys. Klein used her knowledge of adult psychoanalysis as her technical template, especially the principles of free association, transference and interpretation. She believed that the child patient free associated not only with words but also with his play activities and these associations could be interpreted. Moreover, Klein saw that the transference provided clues about the child's past and his unconscious world. She was attuned to the importance of selecting toys which were not function-specific but instead could be used by the child in a variety of ways. This concept has of course, stood the test of time and remains a technical underpinning of play therapy today [3].

While Anna Freud never published a monograph exclusively on the subject of play, many of her writings focused on the development of ego capacities and defenses which make play possible [4]. She postulated

Clinical Child Psychiatry, Second Edition. Edited by W.M. Klykylo and J.L. Kay
© 2005 John Wiley & Sons Ltd.

that the seeds of the ability to play are planted in the early interactions between a baby and his mother. Through play with his body and hers, the baby learns the rudiments of self/other differentiation and by extension, reality and fantasy. Anna Freud believed that play both facilitates and reflects the child's growth process which ideally results in personal autonomy, a developed sense of self and the ability to work. Play provides a way to explore and master internal and external conflicts and gives clues about the child's unconscious strivings. Anna Freud's particular interest in the development of the ego and its impact on id and superego functioning is well known. Moreover, her concept of developmental lines illustrates the cumulative nature of child development, how successes or problems in one phase affect growth in the next. This idea remains useful today as child therapists are responsible for identifying where a patient's development went off track and what is needed to return him to a normal developmental point.

In addition to both Freud and Klein, there were a number of early pioneers who have made significant contributions to the theory of play. Robert Waelder [5] echoed Freud's idea about the usefulness of the repetition compulsion in his writings about trauma, how it can be worked through in play by turning passive into active. Waelder also conceptualized that play permits children to break down the whole untoward nature of a traumatic event into manageable pieces. Erik Erikson [6], known for his epigenetic view of development, pointed out that play allows children to prepare for adult life by trying on different roles and identities. In addition to his work with mothers and babies, Winnicott [7] also provided much to the understanding of the origins and purpose of play and its persistence through the life span. In brief, Winnicott conceptualized that the newborn initially makes no differentiation between himself and mother. Next, the infant makes minute movements away from mother, out of this unified position with her. A space is then created that is not mother, not baby but something in between (Figure 8.1) Winnicott termed this important space 'potential space' and identified it as the cradle of creativity, the place which allows for the selection of a transitional object as well as the emergence of the capacity to play. Understanding of this concept is crucial for child therapists whose assessment of a patient must first confirm the patient's ability to play and second, assess its quality and range [8].

Play and Play Therapy

Although many parents are familiar with the clinical term 'play therapy,' few understand the complexity of

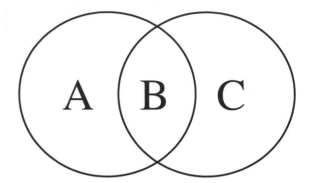

Figure 8.1 Development of play: the cradle of creativity. A, Mother; B, potential space; C, infant.

this simple-sounding treatment. It is therefore incumbent upon the professional to be well informed about the properties of play, how they are therapeutic and to be able to share this information with parents in a clear and cogent manner. Despite this obligation, some professionals find themselves more comfortable doing play therapy rather than explaining what it actually is.

The Function of Play Therapy

Play is marked by a variety of characteristics which, when used in therapy, contribute to an improvement in the child's functioning. Fueling a child's maturation is his innate developmental thrust forward, his built-in ability to progress. Child therapists are able to use this energy as an ally in psychotherapy. Moreover, the natural power of play has been harnessed for treatment by clinicians representing a number of theory bases including psychodynamic, cognitive behavioral, child-centered, Alderian, and short-term play therapy [9]. Despite differences in orientation, there are some shared features including recognition of the value for a strong therapeutic alliance, the need to work with the child patient differently than with the adult patient, the importance of viewing children developmentally, and an appreciation for play as the language of the child [10]. An example of two different concepts of play therapy are as follows. Cognitive behavioral play therapy uses play to subtly communicate cognitive change. It introduces the child to different, more adaptive responses to his difficulties which are then modeled using developmentally appropriate materials. The therapist conveys through play possible solutions to problems which resemble those of the patient [11]. The psychodynamic play therapist relies on four main interventions. Confrontation and then clarification are used to facilitate the growth of the observing ego. The therapist helps the child to understand what is occurring internally and points out defenses before drives. Interpretation is used to help the patient see the history of a problem, the purpose of defenses and to facilitate the working through process. Finally, the psychotherapeutic process itself loosens the child's defensive structure, enabling more adaptive defenses to emerge, as well as providing increased drive satisfaction in a healthier fashion [12,13].

The Properties of Play

The process of play therapy, made possible because of the relationship between the therapist and the patient, builds on the properties of play. Four properties of play are as follows.

First, play is fun; it provides not only pleasure for the child but also a sense of internal satisfaction. It is the external manifestation of a child's imagination and in this way, straddles the boundary between fantasy and reality. Creativity is both nurtured and expressed by play. It is a medium for self-definition and expression and valuable for the unfettered freedom it provides. Play is a process through which a child acquires self-confidence and a sense of efficacy as he finds solutions to problems in his own time and on his own terms. It provides an outlet for the child's creativity. These features are implicit in the therapeutic process. While play certainly has elements of frivolity and excitement, it is also intense and serious. It is meaningful for the child and loaded with affect. It is often helpful for the therapist to follow the lead of a child in play, to include asking the child what he would have the therapist do or say.

CLINICAL EXAMPLE: CHILD-LED PLAY

Child, age nine, is being treated for adjustment difficulties stemming from a move to a new city. She has set up an elaborate scenario using the dolls and doll house, a game she informs that therapist, she often plays with her eight-year-old sister. The patient gives the therapist a doll. The therapist then asks if the patient wishes she had more friends to play with in her new neighborhood. However, in response the child suddenly shrieks 'What are you saying? You don't know how to play!'

In this example, the therapist appears to have associated the patient's description of the game and subsequent attempt to include her as a possible indication of loneliness. The patient's sharp response

clearly showed that the therapist had departed from the child's line of thinking. It would have been more effective for the therapist to have instead remained silent, accepted the doll from the patient, and awaited what came next. In this way, the therapist would have followed the child's lead and allowed the play to unfold in a more natural fashion.

Second, play is absorbing. It can be so encompassing for a child that he can appear to be oblivious to other activities around him and have difficulty stopping his play before he is ready. The play activity can be complete in and of itself and it is not necessarily something a child does in order to accomplish something else. This qualifier does not mean that play cannot be goal-directed, (e.g., build a fort, set up a doll house) but rather, that these goals are part of the larger play activity in general. The process of abreaction is also accomplished through play; the child relives painful situations and experiences the affect belonging to them.

CLINICAL EXAMPLE: ABSORPTION IN PLAY

A child, age eight, with significant concerns about his place in his family has been working on a huge, multifaceted Lego® scene with his therapist for a number of sessions. The particular structure is a castle which houses the orphaned but determined child 'hero' of the game. Great attention is given to the assembly of this structure and is accompanied by a rich narration of the hero's struggles. Aware of the child's absorption in his play, the therapist provides him a five minute reminder of the session's end. He responds with dismay 'but I just got here!'

The above example describes a clinical situation where the patient is intensely invested in his play. Attention to the aspects of 'real life' such as the passage of time are therefore temporarily suspended. Being so immersed in the play scene, the patient is caught off guard by the session's approaching end. The therapist has anticipated this response and thus announces the time but the child is still surprised.

Third, displacement is operative in child's play. Due to the child's ability to combine reality and fantasy without conflict, he can transfer his own affect and personal situation into the play arena. A child changes passive into active; he can be the initiator of events rather than the reactor he may feel himself to be in real life. Displacement permits distance from the original problem as well as from uncomfortable emotions that go along with it. It prevents the child from becoming overwhelmed by his feelings or needing to overly inhibit them to keep them in check. Displacement also allows the child patient to talk or act in ways that are not possible without the protection the defense provides. Another important function of displacement is that it permits the child's ego to balance id and superego influences and to be employed in resolution of the difficulty.

CLINICAL EXAMPLE: DISPLACEMENT IN PLAY

A six-year-old boy is being seen by a child therapist following removal from his home due to child endangerment. While he has been quite laconic with the therapist about the events in his life, his play is very expressive. Using the doll house, the patient acts out scenes of parental violence. A mother doll is shown threatening a child doll whom the patient has hidden behind a piece of doll furniture. Suddenly, the patient moves the child doll out into the open and forcefully tells the mother to stop or he will put her in jail.

In this example, displacement allows the child to behave in a way that is not possible in his day-to-day life. Feelings or fears that cannot be otherwise released can be expressed in play, giving the child access to them in a safe, manageable dose.

Fourth, a child's capacity for imaginative play dovetails with his cognitive growth. Piaget [14] postulated that there are four periods of intellectual development: sensorimotor (birth to the age of two years), preoperational (2–7 years), concrete operational (7–11 years) and formal operational (11 years and after). According to Piaget, between the ages of two and four years, a child acquires the ability to form symbols. Through symbolism, mental representations are created of experiences, people and objects and remain in the child's mind. Such representation frees the child from having to see an object to know it exists; a mental image or a word is sufficient. Through symbolic play, a child can bridge the gap between the concrete and abstract. Symbolism gives a child's play its distinctly individualized flavor because the child can manipulate the play to reflect his own particular needs and wishes. Piaget's study of the cognitive development of older children (ages 4–11 years) included the use of language, communication, the meaning of rules and moral judgments [14]. Again, cognitive maturation will be reflected in the increasingly complex play of older child patients.

CLINICAL EXAMPLE: SYMBOLISM IN PLAY

A patient, aged four years, was recently adopted, having lived with his maternal grandmother for most of his life. His mother, a drug addict with occasional periods of abstinence, came and left the home unpredictably. During his first treatment session the child exhibited little interest in the toys, with the exception of several puppets which he named 'the monster catchers.' He kept one puppet and gave the other to the therapist and pointed to the space under the couch. The patient declared that it was the hiding spot for the monster, a monster who came and went and repeatedly evaded our attempts, as monster catchers, to get him.

The Child Therapist

In psychotherapy with both adults and children, the therapist's warmth, sensitivity, and nonjudgmental attitude are the basis for the therapeutic alliance and critical to therapeutic success. However, due to the immaturity of the child's cognitive and psychic development, the therapist must possess a unique set of behavioral and emotional traits to effectively work with a child. Most importantly, the therapist must genuinely enjoy children, have the capacity to be authentic and to be at ease in the child's presence [3]. It is beneficial for the therapist to have had a personal psychotherapy so that his own life experiences do not unduly influence his interactions with the child. Accordingly, the therapist should have easy access to his own imagination and to be comfortable playing while simultaneously watching and reflecting upon the child's particular situation. To be able to enter the child's world through play yet also remain outside of it requires a great deal of mental elasticity, but without it, the therapist is likely to be more of an observer of rather than a participant in the therapy. Empathy, the capacity to feel what the patient feels, is of course vital to any sound therapeutic relationship. With a child patient, it may be easier to feel sympathy for his situation rather than empathy with his feelings unless the therapist is able to tolerate and give veracity to his own childhood experiences and residual childlike emotions. Further, empathy enables the therapist to respect the reality of the patient's struggles as well as his attempts, however imperfect, to deal with them [15].

Consistency in technique, acceptance of the patient and flexibility are essential as the child patient can be very attuned to clinical variations or insincerities. The therapist should be patient, tolerant and honest with the child which will enhance the patient's ability to be that way with himself; the therapist in this way serves as an ego ideal. Children most often have not requested psychotherapy and can therefore be suspicious, withdrawn or concerned that the therapy is a punishment or a consequence of their behavior. Also, the child may not necessarily feel troubled or believe he needs help despite the concerns of others. The therapist thus needs to be able to convey the helpful intent of the therapy to the patient and to develop a shared understanding of the problem to be addressed. The therapist needs to assure the child patient that their interactions will take place in a safe, confidential atmosphere. This particular issue can be challenging as the therapist must know how to inform the parents about the treatment but also protect the child's confidences. Most research about the role and characteristics of the therapist has been done by those who work with children; there has been minimal study about how children themselves view the therapist. Ethical considerations and difficulty obtaining a sufficient sample size obviously have hampered this type of research. However, the available data suggest that children most valued kindness, helpfulness, and the therapist's ability to understand and reflect back feelings [16].

Play Materials and the Play Space

Beginning therapists are often unsure about both the materials needed to equip the playroom as well as the rationale behind the selection. Toys or play, in and of themselves, are not therapeutic. Rather it is the way in which they are used in treatment that make them effective. It is suggested that from the onset that the therapist refer to the toys in the office as 'play equipment' or 'play materials.' In this way, through both words and actions, the child starts to see that toys and play have different meanings and purposes than they do outside of the office. The toys chosen by the therapist should be interesting and intriguing; they should capture the child's attention and imagination. They need to be capable of being used symbolically as this how the child

communities thoughts, fantasies and wishes. In short, the toys used in therapy should facilitate the child's self expression. These criteria contraindicate, for example, theme toys or toys of well-known television or movie characters which might have a fixed identify rather than one created by the child. The toys should be in good repair and clean; a worn-out toy could leave the patient feeling devalued. While a therapist may see a number of children in the same office, it can be helpful for the individual patient to have his own container in which to place special items or projects. This move contributes to the child's sense of place and belonging in the office as well as to a positive therapeutic atmosphere of safety, containment and continuity.

Toys that are useful in therapy can be divided into three categories: toys that draw out real life experiences; those that elicit or reflect anger or aggressive emotions; and those material that facilitate creative expression [17]. Real life toys include a doll house and a doll family, cars, airplanes, stuffed animals, zoo animals; as well as a toy telephone, puppets, a doctor's/first aid kit and a few soft baby dolls with bottles. These items naturally appeal, both consciously and unconsciously, to the child's experiences and relationships in daily life and provide a means for exploration and expression. This basic inventory of real life toys is quite sufficient for most play therapies. However, if the patient has a particular situation which calls for the addition of specific toys, the therapist could provide them.

CLINICAL EXAMPLE: PLAY MATERIALS FOR A SPECIFIC SITUATION

A seven-year-old girl was seen due to anxiety after witnessing her mother being injured in an accident. The patient and her mother were riding bicycles when the mother accidentally rode off the sidewalk and suffered serious injuries. She was taken by ambulance to the hospital in the presence of the patient and remained in a coma for several days. Aware of this situation, the therapist added a doll-sized bicycle to her toy supply before meeting with the child. The patient used the doll bicycle during the first session in her play.

All children have aggressive feelings, including those who are referred for very different reasons. However, because they have a limited ability to fully express emotions with words, children can be helped by having aggressive toys with which to play out these feelings. Moreover, the child patient may feel safer engaging these feelings in a displaced way with the therapist than in other settings; this is true especially for inhibited children. Aggressive-type toys include army men and related equipment (e.g., tanks, fighter jets,) wild animals – especially with mouths open, teeth exposed – angry-appearing puppets, and police cars. Some therapists provide punching bags or foam balls and bats for a physical release of aggression or energy. With these types of toys, a child's aggression can be easily visible to the therapies. However, the expression of a particular affect is not dependent on having a corresponding toy in reality; anger can be expressed through other means than through, per se, army men or dinosaurs. Children will use materials in nonconventional ways to reveal themselves and therapists need to be alert to the wide variety of meanings a particular action or toy may have.

CLINICAL EXAMPLE

A four-year-old girl with an unstable, chaotic family history (i.e., exposure to continual parental arguments, mother often absent from home) presented for an evaluation due to noncompliance and aggressive behavior at preschool and home. During the second diagnostic session, the child used the doll family and house to play out a very angry scene between family members. Later in the hour, she took the marble game and very carefully arranged them in an intricate pattern. Suddenly, the patient took another marble and obliterated the design while muttering 'crash' and 'bonk.' The patient then commented sadly, 'all the crashing and bonking has wrecked what I worked so hard on.'

The above vignette raises several points. First, aggressive affect can be expressed through many mediums, not just with 'aggressive' looking objects. Here, it is expressed with the dolls and marbles. Second, more meaning can be attributed to the patient's sadness than just the destruction of her marble design. It is possible that the ruin of her arrangement is also a reference to the damage she experienced as a result of the constant fighting (crashing and bonking) at home or a reaction formation to minimize unconscious guilt she may have felt about her contribution to the parents' problems. These addi-

tional, possible interpretations demonstrate the need for therapists to remain attuned to more than the play scenes surface meaning.

The final category of toys refers to tactile and creative materials such as crayons, markers, colored pencils, tape and paper, modeling clay or Play-Doh®. Some therapists use sand and water tables with child patients but this type of equipment clearly requires a large office space and therapist tolerance for potential spills. Additionally, blocks and Legos® of a wide variety of shape and sizes can be useful in several ways. First, they offer the patient a chance to build, disassemble and recreate new structures. Although concrete, the use of blocks can metaphorically mirror treatment, a process which builds, takes apart and recreates new ways of thinking and being in the world. Second, they can easily be used in conjunction with many other toys; they are not function-specific. Third, they are appealing to a wide age group, from preschooler through elementary school-aged patients.

CLINICAL EXAMPLE

A seven-year-old boy, who was reported to be an excellent student and well-behaved child at school, was referred due to his explosive rages and out-of-control behavior at home. The patient was an avid race car fan and during an early session in the treatment, constructed an elaborate race track out of blocks. Special attention was given to reinforcing the walls with extra blocks in case of a car crash. The therapist noted how race car drivers who were concerned about spinning out of control and crashing might find these well constructed walls both necessary and valuable.

While not undoing the displacement, the therapist responded to one of the likely meanings the patient had communicated with blocks.

The above listing of toy possibilities is not exhaustive; other materials such as books, bendable figures, board games, flashlights, and cards can useful. Board games can be particularly useful when working with older children, latency-age and adolescents who are too old for 'pretend' play. The elements of board games – turn taking, following rules, winning or losing – simulate aspects of real life. To conclude, individual therapists may find through their own experience and experimentation, additional toys which enrich their therapy with children. It is how the toys are used and how the play is developed and understood by the child that is therapeutically valuable. The child patient uses the toys to express his inner world and to make sense of his experiences in the presence of the therapist; this combination is what is mutative.

Conducting Child Psychotherapy

Getting Started: The Evaluation Period

The Therapist's Relationship with Parents

While evaluation is an ongoing part of therapy, a thorough diagnostic assessment is vital for effective treatment planning. The first step in the assessment of a child is to meet with the parents. As previously noted, it is not often the child who has sought treatment, but rather the parents due to either their own concerns or those that have been brought to their attention by others, such as the school or neighbors. Moreover, the child is obviously having some developmental difficulty which is troubling to the parents even if it is not ostensibly bothersome to the child. It is therefore important for the therapist to remember the vulnerable position parents are in when they seek help and to respond to them in a nonjudgmental fashion. It is essential that from the initial contact forward, the parents view the therapist as accepting, helpful and trustworthy; there can be no treatment of the child without ongoing support from the parents.

During the 1960s and 1970s, young patients were most frequently seen in hospital settings or child guidance clinics which were equipped to simultaneously work with the parents. While this model is not often practiced today, treatment of children is still indisputably more effective when the problems of the parents are addressed as well [18]. The treatment plan of a child patient should include provision for parental contact. Additionally, the therapist should be prepared to recommend additional services for the parents if needed to support the child's progress.

The therapist first meets with both parents to explain the diagnostic assessment procedure. Depending on the setting (e.g., clinic, private office), this process will take between one and four sessions. The first is generally with parents alone, the following one(s) with the child and the final one with the parents to explain treatment recommendations. If the parents are divorced or separated, it is still highly preferable to have both parents present during the first session. Inclusion of both parents reduces the risk that the therapist becomes aligned primarily with one parent or hears only 'one side of the story.' Such a lopsided arrangement will certainly weaken the alliance with the more distant parent and potentially have a negative impact on the child as well. In some cases, regardless of marital status, one parent may refuse to participate or to support the treatment. The therapist should continue to invite that parent to meetings and most importantly, try to discuss the reasons for opposition to the treatment. This action is derived from Freud's original advice to address the negative transference in treatment while leaving intact the 'unobjectionable positive transference' [2].

During the first session, the therapist should also obtain certain information about the child including:

(1) both parents' perception of the (child's) presenting problem;
(2) precipitant of/background to presenting problem;
(3) BASIC developmental and medical history;
(4) significant family history;
(5) family history of mental illness, drug and/or alcohol addiction;
(6) history of school progress including peer relationships;
(7) description of personality, fears, interests;
(8) reason for seeking treatment at this time;
(9) prior treatment/attempts to solve problem;
(10) parents' perception of child's strengths and weaknesses;
(11) parents' long-term hopes for and fears about the child.

Additionally, the basic administrative aspects of psychotherapy such as fees, cancellation policy, and confidentiality are reviewed in this initial meeting. The therapist also discusses ways to prepare the child for his first visit, something which parents are often uncertain how to do. Briefly, parents need to simply inform the child that they have made an appointment with a special type of doctor, one who helps to figure out problems but who does not administer familiar types of medical care, such as giving shots. The parents indicate that it is their belief that the therapist can assist the child and them with the current difficulties. They can also state that this type of doctor uses toys and games as the treatment equipment and that the child will have a chance to investigate these during the appointment. While parents should answer if the child has additional questions, it is not necessary to inundate him with a detailed description of the play therapy process. Such an explanation could both confuse the child and generate anxiety. More information about therapy can be furnished in a natural way as the sessions go along.

Meeting the child patient

Regardless of the child's age, upon meeting the child, the therapist should greet the child by name before the parents. This action makes it evident to both child and parent who the patient is and where the therapist's focus will be. Some children may be apprehensive about separating from the parent. It is not recommended that the child be 'forced' to separate but rather, that the therapist acknowledge the child's concern, and if need be, suggest that the parent accompany the therapist and child to the office. In this way, the child is certain that the parent knows where he is and vice versa. If the child continues to be uncomfortable, the parent should be permitted to stay. Preschoolers may initially need for the parent to remain for the entire session but the therapist needs to ensure that the attention is fixed on the child. Having a parent in the room may pose an extra challenge for some therapists (particularly new ones) as feelings of inhibition, self-consciousness and professional uncertainty may surface. It is helpful for the therapist to keep in mind that despite his discomfort, the parent is undoubtedly feeling more nervous and that the parental focus is probably on the child.

The First Session

How to proceed during the first session will depend to some degree on the therapist's theoretical orientation. Nondirective play therapy recommends following the child's thoughts and actions and refraining from doing more than reflecting back to the child. Brief psychodynamic therapy starts with the identification of general treatment goals [19]. However, the common denominator among all theory bases is the requirement for a therapeutic alliance and the therapist's actions and comments should be made with this end point in mind. Acceptance and respect for the patient, essential components of the alliance, need to be conveyed to the patient early in the therapy. Like other aspects of psychotherapy, these features will be communicated to the child patient somewhat differently than to the adult. The question of acceptance, which may be raised in subtle ways by adults, is often more apparent with children and may call for a more direct response.

CLINICAL EXAMPLE

Mary, aged six years, reluctantly entered the therapist's office having been referred for difficulties with anger. She had lived in multiple foster homes and had grown used to new settings and new rules; her outbursts seemed to have become worse with each change. She announced to the therapist that she was a tornado, that tornadoes were dangerous and happened outside and wondered if the therapist 'planned to put her and her tornado-self outside where she belonged.' The therapist responded that it sounded as if Mary knew a lot about tornadoes but also that it might be scary to be outside alone with such a powerful tornado swirling so close to her. Perhaps it would be the best idea to have Mary stay in the office where they could learn more about tornadoes and tornado-feelings together.

In this example, Mary clearly is concerned about the destructiveness of her anger and the potential impact it might have on the therapist. Respect for Mary and acceptance of her anger is communicated by the therapist in the following ways:

(1) The therapist does not un-do the displacement. She stays with Mary's language and talks about tornado-feelings, not Mary's actual anger. She accepts the patient's need for the defense.
(2) The therapist's statement to remain in the office and work together obviously conveys acceptance of Mary and her feelings. It also suggests to Mary, perhaps unconsciously, that the therapist will be able to 'weather her storms.'
(3) The therapist's statement confirming Mary's knowledge of 'tornadoes' shows awareness and respect for Mary's experiences.

Many children will look for some direction from the therapist in the first several sessions as they might from the adults at home or school. It can therefore be helpful to familiarize him/her with the office and any relevant limitations, such as the therapist's desk or file cabinet. When showing the toys, it is important to include a statement about the unique role they play in therapy. For instance, the therapist might say 'Here is where I keep the play materials. We will use them as we play and work together to help us better understand your feelings.' This type of introduction makes the point to the child, right from the start, that toys are used differently in therapy than in other settings. It also identifies the therapist as a person who will work with him/her, rather than instruct him/her. During the initial sessions, the therapist's task is to provide an atmosphere of safety and acceptance, as well as to note the emergence of play themes. The concerns and conflicts of most children can be expressed through play even when they are not or cannot be discussed verbally [17]. The therapist's remarks should be tailored to the child's developmental level. Without probing or pressing, the therapist's statements should correspond to the child's moves and comments.

CLINICAL EXAMPLE

A three-year, six-month old boy was referred for an evaluation due to aggressive behavior. The therapist and the boy's mother agreed that the mother could remain in the office for the first several sessions although she was advised to be as unobtrusive as possible. The patient quickly left mother's side and easily explored the office, looking under chairs and eyeing toys which were quite visible on the shelf. The therapist commented 'there are so many new things to look at in this place. You do not need mother right now; you can be an explorer on your own.' The boy found a foam ball and threw it to the therapist who returned the pitch stating: 'we can play something together, now that you've found the ball!'. The patient then went to the doll house and threw the baby doll out the window, and said that 'the family did not need that baby anyway.' The therapist, knowing about the recent birth of a sibling added 'the family seemed fine the way it was before baby sister was born.'

In this example, the therapist pulled out what appeared to be the main threads in the interaction between herself and the patient without over-interpreting or patronizing. First, the therapist noticed that the child is able to leave mother's side to investigate the new place. Such curiosity is both desirable and developmentally appropriate; the therapist's comment speaks to this achievement. Second, the therapist noted the patient's effort to initiate contact with her. Her subsequent action and comment demonstrated her willingness to reciprocate. Third, the therapist slightly extended and thereby perhaps, clarified the child's comment. Fourth, the therapist did not make a link between the patient's action and his real-life sibling. To have made a direct connection between the patient's action and his home situation would have been premature for several reasons. This particular session was

diagnostic in which the purpose leans more toward observation and formulation than interpretation. Second, such a remark would have undone the displacement, potentially leaving the child inadequately defended. Third, the child might have been made anxious by the comment and inhibit his play as a result.

Continuing Therapy

One of the basic precepts of psychotherapy is to begin 'where the patient is.' The child patient will respond to the therapist with emotions and behaviors that reflect not only where his/her development has been derailed but also the defenses with which he/she has protected himself/herself. In the beginning period of treatment, the child patient learns that the therapist is a person whom he/she can trust and who can accept his/her needs, wishes and fears. A connection then forms between patient and therapist which in turn, enables the child to invest in the therapy. During the middle phase of treatment, the therapist and child work together to achieve a sense of a more organized self. The patient has an idea of his/her conflicts and can safely explore them with the therapist. The final stage of treatment brings resolution to or a reduction of the child's difficulties and acceptance of the change that has occurred. It is not uncommon at this time to see the reappearance of original issues as the child deals with separating from the therapist, a person who has become very meaningful to him.

Limit Setting

Psychotherapy with both adults and children involves the setting of limits. Indeed, from the outset, limits are demarcated by the therapist as he/she establishes the frame with the patient and details the conditions of therapy [20]. These requirements include at a minimum, the therapist's payment and cancellation policy, informed consent and the limits of confidentiality. While most therapists are comfortable establishing limits, there is far more uncertainty when it comes to the testing or the enforcing of them. With child patients, whose behavior might result in damage to the office or therapist, limits are clearly necessary. There is agreement among most therapists that the office space, the therapist and the patient cannot be hurt and these rules must be clearly established and enforced. Otherwise, it is not necessary or even possible for the therapist to spell out every limit that might be required. It is more practical to instead to limit the problematic behavior as it arises. Nonetheless, some therapists are uncomfortable with such ambiguity and it is beneficial to know at what point the child's behavior exceeds one's own limit of acceptable behavior. The following guidelines can be used to set limits [21].

First, the therapist provides a verbal reflection to the child of his/her attitudes or wishes.
Example: I see that you want to take the puppets home with you and that is why you are trying to put them in your bag.
Second, the therapist verbally states the limit.
Example: I can tell that you want to the puppets home very much, so much that you are trying to take them out of the office. But the play materials must stay here and you can use them when you are here.
Third, the therapist intervenes physically to control the child's behavior.
Example: While I know how much you want to take the puppets with you, they must stay here until next time. (Therapist removes them from the child)

It can be very frightening to a child to feel that the adult is unable or unwilling to maintain adequate control. By defining and enforcing the limits of safe and acceptable behavior, the therapist assures the child that his/her impulses can be tolerated and contained.

Conclusion

Although methods of play therapy have both evolved and expanded over time, its value as a clinical intervention remains [22]. Play therapy provides a way for the child patient to define and understand personal struggles within a developmentally appropriate context.

References

1. Elkind D: *The Hurried Child.* 3rd ed. Cambridge, MA: Perseus Books, 2001.
2. Freud S: *The Dynamics of Transference.* Standard Edition (12), 1912.
3. Axline V: *Play Therapy.* New York: Ballantine Books, 1947.
4. Marans S, Mayes L, Colonna A: Psychoanalytic views of children's play. In: *The Many Meanings of Play.* Solnit AJ, Cohen DJ, Neubauer PB, eds. New Haven, CN: Yale University Press, 1993.5.
5. Waelder R: The psychoanalytic theory of play. *Psychoanal Quarterly* 1933; **2**.
6. Erikson EH: *Childhood and Society.* New York: Norton, 1950.
7. Winnicott DW: *Playing and Reality.* London: Routledge, 1971.
8. Landreth G, Baggerly J, Tyndall-Lind A: Beyond adapting adult counseling skills for use with children: The paradigm shift to child-centered play therapy. *J Individ Psychol* 1999; **55**:272–287.
9. Kottman T: Integrating the Crucial Cs into Alderian Play Therapy. *J Individ Psychol* 1999; **55**(3):288–297.
10. Solnit A, *et al.*: *The Many Meanings of Play.* New Haven: Yale University Press, 1993.
11. Knell S: (1999) Cognitive-Behavioral Play Therapy. *J Clin Child Psych* 1999; **27**:(1)28–33.
12. Kottman T, Schaefer C: *Play Therapy in Action: A Casebook for Practitioners.* New Jersey: Jason Aronson, Inc.
13. Prat R: Imaginary hide and seek, A technique for opening psychic space in child psychotherapy. *J Child Psychotherapy* 2001; **27**:2.
14. Ginsburg H, Opper S: *Piaget's theory of intellectual development: An Introduction.* Englewood Cliffs, New Jersey: Prentice-Hall, Inc., 1969.
15. McWilliams N: *Psychoanalytic Psychotherapy.* New York: The Guilford Press, 2004.
16. Caroll J: Play therapy: the children's views. *Child and Family Social Work* 2002; **7**:177–187.
17. Schaefer C: *The Therapeutic Powers of Play.* New Jersey: Jason Aronson, Inc., 1993.
18. Wilson K, Ryan V: Helping parents by working with their children in individual child therapy. *Child and Fam Social Work* 2001; **6**:209–218.
19. Racusin R: Brief psychodynamic psychotherapy with young children, *J Am Acad Child Adolesc Psychiatry* 2000; **39**:6.
20. Luborsky L: *The Principles of Psychoanalytic Psychotherapy.* Basic Books, Inc., 1984.
21. Schaefer C: *The Therapeutic Use of Child's Play.* New Jersey: Jason Aronson Inc., 1979.
22. LeBlanc M, Ritchie M: A meta-analysis of play therapy outcomes. *Counseling Psychology Quarterly* 2001; **14**:2.

9

Cognitive Behavioral Therapy

Christina C. Clark

Overview

Mental health providers serving the needs of children, adolescents, and their families find themselves in the midst of challenging and exciting times: challenging because current prevalence rates of significant psychiatric problems (behavioral, emotional or developmental) within this historically underserved population are between 17% and 22% [1,2], exciting because there has been increased focus on expanding the knowledge base and developing effective treatments for this population.

Indeed, it is remarkable to reflect on the fact that the initial publication of the *Diagnostic and Statistical Manual* (DSM-I) in 1952 contained only one childhood disorder while the current version (DSM-IV-TR) has expanded to more than 20 childhood diagnostic categories that include research findings as well as beginning to include developmental and contextual aspects. Furthermore, there has been an explosion of information within the past 10 years regarding child development and psychopathology [3].

At the same time, a number of forces including managed care, have created a climate of accountability to ensure that mental health providers are providing empirically supported treatment (EST) [4], evidence-based medicine (EBM) [5] or evidence-based treatment (EBT) [2].

Clinicians and researchers utilizing cognitive-behavioral therapy (CBT) have responded to these forces by expanding the model downward (i.e., treatments originally designed for use with adults were adapted for use with youth) and subjecting treatment outcome to evaluation of effectiveness. Although much more investigation regarding the effectiveness of CBT with children and adolescents remains to be done, thus far CBT has been shown to be effective for internalizing disorders, including anxiety [6–9], social phobia [10], obsessive–compulsive disorder [11,12], depression [13–17] and externalizing disorders [18], including a parent training component to address childhood attention deficit/hyperactivity disorder (ADHD) [19], aggression [20], conduct disorder [21], and anger [22,23]. Reviewing treatment effectiveness from an EBM perspective, Compton *et al.* [5] stated that CBT is the 'treatment of choice' for children and adolescents with internalizing (anxiety and depression) disorders.

This chapter is intended to be used as a resource for clinicians interested in delivering CBT to children and adolescents. Before discussing CBT specific information, a brief overview of important issues that should be considered regardless of theoretical approach is mentioned. This is followed by specific CBT-oriented information, including a brief description of the CBT model and its principles. Following that, treatment will be discussed. Finally, a set of guidelines that can help clinicians integrate theory and research into daily use with children and adolescents will be presented.

Special Issues

Children and adolescents constitute a 'special population,' and as such, require the clinician to pay particular attention to certain aspects of treatment. These considerations are not unique to CBT; however, as they are integral to clinical work with this population they will be briefly highlighted here. Included are ethical considerations, developmental factors, family involvement, and cultural factors. These issues are not discrete 'entities,' in other words, these considerations often interact or overlap.

Mental health professionals serving children, adolescents, and their families need to remain mindful of the complex nature of serving various family members and of the fact that children are still developing, i.e.,

Clinical Child Psychiatry, Second Edition. Edited by W.M. Klykylo and J.L. Kay
© 2005 John Wiley & Sons Ltd.

they are vulnerable [24,25]. Ethical considerations include, but are not limited to, issues related to referral, informed consent, and provision of effective treatment. Children and adolescents are typically brought to treatment by adults, usually parents [26,27]. Although the child may be identified as the 'patient' it is the adults who are typically stating what they would like treatment to address. Mental health providers consider the perspectives of all parties and attempt to determine what is likely to be in the best interest of the child [25] – which at times may be in direct opposition to what the parents are requesting, resulting in potential conflicts of interest [26]. However, the mental health provider who has followed ethical and legal guidelines regarding informed consent (for example, encouraging participation and providing information in developmentally appropriate language [25] has made it a habit to discuss expectations, responsibilities, risks/benefits and outcome at the outset of treatment and as needed. Best practices for obtaining informed consent with children are briefly outlined by Fisher, Hatashita-Wong, and Greene [24]. Regarding provision of effective treatment, Lyddon [4] states that 'practitioners are obligated us use empirically supported treatments to guide their work as a matter of ethical accountability.'

Special attention to developmental factors, on the part of the clinician, is required throughout the therapy process. Doing so increases the likelihood that developmentally appropriate communication and assessment procedures occur, leading to developmentally titrated goals and selection of interventions. As a result, clinicians report that the child is often more engaged [28–31]. Furthermore, it would appear that the likelihood of progress is increased because, according to Holmbeck et al. [32] developmental sensitivity is thought to increase quality of treatment, though more developmentally oriented research is needed to determine whether this is true. In the meantime, Holmbeck and colleagues [32], in a chapter discussing the relevance of developmental issues for therapists and researchers, have included a table of developmental milestones (Table 9.1) for child/adolescent therapists to integrate into treatment. Finally, it is useful to distinguish between 'deficiency' and 'distortion' [33–35] when working with children, and to recognize that either or both can occur. That is to say, the therapist needs to determine whether a child is engaging in inaccurate thinking or simply lacks skills/experience and aim interventions accordingly.

Generally speaking, the younger the child, the more likely it is that parents may become involved in treatment. This is because the child is still in the process of developing; therefore, they are dependent on parents for guidance and support. Furthermore, the younger the child, the more likely it is that problems are occurring within the family setting. Therefore, taking into account the interactions between the family and the child/adolescent will be an important part of understanding the child and delivering treatment. In most cases, the therapist should work to ensure that adults(s) involved have a good understanding of appropriate developmental expectations, as recommended by Holmbeck et al. [32]. In addition, the clinician facilitates parents' exploration of their own beliefs [36,37] regarding developmental expectations and helps them to recognize when their own beliefs (thinking), feelings, and/or behavior may contribute to the child's problems.

The mention of parents elicits a parenthetical remark: Although many texts use the word 'parent' to denote adults involved in the child's life, throughout this chapter the terms 'parent' and 'caregiver' will be used interchangeably to describe any adult who would live with and/or have major day-to-day responsibility for the child including biological and/or step-parents, grandparents, other biological relatives, foster-parents, adoptive parents, or other adults.

Other contextual areas that should be attended to by the clinician include school, peer group, religion, sexual orientation, social class, and ethnicity/culture [38]. To aid clinicians pay particular attention to these important areas, Friedberg and McClure [30] compiled a table of culturally sensitive questions (Table 9.2) and Fisher, Hatashita-Wong and Greene [24] briefly outline a set of best practices for culturally valid assessment and treatment.

Principles of Cognitive-Behavioral Therapy

Cognitive therapists remain mindful of the basic principles regarding the process of cognitive therapy as they work with clients. These principles as outlined by Beck [39] include the idea that the process is collaborative, structured, active, time-limited, and goal-oriented. The conceptualization of the client evolves continually as new information comes to light. Based on that conceptualization, numerous cognitive and/or behavioral techniques are suggested to aid the client in exploring and changing cognitions and/or behaviors. Typically, at the beginning the therapist takes on more of the responsibility for the content and direction of therapy; however, another principle holds that the ultimate goal is for the therapist to educate the client to become their own cognitive therapist.

Table 9.1 Developmental milestones and stages across childhood, adolescence, and emerging adulthood.

Infancy (0–2 years)	• Infants explore world via direct sensory–motor contact • Emergence of emotions • Object permanence and separation anxiety develop • Critical attachment period: secure parent–infant bond promotes trust and healthy growth of infant; insecure bonds create distrust and distress for infant • Initial use of sounds and words to communicate • Piaget's Sensorimotor stage
Toddler/preschool years (2–6 years)	• Use of multiple words and symbols to communicate • Learns self-care skills • Mainly characterized by egocentricity, but preschoolers appreciate differences in perspectives of others • Use of imagination, engagement in 'pretend' play • Increasing sense of autonomy and control of environment • Develop school readiness skills • Piaget's Preoperational stage
Middle childhood (6–10 years)	• Social, physical, and academic skills develop • Logical thinking and reasoning develops • Increased interaction with peers • Increasing self-control and emotion regulation • Piaget's Concrete Operational stage
Adolescence (10–18 years)	• Pubertal development; sexual development • Development of metacognition (i.e., use of higher-order strategizing in learning; thinking about one's own thinking) • Higher cognitive skills develop, including abstraction, consequential thinking, hypothetical reasoning, and perspective taking • Transformations in parent–child relationships; increase in family conflicts • Peer relationships increasingly important and intimate • Making transition from childhood to adulthood • Developing sense of identity and autonomous functioning • Piaget's Formal Operations stage
Emerging adulthood (18–25 years)	• Establishment of meaningful and enduring interpersonal relationships • Identity explorations in areas of love, work, and worldviews • Peak of certain risk behaviors • Obtaining education and training for long-term adult occupation

Collaboration includes the notion of a positive therapeutic alliance with the client and is most likely achieved when the therapist demonstrates the well-known common factors including skills of 'accurate empathy.' This can be a particularly demanding and challenging task when working with children and adolescents, because it is not uncommon for caregivers to be involved in the treatment, in which case the therapist needs to consider how to work collaboratively with various members of the system without alienating or favoring anyone.

Sessions are structured (with mood-check, review of homework, agenda setting, addressing issues, feedback, and setting new homework) [30,39]. While it may seem obvious, again, it is important to keep in mind what is developmentally appropriate with regard to structure. Therefore, as long as each of the session elements gets addressed during the therapy hour, younger children may require a greater amount of flexibility.

Content of the session (as well as 'homework') needs to engage the child or adolescent. How is this done? We return to the theme of developmental 'fit.' In

Table 9.2 Sample questions addressing cultural context issues.

- What is the level of acculturation in the family?
- How does the level of acculturation shape symptom expression?
- What characterizes the child's ethnocultural identity?
- How does this identity influence symptom expression?
- What are the child and family thinking and feeling as a member of this culture?
- How do ethnocultural beliefs, values, and practices shape problem expression?
- How representative or typical is this family of the culture?
- What feelings and thoughts are proscribed as taboo?
- What feelings and thoughts are facilitated and promoted as a function of ethnocultural context?
- What ethnocultural specific socialization processes selectively reinforce some thoughts, feelings, and behaviors but not others?
- What types of prejudice and marginalization has the child/family encountered?
- How have these experiences shaped symptom expression?
- What beliefs about oneself, the world, and the future have developed as a result of these experiences?

---

general, the younger the child, the more active and play-oriented treatment will be. Preschoolers may need toys, games, books, and/or a sandbox as, generally speaking, play is their 'language.' Relaxation skills can be delivered in a playful way, for example, using games like Simon Says or using soap bubbles to teach them to moderate their breathing. School-age children enjoy activities such as drawing, crafts, games, books, and age-appropriate workbooks, such as *Therapeutic Exercises for Children* [40]. Adolescents are frequently able to engage in talk therapy similar to that of adults but homework might involve journaling, poetry, or artwork. The therapist uses 'guided discovery' to help the child, adolescent and/or caregivers to increase understanding and to learn/practice new ways of thinking and behaving.

Setting goals is an opportunity for collaboration as well as for the therapist to gain additional understanding of beliefs and expectations of the child/adolescent, as well as the caregivers. Input from the child/adolescent should be solicited at the level at which is judged to be developmentally appropriate.

In addition to helping the client with his/her current concerns, cognitive therapy takes an educative approach, that is, to prepare them to learn skills and general concepts that can be extended to their life after therapy. CBT attempts to help the client 'become their own cognitive therapist' [39] by teaching the client skills to apply to current problems while simultaneously teaching them about the CBT model and learning to formulate a coherent 'picture' (conceptualization) of themselves. Therefore, the therapist is not doing something to the client, but is teaching the client how to understand themselves and what to do to help themselves, both now and, hopefully, in the future. The therapist attempts to establish alliances with all participants and explains the conceptualization to individuals within the system at the level that is developmentally appropriate for each member.

The Model

Cognitive behavioral therapy (CBT) is based on a combination [5,41] of behavioral principles such as classical and operant conditioning combined with concepts from social learning theory [30]. Cognitive therapy emphasizes the role of thinking (i.e., cognitive mediation) which mutually interacts with three other aspects of a person, namely, behavior, emotions, and physical reactions [42–44]. In turn, a person affects and is affected by, his/her environment [44]. Environment or context, which is particularly relevant for children and adolescents, includes peers, family, and teachers.

Given the emphasis on cognition as playing a major role in influencing emotions, behavior, and physical reactions, several points are relevant here. First, thinking is not a unitary concept: cognition is an information-processing system [28,45]. This system is comprised of different levels of thinking, structures, and processes including automatic thoughts, intermediate beliefs (rules, attitudes, assumptions), schemas, and compensatory strategies [28,39,43]. Automatic thoughts are the most accessible level of thinking, which can be thought of as the running commentary that goes through your head during your daily activities. Intermediate beliefs are conditional and reveal assumptions or rules used by the patient to organize his/her experience. For example, a child who receives praise only when achieving may come to believe 'If I work hard enough, I will be loved.' Schemas or core beliefs are typically absolute, such as 'I am unlovable' and are usually brought to light over time by the therapist. Compensatory strategies refer to the behaviors

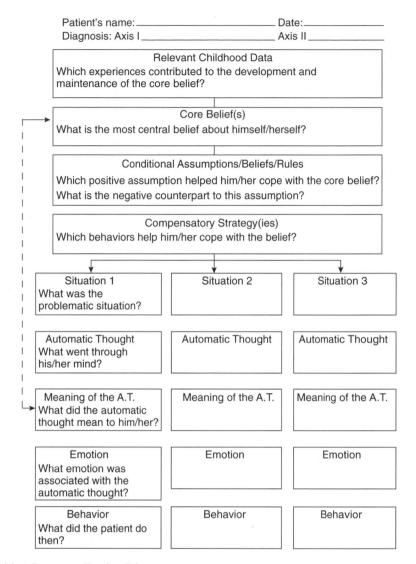

Figure 9.1 Cognitive Conceptualization Diagram.

that help the patient deal with their beliefs [39]. Continuing with the example above, a compensatory strategy for a child with these beliefs would be for him/her to work to achieve what is expected by those whose love he/she wants. These levels of thinking are captured on the Cognitive Conceptualization Diagram [39] shown in Figure 9.1. Beck [39] provides detailed explanation of these structures and gives strategies for eliciting client cognitions as well as modifying them, although not geared specifically to children and adolescents. Stallard [46] demonstrates the application of some of these concepts with children and adolescents.

Second, according to the content-specificity hypothesis proposed by Beck [45], cognitive content will reflect themes that correlate with specific disorders [43]. For example, anxiety disorders are characterized by cognitions related to themes of threat whereas depression is characterized by themes of loss. A recent study including children and adolescents aged 7–16 years demonstrated support for the content-specificity hypothesis, for both internalizing and externalizing disorders [47]. Finally, the distinction of 'deficiency versus distortion' [27] is particularly relevant for the therapist working with children and adolescents because the distinction will influence intervention selection.

Adaptations

Overall, the cognitive behavioral model has appeared to produce efficacious treatment results when adapted for children and adolescents. However, much more work is needed to fine-tune the model and treatment for this population. The process is underway. There are attempts to continue to adapt the CBT model to even younger children. One study [48] using randomized controlled treatment (RCT) involved children aged 4–12 years diagnosed with disruptive behavior disorders. Those treated with a manualized CBT-intervention called 'collaborative problem solving' (CPS), involving parent–child problem solving, experienced significant improvement.

Other extensions to young children include cognitive developmental therapy [31] (CDT) and cognitive behavioral play therapy [49,50] (CBPT). Although CDT and CBPT have not been subjected to RCT studies, case studies are available to illustrate their principles. Both CDT and CBPT utilize play techniques. Although play has long been used as technique in child-oriented therapy, there are few RCT studies to evaluate its effectiveness. Russ [51], apparently in an attempt to encourage the integration of play (in ways that are empirically supported) has compiled information that could be valuable to practitioners working with young children.

Developing the Conceptualization

Conceptualization is an essential cornerstone for effective delivery of CBT and refers to the process by which the therapist gathers and integrates information from several sources [30,39,52,53] including: (1) knowledge of child/adolescent normal biopsychosocial development [32]; (2) knowledge of child/adolescent psychopathology; (3) knowledge of the cognitive-behavioral model, including generic models of pathology and the content-specificity hypothesis; and (4) specific presenting symptoms, including the background of the child/adolescent and his/her family. Once integrated, this information creates a 'picture' of the client allowing the therapist to understand and make predictions (i.e., generate hypotheses) about the client and his/her family.

The rationale for developing a conceptualization is that, simply put, it leads to effective treatment [52]. Why? Because a cogent conceptualization that accounts for the client's problems and proposes to understand the underlying mechanisms will aid the therapist in delivering appropriate treatment, including selecting, timing, and tailoring interventions [52–54].

Once the initial conceptualization is developed, the therapist uses the model to generate and test hypotheses regarding treatment approaches and specific interventions. As treatment progresses the therapist continues to collect information about the client while also deciding whether hypotheses are supported or disconfirmed. Therapists are not tied to their original ideas, because as scientist–practitioners, they revise the conceptualization in an iterative fashion [30,39]. With each 'successive approximation', however, the model should become clearer and more accurate, forming the basis for both within-session and extra-session [54] decisions about the client.

A second use for the conceptualization is to promote client self-awareness, leading to generalization of skills. This is accomplished by sharing the working model of the client with him/her. That being said, it is paramount that the therapist considers the capacity of the client to receive and process information. Expectations for the level of sophistication regarding the conceptualization would be based on the client's developmental level. For example, a young child may have the capacity to recognize and label feelings along with a recent situation whereas a school age child may be able to begin to identify themes like 'I always get mad when my Mom tells me no but not when my teacher tells me no.' Adolescents, if motivated, may want to link their formative experiences with current patterns, 'I was always worried that I would disappoint my Dad so I never tried new things to keep from failing at them.' Clinicians could make use of the Cognitive Conceptualization Diagram [39] for adolescents and, with some adaptation/assistance from the therapist, may be able to have the teen complete it also. From the foundation of the well-developed conceptualization, the therapist begins to make use of it for treatment.

Treatment

A typical outline for an episode of CBT treatment is shown in Table 9.3 [55]. Generally speaking, while making initial treatment recommendations, I explain that frequently each family member may need to do their own changing to help the child or adolescent who has been brought in for treatment. In addition, I provide the rationale for my decisions to the client (titrated to their developmental level) and his/her parents as well as expectations for therapy. Whenever possible, I prefer to hold this meeting with everyone involved; however, in cases where it appears it may be counter-therapeutic (for example, the parent's actions cause the child to 'shut down'), I meet individually with separate parties. Expectations include responsi-

Table 9.3 Outline of standard course of cognitive behavioral therapy.

---

1. Therapist elicits information regarding the development of specific symptoms, as well as situational determinants and temporal course. Objective and subjective data are collected (preferably from multiple informants) regarding the nature of the presenting problem.
2. A goal list is developed with the child and the parents or other caregiver. Cognitive behavioral formulation and treatment recommendations are shared with the child and his or her parents.
3. Underlying beliefs, attitudes, assumptions, expectations, attributions, goals, and self-statements or automatic thoughts are identified. Patients learn to monitor negative or maladaptive thoughts and emotions. Attempts at self-monitoring are rewarded.
4. Specific behavioral and interpersonal skills deficits are identified.
5. Medical, social, and environmental factors maintaining the symptoms are identified. The latter may include stressful life events (both major and minor, short-term and chronic) or the modeling and reinforcement of the symptoms by others in the child's life.
6. Cognitive and behavioral interventions are selected and introduced based upon the specific needs of the child.
7. Homework is assigned. The patient practices the cognitive or behavioral skills during the session. Attempts are made to ensure that the interventions are clearly understood, that the child is motivated to attempt the assignment, and that they expect the intervention to be helpful. Factors that may interfere with the successful completion of the homework assignment are identified and addressed.
8. Effectiveness of the intervention is evaluated through objective ratings, behavioral observations, and subjective reports.
9. Relapse prevention interventions are introduced. Follow-up or booster sessions are scheduled.

---

bilities of both parties and an overview of the anticipated treatment process. For example, families who have a child with symptoms of obsessive–compulsive disorder (OCD) should understand that exposure with response prevention (E/RP) will likely be a significant aspect of treatment. At the beginning of treatment, however, the details of how E/RP will be carried out are not yet known for that particular child.

Treatment focuses simultaneously on two levels of intervention: addressing the specific here-and-now problems of the client and secondly, teaching the client skills and concepts that would prevent relapse as well as deal with future problems [39].

Research on how best to involve parents in CBT treatment has been limited, what is meant by a parental or family component to treatment has not been well-defined in the research studies and adding parents to the treatment can present challenges. However, based on the number of EBTs that include parents and appear to be effective, clinicians need to routinely consider including parents. There are several reasons for this. Involving parents in treatment can help support the child, by acting as a 'coach,' to remind them of what they've learned and help them to use it between sessions or after termination. A second advantage of involving parents in treatment is the opportunity for the clinician to assess and address, if necessary, the parent–child relationship and its impact on the child's symptoms, parental beliefs and expectations.

Typically treatment will consist of interventions that combine both behavioral and cognitive techniques [56] that have been selected by the therapist to fit that specific individual [39], as well as taking into account the client's developmental capacity [31]. Independent of technique, however, it is paramount that the therapist ensure that the child or adolescent understand the CBT model, i.e., the link between thinking and feelings. Friedberg and McClure [30] suggest that clinicians select techniques based on the stage of therapy, i.e., make sure that the client can identify/distinguish thoughts and feelings before the therapist implements more complex techniques.

Determining whether the treatment strategy is effective should be evaluated on an ongoing basis by having the client explain their understanding as well as determining what mood or behavioral changes are occurring. If the therapist sees that a particular intervention is not working, the therapist will attempt to determine the source of difficulty so as to modify some aspect of the current approach or to select a new intervention. All these decisions are made based upon the revised conceptualization.

Examples of Treatment

Let us turn to some examples to illustrate, in particular, adapting CBT interventions to children at different stages of development. Consider a male who has been brought to treatment by his mother, who reports he has been having behavioral problems at school (arguing and fighting with peers). During the first interview, the mother provides information that supports a diagnosis of oppositional defiant disorder (ODD). Furthermore, you have decided that the child may be depressed based on your observation of him and his responses to some questions. During a later session, while the therapist and his mother are discussing an incident that occurred at school (he is present in the room), he wants to speak with his mother. He tries getting her attention twice, then yells, picks up an object, preparing to throw it at her.

Preschool Age (age four years six months)

Mother: (angrily) That is not nice! You could hurt someone doing that!

Child: But mommy . . .

Therapist: What made you get ready to throw that?

Child: She wouldn't listen to me.

Therapist: And how did you feel when she didn't listen?

Child: Huh?

Therapist: (changing strategies to labeling) I wonder if you felt mad.

Child: No.

Therapist: Well I heard your voice get loud, like a tiger growling, and your face got red. I think that goes with being mad. You got mad when she kept on talking.

Child: (nods)

Therapist: I wonder what else you could have done?

Child: I dunno.

Therapist: Here, let me show you. Well, you could just 'zip your lip' (making zipping gesture and funny face, child smiles) until mommy stopped talking, or you could have tried staying still and raising your hand, or if it was real real important (like having to go the restroom), you could even flap your hand around like a flag like this! And that would let us know you can't wait for us to stop talking. But that's only something you do once in a while. Understand?

Child: Nods yes.

Therapist: OK, let's practice with mommy right now.

School Age (age nine years)

Mother: (angrily) That is not nice! You could hurt someone doing that!

Child: But . . .

Therapist: What made you get ready to throw that?

Child: She wouldn't listen to me.

Therapist: And how did you feel when she didn't listen?

Child: Mad.

Therapist: Yeah, I can see how mad you must feel because I heard your voice getting louder and louder.

Child: Yep.

Therapist: I wonder what you said to yourself inside your head when she didn't listen.

Child: She never listens to me. All she ever does is yell. (Starts to cry and mother starts to comfort him).

Therapist: I wonder if there was anything else in your head about you mom. . . .

Child: Maybe she loves my sister more.

Adolescence (14 years)

Mother: (angrily) That is not nice! You could hurt someone doing that!

Child: But . . . I didn't throw it.

Therapist: What made you get ready to throw that?

Child: She wouldn't listen to me.

Therapist: And how did you feel when she didn't listen?

Child: Frustrated.

Therapist: And what was going through your mind?

Child: Parents never listen to their kids because they think they know everything!

Therapist: How often do you get as mad as today?

Child: Almost every time we talk about school, because all they ever do is get on my back!

CASE ONE: PRESCHOOL AGE

Danny, age five years six months, was brought to treatment by his mother who was concerned about his growing oppositional and defiant behaviors, which occurred primarily in the home setting but had also started to manifest in kindergarten. Initially, the therapist recommended that mom use a behavioral chart with three daily tasks, two that were already occurring (so she could practice praise and positive reinforcement) and one challenging task that tended to elicit opposition. After two weeks of using the chart, an exasperated mom said that the client's behavior had actually become more oppositional, not less. In the meantime, the therapist asked mother to note any patterns related to opposition. The only pattern she could see was that when Danny cried, he became more oppositional. Further discussion of recent events revealed that when Danny was asked to do the difficult task, he would frequently cry to which mom responded by saying it wasn't so hard or that it wouldn't take very long. When asked if she talked with him about his crying or attempted to comfort him, she expressed concerns that this would make him into a cry-baby and he would try to get out of doing things. Two interventions took place over time to address the interaction between Danny and his mother. First, the therapist explained that expressing understanding of children's feelings does not mean that the parent has to 'cave' to whatever the child wants. To gain a more in-depth understanding of how to deal with Danny's negative feelings, mother was asked to read a parenting book that explains the role of parent as 'coach' [57]. At the same time, the therapist gathered information from play with Danny, then modeled for mother how to 'coach' Danny through difficult feelings. Due to his age, a small sandbox with plastic animals (he chose horses) was used to facilitate the play. The following example shows how information was collected:

Therapist: So, this horse here (pointing to smaller horse). Is it a boy or girl horse?
Danny: A boy.
Therapist: I wonder how old he is . . .
Danny: Five and a half!
Therapist: And I see that the Mommy horse just asked him to take his nap.
Danny: Yep, and he doesn't want to.
Therapist: How do you know?
Danny: Because he wants to play.
Therapist: So he wants to play – oh, and I think I hear him crying.
Danny: Yup (frown).
Therapist: Hmmm. I wonder what the Mommy horse could do to help him.
Danny: Tell him he can play.
Therapist: Well, but Mommy horse wants him to have his nap. I know, she can tell him he can take his favorite book to read while he goes to sleep and then he can play when he wakes up. Or . . . Mommy horse can say 'It isn't that hard to take a nap.'
Danny: No, it's better if she says it's OK for him to take a book into his room.
Therapist: OK, so he goes and finds his favorite book – do you think he is still crying?

Danny: No, I don't hear him crying but he still would like to play.
Therapist: I know.

Comment: Although all of the oppositional behavior did not disappear, through the combination of mother reading and learning how to interact in a more positive fashion with Danny, about eight weeks into treatment, she stated, 'You know, after reading that book, I realize that I was a big part of the problem.' Over time, Danny continued to reveal more of his feelings and thoughts to his mother, who learned to tolerate negative affect and 'coach' him. This example illustrates how a parent's beliefs about developmental expectations can interact with and influence a child's behavior. It also demonstrates that the child was most likely operating from 'deficits' that were addressed when his mother learned how to respond to him. Finally, the 'coaching' stance of the parent is a good example of a parent modeling emotional regulation and problem-solving for the child.

CASE TWO: MIDDLE CHILDHOOD

Alonzo, a nine year four month old Latino male, was brought for treatment by his single mother, who explained that he was being treated for ADHD by a psychiatrist, who advised the mother to seek psychological services to help her manage her son's temper outbursts. His mother has been working with his teacher to track his daily in-school behaviors, including turning in assignments, paying attention, transitioning, and not interrupting. The daily goal was to obtain an OK in each area, thereby earning points that he could 'cash in' at school for rewards. Furthermore, his mother based home privileges on his school behaviors, as reported by his teacher. As long as Alonzo's behavior was in the acceptable range, all was fine. When it didn't, however, he would receive a 'warning' from the teacher with the purpose of giving him feedback to help him get back on track. In most cases, after he received a warning, he became angry, upset and uncooperative, leading to more difficulties for the rest of the day. At a session with Alonzo and his mother,

I asked Alonzo to explain what he thought was making it so difficult for him to meet his goal, leading to the following dialogue:

Alonzo: Well, when I hear the 'warning' I think that my teacher is just trying to make me fail and once I miss my goal for the day, I can't have any fun at home.

Therapist: Wow, that sounds like a lot of pressure and like you feel the grown ups are out to get you.

Alonzo: Right! Like last week – mom told me that if I could get a perfect week, then I could buy a new computer game.

Therapist: So you were probably trying your hardest because I know how much you like computer games.

Alonzo: Yeah, and then I get a warning on Thursday! And it wasn't even my fault but the teacher wouldn't listen.

Therapist: So, when you get a 'warning' – what does that mean?

Alonzo: It means I am probably not going to make my goal for the day OR the week.

Therapist: Sounds like you worry a lot about not meeting your goal.

Alonzo: Yeah and I get mad thinking about how they don't want me to earn my points.

Therapist: I wonder what would happen if you think of your warnings as strikes, like in baseball – you know, three strikes and you're out. Only your teacher gives you two strikes.

Alonzo: You mean like chances?

Therapist: Yep. It seems like you've been thinking that a warning is an out.

Alonzo: I do and then I just feel like giving up because it's too hard.

At this point, the therapist spoke with Alonzo's mother privately to set up a way that he could earn some privileges even if his day wasn't 'perfect.' She expressed concern that 'if you give him an inch, he will take a mile' but we worked out a 'graduated' system that would allow her to give him basic privileges for 70% achievement, better privileges for 80% achievement and 'deluxe' privileges for 90% and above. Any day with achievement below 60% would result in a loss of all privileges at home for that day. We included Alonzo in the discussion by asking him to rate his favorite privilege as a '1' and so on. Mom agreed to remind Alonzo to think of warnings as chances and we implemented the graduated reward system, to discourage the all-or-nothing thinking of both the adults and Alonzo. As soon as these two interventions were put into place, the conflict level between Alonzo and his mother was greatly reduced though not absent by any means.

Comment: In this case, it is clear that the parent's beliefs and expectations were influencing the child's feelings and beliefs. The intervention modified beliefs of the parent and child as well as teaching them the skill of collaborative problem-solving.

Guidelines for CBT-Oriented Treatment

Mental health providers may wish to consider the following guidelines to for a CBT-oriented approach in their work with children, adolescents, and their families.

Using CBT Principles

Familiarize oneself with, and utilize in each session, the principles of the CBT model. Cognitive therapists are active and directive, while creating an atmosphere that conveys a sense of 'teamwork' comprised of the therapist, the client, and if applicable, family members. That team utilizes structure (agenda and homework, for example) to work together cooperatively to explore existing beliefs and behaviors (collaborative empiricism), as well as to create new ones (skill-building and/or correcting distorted beliefs).

Assessment

Conduct assessment that includes instruments that will lead to a conceptualization that is specifically CBT-oriented and/or that are conducive to evidence-based practice, for example, semistructured interviews that have been used by researchers [58]. Semistructured interviews, in comparison to unstructured interviews, generally produce more reliable and valid diagnoses, as well as sometimes collecting broad-based information for the case conceptualization, leading to decisions about treatment [58] including the choice and timing of specific techniques or interventions. Specifically, as information is collected related to presenting problems and symptoms, the mental health provider frames the information according to the CBT model of the person (thinking–feeling–behavior–body). Similar to other models, assessment will also include the mutual inter-action between the person (child or adolescent) and the child's context, including family, school, culture, etc. Here, what distinguishes the CBT approach from other models is that the cognitive therapist listens for beliefs and observes behaviors (while connecting them to affect and physiological symptoms), so that the data can be organized into a CBT conceptualization. Thinking or cognition is further organized, to the degree that it is developmentally appropriate, into a system that reflects the way in which the client constructs his/her world. Common terms comprising this system include automatic thoughts, conditional beliefs/values/rules, and core beliefs/schemas.

A brief example may serve to clarify. Using three different scenarios that could occur, let's look at how different responses on the part of the caregiver may contribute to a difference in how interventions would be planned. Suppose a mother, Julie, brings her seven-year-old son, Danny, to see you because he has started to have nightmares within the past three months, around the same time she returned to full-time employment outside the home. The therapist, using collaboration, asks Julie if she has any ideas about what has triggered this episode and (to assess problem-solving ability) what she typically does to help him. Note that although this appears casual and conversational, the therapist is gathering information about the 'world view' (cognitions, beliefs, values, rules) of the caregiver and the caregiver's coping strategies (behaviors, skills, problem-solving abilities). This information is key, as children and adolescents are affected by and influenced by the cognitions and behaviors of their caregivers.

Scenario One

Julie: I think Danny is angry with me and spoiled. He always has to have things his way, I don't really think he wants me to work.
Therapist: And what do you do to help him when he wakes up?
Julie: I tell him to go back to bed and stop feeling sorry for himself. He's in first grade now and it's time to start growing up.

Scenario Two

Julie: I feel so guilty because I can't be there for him to be a good mom.
Therapist: And what do you do to help him when he wakes up?
Julie: I hold him for a few minutes and comfort him. And then after I tuck him in I can't get back to sleep

myself because I wonder if I'm permanently damaging him by sending him to daycare.

Scenario Three

Julie: I'm not really sure. Maybe it is just a phase.
Therapist: And what do you do to help him when he wakes up?
Julie: I don't really do anything, I mean, I try to console him by telling him we all have bad dreams sometimes but he just cries. I don't know if anything can really help. Won't he just grow out of it?

Admittedly, before knowing additional details about this child and family, one would not make major treatment decisions. However, after just two questions posed by the therapist, we see three very diverse responses that exemplify the worldviews of the caregivers and give important clues (evidence) which will be used by the therapist to add to the case formulation, eventually leading to hypotheses. As information from caregivers is collected, the therapist fits it with what is known about the child (organizing it according to thinking–feeling–behavior–body domains) and imagines (hypothesizes) the dynamic interplay both intrapersonally and interpersonally.

Quite possibly, the same cognitive techniques would eventually be used in all three scenarios, though perhaps in a different sequence. For example, education about development, education about anxiety, helping the caregiver learn how to soothe the child, or intervening directly with the child. However, the starting point would depend on the conceptualization. In scenario one, Julie is stressed and angry, while also not understanding how to be of comfort to Danny. She is likely to be defensive if told that her stress and statements to him may be exacerbating the problem. Therefore, I would start with the child as the focus (since she sees him as the 'problem'). I would explain to mom that he may benefit from learning how to help himself by learning relaxation exercises. For younger children, like Danny, I request that the caregiver learn the skills simultaneously so that they can support the child by helping them to remember homework assignments (practicing the skills) or in case the child 'forgets' something about the procedure between sessions. While explaining the skill to them both, I routinely mention that adults get stressed too, so can benefit from learning relaxation techniques. Rarely have I had an instance where a parent resisted this approach. Instead, parents express relief that someone recognizes their stress and doesn't blame them for it, yet gently encourages them to address it. If this aspect of treatment goes smoothly, and a solid relationship between myself and the caregiver begins to blossom, I then consider addressing parent beliefs. Specifically, for caregivers who are angry and stressed, it should be a gradual approach (maybe just addressing one of their beliefs as part of a session focused on the child) and one that conveys empathy. As the relationship becomes more well-established a more formal and direct focus on parent beliefs may be pursued.

Assessment procedures should be developmentally sensitive. As information is collected, the therapist organizes it within a CBT-oriented conceptualization. There are many assessment instruments available, and for young children, assessment will be done via interview and observation (probably during play or interacting with the caregiver). For school-age and younger adolescents, I prefer instruments that are particularly 'CBT-friendly.' For instance, the Beck Youth Inventories of Emotional and Social Impairment (BYI) [59], which were developed and normed for children aged 8–14 years, consists of five separate self-report inventories that measure levels of depression, anxiety, anger, disruptive behavior and self-concept. A 'combination' inventory is also available. Each 20-item inventory is written at the second grade reading level, can be completed within 5–10 minutes and scored easily by the therapist during the session, providing an opportunity for discussion of specific items and conveying information to the client and/or family members. I typically ask additional details about items, adding brief notes. A recent review [60] of the BYI notes its limitations, including insufficient evidence for their use by themselves to measure treatment effects. However, clinicians are well advised to consider assessment data, including results from self-report instruments, within the context of other information [61] about the child/adolescent and their functioning.

For assessing anger (ages 7–12 years), I have also used the Children's Anger Response Checklist (CARC) [62]. Features of the CARC that were particularly useful were the Likert-scale (operationalized using faces depicting different degrees of anger) and the fact that the scale uses 10 stories illustrating potentially frustrating situations. As the clinician and child explore the child's anger reaction to each situation, responses are organized according to the domains B, C, E, or P (behavioral, cognitive, emotional, and physiological). Although the 10 vignettes give a sense of the child's anger, in general, sometimes I wanted to gather information about events specific to a child. Therefore, using the general CARC format, I included vignettes based on issues that a particular child was grappling

with. Personally, I found the scoring to be time-consuming but clinically, the CARC yielded valuable qualitative information. For example, some children had absolutely no awareness of any physiological signs of anger (but their parents did!). Some children were eager to discuss their feelings, others became so upset during the CARC administration that we had to take a break and use coping skills before continuing.

As the therapist conducts the assessment, several questions (not necessarily mutually exclusive) the therapist wants to be able to answer fairly quickly (one to two visits) include:

- Are these child's presenting problem(s) due to deficiency or distortion?
- What is this child's 'system of thinking' (how has this child constructed his/her world and how well can the child articulate/understand information about feelings, thinking, behavior, and bodily symptoms?)
- Will it be helpful/necessary for the child's caregiver to be involved in treatment? If so, what will be their role?

The Working Model

Formulate your own 'working model' of the client that reflects a CBT orientation. In other words, the information about a child (or adolescent and their family) can be organized such that the child's thinking, feelings, behavior, and physical functioning present an internally consistent 'picture.' Furthermore, to the degree that it is possible (depending on developmental level), the formulation should include various levels of cognition (automatic thoughts, beliefs, conditional assumptions, rules, schemas) that comprise the client's 'system of thinking' about themselves, others (particularly significant people and events), and the future. For adolescents and some school-age children, the clinician can make use of Beck's Cognitive Conceptualization Diagram [39] to organize the material in a one-page format. Key would be the child's ability to articulate automatic thoughts as well as the accompanying feelings, etc.

Clearly, the more cognitively developed a child is, the more ability he/she will have to articulate such information. When that is not the case, however, the therapist makes inferences through observation and attempts to examine the evidence to for/against the inference. For example, the cardinal question of CBT, 'What was just now going through your mind?' in the presence of heightened affect is not generally developmentally appropriate for a five-year-old. Instead, information would be gathered during story telling or a structured play that touches on areas of difficulty for the child.

In my own experience, I have discovered several benefits of a well-developed (but continuously revised) conceptualization. First, even as this CBT-oriented 'picture' of the client continues to be refined, it provides a sense of continuity in my own thinking about the client, leading to an increased ability to recall details of the client's experiences as well as the ability to identify and explore recurrent themes. It can be quite comforting for client (and their caregivers) to find that they 'make sense' to someone else, even when they haven't been able to put the pieces together yet themselves. Second, the formulation allows for a quick guide to the timing and selection of intervention techniques, as well as how to tailor them to the individual. Finally, the conceptualization even guides the sharing of the conceptualization with the client (and/or caregiver). Why is this important? Because CBT is focused at two levels simultaneously: addressing current concerns while at the same time teaching skills that the client can utilize throughout the lifespan.

Blending Creative and Scientific Aspects

Integrate the creative and scientific aspects of treatment. The creative portion comes naturally to most practitioners in the caring professions and consists of the collaborative, warm, caring relationship which demonstrates to the client the humanity of the therapist. Without this foundation, even the most sophisticated, accurate and brilliant CBT intervention is likely to have minimal impact.

The scientific aspect of treatment includes using outcome measures and incorporating research findings, protocols or manuals and standard CBT techniques, as well as using a scientific approach to treatment. Some outcome measures have already been mentioned above, the results of which should be considered as data [61] in context of the overall picture of the child/adolescent. Frequency of administration of outcome measures can be adjusted depending on the severity of the client's symptoms, the number of measures and length of each, as well as time to score and interpret. Other factors that may influence the therapist's decision to have a client complete outcome measures over the course of treatment could be when there appears to be a significant change in symptom severity (increase or decrease), to help guide decisions regarding changes in frequency of sessions or when deciding to end treatment, and prior to reporting to a third party. For instance, when clients have been given

medication by another provider, it can be helpful feedback to the prescriber to have specific information. For example, 'When I saw this client at intake, the score they obtained on the Beck Depression Inventory for Youth [59] (BDI-Y) fell at the 88th percentile. Now, two months later, they have seen me for six sessions and because I knew they were coming to see you next Tuesday, I had them take the BDI-Y again, with a current score at the 67th percentile.' On the other hand, the conversation could go like this: 'When I saw this client at intake, the score they obtained on the BDI-Y fell at the 88th percentile. Their parent tells me they aren't due to see you again for another six weeks; however, today, when meeting with the family for the third session, the client completed the BDI-Y again and obtained a score at the 95th percentile.'

Empirical literature should be regularly reviewed in order for the clinician to stay familiar with what treatments appear to be the most effective, usually termed EST or EBT. Two recent collections of empirically based practices for children and adolescents [63,64] contain numerous CBT-oriented treatments, including information about specific disorders, age range treated, and parental involvement (whether and how much). Furthermore, specific and practical information about program protocols (delineated by sessions or steps) and manuals (for both therapist and clients) or assessment instruments are included. Treatment guidelines included in these resources address ADHD, anger for school age children, firesetting, OCD, ODD/CD, and anxiety, among others.

For example, the Coping Cat program developed at the Temple University Child and Adolescent Anxiety Disorders Clinic (CAADC) [9] is designed for children aged 7–13 years who have been diagnosed with anxiety disorders, including social phobia, generalized anxiety disorder, and separation anxiety. A total of 16–18 sessions (including two parent sessions) is divided into two phases. Phase one is oriented toward helping the client first acquire coping skills to deal with anxiety, then to practice the skills in phase two. Clients utilize the *Coping Cat Workbook* [65] in parallel with the treatment sessions. Therapists model the skills and assist with practice (exposure tasks).

Because a number of these treatment protocols were found to have effective treatment outcomes, therapists should use them. However, the manuals should be used in a flexible fashion. Doing so provides benefit to both therapist and client, as the therapist retains the freedom to utilize clinical skills to 'fit' the treatment to the client and his/her needs. This is best done based on the conceptualization of the client the therapist has developed. Furthermore, the client benefits as they get the 'best of both worlds' – treatment that has been shown to be effective for other children with similar problems but tailored specifically for him/her by a person who cares about and understands their particular situation. Since many of the evidence-based treatments or manuals use techniques that would be considered part of the standard CBT repertoire, therapists should be familiar with these techniques, the rationale for using them, and the general procedure for implementing them.

No matter whether a therapist is using EBT, adapting a manual, or individualizing CBT techniques and methods in treatment, it goes (almost) without saying that the therapist will combine their interpersonal skills with analytic skills to make clinical decisions and to evaluate progress. The standard way in which this is done is to use the scientific method that consists of the following feedback loop: data collection, development of hypothesis, testing of the hypothesis, then evaluating (i.e., data collection) leading to a revision of the hypothesis. This process occurs throughout each session as the clinician interacts with the client, makes choices about when and how to intervene, and then judges the outcome. An example will serve to illustrate how 'second-nature' this way of thinking becomes for the clinician.

EXAMPLE

Janine is a 13-year-old female who presented due to sleep problems once a week and anxiety in several domains of her life: school, appearance, and her mother who is having some medical issues but are not serious. Until the past quarter, she had always been on the Honor Roll. Being so bright and motivated to feel better, she easily grasped the CBT model, could identify her feelings and bodily symptoms, as well as articulate her automatic thoughts. By session 2, the therapist observes that Janine has many of the foundational abilities that are needed for her to learn about Thought Records thus plans to introduce them to her in session 3. For homework, the therapist suggests that Janine record anxious thoughts and rate how much they bother her, using a numeric rating from 1 to 10, 10 being the highest. When Janine returns to session 3, she reports that her sleep problems have worsened. At this point, the therapist wants to collect information so she can decide how best to proceed with the session:

Scenario One

Therapist: So, was there anything upsetting that happened during the week?

Janine: Well, my mom told me she has to get another medical test – for high blood pressure.

Therapist: And that made you feel?

Janine: Basically terrified.

Therapist: And did you write something about this on your list of anxious thoughts?

Janine: Yes, 'My mother might die.'

Therapist: Well that sounds pretty upsetting. Do you think that had anything to do with you having more sleep problems this week?

Janine: Yeah, I guess I hadn't really thought about it.

Therapist: Did you get a chance to talk with your mom yet?

Janine: No, I'm afraid to bring it up, could you help me talk with her?

Therapist: Sure, let's ask her to come into the session.

Comment: In this case, the therapist has enough information to hypothesize that Janine's anxiety about her mother may have exacerbated the sleep problems. By having her mother come into the session, the therapist shows empathy, support, and caring yet simultaneously plans to model for Janine how to talk with her mother about her concerns. Furthermore, in a sense, the information that will be discussed will be a variation of the Thought Record, as the therapist plans on showing the client how to gather evidence that will dispute her anxious thoughts about her mother dying. After they've first discussed it all, the therapist can assist Janine to write it down in a way that makes sense to her and that she can access again in the future.

Scenario Two

Therapist: So, was there anything upsetting that happened during the week?

Janine: Not really – just sort of the same.

Therapist: When did your sleep problems seem to get worse?

Janine: Well, maybe a couple days after I came here.

Therapist: What would be happening when you were sleeping?

Janine: Well, I was working on making that list of worries after I did my homework – like right before bed.

Therapist: Yes?

Janine: Well, then when I would wake up that was all that I kept thinking about.

Therapist: Your list? You mean, like 'I better get up and add something to it?'

Janine: No, more like everything that was on the list kept coming back into my head. Kind of how it was before – only worse.

Therapist: I see. And then it was hard for you to get back to sleep.

Janine: Yes.

Therapist: OK, tell you what. Would it be alright with you if I keep your list because I know you worked hard on it but I have something else that I want us to do today and we'll come back to the list later.

Janine: Sure.

Comment: In this case, the therapist hypothesizes that the sleep problems were exacerbated due to the client focusing on anxious thoughts. Therefore, although the client appears to have excellent cognitive abilities to engage in Thought Records, the therapist is going to switch temporarily to behavioral techniques (relaxation techniques such as abdominal breathing, progressive muscle relaxation, and distraction – music, for example) to help the client cope. Within a session or two, the therapist believes they will return to Thought Records, but she will take one thought at a time off the list that the client has allowed her to keep in the file in the therapy office. While the scientific method is not unique to CBT practitioners, the way in which the CBT practitioner collects (assessment instruments, the way in which questions are asked, etc.) and organizes information takes place within the context of a CBT framework.

Using Standard CBT Intervention

Familiarize yourself with standard CBT interventions while remembering to adapt them to the developmental level of the child or adolescent. Details of CBT interventions and techniques are described elsewhere; however, the CBT therapist would have in their 'toolbox' a collection of both behavioral and cognitive techniques. Typical behavioral techniques include relaxation training, distraction, systematic desensitization, modeling, role-playing, pleasant activity scheduling, graduated exposure (imaginal and *in vivo*), behavioral experiments, and contingency management (including shaping, extinction, positive reinforcement and punishment). Typical cognitive techniques include guided discovery using Socratic questioning, examining the evidence to address cognitive distortions, self-instruction, and problem solving. Frequently, both cognitive and behavioral techniques may be combined in a single intervention, for example, into a 'lesson' or module [66,67]. In fact, clinicians are advised to consider collecting 'empirically supported treatment modules' [32].

The therapist, then, instead of thinking of treatment as a string of interventions, considers the overall stages of components of treatment needed in order to address the child's problems. A good example of this is described by Kendall and colleagues [66] in working with anxious children. Although the Coping Cat program uses a treatment protocol, with two phases: education and exposure, the overall strategy of treatment could be conceptualized in 'modules' consisting of somatic education, relaxation, self-talk, exposure, self-reward, and consolidation. Each module may consist of several cognitive and/or behavioral interventions. For example, a goal of the self-talk 'module' would be to help the child identify his anxious feelings and related anxious thought(s), but then to generate an alternative thought that would help reduce anxiety level. During the education phase of treatment, the child may be learning about his/her anxiety as well as how to potentially cope via self-talk. During the exposure phase, the skills are actually put into practice.

One of the most challenging tasks of the CBT practitioner is to adapt standard interventions to a child's developmental level, especially at younger ages. As there is scant empirical information available for younger aged children, the practitioner needs to utilize a scientific approach, as previously described. In general, some rules-of-thumb to follow in this area include:

- the younger the child, the more often caregivers will be involved;
- the younger the child, the more often treatment will consist of behavioral interventions;
- the younger the child, the more often treatment will be activity or play-based;
- the younger the child, the more often treatment will address deficiencies (versus distortions);
- the younger the child, treatment will occur *in vivo* (caregiver would carry out homework assignments or support child to do so);
- the younger the child, the less often the conceptualization is shared (but may be shared with caregiver).

Adapting interventions to the child or adolescent's developmental stage and individual interests appears to increase the effectiveness of the treatment, since it would be relevant and interesting, probably increasing motivation. Let us examine how a cognitive technique – Thought Records – might be developmentally adapted.

In general, adolescents can be treated more similarly to adults in terms of their ability to self-reflect and engage in analysis. Frequently, when I have presented the Thought Record to adolescents and asked them to complete between-session samples, they see it as another homework task. So, instead I find out about their interests – journaling, poetry, art, music – to make use of what they already do as a vehicle of discovery. Amanda, a 17-year-old female, who presented with anger (especially at home) and depression, had experienced a recent breakup. When she told me about the paintings and drawings she enjoyed doing, I asked her to bring some into the session. Seeing such work is a powerful communication to the therapist! As she described her work to me, I asked the cardinal CBT question, 'What was going through your mind?' to obtain information while also assisting her to connect her thoughts and feelings, as well as to address her frequent belief 'I'll never find another boyfriend.'

For school-age children, having brief, engaging, and structured written work is quite similar to school tasks. Therefore, a workbook like *Therapeutic Exercises for Children* [40] (TEC) is ideal. TEC consists of 18 exercises designed for children aged 8–12 years who are struggling with anxiety or depression. Each exercise has a name, guidelines for the therapist, tips for children, and a sample. Specifically, the Thought Record has been developmentally adapted with the exercise Catching Feelings and Thoughts, making use of illustrations, coloring, and thought bubbles. Another workbook available online (electronic book available at *www.netLibrary.com*), *Think Good, Feel Good: A Comprehensive Behaviour Therapy Workbook for Children and Young People* [46] contains CBT-oriented exercises and worksheets.

It would be unlikely that I would attempt to adapt a Thought Record for a child under the age of eight years because Thought Records assume the presence of a 'distortion' and has the goal of refuting it with a logical analysis by examining the evidence. At this age, treatment occurs more often in the here-and-now (*in vivo*). Therefore, I would typically use play, drawing, storytelling, puppets, games with or without parent participation. Depending on the presenting issue, I would try to design the session so that it would bring to light issues that need to be addressed. For example, suppose a six-year-old girl, Janie, tells you that nobody likes her or ever wants to play with her. You find from talking with her teacher that other children do keep a bit distant from her since she tends to be somewhat 'bossy.' Play in the sessions can be set up to help her learn turn-taking and/or problem-solving. This can be accomplished first by reading a book [68] about the difficulties of sharing

and assessing the child's ability to recognize affect (her own and others') or by the therapist putting on a puppet show. Sharing skills could then be modeled by the puppets, then practiced by the client in the session.

Role of Psychoeducation

Use client and/or parent education to promote understanding of the CBT model and CBT techniques, as well as their relevance to the client in his/her life. This process actually starts with the initial contact and continues throughout treatment. An obvious way in which education occurs is with the CBT interventions themselves. Suppose the treatment of an anxious child, Dee, is going to involve relaxation and distraction techniques, cognitive restructuring, and exposure. Unless contraindicated, I prefer to have the parent and child together when I am explaining general treatment approach (except in the case of very young children) and usually direct my conversation to the child at their level with the parent observing. Several benefits follow. The child receives treatment aimed at their capacity and the parent has the opportunity to observe how I will be interacting with their child. Furthermore, the parent becomes familiar with the content so they can understand and support their child's treatment.

A second way in which education occurs is whenever the conceptualization is explained. Again, depending on the circumstances, the way in which I share the conceptualization is individualized for each client. Generally speaking, when treatment goals are initially formulated and we decide to focus on particular skills or interventions, I provide the rationale framed in CBT terms. As treatment progresses, I have found that other parts of the conceptualization may come to light. At a later point in treatment, different parts of the conceptualization may be able to be linked together.

A third aspect of education concerns homework or between-session assignments to help the child practice the skills, whether behavioral or cognitive. The explanation I usually give for the assignments is that it will be hard to feel much better if the only time they practice new ways of thinking and feeling is in my office. Homework assignments, like interventions within sessions, are fit to the developmental level of the child. For example, school age children can use structured workbooks but adolescents may prefer to write poems or keep journals to explore their feelings and thoughts.

A final (last but definitely not least) way to utilize education is to assist parents in exploring general issues like development or to find additional information about the particular issues their child might be dealing with, such as anxiety or depression. Education is not particular to CBT providers; however, as a CBT-oriented provider, I prefer to recommend materials that are consistent with the model and that fit the interests and time constraints of the parents. Two general development books I frequently recommend are *Your Child* [69] and *Your Adolescent* [70], both edited by a past-president of the American Academy of Child and Adolescent Psychiatry. For knowledge about emotional development, the books by the Philadelphia Child Guidance Center (covering young children [71], childhood [72], and adolescence [73]) are beneficial. A good source for helping parents to understand how to handle their child's (unpleasant) emotions is *The Heart of Parenting* [74] audiotape with or without its companion book [57]. For parents who want to examine and alter beliefs about themselves and their children, I recommend *Why Can't I Be The Parent I Want to Be?* [75]. Parents of anxious children may want to review *Helping Your Anxious Child* [76] or *Worried No More* [77]. For parents whose children struggle with OCD, *Freeing Your Child From Obsessive–Compulsive Disorder* [78] and *What To Do When your Child has Obsessive–Compulsive Disorder* [79] may be helpful . . . *More Than Moody* [80] describes and explains depression in adolescence, while *Helping Your Teen Beat Depression* [81] takes a problem-solving stance. For parents who want online, easy to access information, sites such as *www.aboutourkids.org* are extremely useful, covering a wide array of topics.

Importance of Feedback

Seek feedback from the client and/or caregivers, both informally and formally. Some agencies have used a written feedback form that can be completed periodically, as often as after each therapy session. In addition, as part of the CBT session structure, feedback is given/asked for toward the end of the session. Feedback is likely to be part of any therapist's work, so what is different about this process for a CBT provider?

As a CBT therapist, I view feedback (especially negative) as absolutely vital! That is why I have learned to encourage it and welcome it. Numerous benefits occur when the client is encouraged in this direction. First, it adds to the sense of collaboration and to the therapeutic relationship. Second, since feedback is seen as a two-way exchange, it reduces (though probably does not eliminate) the power-differential inherent in the therapist–client relationship. Third, the therapist can get a sense of client (or caregiver) beliefs, always adding this information to expand the conceptualization.

Although part of the CBT session structure is to solicit feedback, in my experience, I have found that clients seemed to give me responses like 'fine' or 'Everything was good.' Instead, I have developed several ways of making sure to give the client the message that the sessions are a safe place to give feedback (including negative) by doing the following.

During the session (usually session 2) when I socialize the client to the CBT model, I explain that we will be working together 'like a team, to help you/your child with your problems. Therefore, it is really important and helpful if you tell me when something I say doesn't make sense or if you don't agree with it. Do you think you can do that?' Frequently, this begins to elicit client beliefs. For example, if the response is, 'But I don't want to hurt your feelings,' then I might ask for an example of what would be 'horrible enough' to hurt my feelings and address their concerns. If the response is more like, 'But you are the expert and I should not be questioning you' I give them permission to do so, explaining that their concerns may not have anything to do with my expertise.

However, having such conversations only at the outset of treatment is not enough. Therefore, I have incorporated listening for feedback or asking for it once or twice (or at key points) during a session. That way it becomes second-nature to the client and is part of our ongoing 'dialogue.' Key points have become fairly clear to me by attending to client affect, then asking the cardinal question, 'What just went through your mind?' For example, when working with a mother of a four-year-old female who was having trouble with transitions and complying with commands, I had spent several sessions modeling behavioral techniques like ignoring and redirection. As I 'coached' the mother, preparing her to use these techniques for a few minutes at the next session, her affect shifted, getting 'cloudy.' As I asked 'What was going through your mind?' she hesitantly responded by saying 'You are asking me to do something before I am ready' related to her feeling irritable and anxious. With this information, I was able to find out more about how to support her and to address her concerns. This brief interaction strengthened our relationship but alerted me to her belief that she lacked a skill, a concern which could be addressed.

Finally, another method for obtaining feedback is via written forms. Some practitioners use brief client self-report measures that specifically assess the strength of the therapeutic relationship [82]. These would likely be most appropriate for adolescents or parents involved in treatment. In addition, Friedberg *et al.* [83] developed written feedback forms specifically for children aged 8–11 and 12–16 years to measure engagement as well as what was helpful (or not) to the client.

Promoting Professional Growth

Monitor and expand your development as a cognitive therapist. Development occurs at two frequently overlapping levels, personal and professional. At the personal level, CBT practitioners can learn much from paying attention to their own automatic thoughts [54] during the therapy process and about various issues concerning clients. In fact, completing Thought Records to examine one's own automatic thoughts and related emotions, as well as completing a self-conceptualization using the Cognitive Conceptualization Diagram [39] can be quite informative. As one gets in the habit of reflecting on the cardinal question 'What just went through my mind?' there is an ever-increasing awareness of the connection between one's own thoughts and feelings, and this information can be used during sessions. In fact, at times it may be appropriate to self-disclose (for the benefit of the client) automatic thoughts or feelings. For example, Jake, a 14-year-old male, who presented for depression comes in for the sixth session, and once again, 'forgot' to bring his homework. You notice you feel irritated but don't realize it shows until he tentatively asks 'Are you mad at me?' At that point, you can deny it (and deprive him of his accurate perception) or you can acknowledge the truth, explaining, 'Yeah, I noticed that I am kind of frustrated and what was going through my mind is that you must feel real overwhelmed and it's hard to do anything because the last time you were here we tried to make your homework as easy as possible. It is more that I want to see you start to feel better and be able to do start to do things to help yourself.' This very brief self-disclosure accomplishes a number of objectives: it builds rapport by being open to feedback from the client and showing one's own humanity, it models the ability to connect feeling and thought, and demonstrates that the therapist both understands the depth of the client's distress without criticizing him and believes that the client will be able to help himself at some point in the future.

To enhance your professional development as a CBT practitioner, seek consultation or supervision from a well-trained cognitive behavioral therapist (see *www.academyofct.org* to locate someone in your area), attend workshops that are presented by well-known child and adolescent CBT-practitioners, and make use of the Cognitive Therapy Rating Scale (CTRS) [84]. The CTRS, available from the Beck Institute, is a tool that can be used to evaluate the strengths and weakness of a cognitive therapist. Join organizations such as the Academy of Cognitive Therapy (ACT) and Association for Behavioral and Cognitive Therapy (ABCT, formerly known as AABT – Association for Advancement of Behavior Therapy). ABCT has an annual convention during which you can find workshops by leaders in CBT. Finally, read CBT-oriented literature, particularly *Cognitive Therapy: Basics and Beyond* [39], especially the sections covering guidelines in treatment planning and problems encountered in therapy. For information specific to children and adolescents, read *Clinical Practice of Cognitive Therapy with Children and Adolescents: The Nuts and Bolts* [30] for a source that is loyal to the basic CBT theory as well as including many practical suggestions that can be applied in daily practice. Finally, add CBT-oriented websites (*www.beckinstitute.org* and *www.academyofct.org*) to your Favorites list on your computer and review them regularly.

Summary

The CBT model has shown to be a promising approach to ameliorating the psychological problems of adults and more recently, to those of children and adolescents. Although much more work needs to be done to extend the model further 'downward' and 'outward' to culturally diverse groups, the hard work of various groups (researchers, clinicians, developmental experts) has come together in a confluence that is having an enormous positive impact on the course of mental health treatment for youth.

References

1. Hibbs ED, Jensen PS, eds: *Psychosocial Treatments for Child and Adolescent Disorders: Empirically Based Strategies for Clinical Practice.* Washington, DC, American Psychological Association, 1996.
2. Kazdin AE, Weisz JR: Introduction: Context and background of evidence-based psychotherapies for children and adolescents. In: Kazdin AE, Weisz JR, eds. *Evidence-Based Psychotherapies for Children and Adolescents.* New York: Guilford, 2003:3–20.
3. Mash EJ, Dozois DJA: Child psychopathology: A developmental-systems perspective. In: Mash EJ, Barkley RA, eds. *Child Psychopathology.* 2nd ed. New York: Guilford, 2003:3–71.
4. Lyddon WJ, Jones Jr. JV, eds: *Empirically Supported Cognitive Therapies: Current and Future Applications.* New York: Springer: 2001.
5 Compton SN, March JS, Brent D, Albano AM, Weersing R, Curry J: Cognitive-behavioral psychotherapy for anxiety and depressive disorders in children and

adolescents: An evidence-based medicine review. *J Am Acad Child Adolesc Psychiatry* 2004; **43**(8): 930–959.

6. Christophersen ER, Mortweet SL: *Treatments That Work With Children: Empirically Supported Strategies for Managing Childhood Problems.* Washington, DC: American Psychological Association, 2001.

7. Daleiden EL, Vasey MW, Brown LM: Internalizing disorders. In: Silverman WK, Ollendick TH, eds. *Developmental Issues in the Clinical Treatment of Children.* Boston: Allyn and Bacon, 1999:261–278.

8. D'Eramo KS, Francis G: Cognitive-behavioral psychotherapy. In: Morris TL, March JS, eds. *Anxiety Disorders in Children and Adolescents,* 2nd ed. New York: Guilford, 2004:305–328.

9. Kendall PC, Aschenbrand SG, Hudson JL: Child-focused treatment of anxiety. In: Kazdin AE, Weisz JR, eds. *Evidence-Based Psychotherapies for Children and Adolescents.* New York: Guilford, 2003:81–100.

10. Albano AM, Detweiler MF, Logsdon-Conradsen S: Cognitive-behavioral interventions with socially phobic children. In: Russ SW, Ollendick TH, eds. *Handbook of Psychotherapies with Children and Families.* New York: Plenum Publishers, 1999:255–280.

11. Albano AM, March JS, Piacentini J: Obsessive-compulsive disorder. In: Ammerman RT, Hersen M, Last CG, eds. *Handbook of Prescriptive Treatments for Children and Adolescents.* 2nd ed. Boston: Allyn & Bacon, 1999:193–213.

12. March JS, Mulle K: *OCD in Children and Adolescents: A Cognitive-Behavioral Treatment Manual.* New York: Guilford, 1998.

13. Clarke GN, DeBar LL, Lewinsohn PM: Cognitive-behavioral group treatment for adolescent depression. In: Kazdin AE, Weisz JR, eds. *Evidence-Based Psychotherapies for Children and Adolescents.* New York: Guilford, 2003:120–134.

14. Stark KD, Vaughn C, Doxey M, Luss L: Depressive disorders. In: Ammerman RT, Hersen M, Last CG, eds. *Handbook of Prescriptive Treatments for Children and Adolescents,* 2nd ed. Boston: Allyn & Bacon, 1999:114–140.

15. Weersing VR, Brent DA: Cognitive-behavioral therapy for adolescent depression: Comparative efficacy, mediation, moderation, and effectiveness. In: Kazdin AE, Weisz JR, eds. *Evidence-Based Psychotherapies for Children and Adolescents.* New York: Guilford, 2003:135–147.

16. Weissman MM, Sanderson WC: Promises and problems in modern psychotherapy: The need for increased training in evidence based treatments. In *Josiah Macy, Jr. Foundation Conference, Modern Psychiatry: Challenges in Educating Health Professionals to Meet New Needs'* October 2001, Toronto, Canada.

17. Weisz JR, Southam-Gerow MA, Gordis EB, Connor-Smith J: Primary and secondary enhancement training for youth depression. In: Kazdin AE, Weisz JR, eds. *Evidence-Based Psychotherapies for Children and Adolescents.* New York: Guilford, 2003:165–183.

18. Ammerman RT, Hersen M, Last CG, eds: *Handbook of Prescriptive Treatments for Children and Adolescents,* 2nd ed. Boston: Allyn & Bacon, 1999.

19. Anastapoulos AD, Farley SE. A cognitive-behavioral training program for parents of children with attention-deficit/hyperactivity disorder. In: Kazdin AE, Weisz JR,

eds. *Evidence-Based Psychotherapies for Children and Adolescents.* New York: Guilford, 2003:187–203.

20. Kazdin AE: Child, parent, and family-based treatment of aggressive and antisocial child behavior. In: Hibbs ED, Jensen PS, eds. *Psychosocial Treatments for Child and Adolescent Disorders: Empirically Based Strategies for Clinical Practice,* 2nd ed. Washington, DC: American Psychological Association, 2005:445–476.

21. Kazdin AE: Problem-solving skills training and parent management training for conduct disorder. In: Kazdin AE, Weisz JR, eds. *Evidence-Based Psychotherapies for Children and Adolescents.* New York: Guilford, 2003:241–262.

22. Larson J, Lochman JE: *Helping Schoolchildren Cope with Anger: A Cognitive-Behavioral Intervention.* New York: Guilford, 2002.

23. Lochman JE, Barry TD, Pardini DA. Anger control training for aggressive youth. In: Kazdin AE, Weisz JR, eds. *Evidence-Based Psychotherapies for Children and Adolescents.* New York: Guilford, 2003:263–281.

24. Fisher CB, Hatashita-Wong M, Greene LI: Ethical and legal issues. In: Silverman WK, Ollendick TH, eds. *Developmental Issues in the Clinical Treatment of Children.* Boston: Allyn and Bacon, 1999:470–486.

25. Rae WA, Fournier CJ: Ethical and legal issues in the treatment of children and families. In: Russ SW, Ollendick TH, eds. *Handbook of Psychotherapies with Children and Families.* New York: Plenum Publishers, 1999:67–83.

26. DeKraai MB, Sales BD, Hall SR: Informed consent, confidentiality, and duty to report laws in the conduct of child therapy. In: Morris RJ, Kratochwill TR, eds. *The Practice of Child Therapy*, 3rd ed. Boston: Allyn and Bacon, 1998,540–559.

27. Kendall PC: Guiding theory for therapy with children and adolescents. In: Kendall PC, ed. *Child and Adolescent Therapy: Cognitive-Behavioral Procedures.* New York: Guilford, 2000:3–27.

28. Kendall PC, Warman MJ: Emotional disorders in youth. In: Salkovskis PM, ed. *Frontiers of Cognitive Therapy.* New York: Guilford, 1996:509–530.

29. Friedberg RD, Crosby LE, Friedberg BA, Rutter JG, Knight KR: Making cognitive behavioral therapy user-friendly to children. *Cognit Behav Pract* 1999; **6**(3):189–200.

30. Friedberg RD, McClure JM. *Clinical Practice of Cognitive Therapy with Children and Adolescents: The Nuts and Bolts.* New York: Guilford, 2002.

31. Ronen T. *Cognitive Developmental Therapy with Children.* New York: Wiley, 1997.

32. Holmbeck GN, Greenley RN, Franks EA: Developmental issues and considerations in research and practice. In: Kazdin AE, Weisz JR, eds. *Evidence-Based Psychotherapies for Children and Adolescents.* New York: Guilford, 2003:21–41.

33. Kendall PC: *Child and Adolescent Therapy: Cognitive-Behavioral Procedures.* New York: Guilford, 2000.

34. Kendall PC, MacDonald JP: Cognition in the psychopathology of youth and implications for treatment. In: Dobson KS, Kendall PC, eds. *Psychopathology and Cognition.* San Diego: Academic Press, 1993: 387–427.

35. Kendall PC, Stark KD, Adam T: Cognitive deficit or cognitive distortion of childhood depression. *J Abnorm Child Psychol* 1990; **18**:255–270.

36. Shirk S: Development and cognitive therapy. *J Cognit Psychother* 2001; **15**:155–163.

37. Siqueland L, Diamond GS: Engaging parents in cognitive behavioral treatment for children with anxiety disorders. *Cognit Behav Pract* 1998; **5**:81–102.

38. Silverman WK, Ollendick TH, eds. *Developmental Issues in the Clinical Treatment of Children.* Boston: Allyn and Bacon, 1991.

39. Beck JS: *Cognitive Therapy: Basics and Beyond.* New York: Guilford, 1995.

40. Friedberg RD, Friedberg BA, Friedberg RJ: *Therapeutic Exercises for Children: Guided Discovery Using Cognitive-Behavioral Techniques.* Sarasota, FL: Professional Resource Press, 2001.

41. Krain AL, Kendall PC: Cognitive-behavioral therapy. In: Russ SW, Ollendick TH, eds. *Handbook of Psychotherapies with Children and Families.* New York: Plenum Publishers, 1999:121–135.

42. Beck AT, Rush AJ, Shaw BF, Emery G: *Cognitive Therapy of Depression.* New York: Guilford, 1979.

43. Clark D A, Steer RA: Empirical status of the cognitive model of anxiety and depression. In: Salkovskis PM, ed. *Frontiers of Cognitive Therapy.* New York: Guilford, 1996:75–96.

44. Greenberger D, Padesky CA: *Mind Over Mood: A Cognitive Therapy Treatment Manual for Clients.* New York: Guilford, 1995.

45. Beck AT: *Cognitive Therapy and the Emotional Disorders.* New York: International Universities Press, 1976.

46. Stallard P: *Think Good, Feel Good [Electronic Resource]: a Cognitive Behaviour Therapy Workbook for Children and Young People.* Chichester: West Sussex: John Wiley & Sons, 2002.

47. Schniering CA, Rapee RM: The relationship between automatic thoughts and negative emotions in children and adolescents: A test of cognitive content-specificity hypothesis. *J Abnorm Psychol* 2004; **113**:464–470.

48. Greene RW, Ablon JS, Monuteaux MC, Goring JC, Henin A, Raezer-Blakely L, *et al.*: Effectiveness of collaborative problem solving in affectively dysregulated children with oppositional-defiant disorder: Initial findings. *J Consul Clin Psychol* 2004; **72**:1157–1164.

49. Knell SM: *Cognitive-Behavioral Play Therapy.* Northvale, New Jersey: Jason Aronson, Inc., 1993.

50. Knell SM: Cognitive-behavioral play therapy. In: Russ SW, Ollendick TH, eds. *Handbook of Psychotherapies with Children and Families.* New York: Plenum Press, 1999:385–404.

51. Russ SW: *Play in Child Development and Psychotherapy: Toward Empirically Supported Practice.* Mahwah, NJ: Lawrence Erlbaum Associates, 2004.

52. Needleman LD: *Cognitive Case Conceptualization: A Guidebook for Practitioners.* Mahwah, NJ: Lawrence Erlbaum Associates, 1999.

53. Padesky CA: Developing cognitive therapist competency: Teaching and supervision models. In: Salkovskis PM, ed. *Frontiers of Cognitive Therapy.* New York: Guilford, 1996:266–292.

54. Persons JB: *Cognitive Therapy in Practice: A Case Formulation Approach.* New York: Norton, 1989.

55. Reinecke MA, Dattilio FM, Freeman A: What makes for an effective treatment? In: Reinecke MA, Dattilio FM, Freeman A, eds. *Cognitive Therapy with Children and Adolescents: A Casebook for Clinical Practice,* 2nd ed. New York: Guilford, 2003:1–18.

56. Kendall PC, Panichelli-Mindel SM: Cognitive-behavioral treatments. *J Abnorm Child Psychol* 1995; **23**:107–124.

57. Gottman JM: *The Heart of Parenting: How to Raise an Emotionally Intelligent Child.* New York, NY: Simon & Schuster, 1997.

58. Silverman WK, Kurtines WM: Progress in developing an exposure-based transfer-of-control approach to treating internalizing disorders in youth. In: Hibbs ED, Jensen PS, eds. *Psychosocial Treatments for Child and Adolescent Disorders: Empirically Based Strategies for Clinical Practice,* 2nd ed. Washington, DC: American Psychological Association, 2005:445–476.

59. Beck JS, Beck AT, Jolly JB: *Beck Youth Inventories of Emotional & Social Impairment (BYI).* San Antonio, TX: Psychological Corporation, 2001.

60. Bose-Deakins JE, Floyd RG: A review of the Beck youth inventories of emotional and social impairment. *J Sch Psychol* 2004; **42**:333–340.

61. Seligman LD, Ollendick TH, Langley AK, Baldacci HB: The utility of measures of child and adolescent anxiety. *J Clin Child Adolesc Psychol* 2004; **33**:557–565.

62. Feindler EL, Adler N, Brooks D, Bhumitra E: The children's anger response checklist: CARC. In: VandeCreek L, ed. *Innovations in Clinical Practice: A Sourcebook.* Sarasota, FL: Professional Resource Press, 1993, Vol. **12**:337–362.

63. Hibbs ED, Jensen PS, eds. *Psychosocial Treatments for Child and Adolescent Disorders: Empirically Based Strategies for Clinical Practice,* 2nd ed. Washington, DC: American Psychological Association, 2005.

64. Kazdin AE, Weisz JR, eds. *Evidence-Based Psychotherapies for Children and Adolescents.* New York: Guilford, 2003.

65. Kendall PC: *Coping Cat Workbook.* Ardmore, PA: Workbook Publishing, 1990.

66. Kendall PC, Chu B, Gifford A, Hayes C, Nauta M: Breathing life into a manual: Flexibility and creativity with manual-based treatments. *Cognit Behav Pract* 1998; **5**:177–198.

67. Curry JF, Reinecke MA: Modular therapy for adolescents with major depression. In: Reinecke MA, Dattilio FM, Freeman A, eds. *Cognitive Therapy with Children and Adolescents.* 2nd ed. New York: Guilford, 2003: 95–127.

68. Ginns-Gruenberg D, Zacks A: Bibliotherapy: The use of children's literature as a therapeutic tool. In: Schaefer C, ed. *Innovative Psychotherapy Techniques in Child and Adolescent Therapy.* 2nd ed. New York: John Wiley & Sons, Inc., 1999:454–490.

69. Pruitt DB, ed. *Your Child: What Every Parent Needs to Know About Childhood Development from Birth to Preadolescence.* New York: HarperCollins Publishers, 1998.

70. Pruitt DB, ed. *Your Adolescent: Emotional, Behavioral, and Cognitive Development from Early Adolescence Through the Teen Years.* New York: HarperCollins Publishers, 1999.

71. Philadelphia Child Guidance Center, Maguire J: *Your Child's Emotional Health: The Early Years.* New York: Macmillan, 1994.

72. Philadelphia Child Guidance Center, Maguire J: *Your Child's Emotional Health: The Middle Years.* New York: Macmillan, 1994.

73. Philadelphia Child Guidance Center, Maguire J: *Your Child's Emotional Health: Adolescence.* New York: Macmillan, 1994.

74. Gottman J: *The Heart of Parenting: Raising an Emotionally Intelligent Child.* Los Angeles: Audio Renaissance Tapes, 1997.

75. Elliott CH, Smith LL: *Why Can't I be the Parent I Want to be?* Oakland, CA: New Harbinger, 1999.

76. Rapee RM, Spence SH, Cobham V, Wignall A: *Helping Your Anxious Child: A Step-by-Step Guide for Parents.* Oakland, CA: New Harbinger Publications, Inc., 2000.

77. Wagner AP: *Worried No More: Help and Hope for Anxious Children.* Rochester, NY: Lighthouse Press, Inc., 2002.

78. Chansky TE: *Freeing Your Child from Obsessive-Compulsive Disorder.* New York: Crown Publishers, 2000.

79. Wagner AP: *What to do When Your Child has Obsessive-Compulsive Disorder: Strategies and Solutions.* Rochester, NY: Lighthouse Press, Inc., 2002.

80. Koplewicz HS. *More than Moody: Recognizing and Treating Adolescent Depression.* New York: G.P. Putnam's & Sons, 2002.

81. Manassis K, Levac AM: *Helping your Teenager Beat Depression.* Bethesda, MD: Woodbine House, Inc., 2004.

82. Burns DD: *Therapist's Toolkit: Comprehensive Assessment and Treatment Tools for the Mental Health Professional.* Los Altos Hills, CA: David D. Burns MD, 1995.

83. Friedberg RD, Miller R, Perymon A, Bottoms J, Aatre G: Using a session feedback form in cognitive therapy with children. *J Rational-Emotive Cognitive Behav Ther* 2004; **22**(3):219–230.

84. Young J, Beck AT: *Cognitive Therapy Scale: Rating Manual.* Unpublished manuscript. Philadelphia: University of Pennsylvania, 1980.

Section II
Common Child and Adolescent Psychiatric Disorders

10

Attention Deficit Hyperactivity Disorder

David Rube, Dorothy P. Reddy

Introduction

Attention deficit hyperactivity disorder (ADHD) is one of the most common neuropsychiatric conditions of childhood and adolescence, accounting for as much as 50% of child psychiatry clinic populations [1]. ADHD is a persistent problem, manifesting its core symptoms throughout the life cycle, from preschool through adult life. ADHD symptoms interfere with a child's family and peer interactions, academic attainment, emotional development and self-esteem and in overall quality of life. Given the high prevalence, impairment and societal cost of ADHD, treatment is essential.

ADHD is the most highly studied child psychiatric disorder and fortunately, there are a multitude of evidence-based medication and psychosocial treatments available. The American Academy of Child and Adolescent Psychiatry recently established practice parameters for ADHD [2]. There are more than 400 references for those parameters. Thousands of papers have been published in journals by practitioners of all the disciplines that care for children – pediatricians, child and adolescent psychiatrists, developmental and behavioral pediatricians, and child psychologists.

The purpose of this chapter is to provide the reader with an overview of the history of this disorder, its diagnostic criteria and presentation, epidemiology and etiology, and a brief description of the developmental differences in the child, adolescent, and adult. In an overview of the assessment process, based on the practice parameters established by the American Academy of Child and Adolescent Psychiatry, differential diagnosis including comorbidity, treatment planning, and prognosis and outcome are described. The goal is to provide the reader with a hands-on approach to this very common yet potentially devastating problem for children and their families.

History

References to individuals having problems with inattention, hyperactivity, and impulsivity can be found as early as the Renaissance when Shakespeare made reference to an 'attention deficit' in one of his characters in *Henry VIII*. A poem entitled 'Fidgety Phil' was written by a German physician, Heinrich Hoffman [3]. William James, in his *Principles of Psychology*, described a normal variant of character that resembles the difficulty experienced by children today who are diagnosed with ADHD [4].

Clinical interests expanded when an English physician, George Still, reported on a group of 20 children whom he described as having a deficit in 'volitional inhibition' [5]. He described them as 'aggressive, passionate, lawless, inattentive, impulsive, and overactive.' He reported that there was an overrepresentation of male subjects, a family history of alcoholism, criminal conduct, and depression, a family predisposition, and the possibility that the condition may arise from an injury to the nervous system. Still's observations are quite common and have been corroborated in later research.

In North America, children who survived the great encephalitis epidemics of 1917 and 1918 were noted to have many behavioral problems similar to those constituting what we call ADHD [6–8]. The cases that were reported and others that have arisen due to birth trauma, head injury, exposure, or infections gave rise to the idea of a 'brain injured child syndrome.' This concept evolved into that of minimal brain damage and eventually minimal brain dysfunction. Many challenges were raised to this label, however, because of the lack of evidence of brain injury in many of the children who exhibited the symptoms.

In the late 1950s and early 1960s, the 'hyperactive child syndrome' was described by Burks [9,10] and

---

Clinical Child Psychiatry, Second Edition. Edited by W.M. Klykylo and J.L. Kay

Chess [11]. That syndrome was typified by daily movement that was greater than that of normal children of the same age. In the late 1960s, under the influence of the psychoanalytic movement, the second edition [11] of the *Diagnostic and Statistical Manual of Mental Disorders* (DSM-II) described all childhood disorders as 'reactions,' and the hyperactive child syndrome became the 'hyperkinetic reaction of childhood.' It was defined as a disorder of overactivity, restlessness, distractibility, and short attention span. It was asserted that the behavior usually diminishes in adolescence, leading to the ongoing myth that ADHD 'disappears in adolescence.' DSM-II included for the first time symptoms of inattention, and by the 1970s research emphasized the problem of inattention and poor impulse control in addition to hyperactivity. Douglas [12–14] theorized that the disorder consisted of four major deficits in the following areas: (1) the maintenance of attention and effort; (2) the ability to inhibit impulse control; (3) the ability to modulate arousal levels to meet situational demands; and (4) the ability to delay immediate gratification. Eventually, Douglas' work and other work like it led to a renaming of the disorder as attention deficit disorder (ADD) in 1980 in DSM-III, [15] in which it was noted that it was not simply a behavioral reaction of childhood. The cognitive and developmental nature of the disorder was emphasized, and specific symptom lists and cut-off scores were recommended for each of the three major symptom clusters (inattention measurements, hyperactivity, and impulsivity) to assist with the identification of the disorder. DSM-III distinguished two types of ADD, that with hyperactivity (H) and that without it.

In the DSM-III-R, [16] the disorder was renamed ADHD (attention deficit hyperactivity disorder), with a single list of items incorporating all three symptoms and a single threshold for diagnosis. At that time, there was insufficient research to verify the existence of attention deficit disorder without hyperactivity. In DSMIII-R, ADD without H is relegated to the category named undifferentiated attention deficit disorder, with the specification that insufficient research existed to construct diagnostic criteria. Since the publication of the DSM-III-R, researchers have found that the problems with hyperactivity and impulsivity were not separate but formed a single dimension of behavior. These conclusions led to the creation of two separate symptom lists when DSM-IV was published in 1994 [17]. The establishment of the inattention list once again permitted the diagnosis of a subtype of ADHD. The DSM-IV currently permits diagnosis of subtypes of attention deficit hyperactivity disorder: inattentive type, hyperactive impulsive type, and, for children with problems from both lists, ADHD combined type. As one can plainly see from numerous articles, lengthy history, and controversies surrounding this disorder, much more work must be done to elucidate the core clinical problems of ADHD.

Core Clinical Criteria

As mentioned earlier, DSM-III, DSM-III-R, and DSM-IV differ on how the core symptoms of ADHD are arranged; however, they are consistent in their overall descriptions [15–17]. There is agreement that the core symptoms consist of inattention and hyperactivity and impulsivity. DSM-III arranged these domains into three separate symptom areas, DSM-III-R into one symptom list, and DSM-IV as two core dimensions (inattention and hyperactivity/impulsivity). DSM-IV maintains the requirements of an early age of onset (prior to age seven years), the presence of impairment for six months or longer, and the presence of impairment in two or more settings. Inattention includes failing to give close attention to details, difficulty sustaining attention, not listening, not following through, difficulty organizing, losing things, easily becoming distracted, and forgetfulness. Hyperactivity includes fidgeting, being out of seat, running or climbing excessively, having difficulty playing quietly, being 'on the go' or as if 'driven by a motor,' and talking excessively. The impulsivity symptom criteria include blurting out answers, having difficulty awaiting a turn, and often interrupting or intruding on others [17]. Core deficits include impairment in rule-governed behavior across a variety of settings and relative difficulty for age in inhibiting an impulsive response to internal wishes, needs, or external stimuli.

Most studies have concentrated on hyperactive elementary school children between the ages of six and nine years. The syndrome may manifest itself differently throughout the life cycle; however, school-age children are the most common presenting population to pediatricians, child psychiatrists, and psychologists. Weiss [19,22] points out that these children typically present with:

- inappropriate or excessive activity, unrelated to the task at hand, which generally has an intrusive or annoying quality;
- poor sustained attention;
- difficulties in inhibiting impulses in social behavior and cognitive tasks;
- difficulties getting along with others;
- school underachievement;

- poor self-esteem secondary to difficulties getting along with others and school underachievement;
- other behavior disorders, learning disabilities, anxiety disorders, and depression.

Restlessness is measured by well-standardized rating scales and direct and indirect observation [38–40]. Teachers and parents may not agree with one another, owing to the likelihood that children may act differently in different situations. A child with ADHD may not show his behavior if he likes a teacher or tries harder at home to please his parents. Consequently, a child being evaluated in a physician's office could sit perfectly still during the examination, and the clinician may use rating scales in settings where the child spends the majority of his time. Whalen and Henker [21] suggest that 'each measure reflects a unique child × perceiver × setting example.' Over the course of development, the restlessness described diminishes and changes from running all the time to not being able to sit quietly in a chair or feeling fidgety in adolescence and adulthood. Some hyperactive adults feel 'restless' even when physical restlessness is not observed [22]. Difficulty in sustaining attention contributes to the difficulties children with ADHD have both in school and with their peers. Not paying attention on a given assignment or during class leads to poor school-work. Not paying attention in games and wanting to do something different can contribute to unpopularity with peers.

Bewildered parents will report their child's difficulties with attention. A common complaint is 'he can play Nintendo for hours but to do 20 minutes worth of homework requires 1–2 hours worth of screaming and temper tantrums.' It seems that when a particular activity interests a child, he or she can pay attention for hours. However, these same children can have a poor attention span when attending to tasks they find boring, repetitive, or difficult and that give them no satisfaction. This may be largely a learned behavior, since at school they are constantly told by their teacher to pay attention, to sit up straight, stop fidgeting, and so on, which in and of itself can have a large impact on a child's attention span. Consequently, at home a child, especially around homework or 'task time,' can perceive many negative messages. This can in turn prevent any person, more so a child with ADHD, from paying attention to the task at hand.

Parents and teachers frequently complain that these children do not seem to listen as well as they should for their age, cannot concentrate, are easily distracted, fail to finish assignments, daydream, and change activities more than others [10]. The use of objective measures of attention span research has shown that ADHD children, when compared with normal children, are often recorded as being more off task and less likely to complete as much as others, looking away from the activities they are requested to do, persisting less in correctly performing boring activities such as continuous performance tasks, and being slower and less likely to return to an activity once interrupted [24–26]. These behaviors have also been noted to distinguish them from children with learning disabilities' and other psychiatric disorders [20,27]. Poor attention span should be carefully assessed, as it can also be very similar to the poor concentration seen in anxiety and mood disorders.

Difficulties in Inhibiting Impulses

In DSM-IV, hyperactivity and impulsivity have been linked in a common symptom grouping. Impulsivity is pervasive in everyday tasks in hyperactive children. In school, they have difficulty awaiting their turn, interrupt others, blurt out answers, and engage in physically dangerous activities without considering the consequences. Accidents in children with ADHD are common [22,28,29]. These children are also less able to resist immediate temptations and delay gratification [3]. They tend to respond too quickly and too often when they are required to wait and watch for events to happen [26]. Shopping with these children in a stimulating retail environment is often a challenge.

Impulsivity in ADHD is not only pervasive, it is also likely to be the most enduring symptom as the children grow up [22]. It is the symptom that along with oppositional and aggressive behaviors is most likely to result in rejection by peers. Many adults can present with a chief complaint of inability to get along with authority figures on the job as well as multiple reprimands for not following directions.

Difficulty Getting Along with Others

Peers often quickly reject children with ADHD because of their aggression, impulsivity, and noncompliance with rules [31]. Children with ADHD may be unpopular with their peers and may have difficulties with parents, siblings, and teachers [30,32]. These children may have few 'best friends' and few enduring friendships, and this unpopularity and inability to establish and maintain friendships may be replaced in life by social isolation. This is another characteristic of hyperactive children that is both pervasive and enduring over time [22]. In childhood, sometimes the only person willing to play with a hyperactive child is a younger child or a child with some other similar difficulty.

Sociometric ratings from peers indicate that hyperactive children cause trouble, get others into trouble, bother others, and are not polite which can lead to a negative impact on the ADHD child's sense of self [33]. The negative effect of hyperactive children on others has been observed with respect to their teachers and ability to participate in both dyads and groups of children. Parents may also interact with a hyperactive child in a more negative and intrusive way. When the hyperactive child improves on medication and becomes more cooperative, his relationship with peers, teachers, and parents improve. Studies are in agreement with one another in describing the nature of the difficulties; however, it is not clear whether the cause is a social skills deficit, a performance deficit, or both [3].

School Underachievement

Cantwell and Baker [34] showed that even when intelligence was controlled for, hyperactive children were behind normal children in their grade level in reading, spelling, and arithmetic. The core symptoms of ADHD impair learning. ADHD children have poorer organizational skills, poor sequential memory, deficits in fine and gross motor skills affecting handwriting, and inefficient and unproductive cognitive styles. The more unsuccessful hyperactive children become in their school-work, the less they are motivated to succeed because their efforts at times prove fruitless. All these factors interact to cause school failure or lower levels of academic achievement [37]. It is not uncommon for children to present to clinicians with their parents in the middle to late middle of the school year, when grade retention is a distinct possibility for a given child.

Low Self-Esteem

In general, when children receive praise and acceptance from parents, teachers, and students, their self-esteem and sense of self improves dramatically. However, children with ADHD have multiple difficulties in multiple areas of their lives. They are criticized and embarrassed. At times it is difficult for them to feel liked and successful. It is not uncommon for these children to feel 'demoralized.' With successful treatment, however, some of these symptoms may ameliorate.

Epidemiology of ADHD

Estimates of the prevalence of ADHD in school-age children range from 3% to 5%. In a recent review of six large epidemiologic studies [35] found that the prevalence rates in these studies range from a low of 2% to a high of 6.3%, with most falling within the range of 4.2%–6.3%. The differences in prevalence rates are due at least in part to different methods of solicitation of population selection, difference of nature in the subjects themselves, nationality, ethnicity, urban versus rural status, the sample criteria of ADHD, and the measures used as well as the informants. The Ontario Child Health Study [28] found ADHD prevalent in 10.1% of males and 3.3% of females aged 4–11 years and 7.3% of males and 3.4% of females aged 10–16 years. Cohen and coworkers [36] in a community survey, found ADHD in 8.5% of females and 17.1% of males aged 10–13 years, 6.5% of females and 11.4% of males aged 14–16 years, and 6.2% of females and 5.8% of males aged 17–20 years. In elementary school-age children, the ratio of boys to girls is typically 9 : 1 in a clinical setting, but approximates 4 : 1 in community epidemiologic surveys [36].

The investigators first recognized marked differences in prevalence rates found that when three systems – parent, teacher, and physician – all diagnosed the disorder, the prevalence was far less than when it was diagnosed by one of three sources. Schacher and coworkers [38] in the 1975 study in which they returned to the Isle of Wight to follow up Rutter's original prevalence studies five years earlier, found that 2.2% of the 1500 children about whom questionnaires were complete were still hyperactive. Szatmari [35] found in his review that rates of ADHD tended to increase with lower socioeconomic status.

Teachers typically identify fewer girls than boys with ADHD symptoms. The male-to-female ratio ranges from 4 : 1 for the predominantly impulsive type, to 2 : 1 for the predominantly inattentive type. Even among children rated by teachers as meeting criteria for any subtype of ADHD, fewer girls than boys receive an ADHD diagnosis or stimulant treatment [35]. In clinic-referred samples, the sex ratio can rise to 6 : 1 or 9 : 1 [35] suggesting that boys are much more likely to be referred than girls. A recent meta-analysis found that girls with ADHD have lower rates of oppositional behavior and cognitive problems than do boys in both community and clinical samples [41]. Among clinically referred children with ADHD, girls have greater intellectual impairment than boys. In the general population, girls with ADHD have less inattention, internalizing behavior, peer aggression, and rejection by peers than boys with ADHD. In clinical samples boys and girls have equal levels of impairment. Barkley [18] hypothesizes that these diagnostic criteria were set in a predominantly male distribution, which could create a higher threshold for the diagnosis for female subjects relative to other female populations and for male subjects relative to other male populations. It is our experience that a high percentage of females are not diagnosed with ADHD until they present in middle or late adolescence with a comorbid disorder such as depression, anxiety, or an eating disorder.

Etiology of ADHD

It is unlikely that a simple etiologic factor is responsible for ADHD. There is an interplay of both psychosocial and biologic factors that may lead to a final common pathway syndrome. For example, genetic studies have shown there is a strong hereditary influence in ADHD [42]. However, in addition to the genetic 'passing on of the disorder,' a parent with ADHD may have a poor parenting style, which can affect or exacerbate a child's attention span or behavioral problems.

The etiology of ADHD is unknown. A variety of physical disorders can be mistaken for ADHD and can co-occur. Physical causes of poor attention may include impaired vision or hearing, seizures, sequelae of head trauma, acute or chronic medical illness, poor nutrition, or insufficient sleep due to a sleep disorder. Anxiety disorders, depression, and sequelae of abuse or neglect may interfere with attention as well. Patients with Tourette syndrome may be inattentive because they are distracted by premonitory urges to resist ticking.

Drugs

Some drugs may interfere with attention, including phenobarbital, carbamazepine, and alcohol and illegal drugs. It is possible that there is an effect only on children who already have attentional or achievement problems [43–45] and that parent reports of adverse behavioral side effects may not correspond to more objective data. Some known conditions, such as fragile X syndrome, fetal alcohol syndrome, very low birth weight, and a very rare genetic thyroid disorder, can present behaviorally with the symptoms of ADHD. However, these cases make up only a small portion of the total population of children with the diagnosis [44,45].

Central Nervous System Findings

As mentioned, early theories of the etiology of ADHD attributed it to 'brain damage,' derived from the studies of children who suffered encephalitis in the epidemic of 1917 and 1918. Studies of brain morphology have become more technologically sophisticated. Hynd and coworkers [46] produced magnetic resonance imaging (MRI) findings suggesting that children with ADD had normal planum temporale but abnormal frontal lobes. Giedd and coworkers [47] demonstrated reduced volume in the rostrum and rostral body of the corpus callosum. This finding has been interpreted as consistent with an alteration of functioning of the prefrontal and interior cingulate cortices of the brain [48]. An attempt to replicate this finding, however, failed to show any differences between children with ADHD and control subjects in the size or shape of the entire corpus callosum, with the exception of the region of the splenium, which again was significantly smaller in subjects with ADHD [49].

Studies have demonstrated decreased blood flow in the prefrontal regions of the frontal region [55]. Lou and coworkers [50] and Hynd and coworkers [51] found that children with ADHD had a significantly smaller left caudate nucleus, creating a reversed to normal pattern of left greater than right asymmetry of the caudate nucleus. Looking at structural abnormalities in the basil ganglia in ADHD, Mataro and coworkers [52] studied 11 adolescents with ADHD and 19 healthy control subjects and found that the ADHD group had a larger right caudate nucleus than the control group. In control adolescents, larger caudate nuclear volume were associated with poor performance on tests of attention and higher ratings on the Connors Teachers Rating Scale. These findings, according to the authors [52], provide further evidence of the involvement of the caudate nucleus in the neuropsychologic deficits in behavior problems in ADHD. The larger caudate nucleus found in the ADHD group can be related to a failure of the maturational process that normally results in volume reduction. Lou [53,54] examined the hypoxic and ischemic brain events of premature infants. He demonstrated that the striatum is in a unique position of being highly susceptible to ischemia. He stated that ischemic events are particularly common in premature infants, a fact that seems to explain the high incidence of ADHD in this patient group. The magnitude of the problem is growing with increased survival rates among premature infants. It is not uncommon for an ADHD/psychopharmacologic clinic to see many children who have survived premature births.

The pathophysiology of ADHD has also been investigated using other imaging techniques such as single photon emission computed tomography (SPECT) and positron emission tomography (PET) [57]. Zametkin and colleagues [55] studied 25 biologic parents of children with ADHD. These parents had histories suggestive of ADHD but were never treated. Fifty adults matched for sex, age, and intelligence quotient [IQ] score acted as controls. Glucose metabolism was studied while the subjects were performing an auditory attention task lasting 35 minutes. PET scans were performed during the test and were analyzed. Zametkin and coworkers [56] found an overall glucose metabolism decrease of 8.1% in the cortical areas, affecting 30 of 60 brain regions. The main regions affected were the premotor and prefrontal cortex in the left hemisphere, areas associated with attention. The cause and effect of these findings are not clear, but should prompt further research. In a follow-up study subjects, as compared with the control group, demonstrated less statistical significance. Adolescent females with ADD did have reduced glucose metabolism globally, compared with normal control females and males and compared with males with ADD. Amen and Carmichael [57] compared 54 children and adolescents with ADHD diagnosed by the DSM-III-R and by Connors Teachers Rating Scale criteria as well as a non-ADHD control group. Two imaging studies were done on each group – a resting study and an intellectual stress study, the latter done while the participants were doing a concentration task. Sixty-five percent of the ADHD group exhibited decreased profusion of the prefrontal cortex with intellectual stress, compared to only 5% of the control group. Of the ADHD group who did not show decreased profusion, two-thirds had markedly decreased activity in the prefrontal cortices at rest. Many of the brain imaging studies contained small sample sizes and have yet to be replicated. In considering structural and neuroimaging studies, it is unclear what is cause and what is effect. Are the abnormalities causing symptoms of ADHD or are the symptoms of ADHD causing reduction in glucose metabolism? It is hoped that further studies with larger sample sizes will lead to a clearer understanding of this phenomenon.

The use of stimulants, a cornerstone in the treatment of ADHD, has raised the possibility that the disorder is caused by a dysfunction of the dopaminergic and/or serotonergic systems. Early reports describe brain transmitter metabolites such as MHPG as being lower in the urine of hyperactive children than in normal children's urine; however, these studies have not been replicated. Other studies that measured the urinary amino acids phenylalanine and tyrosine found no differences [58]. Zametkin and Rapoport [58] conclude that the studies comparing ADHD and normal children with respect to monoamines in their metabolism in urine and plasma, cerebrospinal fluid, and platelets have been disappointing. However, these studies conclude that catecholamine function and its modulation are probably involved in the pathogenesis and treatment of ADHD, respectively. Thus, they suggest that the lack of response to one stimulant may predict responsiveness to another.

McCracken [59], in reviewing the current thinking on the neurobiology of ADHD, points out that all medication shown to be effective for this disorder increased dopamine release and inhibition of the noradrenergic locus ceruleus. Mesocortical dopaminergic cells are linked with the prefrontal cortex, which is involved with attention. Children with chromosomal abnormalities such as the excess Y syndrome may show problems with attention, but the chromosomal abnormality shown in that population is uncommon in children with ADHD. However, other evidence suggests that ADHD is highly hereditary in nature [62]. Family genetic factors have been implicated as an etiology for ADHD for over 25 years, and heritability has been estimated to be between 0.55 and 0.92. Concordance was noted as 51% in monozygotic twins and 33% in dizygotic twins in one study [61]. Family aggregation studies have also shown that the ADD syndrome and related problems often occur in closely related family members, and adoption studies have also supported genetic hypotheses [60,63]. Cantwell [63] and Morrison and Stewart [64] reported higher rates of hyperactivity in the biologic parents of hyperactive children than in adoptive parents with hyperactive children. These studies suggest that hyperactive children are more likely to resemble their biologic parents than their adoptive parents. Cadoret and Stewart [65] studied 283 male adoptees and found that if one of the biologic parents had been judged delinquent or to have an adult criminal conviction, the adopted-away sons had a higher likelihood of having ADHD. Twin studies have also demonstrated a high rate of concordance in monozygotic twins when compared with dizygotic twins. Gilger and coworkers [66] found that if one twin was diagnosed with ADHD, the concordance for the disorder was 81% in monozygotic twins and 29% in dizygotic twins. A recent study done by Cook and coworkers [67] implicated the dopamine transporter chain in ADHD: analysis revealed significant association between ADHD and the transporter locus. This study was repeated by Gill and coworkers [68] in 1997. At this time the heritability of ADHD is accepted, but the exact mechanism for this has yet to be determined.

Family and Psychosocial Factors

It is possible to conclude, because of the high heritability of ADHD, that many children will have at least one parent with ADHD. Hence, it is unclear how much of the difficulty the child has in his family comes from parenting, how much from having an ADHD parent, how much from strictly genetics. Hechtman [69] in her follow-up studies of 65 families with ADHD children and 43 families of matched normal control subjects, found that families of children with ADHD have more problems than families of normal children. But these problems improve as the child with ADHD grows up and leaves home. Generally, family interactions with children with ADHD are problematic but improve when the child is on medication and when the child becomes an adult. A relationship between family dysfunction, solo parenting, welfare status, and urban living in hyperactivity was found in the Ontario Health Study [28].

Environmental Toxins and Dietary Findings

A study of 501 children in Edinburgh reported a dose–response relationship between high blood levels of lead and ratings on the Rutter's Teachers Rating Scale, most notably on the aggressive antisocial hyperactive subscores. Thompson and coworkers [70] concluded that high blood levels of lead produce behavior and cognitive disorders in some children. Ferguson and his group [71] found a small but significant correlation in their longitudinal study of lead in dentin levels, intelligence, school performance and behavior.

It is possible to conclude then that children of low socioeconomic status are the ones likely to have high blood levels of lead and may thus be a group at risk. This is an important factor, especially in urban or metropolitan centers. Fetal alcohol syndrome, which results from exposure to alcohol while *in utero*, may present with similar syndromes to ADHD. It is possible that the known craniofacial features associated with fetal alcohol syndrome are one form of the minor physical anomalies known to be associated with ADHD [72].

In the 1970s, the 'Feingold Diet' written by Dr. Ben Feingold claimed that half of all children with ADHD could be cured by a diet that eliminated all food additives. Connors [73] summarized both positive uncontrolled studies and mainly negative controlled studies and concluded that, in general, food additives were not a significant cause of the syndrome, except possibly in an occasional child. Parents also began to believe that sugar may cause the syndrome and many parents still limit sugar and food rich in sugar to children with ADHD. A controlled study carried out by Behar and coworkers [74] was designed to maximize any possible effect of sugar by selecting as probands 28 hyperactive children whose parents claimed they became hyperactive after ingesting an excessive amount of sugar. No differences were found in this study in behavior or attention between children given sucrose, glucose, or saccharine-flavored placebo. Recent studies have confirmed this. Again, however, any particular child could be susceptible to the effects of sugar.

Comorbidity

Children and adolescents diagnosed with ADHD commonly have other diagnosable psychiatric disorders [77]. As many as two-thirds of elementary school age children with ADHD referred for a clinical evaluation have at least one other psychiatric disorder [75]. It is therefore incumbent upon the evaluating clinician to assess a child with ADHD and to evaluate as well for the presence of other conditions [78].

In general, the presence of a second or third comorbid disorder indicates a more serious problem with a worse prognosis [22,76]. If a comorbid condition is found, this will obviously affect the treatment plan, including medication choices, psychotherapy treatment, school consultation, and placement options.

Gaining an understanding of comorbidity in ADHD can potentially lead to a greater understanding of the syndrome. Weiss [22], citing Biederman, points out that it is possible that comorbid disorders do not represent distinct entities but are different expressions of the same disorder; or that they may represent distinct disorders, sharing a common vulnerability and representing subtypes of ADHD. It is also possible that ADHD may be an early manifestation of the comorbid disorder or that ADHD may put a child at risk for the development of another disorder. In considering comorbidity, one must be careful to assess the population being studied. Clinical samples may suffer from what is called 'Berkson's bias,' which means that comorbidity seen in clinical settings may be artifactual, since that population may represent children with more severe psychopathology and more substantial impairment in their functioning, leading to higher rates of comorbidity [77,78].

The prevalence of comorbid conditions in ADHD appears to be high. In a community study, Bird and coworkers [79,80] carried out a probability sample of the population aged 4–16 years in Puerto Rico. They found that among children with ADHD, 93% had comorbid conduct and oppositional disorders. Comorbid internalizing disorders ranged from 50.8% for anxiety disorders to 26.8% for depressive disorders. Cohen and coworkers [81] conducted a longitudinal study of 776 children and adolescents aged 9–18 years using the child and parent Diagnostic Interview Schedule for Children (DISC). They noted that of children with ADHD, 56% had comorbid conduct disorder, 54% had oppositional defiant disorder, 23% had overanxious disorder, 24% had separation anxiety, and 13% had major depressive disorder. The Ontario Child Health Study [82,83] found similar high rates of comorbidity using DSM-III criteria. The investigators found that among children with ADHD, 42.7% had comorbid conduct disorder, whereas the comorbid internalizing disorders among children with ADD were less common – 17.3% for somatization disorder and 19.3% for depressive disorder. Substantiating Berkson's bias, McConaughy and Achenbach [84] compared comorbidity rates based on parent/teacher and subject reports, comparing matched community and clinical samples. They found that the comorbidity rates in the clinical sample were significantly higher than the population sample, regardless of the informant and instrument. The odds ratios showed high comorbidity of aggressive behavior with attention problems, and attention problems with social problems. On the Child Behavior Checklist in the youth self-report, the odds ratio was also high for anxious or depressed state with attention problems.

Comorbid Oppositional Defiant and Conduct Disorders

Barkley and coworkers [85] prospectively studied the psychosocial outcome of 123 hyperactive children and 66 normal control subjects, eight years after initial assessment. They found that more than 80% of the hyperactive children continued to qualify for an ADHD diagnosis, with 60% qualifying for oppositional defiant disorder (ODD) and conduct disorder (CD). ODD and CD can occur with ADHD in about 40% of hyperactive children [80]. Between 35% and 60% of clinic-referred children with ADHD meet the criteria for a diagnosis of ODD by seven years of age or older, and 30%–50% eventually meet the criteria for CD [80,85]. A substantial percentage of clinic-referred children with ADHD also qualify for diagnosis of antisocial personality disorder in adulthood [22,86,87].

Mood and Anxiety Disorders

Angold and Costello [88] reviewed epidemiologic studies using DSM-III or III-R criteria that dealt with depressive comorbidity in children and adolescents with ADHD. Five of the seven studies found significant associations between ADHD and depression, indicating that ADHD appears to be more prevalent in depressed children than in children without depression. It has been reported that 15%–75% of children with ADHD also have mood disorders. Gittelman and coworkers [76] did not confirm that major depression occurred more frequently in the adolescence and adulthood of ADHD-diagnosed children compared with normal control subjects.

There is some evidence, however, that suggests that these disorders may be related to each other, in that familial risk for one increases the risk for the other [89]. Faraone and coworkers [90] began to examine the finding that ADHD is more common in children with child-onset mania as compared with adolescent-onset cases of bipolar disorder. They hypothesize that ADHD may signal a very early onset of bipolar disorder. There are children who, in addition to their symptoms of ADHD, suffer from extreme irritability, violence, and decompensation. The authors suggest, that these children, when they present with or are diagnosed with ADHD, may have a subclinical case of child-onset mania. Clinical experience suggests that a substantial number of children with ADHD may benefit from a trial of a mood stabilizer in addition to psychostimulants. Wozniak and coworkers [91] and Pliszka [92] found that children with mania plus ADHD had an excess of relatives with both disorders and that both disorders co-segregated in these families. A comorbid association between ADHD and anxiety disorders has been found to be between 25% and 40% in clinic-referred children. Pliszka [93], in replicating his own previous study, looked at three groups – one with ADHD alone, one with ADHD and anxiety, and a control group – and found that the groups were significantly different across the spectrum of ADHD behaviors. The ADHD-only group had the most abnormal behaviors, followed by the ADHD plus anxiety group, and then the control group. He also found that the association of anxiety disorders with ADHD seemed to reduce the degree of impulsiveness in subjects compared with those with ADHD without anxiety disorders.

Tic Disorders (Including Tourette Disorder)

The evaluation of comorbidity of ADHD and Tourette disorder is complicated because the diagnosis of ADHD tends to precede in time the diagnosis of Tourette disorder. ADHD does not appear to elevate the risk for the diagnosis of Tourette disorder; however, among individuals with Tourette disorder, 48% may qualify for the diagnosis of ADHD [94].

Learning Disabilities and Poor Academic Functioning

The vast majority of clinic-referred children with ADHD have difficulties in school performance. They often score below normal or below the scores of controlled groups of children on standardized achievement tests [23,94]. It is not clear what causes this. Academic differences can be found in preschool ADHD children, which may imply that the disorder takes a toll on the acquisition of academic skills and knowledge even before first grade. Between 19% and 26% of children with ADHD are likely to have one type of learning disability, conservatively defined as a significant delay in reading, arithmetic, or spelling relative to intelligence, with achievement in one of these three areas at or below the seventh percentile [18,95]. There is conflicting evidence as to whether children with ADHD are more likely to have learning disabilities. Some subtypes of reading disorders associated with ADHD may share a common genetic etiology [97].

Speech and Language Disorders

An elevated prevalence of speech and language disorders has been documented in many studies of ADHD children, ranging from 30% to 64% of the samples. The converse is also true: children with speech and language disorders have a higher than expected prevalence of ADHD. Cantwell also describes a type of comorbidity as 'lack of social savoir faire' [96]. He describes it as an inability to discern social cues, leading to difficulties in interpersonal relationships. The comorbidity when specific learning disabilities are defined more stringently is probably 10% to 20%.

Diagnosis and Assessment

Diagnostic criteria for ADHD can be found in Table 10.1 that follows. The diagnosis of ADHD is a clinical diagnosis. It is made on the basis of a clinical picture that begins early in life, is persistent over time and pervasive across different settings, and causes functional impairment at home, at school, or in leisure activity.

Table 10.1 Criteria for the diagnosis of ADHD.*

The diagnosis requires evidence of inattention or hyperactivity and impulsivity or both

Inattention

  Six or more of the following symptoms of inattention have persisted for at least six months to a degree that is maladaptive and inconsistent with developmental level:

    Often fails to give close attention to details and makes careless mistakes

    Often has difficulty sustaining attention

    Often does not seem to listen

    Often does not seem to follow through

    Often has difficulty organizing tasks

    Often avoids tasks that require sustained attention

    Often loses things necessary for activities

    Often is easily distracted

    Often is forgetful

Hyperactivity and impulsivity

  Six or more of the following symptoms of hyperactivity and impulsivity have persisted for at least six months to a degree that is maladaptive and inconsistent with developmental level:

    Often fidgets

    Often leaves seat

    Often runs about or climbs excessively

    Often has difficulty with quiet leisure activities

    Often is 'on the go' or 'driven by a motor'

    Often talks excessively

    Often blurts out answers

    Often has difficulty awaiting turn

    Often interrupts or intrudes

Symptoms that cause impairment:

  Are present before seven years of age

  Are present in two or more settings (e.g., home, school, or work)

  Do not occur exclusively during the course of a pervasive developmental disorder, schizophrenia, or another psychotic disorder

  Are not better accounted for by another mental disorder (e.g., a mood disorder or an anxiety disorder)

* The criteria are adapted from the *Diagnostic and Statistical Manual of Mental Disorders*, Fourth Edition, Revised.[17]

CASE ONE

Martin, a six-year-old boy who was diagnosed with ADHD, came in for a clinical visit with his father one afternoon after baseball practice. The father stated that practice began at approximately 5:00 p.m. and that Martin's last dose of methylphenidate was at lunch at school. The father described Martin's performance at baseball practice as 'awful.' Martin saw no reason for his father's concern. The father stated that Martin would sit in the outfield and watch the birds, airplanes, and runners on a nearby track. He failed to pay attention when balls were thrown and hit. Adding an afternoon methylphenidate dose to Martin's regimen helped improve his hitting, his batting average, and his status on the baseball team.

The parent interview is the primary input in the assessment process. Interviewing the child alone can be helpful, but many children lack insight into their own difficulties and are unwilling or unable to report them [97]. This does not preclude a child or adolescent interview, however, and in our clinic, one-hour appointments with the parent and with the child are routine. Structured interviews of the parents or DSM-IV symptom checklists may be helpful in ensuring coverage of ADHD symptoms [2,182]. Rating scales may be helpful in gathering information from parents, teachers, other adults, and, in some cases, even the patient. They can be generally divided into broad- and narrow-based scales. The Child Behaviour Checklist developed by Achenbach [97] contains items in a variety of dimensions beyond inattention and hyperactivity. It is a useful broad-based screener. Connors [98], Swanson [99], and Pelham [100] have developed more specific ADHD rating scales. Clinicians must be careful not to make a diagnosis on the basis of a score on a rating scale alone, but rather to take all information including the interviews into account. During the child interview, it is helpful to put many materials out, such as games, crayons, paper, dolls, and so forth, in an effort to observe the child in a place where he or she feels comfortable. It is also helpful to observe the child in the classroom, as well as in less structured settings such as recess and lunch. A classroom assessment can also assess the teacher's style, as well as the child's social and academic environment.

Specialized tests, such as the Continuous Performance Test, the Wisconsin Card Sorting Test, the Matching Familiar Figures Test, and subtests of the Wechsler Intelligence Scale for Children-Third Edition (WISC-III), should not be considered 'diagnostic of ADD.' There is no specific diagnostic test for ADD, despite the frequent requests of parents and others for discrete psychologic testing in which the conclusion is the diagnosis of ADHD. Psychologic testing can elicit findings that are 'consistent with a child who has the diagnosis of ADHD.'

A medical evaluation should include a complete medical history and a physical examination within the past 12 months. Any effects of medication and vision or hearing deficits should be ruled out. Other medical factors predisposing to ADHD include fragile X syndrome, fetal alcohol syndrome, G6PD deficiency, and phenylketonuria. Risk factors include prenatal influences such as poor maternal health, young age, use of alcohol, smoking, toxemia or eclampsia, postmaturity, and extended labor. Health problems or malnutrition in infancy also appear to contribute.

Speech and language evaluation may be required as suggested by clinical findings. Occupational therapy evaluation may also provide supplementary information regarding motor clumsiness or adaptive skills.

Reiff and coworkers [101] proposed the following diagnostic approach:

(1) A comprehensive interview with all parenting figures. This interview should pinpoint the child's symptoms so that the clinician can discern when, where, with whom, and with what intensity the symptoms occur. This should be complemented by a developmental, medical, school, family, social, and psychiatric history. Informing the parents that the presence of all parenting figures will be necessary to complete the evaluation is helpful, since many children present with step-parents; all should have input into the evaluation.

(2) A developmentally appropriate interview with the child to assess the child's view of the presence of signs and symptoms; the child's awareness of an explanation of any difficulties; and, most important, a screening for symptoms of other disorders, especially anxiety, depression, suicidal ideation, hallucinations, and unusual thinking. Questions that I have found helpful in asking a school-age child or adolescent are 'Are you bored?' and 'Is it easier to pay attention to what's going on outside the classroom or to another child who is leaving the classroom than to what the teacher is teaching?'

(3) An appropriate medical evaluation to determine general health status and to screen for sensory deficits, neurologic problems, or other physical explanations for the observed difficulties.

(4) Appropriate cognitive assessment of ability and achievement.

(5) The use of both broad-spectrum and narrowly ADD focused parent and teacher rating scales.

(6) Appropriate adjunct assessments such as speech, language, and occupational therapy in selected cases.

Differential Diagnosis

The differential diagnosis of ADHD includes a number of medical conditions (Table 10.2). In addition, a number of psychiatric disorders and family issues may resemble ADHD.

Age-Appropriate Overactivity Still Within the Norm

Many parents will bring in the oldest sibling after the second child is 3–5 years old. They state that 'we thought that's what boys do,' that is, they tolerated a child's hyperactivity because they felt that it was normal. Some parents do not know what level of activity, concentration span, and compliance to commands can be expected from a normal child at different ages, particularly in boys.

Specific Learning Disabilities Without ADHD

Learning-disabled children are bored and discouraged at school because of their inability to learn at the same speed or keep up with the class. They may be restless and inattentive as a reaction to inappropriate school placement. A child with a speech and language impairment without ADHD may also be bored and restless and inattentive in the classroom.

Conduct Disorder and Oppositional Defiant Disorder Without ADHD

CD and ODD may also present with some degree of restlessness and inattention. It is important in differentiating the two to obtain a symptom timeline, delineating which symptoms came first and which as a reaction to various problems that the child has at home and at school.

Adjustment Disorder and Post-Traumatic Stress Disorder

These are important diagnoses to differentiate from ADHD. Overactivity can be a 'common denominator' symptom of anxiety or post-traumatic stress disorder.

Differentiating ADHD from anxiety would again be easier given a timeline of the various symptoms.

Affective Disorders, Including Depression and Bipolar Disorder

These conditions can produce hyperactivity and interfere with attention. Poor concentration is a neurovegetative sign of mood disorders.

CASE TWO

Charles, a seven-year-old boy who developed severe side effects from methylphenidate, began a trial of dextroamphetamine, 5 mg twice a day and 2.5 mg at 4:00 p.m. He has had persistent sleep problems, refusing to stay in his bed, wanting to sleep on the floor, and wanting his mother to lie with him. A dose of 1.25 mg dextroamphetamine at bedtime has completely resolved these problems. He now sleeps in his own bed all night. Pharmacologic treatment of ADHD symptoms at bedtime in this case facilitated sleep without creating insomnia.

Stimulants may worsen or improve irritable mood [116]. Persistent dysphoria related to stimulants may respond to a lower dose, but switching to a different medication is almost always indicated. There has been concern about prescribing stimulants for patients with tics because of the risks that new persistent tics may be precipitated. Sixty percent of children with ADHD develop transient, usually subtle tics when prescribed a stimulant [113]. For children who have had Tourette syndrome or chronic tics, low to moderate doses of methylphenidate often improve attention without worsening tics [117]. On the other hand, withdrawal of chronic methylphenidate in children with ADHD and Tourette syndrome may result in a decrease in tic frequency and severity and with an increase occurring later if methylphenidate is reinitiated [117]. If there is a family history or if the patient has a tic disorder, stimulants should be used with caution. The clinician along with the parents and child must weigh the risks versus the benefits of a trial of stimulants when the ADHD symptoms cause functional impairment. If the tics remain problematic, dose reduction or a different stimulant may be tried.

Growth retardation resulting from stimulant use has been raised as a concern. Decreases in expected weight

Table 10.2 Mental health conditions that mimic or coexist with ADHD.

Disorder	Symptoms overlapping with ADHD	Features not characteristic of ADHD	Diagnostic problem
Learning disorders	Underachievement in school Disruptive behavior during academicactivity Refusal to engage in academic tasks and use academic materials	Underachievement and disruptive behavior in academic work, rather than in multiple settings and activities	It can be difficult to determine which to evaluate first – a learning disorder or ADHD (follow the preponderance of symptoms)
Oppositional defiant disorder	Disruptive behavior, especially regarding rules Failure to follow directions	Defiance, rather than unsuccessful attempts to cooperate	Defiant behavior is often associated with a high level of activity It is difficult to determine the child's effort to comply in instances of a negative parent–child or teacher–child relationship
Conduct disorder	Disruptive behavior Encounters with law-enforcement and legal systems	Lack of remorse Intent to harm or do wrong Aggression and hostility Antisocial behavior	Fighting or running away may be reasonable reactions to adverse social circumstances
Anxiety, obsessive–compulsive disorder, or post-traumatic stress disorder	Poor attention Fidgetiness Difficulty with transitions Physical reactivity to stimuli	Excessive worries Fearfulness Obsessions or compulsions Nightmares Reexperiences of trauma	Anxiety may be a source of high activity and inattention
Depression	Irritability Reactive impulsivity Demoralization	Pervasive and persistent feelings of irritability or sadness	It may be difficult to distinguish depression from a reaction to repeated failure, which is associated with ADHD
Bipolar disorder	Poor attention Hyperactivity Impulsivity Irritability	Expansive mood Grandiosity Manic quality	It is difficult to distinguish severe ADHD from early-onset bipolar disorder
Tic disorder	Poor attention Impulsive verbal or motor actions Disruptive activity	Repetitive vocal or motor movements	Tics may not be apparent to the patient, the family, or a casual observer
Adjustment disorder	Poor attention Hyperactivity Disruptive behavior Impulsivity Poor academic performance	Recent onset Precipitating event	Chronic stressors, such as having a sibling with mental illness, or attachment-and-loss issues may produce symptoms of anxiety and depression

Adapted from Rappley [181].

gain are usually quite small, although they may be statistically significant. Pretreatment weight adjusted for age, gender, and height is a significant predictor for weight loss in children with ADHD treated with either methylphenidate or dextroamphetamine. In contrast, pretreatment age, duration of treatment, and weight-adjusted dose have not been found to be significant predictors [123]. The effect on height, a frequently stated concern, is rarely clinically significant. The magnitude is dose related and appears greater with dextroamphetamine than with methylphenidate or pemoline [186]. Preliminary data on early adolescents have shown no significant deviation from expected weight or height growth rates [107] and adult height has not been shown to be reduced following methylphenidate treatment in childhood [169].

Stimulants result in small increases in systolic blood pressure and heart rate. It is thought that these effects were not clinically significant and there have been no reports of adults in whom long-term use of stimulants produced cardiovascular effects. Black male adolescents may be at higher risks for mild chronic elevation in blood pressure [119]. Occasional psychotic reactions in children have been reported in the literature. They are rare and usually take the form of tactile and visual hallucinations; auditory hallucinations are less commonly reported. These side effects require the discontinuation of the stimulant. In no reported case did the psychotic reaction persist after the medication was stopped.

Treatment of Attention Deficit Hyperactivity Disorder

The evaluation and management of the treatments used for ADHD require cooperation from the patient, the parents, and the school. This makes the clinician's role as coordinator or case manager vital to the treatment. Once diagnosed, ADHD has an extended course requiring continuous treatment and treatment monitoring to deal with the ongoing challenges that these children and families face. The treatment plan should be individualized according to the particular symptoms of the patient and his or her family. It should target the symptoms that are presented (personal, family, and academic) and take into account the patient's, family's, and school's strengths and weaknesses. Treatment planning should consist of medical treatment and management and psychosocial interventions, such as environmental modification, behavioral therapy, social skills intervention, and individual psychotherapy. The school and the teacher should be

incorporated into the treatment plan, both as participants and as monitors of the treatment.

Psychoeducational treatment in ADHD is the provision of information to patients, parents, and teachers and is considered standard in both research protocols and clinical practice [102]. The content includes symptoms and consequences of the disorder, etiology, treatment options, medication effects and side effects, expected course and prognostic features, basic principles of behavioral management, legal rights within the public school system, and how to work with the child's school. It is also helpful to address the myths of ADHD and its treatment. For example, 'Does ADHD vanish with puberty?' 'Do stimulant medications act paradoxically, cause drug abuse, or stop working in puberty?' Information may be disseminated in a public group setting, through published books and newsletters, or by referral to support groups such as Children and Adults with Attention Deficit Disorders (CHADD) or the National Attention Deficit Disorder Association (see Appendix 10.2) Parent management training is also a part of the psychosocial interventions with ADHD. Parents may learn to use contingency management techniques in cooperation with schools, such as a school/home daily report card or a point token response-cost system [145].

This comprehensive treatment plan should be outlined in a clear methodic approach to the parents, the schools, and the patients (Table 10.3). It is not uncommon for parents to ask during the consultation hour for a prescription for methylphenidate without having discussed the treatment plan with the child. The child should be included in the presentation of the treatment plan or at least a version of it, since therapeutic alliance between the patient and the treating clinician is a powerful predictor of compliance and outcome. Rating scales such as the Child Attention Profile (CAP) [95], the Home and School Situation Questionnaire, the Iowa Connors' Teachers Rating Scale [103], and the Academic Performance Rating Scale [104] or custom-designed target symptom scales for daily behavioral report cards may be useful in monitoring progress.

Pharmacotherapy

In the past several years, there has been an explosion in the number and type of medications available to treat ADHD. These new medications have changed the nature of ADHD pharmacotherapy, offering new options for patients who previously may not have tolerated or responded to treatment. (With the

Table 10.3 Guidelines for the diagnosis and treatment of patients with ADHD. [181]

Diagnosis
    Comprehensive developmental, social, and family history
    Standardized checklists to assess behaviors
    Consideration of coexisting mental health disorders
    Physical examination, not to diagnose ADHD but to assess genetic and other conditions

Treatment
    Management of ADHD as a chronic health condition
    Establishment of treatment goals agreed on by the child, the family, and school personnel
    Medication with stimulants to manage symptoms (monotherapy)†
    Behavioral therapy for parent–child discord and persistent oppositional behavior

Desired outcomes of treatment
    Improved relationships with family, teachers, and peers
    Decreased frequency of disruptive behavior
    Improved quality of and efficiency in completing academic work, and increased quantity of work completed
    Increased independence in caring for self and carrying out age-appropriate activities
    Improved self-esteem
    Enhanced safety (e.g., care in crossing streets, staying with an adult in public places, and reduced risk-taking behavior)

---

exception of atomoxetine, most are improvements in methylphenidate delivery systems.)

Bradley [105] was first to describe the dramatic effect of the stimulant benzedrine on a group of hospitalized disturbed children. The calming effect of the medication on these children as well as an increase in compliance and in academic performance was noted. Pharmacotherapy is often seen as a primary modality, particularly since the publication of the results of The Multimodal Treatment Study of Children with Attention Deficit Hyperactivity Disorder (MTA) results, which pointed to the superiority of well-delivered medication treatment over psychosocial treatment and community standard care for ADD symptoms [154,155]. Nevertheless, psychosocial treatments can

be used successfully, either as a primary treatment or to augment medication treatment effects and can be tailored to target symptoms of ADHD or comorbid disorders in school or at home [156]. Combined medication–psychosocial treatments are particularly effective for patients with numerous and severe symptoms or with other comorbid disorders. Some parents may be resistant to the use of medication, sometimes because of sensational accounts of medical misadventures in the media. The clinician must explain the risks of medication, the risks of the untreated disorder and the expected benefits of the medication relative to other treatments. Medication should not be used as a substitute for appropriate educational programming or other environmental accommodations. As mentioned previously, the therapeutic alliance between the clinician and the family is the most potent instrument for ensuring medication compliance. Faithful adherence to a prescribed regimen requires the cooperation of the parents [146], the patient, school personnel, and often additional caretakers. The child may have to take medication in a variety of settings, including in day care before school, in school, in after-school care, and at home in the evenings. Children and adolescents should not be responsible for administering their own medication, since they will often forget or refuse outright to take medication. However, as an adolescent approaches adulthood, assisting the patient in assuming responsibility for administering his or her own medication is important. Monitoring the effect and side effects of the medication is part of the responsibility of the clinician. A brief checklist such as the CAP Profile [96] or the Iowa Connors Teachers Rating Scale [103] is invaluable in obtaining teachers' reports of medication effects. Many clinicians use them routinely.

Sudden Deaths in Children with Adderall XR

Health Canada has suspended marketing of Adderall XR products from the Canadian market due to concern about reports of sudden unexplained death (SUD) in children taking Adderall and Adderall XR. SUD has been associated with amphetamine abuse and reported in children with underlying cardiac abnormalities such as taking recommended doses of amphetamines, including Adderall and Adderall XR. In addition, a very small number of cases of SUD has been reported in children without structural cardiac abnormalities taking Adderall. At this time, Food and Drug Administration (FDA) cannot conclude that recommended doses of Adderall can cause SUD, but is continuing to carefully evaluate these data.

Given the number of available treatments, practitioners may be confused about subtle differences between treatments and about how to select among the various options. This section reviews the available medication treatments for ADHD and presents a rational approach for choosing among the many medication options in developing a comprehensive treatment plan for the patient with ADHD. Table 10.4 lists the available medications for ADHD and their dosage ranges and schedules.

Psychostimulants

Psychostimulants have been the mainstay of treatment for youth with ADHD, their efficacy having been established in nearly 200 placebo-controlled trials during the past 40 years [158,159]. Increasingly, they are being used to treat ADHD in adults as well [157,160,161], although only Adderall XR is now labeled for the treatment of adults. In most cases, a stimulant is the first-choice medication. Methylphenidate is the most often prescribed and accounts for more than 90% of stimulant use in the USA [107]. These medications are effective in the short term and, based on a large number of research studies and 60 years of clinical experience, effective in large numbers of patients.

Psychostimulants are controlled substances; prescriptions are restricted to 1–3 months (depending on the state), with no refills and their use is monitored. Dextroamphetamine, amphetamine salts, and methylphenidate are schedule II drugs and pemoline is a schedule IV drug. Although the precise mechanisms of action are not known, the therapeutic activity of the stimulants is often attributed to their blockade of the presynaptic dopamine transporter which decreases reuptake and increases synaptic dopamine in striatum and other brain regions [162]. Stimulants also bind to the norepinephrine transporter in the prefrontal cortex, enhancing both norepinephrine and dopamine as a result [163]. Methylphenidate and dextroamphetamine also increase synaptic catecholamine levels by facilitating release of presynatic dopamine, although dextroamphetamine has more potent dopamine-releasing effects than methylphenidate [164]. Also, dextroamphetamine enhances serotoninergic neurotransmission, although its effects on serotonin are less marked than on the catecholamines and are probably not substantial at clinical doses [165].

Most side effects from stimulants are mild and easily reversed. The onset of action is rapid, the dose is easy to titrate, and positive response can be predicted from a single dose [166]. Despite the well-recognized habituating nature of stimulants when self-administered in large doses, there is no evidence that drug abuse results from properly monitored prescribed stimulants [153]. Certainly stimulants can be misused, and caution is indicated in the presence of conduct disorder, preexisting chemical dependency, or a chaotic family. If the risk of drug abuse by the patient or the patient's peers or family is high, a nonstimulant medication may be preferable to methylphenidate and/or other stimulants.

At least 70% of children have a positive response to one of the major stimulants in a first trial. If a clinician conducts a trial of dextroamphetamine, methylphenidate, and pemoline, the response rate to at least one of these is in the 85%–90% range, depending on how response is defined [109]. Contrary to common assumptions, stimulants have a wide variety of social effects, in addition to improving the core symptoms of inattention, hyperactivity, and impulsivity. Stimulant effects on attentional academic behavioral and social domains, however, are highly variable within and between individuals [107]. Response to medication cannot be predicted by dose alone. For a particular child, a dose that produces improvement in one area of functioning may have no effect or even lead to worsening in another [111,112]. The response may differ between measures even in the same domain. In general, however, both behavioral and cognitive measures improve with increasing dosage, within the therapeutic range. Girls and boys appear to respond similarly to methylphenidate [111], and children with ADD without hyperactivity may also have a positive response to stimulants [112].

There is good evidence to show that ADD children with oppositional and conduct symptomatology and aggressive behaviors also respond positively in these areas. Interactions between the child and peers, family, siblings, teachers, and other adults also improve. In addition, participation in leisure activity such as sports improves [151]. Cantwell believes the message to all child caretakers is that stimulants are not only 'school time drugs'; they may be used throughout the waking day and on weekends as well [1].

There are no patient characteristics that are helpful in suggesting which stimulant is best for a particular child. Minimum ages approved by FDA are not based on clinical or research data. Methylphenidate is the most commonly used and best studied drug and may be more effective in reducing motor activity than any other stimulants. Dextroamphetamine often has a longer duration of action than methylphenidate,

Table 10.4 Available medications for ADHD.

Medication	Daily dose	Dose schedule	Dose forms available	Comment
Methylphenidate (MPH)				
Ritalin	Initial dose 5–10 mg 10–60 mg or 0.6–2 mg/kg	b.i.d. or t.i.d.	5, 10, 20 mg	Most studied and prescribed Pharmacologic activity restricted to threoisomer
MPH Methylin	10–60 mg or 0.6 mg/kg 10–60 mg or 0.6 mg/kg 5–30 mg	b.i.d. or t.i.d. b.i.d. or t.i.d.	5, 10, 20 mg 5, 10, 20 mg	Half-life of **MPH** is 2–2.5 hours
Focalin	Initial dose 2.5–5 mg 2.5–40 mg	b.i.d.	2.5, 5, 10 mg	Focalin may require t.i.d. dosing
MPH-extended duration				
Ritalin SR	20–60 mg or 1.0 mg/kg	q.d. or b.i.d.	20 mg	Likely to require immediate-release supplement if given q.d.
Metadate ER	Initial dose 10 mg 10–60 mg or 1.0 mg/kg	q.d. or b.i.d.	10, 20 mg	Same
Metadate CD	Initial dose 10 mg 10–60 mg or 1.0 mg/kg	q.d. or b.i.d.	10, 20, 30, 40 mg	Same
Ritalin LA	Initial dose 20 mg 20–60 mg or 1.0 mg/kg	q.d.		Immediate-release supplement may be used but is not required May not be suitable for pts with gastric narrowing
Focalin XR	5–20 mg	q.d.	5, 10, 20 mg	Long acting focalin **SODAS** technology, sprinkle option

	Initial dose	Dosing	Available strengths	Comments
Concerta	Initial dose 18–27 mg, 18–72 mg		18, 27, 36, 54 mg	
Amphetamine (AMP)				
Dexedrine	Initial dose 5 mg, 5–10 mg, 10–40 mg or 0.3–1 mg/kg	b.i.d. or t.i.d.	5 mg	
Dextostat	10–40 mg or 0.3–1 mg/kg	b.i.d. or t.i.d.	5, 10 mg	
Adderall	Initial dose 5–10 mg, 10–40 mg or 0.5–1.5 mg/kg	b.i.d. or t.i.d.	5, 7.5, 10, 15, 20, 30 mg	
Amphetamine – extended duration				
Dexedrine Spansule	Initial dose 5–10 mg, 10–40 mg	q.d. or b.i.d	5, 10, 15 mg	Likely to require immediate-release supplement if given q.d.
Adderall XR	Initial dose 5–10 mg, 10–40 mg	q.d.	5, 10, 15, 20, 25, 30 mg	FDA ALERT [2/9/2005] – see below for warning
Pemoline				
Cylert	37.5–112.5 mg	q.d. or b.i.d.	18.75, 37.5, 75 mg	Rare, serious hepatotoxicity SEVERELY limits use
Atomoxetine				
Strattera	1.0–1.4 mg/kg	q.d.	10, 18, 25, 40, 60 mg	Nonstimulant, may be useful b.i.d. FDA is advising health professionals about a new warning for the drug Strattera, with a warning about the potential for severe liver injury in patients

permitting less frequent doses or reducing gaps in medication effect between doses. It is less expensive but is not included in many third-party formularies. Long-acting preparations are appealing for children in whom the standard formulations act briefly, who experience severe rebound (see later discussion), or for whom taking a medication every four hours is inconvenient, stigmatizing, or impossible. This is especially true for adolescents who are not used to taking medication during the day or who wish to avoid a lunchtime dose.

Dosage

Stimulant medication is usually initiated with a low dose. The usual range for methylphenidate is 0.3–0.7 mg/kg per dose, rounded to the nearest 2.5 or 5 mg. Dextroamphetamine doses usually are one-half those of methylphenidate. Greenhill [166] prescribes short-acting methylphenidate in dosing schedules of two to three times, first by adding an afternoon dose, and then increasing the dose to 10 mg twice daily, or until a satisfactory clinical response is obtained. If a third dose is needed, the third is usually half the morning or noon dose. (Dosing three times per day is particularly helpful for providing coverage during homework time and maximizing interactions with parents and peers. The upper recommended dose is 60 mg, although higher doses may be required in certain cases. Dextroamphetamine can be administered in a similar way to methylphenidate. Dextroamphetamine is supplied in 5-mg scored tablets. The starting dose of dextroamphetamine is 2.5 mg in the morning, tapering up every three days at 2.5 mg increments at lunch to a total of 5 mg twice a day. The recommended dose range for dextroamphetamine is 2.5–40 mg. Since dextroamphetamine is somewhat longer acting than methylphenidate, it is possible that twice-daily doses are enough. Longer-acting Spansules are also available, in 5-mg, 10-mg, or 15-mg units.) For ease of administration, the translation of a basic science finding (acute tolerance to clinical doses of methylphenidate) into clinical application led to the selection of a new drug delivery pattern for methylphenidate). This approach produced a new product (OROS-methylphenidate or Concerta), which proved to have the predicted rapid onset (with 1–2 hours) and long duration of efficacy (10–12 hours) after a single administration in the morning. Both Ritalin LA and Concerta are effective, however, the different release profiles of the two formulations can result in distinct differences between the effects on measures of attention and deportment.

Side Effects of Stimulants

Side effects of stimulant medication are similar for all the agents, tend to be brief in duration, and increase linearly with the dose (Table 10.5). In an individual patient, however, side effect severity may differ among the stimulants. Hence, it is possible that if a patient has a side effect to methylphenidate, he or she may not have any side effects with dextroamphetamine. Mild appetite suppression is almost universal and may be managed by giving the medication after breakfast and lunch. It is very important when monitoring the patient to know the schedule of the patient's meals and give the medication accordingly. It is not uncommon for children who have a three-times-daily dosing regimen to have a late dinner or even 'a midnight snack.'

Rebound effects are frequently reported in clinical practice but its existence has been difficult to identify and validate in research studies [166,167]. These effects consist of increased excitability, activity, talkativeness, depressed mood, irritability, and insomnia may begin 4–5 hours after a dose, especially as the last dose of the day wears off, or for up to several days after sudden withdrawal of high daily, doses of stimulants. The condition may resemble a worsening of the original symptoms [114]. Management strategies include increased structure after school, a dose of medication in the afternoon that is smaller than the morning and midday doses, use of long-acting formulations, or the addition of clonidine or guanfacine to the regimen. Sleep difficulties are common in these patients; however, difficulty falling asleep may be caused by direct stimulant effects, ADHD symptoms, oppositional behavior, separation anxiety, drug effect rebound or a pre-existing sleep problem. The remedy should address the cause and may include behavior modification, giving clonidine or a small dose of stimulant before bedtime, decreasing the afternoon stimulant dose or moving it to an earlier time. In a recent review of clonidine in sleep disturbances associated with ADHD, Prince and coworkers [115] concluded that clonidine may be an effective agent for sleep disturbances associated with ADHD. However, because of its short half-life, a percentage of children will develop early morning awakening. If the sleep problems are direct symptoms of ADIID, a small dose of a stimulant may be helpful. Another complaint sometimes associated with stimulant treatment is blunted affect. Patients may appear remote or less responsive than usual while on treatment. Some studies conclude that it does not occur more often in medicated than in unmedicated subjects

Table 10.5 Side effects, management, and contraindications of ADHD medications.

Medication	Side effects	Management for most common side effects	Contraindications

Methylphenidate	Appetite suppression, stomach aches, headaches, irritability, weight loss, deceleration in rate of growth, exacerbation of psychosis, exacerbation of tics, mild increase in blood pressure and pulse	(1) Mild appetite suppression is almost universal and may be managed by giving the medication after breakfast and lunch. Monitor patients schedule of meals and give the medication accordingly
		(2) Rebound effects
		  (a) Increased structure after school
		  (b) Dose of medication in the afternoon that is smaller than the morning and mid-day doses
		  (c) Use of long-acting formulations
		  (d) Addition of cionidine or guanfacine to the regimen
			Marked anxiety, tension, agitation, glaucoma, use of monoamine oxidase inhibitors, seizures, tics

Dextroamphetamine	As above	Blunted affect (may be complaint in all stimulants) (a) Managed by dose reduction	Cardiovascular disease, hypertension, hyperthyroidism, glaucoma, dependence, use of monoamine oxidase inhibitors
Atomoxetine	Appetite suppression, nausea, vomiting, fatigue, weight loss, deceleration in rate of growth, mild increase in blood pressure and pulse		Jaundice or other clinical or laboratory evidence of liver injury, use of monoamine oxidase inhibitors, narrow-angle glaucoma

Bupropion	Weight loss, insomnia, agitation, anxiety, dry mouth, seizures	Insomnia
		  (a) Address the cause which may include behavior modification
		  (b) Giving clonidine or a small dose of stimulant before bedtime
		  (c) Decreasing the afternoon stimulant dose or moving it to an earlier time
		  (d) If sleep problems are direct symptoms of ADHD, a small dose of a stimulant may be helpful
			Seizures, bulima, anorexia nervosa, abrupt discontinuation of alcohol or benzodiazepines, use on monoamine oxidase inhibitors or other buproprion products such as Zyban

[166]. When affective blunting does occur, it is usually a dose-dependent adverse effect that can by successfully managed by dose reduction. There has been some controversy about whether stimulant medication has been associated with decreased growth. The general conclusion has been that while the rate of growth may be slowed, the overall height is unchanged [195,197].

Long-Term Use of Stimulants

The long-term use of stimulants in children with ADHD was examined by Gillberg and coworkers [120] in 62 children meeting DSM-III-R criteria for ADHD. They participated in a parallel group-design, randomized, double-blind, placebo-controlled study of amphetamine treatment. The treatment group received active treatment for 15 months. The authors found that the stimulant effects of amphetamine in the treatment of ADHD remained positive 15 months after the start of treatment.

CASE THREE

Jose, a 10-year-old boy who was brought to the clinic for evaluation of treatment for his ADHD, was prescribed methylphenidate for his symptoms. Within two weeks the patient became increasingly irritable, complained that there were bugs around him that were trying to get him, and at times was afraid and had to hide under the furniture. He was using no other medication and there was no history of psychotic disorders in the family or previous psychotic episodes with the patient. The stimulants were discontinued and his symptoms persisted for two weeks, requiring approximately five days of low-dose thioridazine. Once the hallucinations ended, thioridazine was discontinued and the patient reported no further incidents of hallucinations. Hallucinosis is a rare but reported side effect of psychostimulants.

As mentioned earlier, there has also been much discussion about whether stimulants represent a risk of substance abuse, however, while some studies have reported sensitization following stimulant treatment [166,170], most evidence in humans suggests that stimulants reduce the risk rather than increase the risk [171,172].

Stimulants exert their beneficial effects almost immediately, but these effects wear off rapidly. As a result, steady state is generally not reached, and each day represents a new treatment period. For years, the most effective stimulant formulations were short acting (about four hours), which necessitated multiple administrations each day to maintain the effect. This dosing regimen is considerably impractical, may decrease compliance and may lead to stigmatization of the patient.

In a study of 25 boys with ADHD, sleep duration between children on twice-daily schedules and those on three-times-daily schedules were compared. Total sleep time appeared to decrease slightly in the children on the three-times-daily schedule as compared with those receiving placebo. Stein and coworkers [173] concluded that the dosing regimen should be selected according to the severity and time course of ADHD symptoms rather than in anticipation of dosing schedule-related side effects. More recent studies have pointed to t.i.d dosing for optimal response [173,174].

New, longer-acting stimulants offer more sustained duration of action, more consistent response, increased compliance and decreased risk of patient stigmatization (Table 10.6).

Amphetamine

Amphetamines are naturally occurring psychostimulants available over the last 60 years. Amphetamine is available in both dextro and recemic formulations. Adderall is approximately 75% dextroamphetamine. Amphetamine is approximately twice as potent as methylphenidate. Dextroamphetamine is labeled for use in children three years of age or older.

Amphetamine Preparations

Immediate-release amphetamine preparations include dextroamphetamine and immediate-release Adderall. When used as primary agent, these medications can be given twice or three times daily. Amphetamine can be limited to twice daily administration due to its longer half-life. Dextroamphetamine is available as a spanule, which provides coverage for approximately six hours, making it a good choice for an intermediate-duration formulation.

Since 2002 Adderall XR (extended-release form of Adderall), and Concerta now dominate the stimulant market in the USA, and are said to account for more than 50% of the prescriptions written for ADHD. Adderall XR uses a beaded delivery system to deliver

Table 10.6 Long-acting methylphenidate medication.

Products	Concerta	Metadate CD (continuous duration)	Ritalin LA (long-acting)
Formulation technology	OROS (osmotic release delivery system)	Diffucaps (beaded delivery system)	SODAS (beaded preparation similar to Metadate CD)
Dose	18, 27, 36, 54 mg	10, 20, 30 mg	20, 30, 40 mg
Immediate release	22% 4, 6, 8, 12 mg	30% 3, 6, 9 mg	50% 10, 15, 20 mg
Sustained/second release	78% 14, 21, 28, 42 mg	70% 7, 14, 21 mg	50% 10, 15, 20 mg
Comment	Delivery over 12 hours Consistent and ascending level of medication Most prescribed medication for ADHD Patients with gastric narrowing not suitable candidates	Delivery over 8–9 hours Same ascending dose profile as Concerta but does not provide a continuous release of medication Capsule can be opened for easy administration to younger patients	Delivery over 8 hours For patients with high level of ADHD-related impairments in the morning but do not require larger afternoon dose Good choice for patients with insomnia

a double pulse of the active drug. Similar to methylphenidate preparations, Adderall XR can be opened, which is an advantage for young patients who cannot swallow pills.

Atomoxetine

In January 2003, atomoxetine was released in the USA, becoming the first nonstimulant approved for the treatment of ADHD. Also, atomoxetine is the only ADHD medication that is labeled for use in adults.

Atomoxetine is a potent presynaptic, noradrenergic transport blocker with low affinity for any other receptors or transporters. Studies have found comparable efficacy when the medication is administered once daily [174]. Atomoxetine is labeled for use once- or twice-daily use. It is administered in capsules that cannot be opened. Dosing follows a weight-based schedule because plasma levels vary considerably as a function of body weight. The target dose is 1.2 mg/kg and the FDA-recommended upper dose is 1.4 mg/kg. Although there is some immediate improvement [174], a longer period (approximately two weeks at the most effective tolerated dose) is required before the full effect of treatment is observed. Adverse effects include sedation, nausea and vomiting, decreased appetite, weight loss, and modest increase in pulse and blood pressure (comparable to stimulants). It is uncertain whether atomoxetine affects growth, particularly after the initial effects of decreased appetite are accounted for, although effects appear to be small [175]. No changes were observed in any clinical trials [176]. Recently there have been reports of aggression, mania, and hypomania induction associated with atomoxetine [177]. Also, seizures and prolonged QTc with atomoxetine overdose have been reported [178].

Non-FDA-Approved Medication Treatments

The most frequently used off-label, nonstimulant treatments for ADHD are the noradrenergic tricyclic antidepressants, bupropion, venlafaxine, and the alpha-2 adrenergic agonists. These medications have been found to be effective in ADHD youths with and without comorbidity, although comorbidity has been a frequent focus.

Tricyclic Antidepressants

Tricyclics were the best studied of the antidepressants for ADHD. There are controlled studies for tricyclic antidepressants in both children and adolescents that demonstrate their efficacy in the treatment of ADHD [121]. These drugs may be indicated as second-line options for patients who do not respond to psychostimulants or who develop significant depression or other side effects of stimulants as well as for the treatment of ADHD symptoms in patients with tics or Tourette syndrome [118,122]. However, reports in the 1990s of episodes of sudden death on tricyclic antidepressants have virtually eliminated them from consideration as a stimulant alternative.

Other Antidepressants

Bupropion

More recently, buproprion has become a frequently used second-line agent, with efficacy (not as great as stimulants) having been demonstrated in a large multsite trial, which included a methylphenidate comparator arm [123]. Bupropion is a mixed catecolaminergic agonist that was brought to market as an antidepressant, and it may be particularly useful in the treatment of comorbid ADHD and depression and/or substance abuse or as an alternative treatment of ADHD in adults [179], or to provide a more sustained effect on which to superimpose acute stimulant treatment.

This medication may decrease hyperactivity and aggression and perhaps improve cognitive performance of children with ADHD and CD [123]. Bupropion is an antidepressant that is not a serotonin reuptake inhibitor or a tricyclic. Its side effect profile is very positive and its efficacy in depression has been documented in several studies. One blind controlled crossover study found the efficacy of bupropion statistically equal to that of methylphenidate [123]. It is administered in two or three daily doses beginning with a low dose of 37.5 or 50 mg twice daily with titration over two weeks to a usual maximum of 250 mg per day or 300–400 mg per day in adolescence. An extended-release preparation is available, but its appropriate dose in children and adolescents is not known. The most serious side effect of bupropion is a decrease in the seizure threshold, which is most frequently seen in patients with eating disorders or with doses of greater than 450 mg per day [124]. Clinical experience in our center is that bupropion has been helpful in patients who have had tics, as well as in patients who have been unable to tolerate the mood-related side effects and irritability of psychostimulants.

Selective Serotonin Reuptake Inhibitors/MAO Inhibitors

There are few data to support the use of selective serotonin reuptake inhibitors (SSRIs) in the treatment of

ADHD. The only published studies are an open trial of fluoxetine alone, an open case series in which fluoxetine was added to methylphenidate because of inadequate response in a population of ADHD children with multiple comorbid conditions, and a single case study of the combination of fluoxetine and methylphenidate [125,126]. Findling [183] examined seven pediatric patients and four adult patients whose ADHD and comorbid major depression were treated in a naturalistic open clinical fashion. For all 11 patients, the major depression responded to SSRI monotherapy, but no improvement in their ADHD symptoms were observed during SSRI treatment. Adjunctive treatment with psychostimulants did not provide any antidepressant effects, but did decrease the ADHD effects [183]. Among monoamine oxidase inhibitors, tranylcypromine has been shown in one study to be as effective as dextroamphetamine [127]. However, the dietary restriction required when using this drug makes it impractical for use in children and adolescents. Deprenyl, a monoamine oxidase inhibitor not requiring dietary restriction, showed positive results in an open trial with children with ADHD and Tourette syndrome [187], but these results were not replicated in a controlled trial with adults with ADHD [188]. Some statistically marginal benefits from deprenyl for both the ADHD and tic symptoms were reported, however.

Venlafaxine

This is an antidepressant that has noradrenergic as well as serotonin reuptake inhibition and was thought to be a possible treatment for subjects with ADHD who did not respond to other medication [128]. In a small group of children and adolescents, low doses of venlafaxine appeared to be effective in reducing behavioral but not cognitive symptoms. Adverse effects were not tolerable in 25% of the patients studied. These included three ADHD subjects who displayed a worsening of their hyperactivity and required discontinuation of venlafaxine, and nausea in one patient which also led to drug discontinuation. There was also concern that venlafaxine, because of its serotonergic activity, may aggravate symptoms of hyperactivity. Findling and coworkers [129], in an open clinical trial looking at adults with ADHD treated with venlafaxine, found that seven of the nine patients taking a dose of 37.5 mg twice daily responded with reductions in their ADHD symptomatology.

Modafinil

Modafinil (Provigil) has been examined for efficacy in ADHD. This agent is a schedule IV stimulant, which increases extracellular dopamine by binding to the presynaptic dopamine transporter, although its clinical effects may be linked to alterations in gamma-aminobutyric acid (GABA) and glutamate levels in the hypothalamus [189]. Modafinil increases arousal and alertness and is an approved treatment for narcolepsy. An open-label study, which used once-daily dosing in 11 children and adolescents with ADHD [189], reported improvements on the ADHD Rating Scale, Conners parent and teacher scales, and TOVA continuous performance test. However, lack of a placebo control poses difficulty in interpretation of findings. Another study [180] compared modafinil to dextroamphetamine, each administered twice daily, in 22 adults with ADHD, using a placebo-controlled, cross-over design. The two treatments performed better than placebo on the ADHD checklist and did not differ from each other in their magnitude of effect.

Adrenergic Agents

Clonidine is an alpha-adrenergic agonist. Clinical experience suggests that clonidine may be useful in modulating activity level and improving cooperation and frustration tolerance in a subgroup of children with ADHD, especially those who are highly aroused, hyperactive, impulsive, defiant, and labile. Open trials suggest that it may be useful in combination with a stimulant when the stimulant response is only partial or when the stimulant dose is limited by side effects [130]. The clonidine–methylphenidate combination was associated with three cases of sudden death [131]. Clonidine has been considered as monotherapy in treating patients with behavioral symptoms or treating children with comorbid tic disorders with ADHD; the research, however, is limited. Prior to starting treatment with clonidine, the clinician should obtain a thorough cardiovascular history, vital signs, and the results of a recent physical or cardiac examination. History of syncope is a relative contraindication [131]. Clonidine is initiated at a dose of 0.05 mg at bedtime. This maximizes the usefulness of its sedative effect. It is titrated gradually over several weeks to 0.15–0.3 mg per day in three or four divided doses. Pulse and blood pressure should be monitored for bradycardia and hypotension. The skin patch or transdermal form may be useful in improving compliance and reducing variability in blood level. Allergic skin reactions such as local dermatitis are quite common, however. The most common side effect is sedation, although this tends to decrease after several weeks [132]. Dry mouth, nausea, and photophobia have also been reported. Glucose tolerance may decrease, especially in patients at risk for diabetes. Clonidine should be tapered instead of stopped suddenly to avoid a withdrawal syndrome consisting of motor restlessness, headache, agitation, increased blood pressure and pulse rate, and possible worsening of tics. Erratic compliance can increase the risk of cardiovascular events, and clonidine should not be prescribed unless it can be administered reliably.

Guanfacine hydrochloride is a long-acting alpha-adrenergic agonist with a longer half-life and a more favorable side effect profile than clonidine. Only open trials have been published [133–135], but there may be a use for this medication in ADHD and Tourette syndrome patients who cannot tolerate stimulants because of worsening of tics. It may also be indicated for the children with ADHD who cannot tolerate the sedative side effects of clonidine or in whom clonidine has too short a duration of action, leading to rebound effects.

Combinations of Medication

There are no studies showing that combinations of various medications are particularly effective in treating ADHD. Anecdotal clinical experience supports the usefulness of methylphenidate and clonidine. Four deaths have been reported to the FDA among children who at one time took clonidine and methylphenidate; however, the evidence linking the drugs to the deaths is tenuous at best [136,137]. Extra caution is advised when treating children with cardiac or cardiovascular disease when combining clonidine with additional medication, especially if administration of the medication is inconsistent. Grob and his group [139] suspected adverse methylphenidate–imipramine interactions in two children. In each case, severe adverse effects, including cognitive and mood deterioration, were experienced by the child when treated with a combination of methylphenidate and imipramine. One study found the combination of desipramine and methylphenidate to have more side effects than either drug alone [138]. The combination of imipramine and methylphenidate has been associated with a syndrome of confusion, irritability, marked aggression, and severe agitation [136]. Carlson [140] evaluated the use of desipramine and methylphenidate in a blind controlled crossover study of 16 hospitalized children with ADHD, mood disorder, or both, and either CD or ODD. The combination was statistically significantly better than either drug alone, but the results were modest. The use of combined medications must be done in a highly controlled setting with careful monitoring for side effects including cardiovascular effects.

Neuroleptics

Early studies suggested some usefulness of thioridazine or other major tranquilizers in the treatment of ADHD. However, owing to the long-term risks of tardive dyskinesia and neuroleptic malignant syndrome, as well as the potential for sedation and cognitive dulling, these drugs should be used only in extreme circumstances.

Other Drugs

There are no data to support the use of fenfluramine, benzodiazepines, or lithium in the treatment of ADHD alone. Silva and coworkers [141] in a recent review proposing the use of carbamazepine in ADHD, suggests a use for this drug in highly resistant cases or in patients with symptoms of brain damage or epilepsy.

Psychosocial Interventions

Behavioral and Cognitive Therapies

A variety of psychosocial therapies have been found to be useful for treating children with ADHD. They can be broadly grouped into behavioral therapy and cognitive behavioral therapy. In all cases, family, peer, and school interventions are important [142]. Behaviorial therapy relies primarily on training parents or teachers to be the agents of change, focusing on decreasing the frequency of problem behavior and increasing the rate of desirable behaviors. Techniques for use in schools and at home include token economies (star charts), attention to positive behavior as well as time-out, and response cost programs [143]. Re-enforcers may be dispersed by the teacher or the parent for positive recognition, such as stars on a chart or notes to parents or by the parents through the use of a daily report card [144]. The parents may use daily charts as a way to shape behavior response benefit programs in order to change behavior in school and at home. A homework notebook that is reviewed and signed by the parent and teacher daily is useful in improving organization and compliance with assignments, but the concurrent support of a contingency program is usually also required. The limiting step in an effective behavioral program is the parents' or teachers' willingness to agree to be part of a labor-intensive treatment protocol. In general, behavior modification alone has been found to be less effective than medication alone, although some clinical experience may suggest otherwise. Most controlled studies have been able to demonstrate little additional benefit when behavior modification is added to medication [145]. Attempts to demonstrate empirically that behavior modification can facilitate medication withdrawal have been unsuccessful, although again clinical experience seems to suggest otherwise.

Multimodal Treatment

In the MTA study conducted by Abikoff and colleagues [147], children aged 7–9 years with ADHD were randomly assigned to one of three groups: methylphenidate medication management alone; intensive multimodal treatment consisting of medication, academic skills training, remedial tutoring, individual psychotherapy, social skills training, parent training, family counseling, and a home-based daily report card reinforcement program for school behavior; or medication management with nonspecific education and nondirective support. The aims of the investigators were to determine whether intensive multimodal treatment is additive to stimulant medication in improving functioning and whether after multimodal treatment a greater proportion of children with ADHD are able to function adequately without medication. At the two-year evaluation, medication could not be withdrawn without clinical relapse, however, and multiple outcome measures and various domains of functioning were unable to distinguish children who received medication management alone from those in the other two groups. This study could have far-reaching ramifications for treatment planning for these patients.

Cognitive behavior therapy and approaches are based on the premise that the difficulties experienced by children with ADHD are results of deficient self-control and problem-solving skills. Examples of cognitive behavioral therapy approaches include self-monitoring and anger-management training.

Parent Training

Parent training has been suggested as a way to improve the social functioning of children with ADHD by teaching parents to recognize the importance of peer relationships, to use naturally occurring opportunities to teach social skills and self-evaluation, to take an active role in organizing the child's social life, and to facilitate consistency among adults in the child's environment. During the training, parents are taught to give clear instructions, to positively reinforce good behavior, to ignore some behavior, and to use punishment effectively. One frequently used negative contingency is the time-out, which puts the child in an unstimulating situation in which naturally occurring positive reinforcement is not available. As mentioned earlier in the chapter, since a high number of ADHD children have parents with ADHD, compliance with

training programs and behavioral therapy is often difficult.

Adolescent and Adult Outcomes

Adolescent Outcome

Overall, 30%–80% of diagnosed hyperactive children continue to have features of ADHD persisting into adolescence. Barkley [95] reported that 70% of hyperactive children continue to meet criteria for ADHD as adolescents. A family history of ADHD, psychosocial adversity, and comorbidity with conduct, mood, and anxiety disorders increase the risk of persistence of ADHD symptoms. Lambert and coworkers [148] obtained information on the outcome at age 12 years of hyperactive children. Of this total group, 20% were problem-free and 37% had persistent learning disabilities and behavioral and emotional problems. By age 14 years, 19% showed antisocial behaviors. As a follow-up to this study, Lambert [149] confirmed that the hyperactive group continued to manifest lower educational status and significantly more antisocial behavior. This study, like many others, found that the interaction of both child variables and family characteristics predicted good or bad outcomes. Satterfield's work [150] is frequently mentioned because of the high percentage of felonies committed by his subjects. About 50% of 110 hyperactive boys had committed at least one felony, compared to 10% of 88 matched control subjects. Barkley and coworkers [151] reported a prospective study on adolescent outcomes carried out with 123 hyperactive children who were followed for eight years and compared with 60 community control subjects: The average age at follow-up was 15 years and 14 years, respectively. At follow-up, 71.5% of the hyperactive adolescents and 3% of the control subjects met DSM-III-R diagnostic criteria for ADHD and 60% of the hyperactive and 11% of the control subjects also had diagnostic criteria for ODD. Forty percent of the hyperactive and 1.6% of the control subjects also met criteria for CD. CD adolescents used more cigarettes and marijuana and were expelled from school more frequently. Families of the hyperactive subjects were less stable and had higher divorce rates, more frequent moves and, among the parents, more job changes. Fathers of hyperactive children showed more antisocial behavior. ADHD adolescents were more likely to experience auto crashes and more bodily injuries associated with auto crashes, and were more frequently at fault in the crashes. They also received more speeding tickets. Barkley [19,24] concludes that the persistence of ADHD symptoms into adolescence is associated with the initial degree of hyperactive and impulsive behavior as well as the coexistence of conduct problems, ODD, poor family relations, and, specifically, conflict in parent–child interactions, as well as maternal depression and duration of mental health interventions. Children with ADHD are more likely to experiment with drugs and to use cigarettes in adolescence.

Adult Outcome

Weiss and Hechtman [23] summarized the findings of their prospective, controlled, 15-year follow-up study of hyperactive children. In the final follow-up assessment, only 64 children of the original 103 appeared for complete comprehensive evaluation. The results of the study are as follows. Two-thirds of the group continued to be troubled by at least one core symptom of the original syndrome. Twenty-three percent had antisocial personality disorder. The hyperactive adults had more evidence of psychopathology, including more suicide attempts, low self-esteem, poor social skills, more difficulty on the job, and a final level of education inferior to that of normal control subjects. Mannuzza and coworkers [152,185] had similar findings; however, their percentage of adults meeting all criteria for ADHD was significantly lower, In their study, only 11% of the subjects met diagnostic criteria for full ADHD in adulthood, as compared with the Weiss–Hechtman study in which 66% of the adults had one disabling core syndrome. These differences, although similar in the fact that the ADHD adult outcomes were significantly different from those of the normal control subjects, can be explained by the sample, the raters, and the type of criteria used at follow-up. Findings from the Klein and Mannuzza [160] study confirmed findings from the Weiss and Hechtman study that probands did not show increased risk for major depression, bipolar disorder, schizophrenia, or anxiety disorder. Although girls have been studied far less than boys, limited data suggest a similar outcome.

Weiss [22] presented multiple conclusions about the outcome studies: (1) Hyperactive children continue to be disabled into adulthood by one or more initial core symptoms of the syndrome. Approximately one-third are diagnosed as having a full syndrome at 18 years of age, and hyperactive children are at risk for later development of antisocial personality disorder, shown in about 18%–23% of the follow-up sample. (2) Higher figures reflect hyperactive children who had comorbid conduct disorder. For a child who has ADHD without a conduct disorder in childhood, the risk of developing antisocial behavior in adulthood is much lower. (3) Final educational achievement and work record are inferior to those of matched normal control subjects, although most hyperactive persons are gainfully employed as adults. Mannuzza and coworkers [184] found that proband subjects completed significantly less formal schooling than control subjects by about two years and had lower-ranking occupational positions. These findings were not accounted for by adult mental status. These data demonstrate that ADHD disappears in adulthood is truly a myth. The outcomes need to be used in clinical practice to reinforce to parents the importance of persisting with a treatment protocol. As in any medical illness, untreated problems may continue and lead to a poor outcome. There is no study of a group of probands who have been treated continually and successfully over a period of many years.

Summary and Conclusions

The writings and research on ADHD are voluminous. Thousands of papers have been published on the topic. ADHD continues to be widely studied, and new ideas for treatment, both medical and psychosocial, are being evaluated on a regular basis. As described in this chapter, the potential for a poor outcome is great. This should motivate every clinician to do a thorough assessment and to offer a comprehensive individualized treatment plan, with the expectation that successful treatment may improve outcome. Our knowledge of comorbidity will allow clinicians to be aware of roadblocks to treatment as well as the frequent need for additional and extended treatment plans. Much has been done and there is yet much more to do.

Appendix 10.1

PRACTICE PARAMETERS [2]

(I) **Initial evaluation** (a complete psychiatric assessment is indicated; see Practice Parameters for the Psychiatric Assessment of Children and Adolescents [American Academy of Child and Adolescent Psychiatry, 1995])

(A) Interview with parents
   (1) Child's history
      (a) Developmental history
      (b) DSM-IV symptoms of ADHD
         (i) Presence or absence (may use symptom or criterion checklist)
         (ii) Development and context of symptoms and resulting impairment, including school (learning, academic productivity, and behavior), family, peers
      (c) DSM-IV symptoms of possible alternate or comorbid psychiatric diagnoses
      (d) History of psychiatric, psychologic, pediatric, or neurologic treatment for ADHD; details of medication trials
      (e) Areas of relative strength (e.g., talents and abilities)
      (f) Medical history
         (i) Medical or neurologic primary diagnosis (e.g., fetal alcohol syndrome, lead intoxication, thyroid disease, seizure disorder, migraine, head trauma, genetic or metabolic disorder, primary sleep disorder)
         (ii) Medications that could cause symptoms (e.g., phenobarbital, antihistamines, theophylline, sympathomimetics, steroids)
   (2) Family history
      (a) ADHD, tic disorders, substance use disorders, conduct disorder, personality disorders, mood disorders, obsessive–compulsive disorder and other anxiety disorders, schizophrenia
      (b) Developmental and learning disorders
      (c) Family coping style, level of organization, and resources
      (d) Past and present family stressors, crises, changes in family constellation
      (e) Abuse or neglect
(B) Standardized rating scales completed by parents
(C) School information from as many current and past teachers as possible
   (1) Standardized rating scales
   (2) Verbal reports of learning, academic productivity, and behavior
   (3) Testing reports (e.g., standardized group achievement tests; individual evaluations)
   (4) Grade and attendance records
   (5) Individual educational plan, if applicable
   (6) Observations at school if feasible and if case is complex
(D) Child diagnostic interview: history and mental status examination
   (1) ADHD symptoms (note: may not be observable during interview and may be denied by child)
   (2) Oppositional behavior
   (3) Aggressive behavior
   (4) Mood and affect
   (5) Anxiety
   (6) Obsessions or compulsions
   (7) Form, content, and logic of thinking and perception
   (8) Fine and gross motor coordination
   (9) Tics, stereotypes, or mannerisms
   (10) Speech and language abilities
   (11) Clinical estimate of intelligence
(E) Family diagnostic interview
   (1) Patient's behavior with parents and siblings
   (2) Parental interventions and results
(F) Physical evaluation
   (1) Medical history and examination within 12 months or more recently if clinical condition has changed

       (2)   Documentation of health history, immunizations, screening for lead level, etc.
       (3)   Measurement of lead level (if not done already) only if history suggests pica or environmental exposure
       (4)   Documentation or evaluation of visual acuity
       (5)   Documentation or evaluation of hearing acuity
       (6)   Further medical or neurologic evaluation as indicated
       (7)   In preparation for pharmacotherapy
            (a) Baseline documentation of height, weight, vital signs, abnormal movements
            (b) Electrocardiogram before tricyclic antidepressant or clonidine
            (c) Consider electroencephalogram before tricyclic antidepressant or bupropion, if indicated
            (d) Liver function studies before pemoline
  (G) Referral for additional evaluations if indicated
       (1)   Psychoeducational evaluation (individually administered)
            (a) Intelligence quotient
            (b) Academic achievement
            (c) Learning disorders
       (2)   Neuropsychologic testing
       (3)   Speech and language evaluation
       (4)   Occupational therapy evaluation
       (5)   Recreational therapy evaluation

(II) Psychiatric Differential Diagnosis

  (A) Oppositional defiant disorder
  (B) Conduct disorder
  (C) Mood disorders – depression or mania
  (D) Anxiety disorders
  (E) Tic disorder (including Tourette disorder)
  (F) Pica
  (G) Substance use disorder
  (H) Learning disorder
       (1)   Pervasive developmental disorder
       (2)   Mental retardation or borderline intellectual functioning

(III) Diagnosis

  (A) Establish target symptoms and baseline impairment (rating scales may be useful)
  (B) Consider treatment for comorbid conditions
  (C) Prioritize modalities to fit target symptoms and available resources
       (1)   Education about ADHD
       (2)   Classroom placement and resources
       (3)   Medication
       (4)   Other modalities may assist with remaining target symptoms
  (D) Monitor multiple domains of functioning
       (1)   Learning in key subjects (achievement tests, classroom tests, homework, classwork)
       (2)   Academic productivity (homework, classwork)
       (3)   Emotional functioning
       (4)   Family interactions
       (5)   Peer relationships
       (6)   If on medication, appropriate monitoring of height, weight, vital signs, relevant laboratory parameters
  (E) Re-evaluate efficacy and need for additional interventions
  (F) Maintain long-term supportive contact with patient, family, and school
       (1)   Assure compliance with treatment
       (2)   Address problems at new developmental stages or in response to family or environmental changes

TREATMENT

(A) Education of parents, child, other significant adults B. School interventions
   (1) Ensure appropriate class placement and availability of needed resources (e.g., tutoring)
   (2) Consult or collaborate with teachers and other school personnel
      (a) Information about ADHD
      (b) Educational techniques
      (c) Behavior management
   (3) Direct behavior modification program when possible, and if problems are severe in school setting
(B) Medication
   (1) Stimulants
   (2) Bupropion
   (3) Tricyclic antidepressants
   (4) Other antidepressants
   (5) Clonidine or guanfacine (primarily as an adjunct to a stimulant)
   (6) Neuroleptics – risks usually exceed benefits in treatment of ADHD; consider carefully before use
   (7) Anticonvulsants – few data support use in the absence of seizure disorder or brain damage
(C) Psychosocial interventions
   (1) Parent behavior modification training
   (2) Referral to parent support group, such as CHADD
   (3) Family psychotherapy if family dysfunction is present
   (4) Social skills group therapy for peer problems
   (5) Individual therapy for comorbid problems, not core ADHD
   (6) Summer day treatment
(D) Ancillary treatments
   (1) Speech and language therapy
   (2) Occupational therapy
   (3) Recreational therapy
(F) Dietary treatment rarely useful
(G) Other treatments are outside the realm of the usual practice of child and adolescent psychiatry and are not recommended

CHILDREN AGED 3–5 YEARS

Same protocol as above, except:

(I) Evaluation

   (A) Higher index of suspicion for neglect, abuse, or other environmental factors
   (B) More likely to require lead level evaluation
   (C) More likely to require evaluation of
      (1) Speech and language disorders
      (2) Cognitive development

(II) Treatment

   (A) Increased emphasis on parent training
   (B) Highly structured preschool
   (C) Additive-free diet may occasionally be useful
   (D) If medications are used, exercise more caution, use lower doses, and monitor more frequently

ADOLESCENTS

Same protocol as children aged 6–12 years, except:

(I) Higher index of suspicion for comorbidity with

   (A) Conduct disorder
   (B) Substance use disorder
   (C) Suicidality

(II) Teacher reports less useful in middle and high school than in grammar school

(III) **Patient must participate actively in treatment**

(IV) **Increased risk of medication abuse by patient or peers**

(V)   **Greater need for vocational evaluation, counseling, or training VI. Evaluate patient's safe driving practices**

ADULTS

(I)   **Initial evaluation** (a complete psychiatric assessment is indicated; see APA Practice Guideline for Psychiatric Evaluation of Adults, 1995)
   (A) Interview with patient
      (1) Developmental history
      (2) Present and past DSM-IV symptoms of ADHD (may use symptom or criterion checklist or self-report form)
      (3) History of development and context of symptoms and resulting past and present impairment
         (a) School (learning, academic productivity, and behavior)
         (b) Work
         (c) Family
         (d) Peers
      (4) History of other psychiatric disorders
      (5) History of psychiatric treatment
      (6) DSM-IV symptoms of possible alternate or comorbid psychiatric diagnoses, especially
         (a) Personality disorder
         (b) Mood disorders – depression or mania
         (c) Anxiety disorders
         (d) Dissociative disorder
         (e) Disorder (including Tourette disorder)
         (f) Substance use disorder
         (g) Learning disorders
      (7) Strengths (e.g., talents and abilities)
      (8) Mental status examination
   (B) Standardized rating scales completed by patient's parent
   (C) Medical history
      (1) Medical or neurologic primary diagnosis (e.g., thyroid disease, seizure disorder, migraine, head trauma)
      (2) Medications that could be causing symptoms (e.g., phenobarbital, antihistamines, theophylline, sympathornimetics, steroids)
   (D) Family history
      (1) ADHD, tic disorders, substance use disorders, conduct disorder, personality disorders, mood disorders, anxiety disorders
      (2) Developmental and learning disorders
      (3) Family coping style, level of organization, and resources
      (4) Family stressors
      (5) Abuse or neglect (as victim or perpetrator)
   (E) Interview with significant other or parent, if available
   (F) Physical evaluation
      (1) Examination within 12 months or more recently if clinical condition has changed
      (2) Further medical or neurologic evaluation as indicated
   (G) School information
      (1) Standardized rating scales if done in childhood
      (2) Narrative childhood reports regarding learning, academic productivity, and behavior
      (3) Reports of testing (e.g., standardized group achievement tests and individual evaluations)
      (4) Grades and attendance records
   (H) Referral for additional evaluations if indicated
      (1) Psychoeducational evaluation
         (a) Intelligence quotient
         (b) Academic achievement
         (c) Learning disorders evaluation
      (2) Neuropsychologic testing
      (3) Vocational evaluation

(II) Treatment planning

(A) Establish target symptoms of ADHD and baseline levels of impairment; consider treatment for comorbid conditions (monitor possible drug seeking behavior)

(B) Prioritize modalities to fit target symptoms and available resources

(C) Monitor multiple domains of functioning

    (1) Academic or vocational

    (2) Daily living skills

    (3) Emotional adjustment

    (4) Family interactions

    (5) Social relationships

    (6) Medication response

(D) Re-evaluate periodically the efficacy of and need for additional interventions

(E) Maintain long-term supportive contact with patient and family to ensure compliance with treatment and to address new problems that arise

(III) Treatment

(A) Education for patient, spouse, or other significant adults

(B) Consideration of vocational evaluation, counseling, or training

(C) Medication

    (1) Stimulants

    (2) Tricyclic antidepressants

    (3) Other antidepressants

    (4) Other drugs (buspirone, propranolol)

(D) Psychosocial interventions

    (1) Individual cognitive therapy; 'coaching'

    (2) Family psychotherapy if family dysfunction is present

    (3) Referral to support group, such as CHADD

(E) Other treatments are outside the realm of the usual practice of psychiatry and are not recommended

---

Appendix 10.2

READINGS FOR PARENTS, PATIENTS, AND TEACHERS

Books

1. Barkley RA: *Taking Charge of ADHD: The Complete, Authoritative Guide for Parents*. New York: Guilford Press, 1995.

2. Braswell I, Bloomquist M, Pederson S: *ADHD: A Guide to Understanding and Helping Children with Attention Deficit Hyperactivity Disorder in School Settings*. Minneapolis: University of Minnesota; 1991. (Department of Professional Development and Conference Services, Continuing Education and Extension, 315 Pillsbury Drive S.E., Minneapolis, MN 55455, 612-625-3504.)

3. Clark L: *The Time-Out Solutions: A Parent's Guide for Handling Everyday Behavior Problems*. Chicago: Contemporary Books; 1989. (Lots of detail on using time-out, but also other punishments and positive ways of increasing appropriate behavior. Includes examples, checklists, and tear-out reminder sheets.)

4. Fowler MC: *Maybe You Know My Kid: A Parent's Guide to Identifying, Understanding and Helping Your Child with Attention Deficit Hyperactive Disorder*. New York: Carol Publishing Group, 1990.

5. Garber SW, Garber MD, Spizman RE: *If Your Child is Hyperactive, Inattentive, Impulsive, Distractible . . . Helping the ADD (Attention Deficit Disorder) Hyperactive Child*. New York: Villard Books, 1990. (A practical program for changing behavior with or without medication.)

6. Hallowell E, Ratey J: *Driven to Distraction: Recognizing and Coping with Attention Deficit Disorder from Childhood Through Adulthood*. New York: Pantheon Books, 1994. (Written by two psychiatrists who have ADHD themselves. Especially strong on the diagnosis and treatment of ADHD in adults.)

7. Hallowell EM, Rarey JI: *Answers to Distraction*. New York: Pantheon Books, 1994.

8. Ingersoll B: *Your Hyperactive Child: A Parent's Guide to Coping with Attention Deficit Disorder*. New York: Doubleday, 1988. (A comprehensive book with many examples. Includes brief guidelines for teachers and an appendix with behavioral management programs for classroom use.)

9. Ingersoll B, Goldstein S: *Attention Deficit Disorder and Learning Disabilities: Realities: Myths and Controversial Treatments.* New York: Doubleday Main Street Books, 1993. (An up-to-date review by two psychologists focusing on causes and treatment. Good coverage of common myths and unfounded claims.)
10. Kelly K, Ramundo P: *You Mean I'm Not Lazy, Stupid or Crazy?!.* New York: Fireside Books, 1996.
11. Nadeau KG: *A Comprehensive Guide to Attention Deficit Disorder in Adults: Research, Diagnosis, and Treatment.* New York: Brunner/Mazel, 1995.
12. Nadeau K: *Survival Guide for College Students with ADD or LD.* New York: Magination Press. 1994. (A handy practical guide for the adolescent or young adult student with ADHD.)
13. Wender P: *Hyperactive Child, Adolescent and Adult.* New York: Oxford University Press, 1987.
14. Wender P: *Attention-Deficit Hyperactivity Disorder in Adults.* New York: Oxford University Press, 1995.

Newsletters

1. Attention! The Magazine of Children and Adults with Attention Deficit Disorders, 449 N.W. 70th Avenue, Suite 208, Plantation, FL 33317.
2. The ADHD Report. New York: Guilford Press.
3. Challenge: The First National Newsletter on Attention Deficit (Hyperactivity) Disorder, PO. Box 2001, West Newbury, MA 01985.
4. Adapted from American Association of Child and Adolescent Psychiatry (1997). Practice parameters. *J Am Acad Child Adolesc Psychiatry* 1997; 36(suppl 10):120S–121S.

References

1. Cantwell DP: Attention deficit disorder: A review of the past 10 years. *J Am Acad Child Adolesc Psychiatry* 1996; **35**:978–987.
2. American Association of Child and Adolescent Psychiatry (1977) Practice parameters. *J Am Acad Child Adolesc Psychiatry* 1997; **36**(suppl 10):085S–121S.
3. Stewart MA: Hyperactive children. *Sci Am* 1970; **222**:94–98.
4. James W: *The Principles of Psychology.* London: Dover, 1890.
5. Still GF: Some abnormal physical conditions in children. *Lancet* 1902; **1**:1008–1012, 1077–1082, 1163–1168.
6. Ebaugh FG: Neuropsychiatric sequelae of acute epidemic encephalitis in children. *Am J Dis Child* 1923; **25**:89–97.
7. Holman LB: Post-encephalitic behavior disorders in children. *Johns Hopkins Hosp Bull* 1922; **33**:372–375.
8. Stryker S: Encephalitis lethargica: The behavior residuals. *Training School Bulletin* 1925; **22**:152–157.
9. Burks H: The hyperkinetic child. *Exceptional Children* 1960; **27**:18.
10. Chess S: Diagnosis and treatment of the hyperactive child. *NYS J Med* 1960; **60**:2379–2385.
11. American Psychiatric Association: *Diagnostic and Statistical Manual of Mental Disorders*, 2nd ed. Washington, DC: American Psychiatric Association, 1968.
12. Douglas VI: Stop, look, and listen: The problem of sustained attention and impulse control in hyperactive and normal children. *Can J Behav Sci* 1923; **9**:254–282.
13. Douglas VI: Higher mental processes in hyperactive children: Implications for training. In: Knights R, Bakker D, eds. *Treatment of Hyperactive and Learning Disordered Children.* Baltimore: University Park Press, 1980:65–92.
14. Douglas VI: Attention and cognitive problems. In: Rutter M, ed. *Developmental Neuropsychiatry.* New York: Guilford Press, 1983:329.
15. American Psychiatric Association: *Diagnostic and Statistical Manual of Mental Disorders*, 3rd ed. Washington, DC: American Psychiatric Association, 1980.
16. American Psychiatric Association: *Diagnostic and Statistical Manual of Mental Disorders*, 3rd ed., revised. Washington, DC: American Psychiatric Association, 1987.
17. American Psychiatric Association: *Diagnostic and Statistical Manual of Mental Disorders*, 4th ed. Washington, DC: American Psychiatric Association, 1994.
18. Barkley RA: Attention-deficit hyperactivity disorder. In: Mash EJ, Barkley RA, eds. *Child Psychopathology.* New York: Guilford Press, 1996:63–112.
19. Weiss G: Attention deficit hyperactivity disorder. In: Lewis ML, ed. *Child and Adolescent Psychiatry, A Contemporary Approach*, 2nd ed. Baltimore: Williams and Wilkins, 1996:544–563.
20. Rutter M: Syndromes attributed to 'minimal brain dysfunction' in childhood. *Am J Psychiatry* 1982; **139**: 21–33.
21. Whalen CK, Henker B: Therapies for hyperactive children: Comparisons, combinations, and compromises. *J Consult Clin Psychol* 1991; **91**:126–137.
22. Weiss G, Hechtman L: *Hyperactive Children Grown Up: Empirical Findings and Theoretical Considerations*, 2nd ed. New York: Guilford Press, 1993.
23. Barkley RA, DuPaul GJ, McMurray MB: A comprehensive evaluation of attention deficit disorder with

and without hyperactivity. *J Consult Clin Psychol* 1990; **58**:775–789.

24. Barkley RA, Ullman DG: A comparison of objective measures of activity level and distractibility in hyperactive and non-hyperactive children. *J Abnormal Child Psychol* 1975; **3**:213–244.

25. Corkum PV, Siegel LS: Is the performance task a valuable research tool for use with children with attention deficit hyperactivity disorder? *J Child Psychol Psychiatry* 1993; **34**:1217–1239.

26. Luk S: Direct observations: studies of hyperactive behaviors. *J Am Acad Child Adolesc Psychiatry* 1985; **24**:338–344.

27. Werry JS, Elkind GS, Reeves JS: Attention deficit, conduct, oppositional, and anxiety disorders in children: 111. Laboratory differences. *J Abnormal Child Psychol* 1987; **15**:409–428.

28. Szatmari P, Offord DR, Boyle MN: Ontario Child Health Study: Prevalence of attention deficit disorder with hyperactivity. *J Child Psychol Psychiatry* 1989; **30**:205–218.

29. Barkley RA, Guevremont DC, Anastopoulos AD, *et al.*: Driving-related risks and outcome of attention deficit hyperactivity disorder in adolescents and young adults: A 3–5 year follow-up survey. *Pediatrics* 1993; **92**:212–218.

30. Anderson CA, Hinshaw SP, Simmel C: Mother–child interactions in ADHD and comparison boys: Relationships with overt and covert externalizing behavior. *J Abnormal Child Psychol* 1994; **22**:247–265.

31. Erhardt D, Hinshaw SP: Initial sociometric impressions of attention-deficit hyperactivity disorder and comparison boys: Predictions from social behaviors and from non-behavioral variables. *J Consult Clin Psychol* 1994; **62**:833–842.

32. Pelham W, Bender M: Peer relations in hyperactive children: Description and treatment. In: Gadow K, Slater I, eds. *Advances in Learning and Behavioral Disabilities*, Vol. 1. Greenwich, CT: JAI, 1982.

33. Whalen CK, Henker B: The social profile of attention deficit hyperactivity disorder: Five fundamental facets. *Child Adolesc Psychiatr Clin North Am* 1992; **1**(2):395–410.

34. Cantwell DP, Baker L: Issues in classification of child and adolescent psychopathology. *J Am Acad Child Adolesc Psychiatry* 1988; **27**:521–533.

35. Szatmari P: The epidemiology of attention-deficit hyperactivity disorders. *Child Adolesc Psychiatr Clin North Am* 1992; **1**(2):361–371.

36. Cohen P, Cohen J, Kasen S, *et al.*: An epidemiological study of disorders in late childhood and adolescence; I. Age and gender-specific prevalence. *J Child Psychol Psychiatry* 1993; **34**:851–867.

37. Lambert NM, Sandoval J, Sassone D: Prevalence of hyperactivity in elementary school children as a function of social system definers. *Am J Orthopsychiatry* 1978; **48**:446–463.

38. Schachar R, Rutter M, Smith A: The characteristics of situationally and pervasively hyperactive children: Implications of syndrome definition. *J Child Psychol Psychiatry* 1981; **23**:375–392.

39. Wolraich ML, Hannah JN, Pinnock TY, *et al.*: Comparison of diagnostic criteria for attention deficit hyperactivity disorder in a country-wide sample. *J Am Acad Child Adolesc Psychiatry* 1996; **35**:319–324.

40. Ross DM, Ross SA: *Hyperactivity: Research, Theory and Action.* New York: John Wiley & Sons, 1982.

41. Gaub M, Carlson CL: Gender differences in ADHD: A meta analysis and critical review. *J Am Acad Child Adolesc Psychiatry* 1977; **36**:1036–1045.

42. Faraone SV, Biederman J: Genetics of attention-deficit hyperactivity disorder. *Child Adolesc Psychiatr Clin North Am* 1994; **3**:285–301.

43. Creer LT, Gustafson KE: Psychological problems associated with drug therapy in childhood asthma. *J Pediatrics* 1989; **115**:850–855.

44. Schlieper A, Akock D, Beaudry P, *et al.*: Effect of therapeutic plasma concentrations of theophylline on behavior, cognitive processing, and affect in children with asthma. *J Pediatrics* 1991; **118**:449–455.

45. Bender B, Milgrom H: Theophylline-induced behavior change in children: An objective evaluation of parents' perceptions. *JAMA* 1992; **267**:2621–2624.

46. Hynd GW Semrud-Clikeman M, Lorys AR, *et al.*: Brain morphology in developmental dyslexia and attention deficit disorder with hyperactivity. *Arch Neurol* 1990; **47**:919–926.

47. Giedd JN, Castenalos FX, Korzuch P, *et al.*: Quantitative morphology of the corpus callosum in attention deficit hyperactivity disorder. *Am J Psychiatry* 1994; **151**:665–669.

48. Steere G, Amsten AFT: Corpus callosum morphology in ADHD. *Am J Psychiatry* 1995; **152**:1105–1107.

49. Semrod-Clikeman M, Filepek PA, Biederma J, *et al.*: Attention-deficit hyperactivity disorder: Magnetic resonance imaging morphometric analysis of the corpus callosum. *J Am Acad Child Adolesc Psychiatry* 1994; **33**:875–881.

50. Lou HC, Henriksen L, Bruhn P: Focal cerebral hypoperfusion in children with dysphasia and/or attention deficit disorder. *Arch Neurol* 1984; **41**:825–829.

51. Hynd GW, Hem KL, Novey ES, *et al.*: Attention-deficit hyperactivity disorder and asymmetry of the caudate nucleus. *J Child Neurol* 1993; **8**:359–347.

52. Mataro M, Garcia-Sanchez C, Jurque C, *et al.*: Magnetic resonance imaging measurement of the caudate nucleus in adolescents with attention-deficit hyperactivity disorder and its relationship with neuropsychology and behavior. *Arch Neurol* 1987; **54**:963–968.

53. Lou HC: Etiology and pathogenesis of ADHD: Significance of prematurity and perinatal hypoxichaemodynamic encephalopathy. *Acta Pediatr* 1996; **85**:1266–1271.

54. Lou HC, Henriksen L, Bruhn P, *et al.*: Striatal dysfunction in attention deficit and hyperkinetic disorder. *Arch Neurol* 1989; **46**:48–52.

55. Zametkin AJ, Nordahl TE, Gross M, *et al.*: Cerebral glucose metabolism in adults with hyperactivity of childhood onset. *N Engl J Med* 1990; **323**:1361–1366.

56. Zametkin AJ: Brain metabolism in teenagers with attention-deficit hyperactivity disorder. *Arch Gen Psychiatry* 1993; **50**:333–340.

57. Amen DG, Carmichael RD: High resolution brain SPECT imaging in ADHD. *Am Clin Psychiatry* 1997; **9**:81–86.

58. Zametkin AJ, Rapoport JL: Neurobiology of attention-deficit disorder with hyperactivity: Where have we come in 50 years? *J Am Child Adolesc Psychiatry* 1987; **26**:676–686.

59. McCracken JT: A two part model of stimulant action on ADHD disorder in children. *J Neuropsychol* 1991; **3**:201–209.

60. LaHoste GH, Swanson JM, Wigal SB, *et al.*: Dopamine D4 receptor gene polymorphism is associated with attention deficit hyperactivity disorder. *Mol Psychiatry* 1996; **1**:121–124.

61. Goodman R, Stevenson J: A twin study of hyperactivity: II. The aetiologic role of genes, family relationships, and perinatal adversity. *J Child Psychol Psychiatry* 1989; **30**:691–709.

62. Biederman J, Faraone SW, Keenan K, *et al.*: Further evidence of family genetic risk factors in ADHD: Patterns of comorbidity in probands and relatives in psychiatrically and pediatrically referred samples. *Arch Gen Psychiatry* 1992; **49**:728–732.

63. Cantwell DP: *The Hyperactive Child.* New York: Spectrum, 1975.

64. Morrison J, Stewart M: The psychiatric status of the legal families of adopted hyperactive children. *Arch Gen Psychiatry* 1973; **28**:888–891.

65. Cadoret RJ, Stewart MA: An adoption study of attention deficit/hyperactivity/aggression and their relationship to adult, antisocial personality. *Compr Psychiatry* 1991; **32**:73–82.

66. Gilger JW, Pennington BF, Defries JC: A twin study of the etiology of comorbidity: Attention deficit/hyperactivity disorder and dyslexia. *J Am Acad Child Adolesc Psychiatry* 1992; **31**:343–348.

67. Cook EH, Stein MA, Krasowski MD, *et al.*: Association of attention deficit disorder and the dopamine transporter gene. *Am J Hum Genet* 1995; **56**:993–998.

68. Gill M, Daly G, Heron S, *et al.*: Confirmation of association between attention deficit hyperactivity disorder and a dopamine transporter polymorphism. *Mol Psychiatry* 1997; **2**:311–313.

69. Hechtman L: Families of children with attention deficit hyperactivity disorder: A review. *Can J Psychiatry* 1996; **41**:350–360.

70. Thompson G, Raals GM, Hepburn WS, *et al.*: Blood lead levels and children's behavior: Results from the Edinburgh Lead Study. *J Child Psychol Psychiatry* 1989; **30**:523–528.

71. Ferguson DM, Fergusson FE, Howard, *et al.*: A longitudinal study of dentin lead levels, intelligence, school performance and behavior. *J Child Psychol Psychiatry* 1988; **29**(6):781–792.

72. Pomeroy JC, Spralldn J, Gadow FD: Minor physical anomalies as a biological marker for behavior disorders. *J Am Acad Child Adolesc Psychiatry* 1988; **27**:466–473.

73. Connors CK: *Food Additives and Hyperactive Children.* New York: Plenum, 1980.

74. Behar D, Rapoport FL, Adam AJ, *et al.*: Sugar challenge testing with children considered sugar reactive. *Nutrit Behav* 1984; **1**:277–288.

75. Nottlemann E, Jensen P: Comorbidity of disorders in children and adolescents: Developmental perspectives. In: Lahey B, Kazdin A, eds. *Advances in Clinical Child Psychology*, Vol.17. New York: Plenum, 1995.

76. Gittelman R, Mannuzza S, Slenker R, *et al.*: Hyperactive boys almost grown up. *Arch Gen Psychiatry* 1985; **42**:937–947.

77. Caron C, Rutter M: Comorbidity in child psychopathology: Concepts, issues and research strategies. *J Child Psychol Psychiatry* 1991; **32**:1063–1080.

78. Jensen PS, Martin D, Cantwell DP: Comorbidity in ADHD: Implications for research, practice and DSM-V. *J Am Acad Child Adolesc Psychiatry* 1997; **36**:1065–1079.

79. Bird HR, Canino G, Rubio-Stipec M, *et al.*: Estimates of the prevalence of childhood maladjustment in a community survey in Puerto Rico. *Arch Gen Psychiatry* 1988; **45**:1120–1126.

80. Bird HR, Gould MS, Staghezza BM: Patterns of diagnostic comorbidity in a community sample of children aged 9 through 16 years. *Am Acad Child Adolesc Psychiatry* 1993; **32**:361–368.

81. Cohen P, Cohen J, Kasen, *et al.*: An epidemiological study of disorders in late childhood and adolescence: I. Age and gender specific prevalence. *J Child Psychol Psychiatry* 1993; **34**:851–867.

82. Offord DR, Boyle MH, Racine Y: Ontario Child Study: Correlates of the disorder. *J Am Acad Child Adolesc Psychiatry* 1989; **28**:856–860.

83. Offord DR, Boyle MN, Szatmari P, *et al.*: Ontario Child Health Study: II. Six month prevalence of disorders and rates of service utilization. *Arch Gen Psychiatry* 1989; **44**:832–836.

84. McConaughy SH, Achenbach TM: Comorbidity of empirically based syndromes in matched general population and clinic samples. *J Child Psychol Psychiatry* 1994; **35**:1141–1157.

85. Barkley RA, Fischer M, Edelbrooke, Smallish L: The adolescent outcome of hyperactive children diagnosed by research criteria; I. An 8 year prospective follow-up study. *J Am Acad Child Adolesc Psychiatry* 1990; **29**:546–557.

86. Biederman J, Faraone SW, Lapeg K: Comorbidity of diagnosis in attention deficit hyperactivity disorder. *Child Adolesc Psychiatry Clin North Am* 1992; **3**:335–360.

87. Mannuzza S, Klein R: Predictors of outcome of children with attention deficit hyperactivity disorder. *Child Adolesc Psychiatry of Clin North Am* 1992; **3**:567–578.

88. Angold A, Costello EJ: Depressive comorbidity in children and adolescents: Empirical, theoretical, and methodological issues. *Am J Psychiatry* 1993; **150**:1779–1791.

89. Biederman J, Faraone SV, Feenan K, *et al.*: Evidence of a familial association between attention deficit disorder and major affective disorders. *Arch Gen Psychiatry* 1991; **48**:633–642.

90. Faraone SV, Biederman J, Wozniak J, *et al.*: Is comorbidity with ADHD a marker for juvenile onset mania? *J Am Acad Child Adolesc Psychiatry* 1997; **36**:1046–1055.

91. Wozniak J, Biederman J, Mundy E, *et al.*: A pilot family study of childhood onset mania. *J Am Acad Child Adolesc Psychiatry* 1995; **34**:1577–1583.

92. Pliszka SR: Comorbidity of attention deficit hyperactivity disorder and overanxious disorder. *J Am Acad Child Adolesc Psychiatry* 1992; **31**:197–203.

93. Comings DE, Comings BG: Tourette's syndrome and attention deficit disorder. In: Cohen DI, Brun RD, Leckman JF, eds. *Tourette's Syndrome and Tic Disorders: Clinical Understanding and Treatment.* New York: John Wiley & Sons Ltd, 1988.

94. Cantwell DP, Satterfield JH: The prevalence of academic underachievement in hyperactive children. *J Pediatr Psychol* 1978; **3**:168–171.

95. Barkley RA: *Attention-Deficit Hyperactivity Disorder. A Handbook for Diagnosis and Treatment.* New York: Guilford Press, 1990.

96. Baker L, Cantwell DP, Mattison RE: Behavior problems in children with pure speech disorders and in children with combined speech and language disorders. *J Abnormal Child Psychol* 1980; **8**:245–256.

97. Achenbach TM: *Integrative Guide for the 1991 CBCL/4-18 YSR, and TRF Profiles.* Burlington: University of Vermont, Department of Psychiatry, 1991.

98. Conners K: *Conners Abbreviated Symptom Questionnaire.* North Tonowanda, NY: Multi Health Systems, 1994.

99. Swanson JM: *SNAP-IV Seak.* Irvine, CA: University of California Child Development Center, 1995.

100. Pelham WE: Teacher ratings of DMS-III-R symptoms for the disruptive behavior disorders. *J Am Acad Child Adolesc Psychiatry* 1992; **31**:210–218.

101. Reiff MI, Banex GA, Culbert TP: Children who have attentional disorders: Diagnosis and evaluation. *Pediatr Rev* 1993; **12**:455–461.

102. Weiss M: Psychoeducational intervention with family, school and children with attention-deficit/ hyperactivity disorder. *Child Adolesc Psychiatr Clin North Am* 1992; **1**:467–479.

103. Lorey J, Milich R: Hyperactivity, inattention and aggression in clinical practice. *Adv Dev Behav Pediatr* 1982; **3**:113–147.

104. Dupaul GJ, Rapport MD, Perriello LM: Teacher ratings of academic skills: The development of the Academic Performance Rating Scale. *Sch Psychol Rev* 1991; **20**:284–300.

105. Bradley C: The behavior of children receiving benzedrine. *Am J Psychiatry* 1997; **94**:577–585.

106. Buitelaar JK, Van der Gaag RJ, Swaab-Barnweld H, et al.: Predilection of clinical response to methylphenidate in children with attention deficit hyperactivity disorder. *J Am Acad Child Adolesc Psychiatry* 1995; **34**:1205–1032.

107. Rapport MD, Denny C, Dupaul G, Gardner M: Attention deficit disorder and methylphenidate normalization rates, clinical effectiveness, and response prediction in 76 children. *J Am Acad Child Adolesc Psychiatry* 1994; **33**:882–893.

108. Elia J: Drug treatment for hyperactive children: Therapeutic guidelines. *Drugs* 1973; **46**:863–872.

109. Rapport MD, Stoner G, Dupaul GJ, et al.: Attention deficit disorder and methylphendate: A multilevel analysis of dose response effects on children's impulsivity across settings. *J Am Acad Child Adolesc Psychiatry* 1988; **27**:60–69.

110. Ullman RD, Sleator EK: Attention deficit disorder children with or without hyperactivity: Which behaviors are helped by stimulants? *Clin Pediatr* 1985; **24**:547–551.

111. Pelham NE, Walker JL, Sturges J, Hoza J: Comparative effects of methylphenidate on ADD girls and ADD boys. *J Am Acad Child Adolesc Psychiatry* 1989; **28**: 773–776.

112. Famulara R, Fenton T: The effect of methylphenidate on school grades in children with attention deficit disorder without hyperactivity: A preliminary report. *J Clin Psychiatry* 1987; **48**:112–114.

113. Borcherding BG, Keysor CS, Cooper TB, Rapport JL: Differential effects of methylphenidate and dextroampheemine and the motor activity level of hyperactive children. *Neuropsychopharmacol* 1989; **2**: 255–263.

114. Zahn TP, Rapoport JL, Thomson CL: Autonomic and behavioral of dextroamphetamine and placebo in normal and hyperactive prepuberant boys. *J Abnormal Child Psychol* 1980; **8**:145–160.

115. Prince JB, Wilens TE, Biedeman J, et al.: Clonidine for sleep disturbances associated with attention deficit hyperactive disorder: A systematic chart review of 62 cases. *J Am Acad Child Adolesc Psychiatry* 1996; **35**:599–605.

116. Gudow KD: Pediatric psychopharmacology: A review of recent research. *J Child Psychol Psychiatry* 1992; **33**:153–195.

117. Riddle MA, Lynch KA, Schill L, et al.: Methylphenidate discontinuation and re-initiation during long term treatment of children with Tourettes disorder and attention deficit hyperactivity disorder. A pilot study. *J Child Adolesc Psychopharmacol* 1995; **5**:205–214.

118. Schertz M, Adesman AR, Alfieri NE, et al.: Protectors of weight loss in children with attention deficit hyperactivity disorder treated with stimulant medication. *Pediatrics* 1996; **98**:763–769.

119. Brown RT, Sexson SB: A controlled trial of methylphenidate in black adolescents: Attentional, behavioral, and physiologic effects. *Clin Pediatr* 1988; **27**:74–81.

120. Gillberg C, Melander H, von Knoming AL, et al.: Long term stimulant treatment of children with attention deficit hyperactivity disorder symptoms, randomized, double blind placebo controlled trial. *Arch Gen Psychiatry* 1997; **54**:857–864.

121. Spencer T, Brederman J, Wilens T, et al.: Pharmacotherapy of attention deficit hyperactivity disorder across the life cycle. *J Am Acad Child Adolesc Psychiatry* 1996; **35**:409–432.

122. Riddle MA, Hardin MT, Cho SL, et al.: Desipramine treatment of boys with attention deficit hyperactivity disorder and tics: Preliminary clinical experience. *J Am Acad Child Adolesc Psychiatry* 1988; **27**:811-813.

123. Barrickman LL, Perry PH, Allen AJ, et al.: Buproprion versus methylphenidate in the treatment of attention deficit hyperactivity disorder. *J Am Acad Child Adolesc Psychiatry* 1995; **35**:649–657.

124. Spencer T, Biederman J, Steingard R, Wilens T: Buproprion exacerbation of tics in children with attention deficit hyperactivity disorder and Tourette's syndrome. *J Am Acad Child Adolesc Psychiatry* 1993; **32**:211–214.

125. Barrickman L, Noyes R, Kuperman S, et al.: Treatment of ADHD with fluoxetine: A preliminary trial. *J Am Acad Child Adolesc Psychiatry* 1991; **30**:762–767.

126. Busing R, Levin GM: Methamphetamine-fluoxetine treatment in a child with attention deficit hyperactivity disorder and obsessive compulsive disorder. *J Child Adolesc Psychopharmacol* 1993; **3**:53–58.

127. Zametkin A, Rapoport JL, Murphy DL, et al.: Treatment of hyperactive children with monoamine oxidase inhibitors. *Arch Psychiatry* 1985; **42**:962–966.

128. Olvera RL, Pliszka SR, Luh J, Tatum R: An open trial of venflaxine in the treatment of attention deficit hyperactivity disorder in children and adolescents. *J Child Adolesc Psychopharmacol* 1996; **6**:241–250.

129. Findling RL, Schwartz MA, Flannery DJ, Myers MT: Venlafaxine in adults with attention deficit hyperactivity disorder in an open clinical trail. *J Clin Psychiatry* 1996; **57**:184–189.

130. Hunt RD, Lau S, Ryu J: Alternative therapies for ADHD. In: Greenhill LL, Osman BB, eds. *Ritalin: Theory and Patient Management.* New York: Mary Ann Liebert, 1991:75–95.

131. Cantwell DP, Swanson J, Connor DF: Case study: adverse response to clonidine. *J Am Acad Child Adolesc Psychiatry* 1997; **36**:539–544.

132. Hunt RD, Copper S, O'Connell P: Clonidine in child and adolescent psychiatry. *J Child Adolesc Psychopharmacol* 1990; **1**:87–102.

133. Chappell PB, Ridelle MA, Seahill L, *et al.*: Guanfacine treatment of comorbid attention deficit hyperactivity disorder and Tourettes syndrome: Preliminary clinical experience. *J Am Acad Child Adolesc Psychiatry* 1995; **34**:1140–1146.

134. Harrigan JP, Barnhill LJ: Guanfacine for treatment of attention deficit hyperactivity disorder in boys. *J Child Adolesc Psychopharmacol* 1995; **5**:215–223.

135. Hunt RD, Arnsten AFT, Asbell MD: An open trial of guanfacine in the treatment of attention deficit hyperactivity disorder. *J Am Acad Child Adolesc Psychiatry* 1995; **34**:50–54.

136. Fenichel RR: Continuing methylphenidate and clonidine: The role of post marketing surveillance. *J Child Adolesc Psychopharmacol* 1995; **5**:155–156.

137. Popper CN: Combining methylphenidate and clonidine: Pharmacologic questions and news reports about sudden death. *J Child Adolesc Psychopharmacol* 1995; **5**:157–166.

138. Pataki CS, Carlson GA, Kelley KL, *et al.*: Side effects of methylphenidate and desipramine alone and in combination in children. *J Am Acad Child Adolesc Psychiatry* 1993; **32**:1065–1072.

139. Grob CS, Coyle JT: Suspected adverse methylphenidate-imipramine interactions in children. *J Dev Behav Pediatr* 1986; **7**:265–267.

140. Carlson GA, Rapport MD, Kelly KL, Pataki CS: Methylphenidate and desipramine in hospitalized children with comorbid behavior and mood disorders: Separate and combined effect on behavior and mood. *J Child Adolesc Psychopharmacol* 1995; **5**:191–204.

141. Silva RR, Munoz DM, Alpert M: Carbamazepine use in children and adolescents with features of attention-deficit hyperactivity disorder: A beta analysis. *J Am Acad Child Adolesc Psychiatry* 1996; **35**:352–358.

142. Sharma V, Newcorn JH, Matier-Sharma T, Halperin JM: Attention deficit and disruptive behavior disorders. In: Tasman A, Kay J, Lieberman J, eds. *Psychiatry.* Philadelphia: WB Saunders, 1997:667–682.

143. Abromowitz AJ, O'Leary SG: Behavioral interventions for the classroom: Implications for students with ADHD. *Sch Psychol Rev* 1991; **20**:220–234.

144. Kelley ML, McCain AP: Promoting academic performance in inattentive children: The relative efficacy of school-home notes with and without response cost. *Behav Modif* 1995; **14**:357–375.

145. Cousins LS, Weiss G: Parent training and social skills training for children with attention deficit hyperactivity disorder: How can they be combined for greater effectiveness? *Can J Psychiatry* 1993; **38**:449–457.

146. Anastopoulos AD, Shelton TL, Dupaul GJ, *et al.*: Parent training for attention deficit hyperactivity disorder: Its impact on parent functioning. *J Abnorm Child Psychol* 1993; **21**:581–596.

147. Abikoff H, Hechtman L: Multimodel therapy and stimulants in the treatment of children with ADHD. In: Jensen P, Hibbs ED, eds. *Psychosocial Treatment for Child and Adolescent Disorders: Empirically Based Approvals.* Washington, DC: American Psychological Association, 1996:501–546.

148. Lambert N, Hartbaugh C, Sasson D: Persistance of hyperactivity symptoms from childhood to adolescence. *Am J Orthopsychiatry* 1987; **57**:22–31.

149. Lambert N: Adolescent outcomes of hyperactive children. *Am Psychol* 1988; **43**:786–799.

150. Satterfield JH, Hoppe CM, Schell AM: A prospective study of delinquency in 110 adolescent boys with attention deficit disorder and 88 normal adolescent boys. *Am J Psychiatry* 1982; **139**:795–798.

151. Barkley RA, Fischer M, Edtbrock CS, *et al.*: The adolescent outcome of hyperactive children diagnosed by research criteria: An 8-year prospective follow-up study. *J Am Acad Child Adolesc Psychiatry* 1996; **29**:546–557.

152. Mannuzza S, Gittman-Klein R, Horowitz-Konig P, *et al.*: Hyperactive boys almost grown up: IV. Criminality and its relationship to psychiatric status. *Arch Gen Psychiatry* 1989; **46**:1073–1079.

153. Klein RG, Mannuzza S: Long term outcome of hyperactive children: A review. *J Am Acad Child Adolesc Psychiatry* 1991; **30**:383–387.

154. A 14-month randomized clinical trial of treatment strategies for attention-deficit/hyperactivity disorder. MA Cooperative Group. Multimodal Treatment Study of Children with ADHD. *Arch Gen Psychiatry* 1999; **56**:1073–1086.

155. Moderators and mediators of treatment response for children with attention-deficity/hyperactivity disorder: the Multimodal Treatment Study of children with attention-deficit/hyperactivity disorder. *Arch Gen Psychiatry* 1999; **56**:1088–1096.

156. Pelham WE, Murphy HA: Attention deficit and conduct disorders. In: Herson M, ed. *Pharmacological and Behavioral Treatments: An Integrative Approach.* New York: John Wiley and Sons, 1986:108–148.

157. Newcorn JH: Therapeutic Options and Treatment Algorithms for ADHD. *Mount Sinai School of Medicine Reports on Attention-Deficit/Hyperactivity Disorder* 2003; **1**(1):1–12.

158. Spencer T, Biederman J, Wilens T, *et al.*: Attention-deficit hyperactivity disorder. In: Martin A, Scahill L, Charney DS, *et al.* eds. *Pediatric Psychopharmacology: Principles and Practice.* New York: Oxford University Press, 2003:447–465.

159. Spencer T, Biederman J, Wilens T, *et al.*: Pharmacotherapy of attention-deficit hyperactivity disorder across the life cycle. *J Am Acad Child Adolesc Psychiatry* 1996; **35**:409–432.

160. Spencer T, Wilens T, Biederman J, *et al.*: A double-blind, crossover comparison of methylphenidate and lacebo in adults with childhood-onset attention-deficit hyperactivity disorder. *Arch Gen Psychiatry* 1995; **52**:434–443.

161. Spencer T, Biederman J, Wilens T, *et al.*: Efficacy of a mixed amphetamine salts compound in adult with

attention-deficit/hyperactivity disorder. *Arch Gen Psychiatry* 2001; **58**:775–782.

162. Volkow ND, Wang GJ, Fowler JS, *et al.*: Dopamine transporter occupancies in the human brain induced by therapeutic doses of oral methylphenidate. *Am J Psychiatry* 1998; **155**:1325–1331.

163. Bymaster FP, Katner JS, Nelson DL, *et al.*: Atomoxetine increases extracellular levels of norepinephrine and dopamine in prefrontal cortex of rat: a potential mechanism for efficacy in attention deficit/hyperactivity disorder. *Neuropsychopharmacology* 2002; **27**:699–711.

164. Ford RE, Greenhill LL, Posner K: Stimulants. In: Martin A, Scahill L, Charney DS, *et al.*, eds. *Pediatric Psychopharmacology: Principles and Practice.* New York: Oxford University Press, 2003:255–263.

165. Kuczenski R, Segal DS: Effects of methylphenidate on extracellular dopamine, serotonin and norepinerhrine: comparison with amphetamine. *J Neurochem* 1997; **8**:2032–2037.

166. Greenhill LL: Clinical effects of stimulant medication in ADHD. In: Solanto MV, Arnsten AF, Castellanos FX, eds. *Stimulant Drugs and ADHD:Basic and Clinical Neuroscience.* New York: Oxford University Press, 2001:31–71.

167. Porino L, Rapoport J: A naturalistic assessment of the motor activity of hyperactive boys: I. Comparison with normal controls. *Arch Gen Psychiatry* 1983; **40**:681–687.

168. Spencer TJ, Biederman J, Harding M, *et al.*: Growth deficits in ADHD children revisited: Evidence for disorder-associated growth delays? *J Am Acad Child Adolesc Psychiatry* 1996; **35**:1460–1469.

169. Klein RG, Mannuzza S: Hyperactive boys almost grown up. III. Methylphenidate effects on ultimate height. *Arch Gen Psychiatry* 1988; **45**:1131–1134.

170. Pierce RC, Kalivas PW: Amphetamine produces sensitized increases in locomotion and extracellular dopamine preferentially in the nucleus accumbens shell of rats administered repeated cocaine. *J Pharmacol Exp Ther* 1995; **275**:1019–1029.

171. Wilens TE, Faraone SV, Biederman J, *et al.*: Does stimulant therapy of attention-deficit/hyperactivity disorder predict later substance abuse? A meta-analytic review of the literature. *Pediatrics* 2003; **111**:179–185.

172. Barkley RA, Fischer M, Smallish L: Does the treatment of attention-deficit/hyperactivity disorder with stimulants contribute to drug use/abuse? A 13-year prospective study. *Pediatrics* 2003; **111**:97–109.

173. Stein MA, Blondis TA, Schnitzler ER, *et al.*: Methylphenidate dosing: Twice daily versus three times daily. *Pediatrics* 1996; **98**(4 Pt 1):748–756.

174. Newcorn J: Efficacy trials of atomoxetine for ADHD in children, adolescents, and adults. *Scientific Proceedings of the Annual Meeting of the American Academy of Child and Adolescent Psychiatry*, 2002:66.

175. Wernicke JF, Kratochvil CJ: Safety profile of atomoxetine in the treatment of children and adolescents with ADHD. *J Clin Psychiatry* 2002; **63**(Suppl 12): 50–55.

176. Wernick J, Faries D, Girod D, *et al.*: Cardiovascular effects of atomoxetine in children, adolescents, and adults. *Drug Safety* 2003; **26**:729–740.

177. Henderson TA, Hartman K: Aggression, mania, and hypomania induction associated with atomoxetine. *Pediatrics* 2004; **114**(3):895–896.

178. Sawant S, Daviss SR: Seizures and prolonged QTc with atomoxetine overdose. *Am J Psychiatry* 2004; **161**(4): 757.

179. Riggs PD, Leon SL, Mikulich Sk, *et al.*: An open trial of bupropion for ADHD in adolescents with substance use disorders and conduct disorder. *J Am Acad Child Adolesc Psychiatry* 1998; **37**:1271–1278.

180. Taylor FB, Russo J: Efficacy of modafinil compared to dextroamphetainie for the treatment of attention deficit hyperactivity disorder in adults. *J Child Adolesc Psychopharmacol* 2000; **10**:311–320.

181. Rappley MD: Attention deficit-hyperactivity disorder. *N Engl J Med* 2005; 352, **2**:165–173.

182. Baumgartel A, Wolraich ML, Dietrich M: Comparison of diagnostic criteria for attention deficit disorder in a German elementary school sample. *J Am Acad Child Adolesc Psychiatry* 1995; **34**:629–638.

183. Findling RL: Open label treatment of comorbid depression and attention disorders with coadministration of serotonin reuptake inhibitors and psychostimulants in children, adolescents, and adults. *J Child Adolesc Psychopharmacol* 1996; **7**:165–175.

184. Mannuzza S, Klein RG, Besster A, *et al*: Adult outcome of hyperactive boys: Educational achievement, occupational rank and psychiatric status. *Arch Gen Psychiatry* 1993; **50**:565–576.

185. Mannuzza S, Klein RF, Besifert A, *et al*: Educational and occupational outcome of hyperactive boys grown up. *J Am Acad Child Adolesc Psychiatry* 1997; **36**:1222–1227.

186. Greenhill LL: Stimulant related growth inhibition in children: A review. In: Gittleman M, ed. *Strategic Interventions for Hyperactive Children.* New York: Me Sharp, 1981:33–63.

187. Junkovic J: Deprenyl in attention deficit associated with Tourette's syndrome. *Arch Neurol* 1993; **50**:286–288.

188. Feigin A, Kurlan R, McDermott M, *et al*: A controlled trial of deprenelyl in children with Tourette's syndrome and attention deficit hyperactivity disorder. *Neurology* 1996; **46**:965–968.

189. Rugino, TA, Coley TC: Effects of modafinil in children with attention-deficit hyperactivity disorder: An open-label study. *J Am Acad Child Adolesc Psychiatry* 2001; **40**:230–235.

11

Disruptive Behavior Disorders

Niranjan S. Karnik, Hans Steiner

Introduction

Disruptive spectrum disorders constitute one of the most frequent presenting complaints to mental health professionals who provide care for children [1,2]. These behaviors, as a group, are often seen as signs and symptoms of other illness but can in many instances be primary manifestations of childhood psychopathology. The challenge for the treating clinician, then, is to differentiate normal from abnormal, as well as primary from secondary process. These disorders are challenging to treat and exact a high toll in terms of individual, familial, and societal loss. One of the hallmarks of these disorders, which include conduct disorder, oppositional defiant disorder (ODD), and disruptive behavior disorder not otherwise specified, is that parents and others are usually more distressed by the behavior than is the child. As such, it is often hard to enlist the child's cooperation in the evaluation and treatment process.

This chapter presents the background on disruptive spectrum disorders as well as a method for evaluating and treating a child or adolescent. Beginning with a historical overview and definition of the disorder, it then considers epidemiology, etiology, diagnosis, course and natural history, treatment principles and guidelines, and finally prognosis and outcomes.

Definitions and Nosology

Conduct disorder first appeared in the second edition of the *Diagnostic and Statistical Manual of Mental Disorders* (DSM-II) in 1968 [3]. DSM-I included sociopathic personality, but this classification did not extend to children. Beginning with the DSM-II, disruptive behavior disorders comprised three categories: unsocialized aggressive reaction of childhood or adolescence, the runaway reaction of childhood, and the group delinquent reaction of childhood. DSM-III [4]

expanded these subtypes and first introduced the term conduct disorder into official nomenclature. Building on the DSM-II subtypes, DSM-III outlined four general variants of conduct disorder: socialized, undersocialized, aggressive, and nonaggressive. The 1987 revision, the DSM-III-R, further defined the category of conduct disorder by identifying the three most common variants of the previous classification: solitary aggressive, group type, and undifferentiated [5]. A comparison of these definitions reveals the basic feature of conduct disorder: a pattern of behavior by an individual or group that violates age-appropriate and socially appropriate behavior.

The most recent editions, the 1994 DSM-IV [6] and the 2000 DSM-IV TR [7], cease to differentiate by socialization and aggression, since validation has proved difficult. These versions instead emphasize aspects of the disorder that have been empirically validated. Two subtypes are defined: early- or childhood-onset, and late- or adolescent-onset. There is also a coding for severity.

The essential feature of conduct disorder as defined by DSM-IV is a 'repetitive and persistent pattern of behavior in which the basic rights of others or major age-appropriate societal norms or rules are violated.' These behaviors fall within four categories: (1) aggression to people and animals; (2) destruction of property; (3) deceitfulness or theft; and (4) serious violation of rules (Table 11.1). Of the 15 types of behaviors within these categories, an individual must have had three or more within the past 12 months and at least one within the past 6 months. In addition, the behavior must have caused clinically significant impairment in functioning. The subtypes provide useful diagnostic and prognostic information. Individuals with childhood- or early-onset are more aggressive, show decreased socialization and regard for others, and have poor peer relationships. Their aggression usually shows

Clinical Child Psychiatry, Second Edition. Edited by W.M. Klykylo and J.L. Kay
© 2005 John Wiley & Sons Ltd.

Table 11.1 DSM-IV-TR criteria for conduct disorder. Reprinted with permission from the Diagnostic and Statistical Manual of Mental Disorders, Copyright 2000. American Psychiatric Association.

(A) A repetitive and persistent pattern of behavior in which the basic rights of others or major age-appropriate societal norms or rules are violated, as manifested by the presence of three (or more) of the following criteria in the past 12 months, with at least one criterion present in the past 6 months:

Aggression to people and animals
(1) often bullies, threatens, or intimidates others
(2) often initiates physical fights
(3) has used a weapon that can cause serious physical harm to others (e.g., a bat, brick, broken bottle, knife, gun)
(4) has been physically cruel to people
(5) has been physically cruel to animals
(6) has stolen while confronting a victim (e.g., mugging, purse snatching, extortion, armed robbery)
(7) has forced someone into sexual activity

Destruction of property
(8) has deliberately engaged in fire setting with the intention of causing serious damage
(9) has deliberately destroyed others' property (other than by fire setting)

Deceitfulness or theft
(10) has broken into someone else's house, building, or car
(11) often lies to obtain goods or favors or to avoid obligations (i.e., 'cons' others)
(12) has stolen items of nontrivial value without confronting a victim (e.g., shoplifting, but without breaking and entering; forgery)

Serious violations of rules
(13) often stays out at night despite parental prohibitions, beginning before age 13 years
(14) has run away from home overnight at least twice while living in parental or parental surrogate home (or once without returning for a lengthy period)
(15) is often truant from school, beginning before age 13 years
(B) The disturbance in behavior causes clinically significant impairment in social, academic, or occupational functioning
(C) If the individual is age 18 years or older, criteria are not met for antisocial personality disorder

Specify type based on age at onset:
Childhood-onset type – onset of at least one criterion characteristic of conduct disorder prior to age 10 years
Adolescent-onset type – absence of any criteria characteristic of conduct disorder prior to age 10 years

Specify severity:
Mild – few if any conduct problems in excess of those required to make the diagnosis and conduct problems cause only minor harm to others
Moderate – number of conduct problems and effect on others intermediate between 'mild' and 'severe'
Severe – many conduct problems in excess of those required to make the diagnosis or conduct problems cause considerable harm to others

---

a progression from ODD during early childhood to a persistent course of conduct disorder during adolescence to antisocial personality disorder as adults. Individuals with adolescent- or late-onset are typically less aggressive, show better peer socialization and relationships, and are more often female. Several additional alternative classifications have been proposed. Fergusson and colleagues have suggested a division based on overt (aggression, violence) and covert (theft, dishonesty) behaviors [8,9]. Like the DSM-IV subtypes, these two types show relatively distinct developmental patterns, comorbidities, and prognoses.

ODD is often viewed as a milder form or a precursor of conduct disorder (Table 11.2). As with conduct disorder, the behaviors are more distressing to others than to the individual causing them and often cause a

Table 11.2 DSM-IV-TR criteria for oppositional defiant disorder. Reprinted with permission from the Diagnostic and Statistical Manual of Mental Disorders, Copyright 2000. American Psychiatric Association.

(A) A pattern of negativistic, hostile, and defiant behavior lasting at least six months, during which four (or more) of the following are present:

(1) often loses temper

(2) often argues with adults

(3) often actively defies or refuses to comply with adults' requests or rules

(4) often deliberately annoys people

(5) often blames others for his or her mistakes or misbehavior

(6) is often touchy or easily annoyed by others

(7) is often angry and resentful

(8) is often spiteful or vindictive

Note: Consider a criterion met only if the behavior occurs more frequently than is typically observed in individuals of comparable age and developmental level

(B) The disturbance in behavior causes clinically significant impairment in social, academic, or occupational functioning

(C) The behaviors do not occur exclusively during the course of a psychotic or mood disorder

(D) Criteria are not met for conduct disorder, and, if the individual is age 18 years or older, criteria are not met for antisocial personality disorder

---

significant decrease in family, academic, and social functioning. In addition, the behaviors are normal at certain developmental periods, particularly the toddler and adolescent years. Unlike conduct disorder, however, the behaviors usually do not involve serious violations of others' rights or delinquency.

ODD first appeared in the DSM-III as oppositional disorder. It defined a spectrum of behaviors characterized by hostility, usually toward an authority figure. The DSM-III-R added the term defiant to the disorder and broadened the range of behaviors encompassed by the diagnosis, including the use of obscene language or swearing. The DSM-IV dropped this last behavior but retained the term defiant. The key feature remains a 'pattern of negativistic, hostile, and defiant behavior.' Of the eight types of behavior, an individual must have had four or more that lasted at least six months, and the behavior must have caused clinically significant impairment in functioning.

Increasingly, recent developments in the etiology of disruptive spectrum disorders have led to the under-

standing that there are two major forms of aggression in childhood. There is reactive aggression which is characterized as impulsive and triggered by anger or frustration on the part of the child. More disturbing in nature is the second form of aggression that is understood as proactive or instrumental. This form of aggression is planned and premeditated, and often showing a lack of remorse or morality. Proactive aggression is highly correlated with future delinquency, whereas reactive aggression shows a lack of direct correlation, and appears to have significant connections to other causes of behavioral instability. The neuroscience of aggression has begun to trace out the differences between these forms of aggression at a neuroanatomical level, and that these pathways may have functional impacts [10–13]. More specifically, the medial and orbitofrontal cortical pathways as parts of the five major prefrontal pathways of the mind have been implicated as the potentially mediating aggression and violence [10]. Nevertheless, it is evident that these neurological risk factors are not deterministic and instead act in a dynamic relationship with the social world around the child [14]. For a full summary of the neuroscience literature on maladaptive aggression in youth populations please see a report of the American Academy of Child Adolescent Psychiatry Workgroup on Juvenile Aggression and Impulsivity [15].

Epidemiology

Conduct disorder is generally recognized as the most common form of childhood psychopathology. It represents the most common reason for psychiatric consultation, accounting for 25–90% of consultations in some clinics [16]. The general population prevalence varies from 1.5% to 20%, depending on the method of data collection, time frame of study and the particular site [16]. The male-to-female ratio varies from 3:1 to 5:1, depending on the age range studied; specifically, the gender difference decreases in adolescence because of the increased rate among girls [17]. In addition, it appears that girls exhibit different types of violence and aggression than boys, and that these may have contributed to lower rates among girls [18]. Girls tend to produce less overt aggressive violence, and instead use social networks as a means of violence. That is to say that they will shun or exclude people they wish to harm, and do so in ways that utilize the social and emotional systems rather than using physical means. In addition, due to the difficulty in diagnosing early onset, pervasive antisocial behavior in girls, our current estimates of prevalence in this population may be artificially low [19]. The peak age of onset for all children is in late childhood and early adolescence but ranges from preschool to late adolescence. The impact of conduct disorder extends beyond the above estimates. Because of costs at the familial, community, and state levels (i.e., the involvement of educational and legal systems), the actual impact is greater than that recorded on the individual level.

Etiology

As noted previously, the etiology of conduct disorder is multifactorial. The current model is that of premorbid genetic or neurological liability, which is worsened by psychosocial adversity and finally produced by high environmental risk. From this perspective, one can deduce that there are protective factors as well.

Early theories viewed the development of antisocial behavior in children from two perspectives: an internal deficit and an ecologic adaptation. William Healy, who developed the first view, described these children as having a 'psychic constitutional deficiency' [20]. He stressed having found both mental and physical defects in these children, which supported his belief that the behavior was hereditary. An opposing view was proposed by Aichhorn, who applied psychodynamics to the study of delinquency. He described the 'neurotic delinquent,' a youth who seeks to assuage neurotic guilt by seeking punishment through his or her delinquent deeds [21]. Today, both theories are thought to be components of conduct disorders. Conduct problems are heterogeneous, and multiple pathways need to be considered in their genesis.

Biologic studies show abnormalities in the neurotransmitter systems of people with conduct disorders, including serotonin [22,23], noradrenergic and dopaminergic [24] activity. Among these the best studied and most highly supported neurochemical pathways is serotonin dysregulation. Further research has also supported the notion that the autonomic nervous system shows low reactivity on a variety of parameters (e.g., decreased heart rate and skin conductance) in youth with conduct disorder [25]. Finally, the neuroanatomy of aggression, as mentioned above, is beginning to be better understood and has helped to shaped our etiology of youth aggression [10,11,13,14].

Genetic studies suggest a possible heritable factor to conduct disorders. One study found concordance in monozygotic twins to be higher than in dyzygotic twins [25,26]; however, in a study that examined biologic twins who were later adopted, both genetic and environmental factors were shown to be influential [27,28]. Conduct disorder is perceived as the childhood pre-

cursor of antisocial personality disorder; therefore, estimates of heritability from adults with antisocial personality disorder could be useful to evaluate the genetic contribution to conduct disorder. Yet these studies are difficult to interpret; most children with conduct disorder do not develop antisocial personality disorder in adulthood. Those who do, therefore, may represent a subgroup with more severe pathology. Early constitutional factors such as temperament and restraint may also be genetically mediated. Clearly, genetic studies are presently incomplete; it still seems likely, however, that there is a heritable component that acts as a risk factor for the development of conduct disorder.

The high incidence of neurological abnormalities in children with conduct disorder provides further evidence that neurological factors may be significant. This high incidence, however, may actually represent an increased exposure to accidents, injuries, and illnesses that affect central nervous system (CNS) functioning. Among more seriously disordered youth, there does seem to be a significantly higher incidence of psychomotor seizures. Lewis and colleagues in a small sample of incarcerated youths found a 20-fold higher incidence of seizure disorder in those with conduct disorder over the general population [29]. These youths also show more subtle findings, including learning and communication disorders, impaired memory for behavior, and minor motor abnormalities.

Other forms of psychiatric disability can act as risk factors. Hyperactivity represents a risk [30]. In addition, cognitive deficits and linguistic problems can act as predisposing factors, and chronic illness and disability have also been shown to be risk factors. Children who are chronically ill have three times the incidence of conduct problems as that of healthy peers. Moreover, if the chronic condition affects the CNS, the risk can increase as much as fivefold [31]. Individual personality factors such as aggression and coping style may similarly predispose individuals to later conduct disorder and delinquency [32].

Several familial factors have been found to affect the incidence of conduct disorder. Poor family functioning, poor parenting, marital discord, and child abuse are proven risk factors. More specifically, drug and alcohol abuse [33–35], mood disorders [36,37], psychotic disorders [38,39], attention deficit hyperactivity disorder (ADHD) and learning disorders [33,40–42], intrafamilial trauma [43,44], and parental antisocial personality disorder [45] also increase the risk. Although all of these factors are significant, the risk is highest for parenting practices that are abusive and injurious.

Risk elements also exist at the community and social levels. Socioeconomic disadvantage, poor housing, crowding, and poverty exert negative influences; and poor peer relations, limited role models, and prosocial structures (e.g., schools and churches) and increased antisocial structures (e.g., organized violence and drug sales) represent another layer of risk [46]. These community risk factors are not limited to the development of conduct disorder and delinquency, however, since they can also increase the incidence of other forms of psychopathology such as post-traumatic stress disorder (PTSD) [47–49].

Some attention should be given to protective factors. Increasingly, we find that there is evidence for a positive psychology which defines a set of factors which act to protect and even enhance the lives of young people who may traditionally be seen as at-risk [50,51]. Within the individual domain, an easy temperament, intelligence, good rapport with others, good work habits at school, and areas of competence outside school all offer protection [52]. Within the family domain, a good relationship with at least one parent or another important adult affords a degree of protection; and in the community domain, prosocial peers and a school that promotes empowerment also emerge as protective factors [46]. After some point, however, protection is probably no longer possible, and the disorder arises; at a further point, the disorder becomes unresponsive to even the most concerted treatment effort. The challenge is to diagnose and intervene early in order to stem the progression and improve outcomes.

Diagnosis

The clinical evaluation of a child for disruptive spectrum disorders needs to take place across several dimensions, with multiple informants, with diverse methods, and in different settings. Without this comprehensive approach, it becomes difficult not only to identify disordered behaviors but also to distinguish them from other potential etiologies.

The multidimensional category refers to evaluating individual, family, and community risk and protective factors. The assessment may begin with individual factors. This includes a thorough history and physical examination and appropriate laboratory and diagnostic studies. More than one informant should be consulted: both the child and his or her family should be interviewed as well as teachers and other significant adults who have had the opportunity to observe the child. More than one method of assessment with each informant should be used: interviews, rating scales (e.g., Conners Scale, the Child Behavior Checklist,

Response Evaluation Measure [53] and the child hostility inventory and child version of the Overt Aggression Scale), neuropsychologic testing and school records may be used. In addition, the child's behaviors may require assessment in more than one setting (e.g., office, home, school). This gives the clinician a context in which to consider the behavior as well as an indication of the chronicity and habituation of the behavior. One should assess the familial and community dimension similarly (Figure 11.1).

After a complete assessment, one can begin to look at the number of behaviors (severity), associated factors (comorbidity), and patterns of behavior (subtypes). This allows one to generate a complete differential diagnosis and identify any comorbid conditions.

Comorbidity and Differential Diagnosis

As detailed earlier, conduct disorder is associated with many other psychiatric and non-psychiatric disorders [41,54–59]. The most common associated disorders are other disruptive behavior disorders. Up to 90% of the children diagnosed with early-onset conduct disorder also meet criteria for ODD at an earlier age. In fact, because of the high degree of overlap between conduct disorder and ODD, many believe they are manifestations of the same illness at different levels of severity. Both conduct disorder and ODD are also associated with ADHD: up to 45% of children with either conduct disorder or ODD also have ADHD. The concurrence of conduct disorder and ADHD is highest in the preteen years and decreases slightly in the teen years. There is a significant gender difference; comorbid ADHD seems to predispose girls to the development of conduct disorder and to increase the intensity and chronicity of conduct disorder among boys. Alcohol and drug abuse represent two additional disorders that are significantly higher in individuals with conduct disorder [60–66].

Conduct disorder is associated with other psychiatric disorders. Mood disorders, particularly depressive and unipolar syndromes, occur in up to 50% of individuals with conduct disorder. Anxiety disorders also occur at a higher level for girls with conduct disorder. Learning disabilities, especially dyslexia, show a comorbidity of 20% with conduct disorder. Other developmental disabilities such as mental retardation and personality disorders (usually antisocial in boys and borderline in girls) occur frequently [67]. Head trauma, seizure disorders and other neurologic disorders are also comorbid conditions.

As a result of the frequent comorbidity, the differential diagnosis of conduct disorder is broad and raises

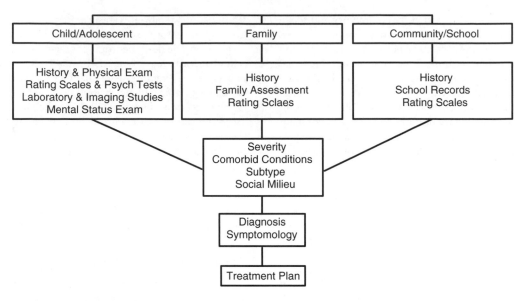

Figure 11.1. Diagnostic assessment.

the question of comorbid (i.e., simply coexisting) versus compound (i.e., complicating each other) psychopathologies. In addition to the comorbidities, the differential diagnosis includes psychotic disorders, intermittent explosive disorder, and other personality disorders. In essence, almost any condition with socially unacceptable behaviors can mimic conduct disorder. Most disorders other than conduct disorder, however, lack the critical determinant of persistently inappropriate behavior that violates the rules and rights of others. A careful family history, qualification of the frequency and severity of behaviors, and a thorough medical evaluation can help differentiate conduct disorder from other distinct and potentially more treatable conditions.

Course and Pattern

Among the disruptive spectrum disorders, ODD is often seen as being the gateway diagnosis. It presents at earlier ages than does conduct disorder, and usually begins as a pattern of behavior which show resistance to authority and parental control. To some extent, all children exhibit some qualities of this behavior because this is the method through which children learn the rules of society. These behaviors enter the diagnostic realm when the pattern has become fixed or the behaviors are escalating, and thereby significantly impacting the child's life.

In contrast, conduct disorder is a relatively stable diagnosis, in fact, untreated it may progress to severe behavioral disturbances and criminality. Conduct disorder with onset in childhood may predispose these children to developing adult antisocial personality disorder: one study found that 30%–50% of affected children showed this developmental course. As noted previously, different subtypes of conduct disorder have different trajectories [68]. Factors that predispose individuals to a more severe case and poor outcome include: (1) childhood-onset and proactive type; (2) comorbid conditions, especially ADHD; (3) individual risk factors such as poor peer relations, labile temperament, and reduced intelligence; and (4) familial risk factors such as family discord and disorganization.

Children with more chronic and severe conduct disorder show impairment across multiple areas: difficulties with social mechanics and the legal system, lower academic and vocation achievement, and retarded interpersonal development. They have a higher risk of suicidal or homicidal behavior and an increased rate of substance abuse. More extreme forms of the disorder may worsen associated comorbid conditions. It is when working with these more disturbed children that one really begins to appreciate the cost of this disease and the importance of skilled, expedient interventions and treatments.

Treatment

Disruptive spectrum disorders should warrant conservative treatment during their early presentation. Particularly for the child who is diagnosed with ODD, family and individual therapy are the recommended interventions. Medications should not play a role at this stage unless there are comorbid conditions such as mood disorder that warrant pharmacological treatment. Should the illness begin to worsen despite these interventions, and the child begins to show early manifestations of conduct disorder by attempt to harm themselves or others, or exhibit marked violence against property or animals, then the clinician can consider expanding the approach.

Because of the multitude of illnesses that can complicate conduct disorder, it is a complex illness to treat. In addition, since the behaviors are more distressing to others, it is difficult for a child or teen with conduct disorder to acknowledge the problem and comply with treatment. As with diagnosis and assessment, treatment should proceed from multiple perspectives on multiple levels and should use a variety of techniques.

The initial task is to decide on the treatment setting (Figure 11.2). This is usually determined by the affected child. Despite the fact that studies on criteria for hospitalization of those with conduct disorder are lacking [69], if the behaviors are severe and pose a danger to either the child or others, the child should be treated as an inpatient. Initial intervention consists of providing a safe, secure environment and pharmacologic treatment as needed. After the child has been stabilized, discharge is recommended as soon as possible. A transition to the outpatient setting allows patients more definitive, long-term treatment while they and their caretakers are still actively involved and committed [70].

With both inpatients and outpatients, it is important to consider the presence of comorbid conditions. If present, these conditions should be treated first, since this type of therapy often decreases the intensity and frequency of antisocial behavior. Usually a combined treatment approach is needed: individual psychotherapy, group psychotherapy, family psychotherapy, community interventions (i.e., educational support and restructuring) [71,72] and medication all should be considered. The recommendations for medication follow traditional guidelines and target other complicating symptoms: (1) psychostimulants, norepinepherine reuptake inhibitors, and clonidine for ADHD; (2) selective serotonin reuptake inhibitors (SSRIs) for

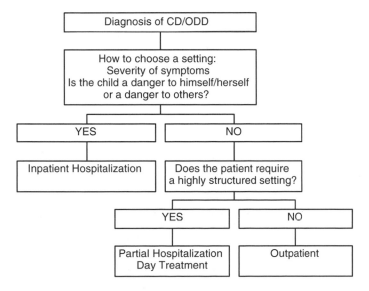

Figure 11.2. Treatment approach.

depression; and (3) diphenhydramine (Benadryl), benzodiazepines, SSRIs, and possibly buspirone (BuSpar) for anxiety [73,74]. Rarely, if ever, is simple psychopharmacology sufficient for treatment; usually a comprehensive and extensive treatment package is needed.

Psychosocial approaches to conduct disorder include individual psychotherapy (behavioral, supportive, and insight-oriented), group psychotherapy, and family psychotherapy. Behavioral and supportive variants of psychotherapy seem to have more success than insight-oriented psychotherapy but there are ongoing investigations in the efficacy of psychoanalytic models [75–77]. Cognitive behavioral therapy can enhance the child's sense of self-control (internal locus of control) and begin to nurture healthy problem-solving skills [78–80]. Insight-oriented therapy, however, may still be useful: those who demonstrate more distress and interest about their behaviors and those subtyped as reactive (responding to external stressors with rapid anger) may benefit from such treatment. Group therapy may be helpful, since many youths are more comfortable discussing issues among peers than adults. Family therapy is usually indicated as well, especially if the child is preadolescent or younger; often the behavior may be reinforced or suppressed by the reactions of family members. By providing a safe place to express these reactions, families may be able to identify ways to alter their reactions and avenues for meaningful family interactions, and family risk factors such as chronic discord, disorganization, and abuse can be addressed. Approaches focused on enhancing attachment to important caregivers have been found to decrease the rate of conduct disordered behaviors. Therapy for couples may also be appropriate if there is significant marital discord and conflicting or dysfunctional and injurious parenting styles.

Psychoeducational approaches to conduct disorder include social skill building and behavior modification for the affected youth, family, and community. Children can be taught more appropriate coping strategies and social skills, for which day treatment programs are particularly beneficial. If indicated, supplemental academic and vocational training can be provided. Parent-directed methods are also effective. Parent management training consists of positively reinforcing prosocial behavior and negatively reinforcing antisocial behavior. The latter refers to nonviolent punishments for previously defined behaviors. The key to this method is consistency, which requires parents to be patient and highly motivated; thus, like many of these treatment methods, it may not apply to every situation.

The combination of child- and parent-directed methods is particularly effective in decreasing the incidence of aggressive and inappropriate behavior. Henggeler has described an intervention that acts at the community level called multisystemic treatment. It combines child- and parent-directed interventions with community case management and family support services. The results are promising, especially for treatment-resistant populations such as violent juvenile delinquents [81,82].

Although pharmacologic interventions have had varying degrees of success, medication should still be considered as part of the comprehensive treatment plan. Divalproex sodium has been found to have good mood stabilizing qualities in children and adolescents, and has expanded in use given its efficacy [73,74]. Other mood stabilizers such as lithium and carbamazepine may help manage aggressive and impulsive behavior. Likewise, neuroleptics such as risperidone, olanzapine and haloperidol may be used, and propranolol has been tried with some success. Stimulants like methylphenidate should be used with extreme caution in this population as they can exacerbate behavioral swings and aggressive patterns. When using pharmacologic treatment, one should first address any comorbid conditions and then define target symptoms and consider potential side effects [74]. All medications require careful consideration of risks and benefits, and increasingly good medical monitoring. Divalproex puts children at risk for major hepatic injury, and careful monitoring of blood levels as well hepatic function is necessary. All atypical antipsychotics now carry a warning on the development of diabetes mellitus, and regular measurements of height, weight, and appropriate laboratory studies are now an expected part of care based on recent recommendations by the American Diabetes Association and the American Psychiatric Association [83].

Prognosis

With appropriate treatment, much can be done to alter the course and outcome of patients with conduct disorder. Clearly, conduct disorders are typical developmental forms of psychopathology: risks accrue over many years, and the combination of multiple risks ultimately produces the disorder. There is ample time, therefore, to intervene prior to the crystallization of a risk into a disorder. Interventions have a chance to work provided they are multifocal, use different methods, and are delivered consistently over extensive periods. Combined treatment approaches can significantly reduce the degree of disordered behaviors and the attendant rate of criminal activity and incarceration. True preventive methods, however, must take place fairly quickly after the onset of behaviors, probably in the first decade of life if not the first five years. Parents represent the first line of defense, followed by other important adults, teachers and the education system, peers, and the larger community. Although conduct disorders currently remain difficult to treat, much progress has been made; many research projects are exploring additional ways to decrease the cost to the individuals, family, and society.

Even with the best interventions, some individuals still fail and eventually enter criminal pathways and delinquency. Prevalence rates of disruptive behavior disorders among adjudicated youths range between 70% and 100% depending on the study [84–89]. This finding may reflect the fact that the criteria for conduct disorder mirror most social rules and laws which children are likely to break. Substance abuse seems to have a special role in this progression: once youngsters develop extensive substance abuse patterns, disorders, or even dependency, it becomes even more difficult to extricate them from a career of crime. Eighty percent of incarcerated juveniles report extensive experimentation, and 25% fulfill diagnostic criteria for dependency. Since drugs are expensive, youngsters are increasingly forced to resort to criminal activity to support their habits, with its resulting risk of arrest and criminal punishment. The clinician should always consider substance abuse and its treatment when dealing with an adjudicated youngster. Such treatment needs to be concomitant with the treatment of learning disabilities and psychosocial deficits.

Our approach to the youngster in the juvenile justice system deserves some special consideration. Many of our conduct-disordered patients ultimately end up in a system in which mental health becomes secondary to criminologic management and considerations. Once a juvenile has been adjudicated, his or her life becomes more complex and difficult, as does access to mental health professionals. Nevertheless, clinicians have a vital role to fulfill, since they can more easily prescribe treatment and rehabilitation that were not previously available. We like to view periods of confinement as an opportunity to deal with the treatment needs of those who for a variety of reasons have failed to respond to previous interventions. There is evidence that youngsters in confinement have high rates of psychopathology, which interferes with rehabilitative programs and has a bearing on their future recidivism after release. The task before us when dealing with juveniles in prison is as follows:

(1) Establish diagnostic profiles and comorbidities, which dictate what interventions are most appropriate for certain youngsters; ADHD, affective disorders and PTSD occur at very high rates and have immediate management implications.
(2) Assist the staff in making appropriate recommendations to the youthful offender parole board regarding dispositions within the system and after release.
(3) Assess crises that arise during confinement that have been triggered by events in prison or by contacts (or lack thereof) with families.
(4) Serve as a consultant to the system regarding the appropriate timing of release of the youngsters and their readiness to face the external world.

Future Directions

The future directions for care of children with disruptive disorders are manifold. The field is changing rapidly as advances in our understanding of the neuropsychology of aggression expand so will the options for interventions using a multiplicity of pharmacological and neurochemical techniques. But even as these choices expand, it is prudent for the treating clinician to be ever mindful of the social and family milieu of the child, and the potential interventions that can be done using the social resources around the child including parents, schools and peers. These options used in concert with judicious pharmacological options are likely to have best and most lasting effects for the child.

References

1. Steiner H: Practice parameters for the assessment and treatment of children and adolescents with conduct disorder. *J Am Acad Child Adolesc Psychiatry* 1997; **36**:122S–139S.
2. Steiner H, Dunne JE: Summary of the practice parameters for the assessment and treatment of children and adolescents with conduct disorder. *J Am Acad Child Adolesc Psychiatry* 1997; **36**:1482–1485.
3. American Psychiatric Association: Committee on Nomenclature and Statistics. *Diagnostic and Statistical Manual of Mental Disorders*. Washington, DC: American Psychiatric Association, 1968.
4. American Psychiatric Association: Task Force on Nomenclature and Statistics. *Diagnostic and Statistical Manual of Mental Disorders*. Washington, DC: American Psychiatric Association, 1978.
5. American Psychiatric Association: Work Group to Revise DSM-III. *Diagnostic and Statistical Manual of Mental Disorders: DSM-III-R*. Washington, DC: American Psychiatric Association, 1987.

6. American Psychiatric Association: Task Force on DSM-IV: *Diagnostic and Statistical Manual of Mental Disorders: DSM-IV*, Washington, DC: American Psychiatric Association, 1994.

7. American Psychiatric Association: Task force on DSM-IV. *Diagnostic and Statistical Manual of Mental Disorders: DSM-IV-TR*. Washington, DC: American Psychiatric Association, 2000.

8. Fergusson DM, Horwood LJ, Lynskey MT: Structure of DSM-III-R criteria for disruptive childhood behaviors: Confirmatory factor models. *J Am Acad Child Adolesc Psychiatry* 1994; **33**:1145–1155; discussion 1155–1157.

9. Fergusson DM, Horwood LJ, Lynskey MT: Prevalence and comorbidity of DSM-III-R diagnoses in a birth cohort of 15 year olds. *J Am Acad Child Adolesc Psychiatry* 1993; **32**:1127–1134.

10. Blair RJ: The roles of orbital frontal cortex in the modulation of antisocial behavior. *Brain Cogn* 2004; **55**:198–208.

11. Blair RJ: Neurocognitive models of aggression, the antisocial personality disorders, and psychopathy. *J Neurol Neurosurg Psychiatry* 2001; **71**:727–731.

12. Richell RA, Mitchell DG, Newman C, Leonard A, Baron-Cohen S, Blair RJ: Theory of mind and psychopathy: Can psychopathic individuals read the 'language of the eyes'? *Neuropsychologia* 2003; **41**:523–526.

13. Blair RJ: Neurobiological basis of psychopathy. *Br J Psychiatry* 2003; **182**:5–7

14. Karnik NS: The social environment. In Steiner H, ed. *Handbook of Mental Health Interventions in Children and Adolescents: An Integrated Developmental Perspective*. San Francisco: Jossey-Bass, 2004.

15. Blair RJ, Coccaro EF, Connor DF and the Members of the AACAP Workgroup on Juvenile Impulsivity and Aggression. The Neuroscience of Maladaptive Aggression. Working Paper of the American Academy of Child & Adolescent Psychiatry. 2005.

16. Connor DF: *Aggression and Antisocial Behavior in Children and Adolescents: Research and Treatment*. New York: Guilford Press, 2002.

17. Cohen P, Cohen J, Kasen S, Velez CN, Hartmark C, Johnson J, Rojas M, Brook J, Streuning EL: An epidemiological study of disorders in late childhood and adolescence–I. Age- and gender-specific prevalence. *J Child Psychol Psychiatry* 1993; **34**:851–867.

18. Hawkins S, Miller S, Steiner H: Aggression, psychopathology and delinquency: Influences of gender and maturation. Where did the good girls go? In: Hayward C, ed. *Gender Differences at Puberty*. London, UK: Cambridge University Press, 2003.

19. Zoccolillo M, Tremblay R, Vitaro F: DSM-III-R and DSM-III criteria for conduct disorder in preadolescent girls: specific but insensitive. *J Am Acad Child Adolesc Psychiatry* 1996; **35**:461–470.

20. Healy W: *The Individual Delinquent*. Boston: Little, Brown, and company, 1915.

21. Aichhorn A: *Wayward Youth*. New York: Viking Press, 1935.

22. Swann AC: Neuroreceptor mechanisms of aggression and its treatment. *J Clin Psychiatry* 2003; **64**:(Suppl 4)26–35.

23. Lee R, Coccaro E: The neuropsychopharmacology of criminality and aggression. *Can J Psychiatry* 2001; **46**:35–44.

24. Pliszka SR, Rogeness GA, Renner P, Sherman J, Broussard T: Plasma neurochemistry in juvenile offenders. *J Am Acad Child Adolesc Psychiatry* 1998; **27**:588–594.

25. Raine A: Biosocial studies of antisocial and violent behavior in children and adults: a review. *J Abnorm Child Psychol* 2002; **30**:311–326.

26. Raine A: *Biosocial Bases of Violence*. New York: Plenum Press, 1997.

27. Riggins-Caspers KM, Cadoret RJ, Knutson JF, Langbehn D: Biology-environment interaction and evocative biology-environment correlation: contributions of harsh discipline and parental psychopathology to problem adolescent behaviors. *Behav Genet* 2003; **33**:205–220.

28. Cadoret RJ, Cain CA, Crowe RR: Evidence for gene-environment interaction in the development of adolescent antisocial behavior. *Behav Genet* 1983; **13**: 301–310.

29. Lewis DO, Pincus JH, Shanok SS, Glaser GH: Psychomotor epilepsy and violence in a group of incarcerated adolescent boys. *Am J Psychiatry* 1982; **139**: 882–887.

30. Offord DR, Boyle MH, Racine YA, Fleming JE, Cadman DT, Blum HM, Byrne C, Links PS, Lipman EL, Macmillan HL: Outcome, prognosis, and risk in a longitudinal follow-up study. *J Am Acad Child Adolesc Psychiatry* 1992; **31**:916–923.

31. Cadman D, Boyle MH, Offord DR, Szatmari P, Rae-Grant NI, Crawford J, Byles J: Chronic illness and functional limitation in Ontario children: findings of the Ontario Child Health Study. *CMAJ* 1986; **135**:761–767.

32. Coon H, Carey G, Corley R, Fulker DW: Identifying children in the Colorado Adoption Project at risk for conduct disorder. *J Am Acad Child Adolesc Psychiatry* 1992; **31**:503–511.

33. Disney ER, Elkins IJ, Mcgue M, Iacono WG: Effects of ADHD, conduct disorder, and gender on substance use and abuse in adolescence. *Am J Psychiatry* 1999; **156**:1515–1521.

34. Myers MG, Stewart DG, Brown SA: Progression from conduct disorder to antisocial personality disorder following treatment for adolescent substance abuse. *Am J Psychiatry* 1998; **155**:479–485.

35. Fisckenscher A, Novins D: Gender differences and conduct disorder among American Indian adolescents in substance abuse treatment. *J Psychoactive Drugs* 2003; **35**:79–84.

36. Marmorstein NR, Iacono WG: Major depression and conduct disorder in a twin sample: gender, functioning, and risk for future psychopathology. *J Am Acad Child Adolesc Psychiatry* 2003; **42**:225–233.

37. Knapp M, McCrone P, Fombonne E, Beecham J, Wostear G: The Maudsley long-term follow-up of child and adolescent depression: 3. Impact of comorbid conduct disorder on service use and costs in adulthood. *Br J Psychiatry* 2002; **180**:19–23.

38. Mueser KT, Drake RE, Ackerson TH, Alterman AI, Miles KM, Noordsy DL: Antisocial personality disorder, conduct disorder, and substance abuse in schizophrenia. *J Abnorm Psychol* 1997; **106**:473–477.

39. Mueser KT, Rosenberg SD, Drake RE, Miles KM, Wolford G, Vidaver R, Carrieri K: Conduct disorder,

antisocial personality disorder and substance use disorders in schizophrenia and major affective disorders. *J Stud Alcohol* 1999; **60**:278–284.

40. Connor DF, Barkley RA, Davis HT: A pilot study of methylphenidate, clonidine, or the combination in ADHD comorbid with aggressive oppositional defiant or conduct disorder. *Clin Pediatr (Philadelphia)* 2000; **39**:15–25.

41. Rothenberger A, Banaschewski T, Heinrich H, Moll GH, Schmidt MH, Van't Klooster B: Comorbidity in ADHD-children: Effects of coexisting conduct disorder or tic disorder on event-related brain potentials in an auditory selective-attention task. *Eur Arch Psychiatry Clin Neurosci* 2000; **250**:101–110.

42. Biederman J, Mick E, Faraone SV, Burback M: Patterns of remission and symptom decline in conduct disorder: a four-year prospective study of an ADHD sample. *J Am Acad Child Adolesc Psychiatry* 2001; **40**:290–298.

43. Plattner B, Silvermann MA, Redlich AD, Carrion VG, Feucht M, Friedrich MH, Steiner H: Pathways to dissociation: intrafamilial versus extrafamilial trauma in juvenile delinquents. *J Nerv Ment Dis* 2003; **191**: 781–788.

44. Steiner H, Carrion V, Plattner B, Koopman C: Dissociative symptoms in posttraumatic stress disorder: diagnosis and treatment. *Child Adolesc Psychiatr Clin N Am* 2003; **12**:231–249.

45. Frick PJ, Lahey BB, Loeber R, Stouthamer-Loeber M, Christ MA, Hanson K: Familial risk factors to oppositional defiant disorder and conduct disorder: Parental psychopathology and maternal parenting. *J Consult Clin Psychol* 1992; **60**:49–55.

46. Bassarath L: Conduct disorder: a biopsychosocial review. *Can J Psychiatry* 2001; **46**:609–616.

47. Ruchkin V, Koposov R, Vermeiren, R, Schwab-Stone M: Psychopathology and age at onset of conduct problems in juvenile delinquents. *J Clin Psychiatry* 2003; **64**:913–920.

48. Steiner H, Garcia IG, Matthews Z: Posttraumatic stress disorder in incarcerated juvenile delinquents. *J Am Acad Child Adolesc Psychiatry* 1997; **36**:357–365.

49. Cauffman E, Feldman SS, Waterman J, Steiner H: Posttraumatic stress disorder among female juvenile offenders. *J Am Acad Child Adolesc Psychiatry* 1998; **37**: 1209–1216.

50. Furstenberg FF: *Managing to Make It: Urban Families and Adolescent Success.* Chicago: University of Chicago Press, 1999.

51. Seligman ME, Csikszentmihalyi M: Positive psychology. An introduction. *Am Psychol* 2000; **55**:5–14.

52. Rae-Grant N, Thomas BH, Offord DR, Boyle MH: Risk, protective factors, and the prevalence of behavioral and emotional disorders in children and adolescents. *J Am Acad Child Adolesc Psychiatry* 1989; **28**: 262–268.

53. Steiner H, Araujo KB, Koopman C: The response evaluation measure (REM-71): A new instrument for the measurement of defenses in adults and adolescents. *Am J Psychiatry* 2001; **158**:467–473.

54. Goodwin RD, Hamilton SP: Lifetime comorbidity of antisocial personality disorder and anxiety disorders among adults in the community. *Psychiatry Res* 2003; **117**:159–166.

55. Lahey BB, Loeber R, Burke J, Rathouz PJ, McBurnett K: Waxing and waning in concert: dynamic comorbidity of conduct disorder with other disruptive and emotional problems over 7 years among clinic-referred boys. *J Abnorm Psychol* 2002; **111**:556–567.

56. Fischer M, Barkley RA, Smallish L, Fletcher K: Young adult follow-up of hyperactive children: self-reported psychiatric disorders, comorbidity, and the role of childhood conduct problems and teen CD. *J Abnorm Child Psychol* 2002; **30**:463–475.

57. Newcorn JH, Halperin JM, Jensen PS, Abikoff HB, Arnold LE, Cantwell DP, Conners CK, Elliott GR, Epstein JN, Greenhill LL, Hechtman L, Hinshaw SP, Hoza B, Kraemer HC, Pelham WE, Severe JB, Swanson JM, Wells KC, Wigal T, Vitiello B: Symptom profiles in children with ADHD: Effects of comorbidity and gender. *J Am Acad Child Adolesc Psychiatry* 2001; **40**: 137–146.

58. Thapar A, Harrington R, McGuffin P: Examining the comorbidity of ADHD-related behaviours and conduct problems using a twin study design. *Br J Psychiatry* 2001; **179**:224–229.

59. Miller-Johnson S, Lochman JE, Coie JD, Terry R, Hyman C: Comorbidity of conduct and depressive problems at sixth grade: substance use outcomes across adolescence. *J Abnorm Child Psychol* 1998; **26**:221–232.

60. Neighbors B, Kempton T, Forehand R: Co-occurrence of substance abuse with conduct, anxiety, and depression disorders in juvenile delinquents. *Addict Behav* 1992; **17**:379–386.

61. Fergusson DM, Lynskey MT, Horwood LJ: Factors associated with continuity and changes in disruptive behavior patterns between childhood and adolescence. *J Abnorm Child Psychol* 1996; **24**:533–553.

62. Fergusson DM, Lynskey MT, Horwood LJ: Origins of comorbidity between conduct and affective disorders. *J Am Acad Child Adolesc Psychiatry* 1996; **35**:451–460.

63. Fergusson DM, Horwood LJ, Lynskey MT: The stability of disruptive childhood behaviors. *J Abnorm Child Psychol* 1995; **23**:379–396.

64. Fergusson DM, Lynskey M, Horwood LJ: The adolescent outcomes of adoption: a 16-year longitudinal study. *J Child Psychol Psychiatry* 1995; **36**:597–615.

65. Fergusson DM, Horwood LJ, Lynskey MT: The comorbidities of adolescent problem behaviors: a latent class model. *J Abnorm Child Psychol* 1994; **22**:339–354.

67. Eppright TD, Kashani JH, Robison BD, Reid JC: Comorbidity of conduct disorder and personality disorders in an incarcerated juvenile population. *Am J Psychiatry* 1993; **150**, 1233–1226.

68. Loeber R: Antisocial behavior: more enduring than changeable? *J Am Acad Child Adolesc Psychiatry* 1991; **30**:393–397.

69. Lock J, Strauss GD: Psychiatric hospitalization of adolescents for conduct disorder. *Hosp Community Psychiatry* 1994; **45**:925–928.

70. Kazdin AE, Whitley MK: Treatment of parental stress to enhance therapeutic change among children referred for aggressive and antisocial behavior. *J Consult Clin Psychol* 2003; **71**:504–515.

71. Kazdin AE, Wassell G: Predictors of barriers to treatment and therapeutic change in outpatient therapy for antisocial children and their families. *Ment Health Serv Res* 2000;**2**:27–40.

72. Kazdin AE: Treatments for aggressive and antisocial children. *Child Adolesc Psychiatr Clin N Am* 2000; **9**:841–858.

73. Steiner H, Petersen ML, Saxena K, Ford S, Matthews Z: Divalproex sodium for the treatment of conduct disorder: A randomized controlled clinical trial. *J Clin Psychiatry* 2003b; **64**:1183–1191.

74. Steiner H, Saxena K, Chang K: Psychopharmacologic strategies for the treatment of aggression in juveniles. *CNS Spectr* 2003; **8**:298–308.

75. Fonagy P, Target M: The efficacy of psychoanalysis for children with disruptive disorders. *J Am Acad Child Adolesc Psychiatry* 1994; **33**:45–55.

76. Fonagy P, Target M: Understanding the violent patient: The use of the body and the role of the father. *Int J Psychoanal* 1995; **76**(Pt 3):487–501.

77. Fonagy P, Target M: The place of psychodynamic theory in developmental psychopathology. *Dev Psychopathol* 2000; **12**:407–425.

78. Rohde P, Clarke GN, Mace DE, Jorgensen JS, Seeley JR: An efficacy/effectiveness study of cognitive-behavioral treatment for adolescents with comorbid major depression and conduct disorder. *J Am Acad Child Adolesc Psychiatry* 2004; **43**:660–668.

79. Kazdin AE, Siegel TC, Bass D: Cognitive problem-solving skills training and parent management training in the treatment of antisocial behavior in children. *J Consult Clin Psychol* 1992; **60**:733–747.

80. Kazdin AE, Bass D, Siegel T, Thomas C: Cognitive-behavioral therapy and relationship therapy in the treatment of children referred for antisocial behavior. *J Consult Clin Psychol* 1989; **57**:522–535.

81. Henggeler SW, Melton GB, Brondino MJ, Scherer DG, Hanley JH: Multisystemic therapy with violent and chronic juvenile offenders and their families: the role of treatment fidelity in successful dissemination. *J Consult Clin Psychol* 1997; **65**:821–833.

82. Henggeler SW, Melton GB, Smith LA: Family preservation using multisystemic therapy: an effective alternative to incarcerating serious juvenile offenders. *J Consult Clin Psychol* 1992; **60**:953–961.

83. Consensus development conference on antipsychotic drugs and obesity and diabetes. *Diabetes Care* 2004; **27**:596–601.

84. Haapasalo J, Hamalainen T: Childhood family problems and current psychiatric problems among young violent and property offenders. *J Am Acad Child Adolesc Psychiatry* 1996; **35**:1394–1401.

85. Pliszka SR, Sherman JO, Barrow MV, Irick S: Affective disorder in juvenile offenders: A preliminary study. *Am J Psychiatry* 2000; **157**:130–132.

86. Ruchkin VV, Schwab-Stone M, Koposov R, Vermeiren R, Steiner H: Violence exposure, posttraumatic stress, and personality in juvenile delinquents. *J Am Acad Child Adolesc Psychiatry* 2002; **41**:322–329.

87. Ulzen TP, Hamilton H: The nature and characteristics of psychiatric comorbidity in incarcerated adolescents. *Can J Psychiatry* 1998; **43**:57–63.

88. Vermeiren R, De Clippele, A, Deboutte D: A descriptive survey of Flemish delinquent adolescents. *J Adolesc* 2000; **23**:277–285.

89. Vermeiren R, Schwab-Stone M, Ruchkin V, De Clippele A, Deboutte D: Predicting recidivism in delinquent adolescents from psychological and psychiatric assessment. *Compr Psychiatry* 2002; **43**:142–149.

12

Child and Adolescent Affective Disorders and their Treatment

Rick T. Bowers

Introduction

This chapter on affective disorders was written primarily with the clinician in mind and attempts to address the current diagnostic uncertainties in identifying and treating affective disorders in children and adolescents. Research provides hope that current diagnostic and treatment obstacles can be overcome.

While research in child/adolescent psychiatry has made rather commendable progress in the last decade or so, it still has lagged behind research in adult psychiatry. This will probably always be the case due to the limited support from pharmaceutical companies to test medications in children once they have been approved for adults. However, the US Food and Drugs Administration (FDA) is now incentivizing and requiring, in some instances, pharmaceutical companies to do more drug research in children of their products. Despite this advancement clinicians are presently often left to extrapolate findings from adult studies and make adjustments given the developmental differences for children.

Depressive Disorders

Historical Perspectives

The 1930s were influenced by the psychoanalytic school of thought which held that children were basically incapable of experiencing a major depressive episode similar to those experienced by adults. In essence, depression was felt to be the result of an intrapsychic conflict between the ego and persecutory superego. However, it was felt that the young child had not yet developed a superego, which was theorized to evolve with resolution of the Oedipal conflict and

formalize by late adolescence. Thus, on theoretical grounds, if no superego was present, there could be no intrapsychic conflict and thus no depression. This view was widely accepted despite the numerous prior clinical descriptions by therapists of children who, by present day terminology, would appear to have been experiencing a severe major depression. Today, it seems almost amazing that it was only 20 years ago when depression in children was officially recognized in the US at the 1975 National Institute of Mental Health (NIMH) Conference on Depression in Childhood [1]. Indeed, a similar phenomenon occurred in the debate as to whether children could experience mania, which may have been missed in the past in a significant fashion due to the fact that the adult criteria were used to diagnose mania and were not appropriate to diagnose children. This diagnostic deficit persisted despite reports by respected clinicians such as Kraepelin [2] in 1921 that 4% of manic-depressives first exhibited their symptomatology before puberty. Thus, one of the major tenets of child and adolescent psychiatry is that the therapist must always take into account the developmental level of the child in question. As such it is now fairly well accepted that even prepubertal children can experience unipolar and bipolar affective disorders.

Clinical Description

Although the *Diagnostic and Statistical Manual of Mental Disorders* (DSM-IV-TR) generally uses the same criteria to diagnose mood disorders for both children and adolescents, the developmental continuum through which children and adolescents progress will to some degree dictate the clinical presentation and

Clinical Child Psychiatry, Second Edition. Edited by W.M. Klykylo and J.L. Kay
© 2005 John Wiley & Sons Ltd.

expression of depressive symptoms [3]. Children's levels of intellectual and emotional maturity indeed affect the way they communicate their innermost feelings as well as the way adults perceive them. Although parents are especially helpful in making a diagnosis in younger children, parental reports cannot serve as the sole source of information. Studies that compare self- versus parental reports demonstrate clearly that parents effectively detect and reporting externalizing disorders such as oppositional defiant disorder (ODD) or attention deficit hyperactivity disorder (ADHD) in their children but they tend to miss internalizing disorders such as a major depressive disorder (MDD) or anxiety disorders [4–7]. When it comes to pediatric bipolar disorder (PBD) however, Youngstrom *et al.* [8] found that when using bipolar disorder screening instruments parental report was more useful than teacher report or adolescent self-report at identifying bipolar disorder. While the core DSM-IV-TR depression criteria symptoms have similar occurrence rates across the life span, neurovegetative and cognitive impairment (increasing with age) do seem to have different age-related rates of occurrence. Table 12.1 (adapted from Kovacs) describes some of the developmental differences in clinical presentation of children and adolescents versus adults in symptom expression of an affective disturbance.

The diagnostic criteria for affective mental disorders are listed in the DSM-IV-TR. It is expected that the reader is familiar with DSM-IV-TR and thus references will be made to it rather than citing from it extensively.

Depressive Disorders

Major Depressive Disorder

The DSM-IV-TR defines major depression as the presence of a single major depressive episode, with five or more of the following symptoms present during the same two-week period, and at least one of the symptoms being either depressed mood or loss of interest or pleasure. Symptoms include the following [9]:

(1) depressed mood for most of the day and nearly every day;
(2) markedly diminished interest or pleasure in almost all activities nearly every day;
(3) significant weight loss or gain due to decrease or increase in appetite resulting in a 5% change in body weight in a month;
(4) insomnia or hypersomnia nearly every day;
(5) psychomotor agitation or retardation nearly every day;
(6) fatigue or loss of energy nearly every day;
(7) feelings of excessive worthlessness or guilt;
(8) diminished ability to think or concentrate;
(9) current thoughts of death and/or suicidal ideation that may include a plan or an actual suicide attempt.

The DSM-IV-TR specifies several exclusionary criteria and should be referred to in making the diagnosis. For every one of the major inclusion area criteria, the symptoms must cause clinically significant distress or impairment in the child/adolescent's academic, social, or other important areas of functioning. Melancholia is a type of depression that appears to indicate a more severe form. Because the criteria cited in DSM-IV-TR are most appropriate for adults, it is often difficult for children to meet the minimum number of five symptoms for diagnosis as required in DSM-IV-TR.

Preschool age children who have not yet developed good language skills make it more difficult to utilize them as informants of their mood state and as a corollary their parents may be the primary sources in making the diagnosis. These young children tend to exhibit more anxiety, irritability, somatic complaints, temper tantrums and other behavior problems instead of verbalizing their inner feelings. While this type of

Table 12.1 Developmental differences in clinical presentation of children and adolescents versus adults in symptom expression of an affective disturbance.

Symptoms	Children	Adolescents	Young/middle-aged adults	Elderly
Hypersomnia	+/−	+	+++	++
Appetite/Weight loss	+	+	++	+++
Delusions	+	+	++	+++

+/−, rare; +, very infrequent; ++, infrequent; +++, common.
Adapted from Kovacs M: Presentation and course of major depressive disorder during childhood and later years of the life span. *J Am Acad Child Adolesc Psychiatry* 1996; **35**:707 [126].

'masked depression' does occur, particularly in younger children, many children exhibit sadness and mood changes similar to adults.

Signs and Symptoms of Depression in Children [10]

(1) Complain of sadness or report a negative self-concept when it pertains to their behavior, intelligence, appearance, or acceptance by peers.
(2) Complain of frequent somatic complaints such as fatigue, stomachache or headache (often to miss school) that do not respond to treatment.
(3) Social withdrawal typified by refusal to engage with friends or participate in extracurricular activities, hobbies or other interests with a general sense of anhedonia.
(4) Isolation – opting to stay in their rooms, sleep extensively and are more irritable or moody in their interactions with family.
(5) Increased sensitivity to perceived criticism or rejection with vocal outbursts or crying.
(6) Behavioral problems with anger outbursts.
(7) Thoughts of death or suicide (rare completions in children under the age of 12 years).
(8) Rarely complains of auditory hallucinations but this type of psychotic depression needs to be differentiated from other conditions such as PBD [11].

Older adolescents may be better able to report actual feeling states and neurovegetative disturbances but some clinical sophistication is often necessary to translate a teenagers symptoms into clinically relevant data. One must also distinguish these symptoms from a transient period of adolescent turmoil where emotional upheaval is not uncommon. Collateral information provided by parents, friends and their parents, teachers, coaches, etc., may be invaluable in making a proper diagnosis. This is crucial as teenagers may have more feelings of hopelessness, suicidal ideation and engage more frequently in suicide attempts with higher rates of completed suicides than younger children.

Signs and Symptoms of Depression in Adolescents [12,13]

(1) Boredom, irritability, anxiety or a feeling of hopelessness.
(2) Withdrawal from friends and isolation from family when at home.
(3) Sadness may be exemplified by wearing black clothes, writing poetry with morbid themes or a preoccupation with music that has nihilistic themes.

(4) Sleep disturbance manifested by staying awake all night watching TV, difficulty getting up for school and sleeping during the day.
(5) Lack of motivation resulting in skipped classes, inability to concentrate and lowered grades.
(6) Loss of appetite or compulsive eating may become anorexia or bulimia.
(7) Rebellious behavior, alcohol or drug use, and promiscuous sexual activity.
(8) Somatic complaints or chronic fatigue.
(9) Preoccupation with death and dying.

Besides melancholia, another specifier is the seasonal pattern affective disorder. This occurs when there is a regular temporal relationship between the onset of a depression, either in the context of a major depressive episode or bipolar disorder within a particular time of the year. This must have been duplicated in three separate years. Once again, developmental issues need to be taken into account such as the fact that many children start to school in late summer and fall, which is known to provide a significant stressor. For some this may result in a depressed mood as the winter quarter is often a time when final grades are realized.

Dysthymia

This is one of the mood disorders in which the DSM-IV-TR criteria are altered for children and adolescents. The major exception allowed is that for children and adolescents the mood can be primarily irritable with duration of at least one year compared with duration of two years in adults. This depressed mood must occur most days or more days than not, and the person must never have been without symptoms for more than two months at a time. These symptoms are similar to those of a major depression but of a lesser severity and degree of impairment in daily living. In about 30% of children and adolescents MDD coexists with a dysthymic disorder, often referred to as a 'double depression' or an anxiety disorder [14]. An anxiety disorder foreshadows the MDD two-thirds of the time in fact, which is the exact converse of what is observed in adults. Kovacs *et al.* [15] reported dysthymic children to be at risk for developing depression and mania on follow-up. About 15% of depressed juveniles have comorbid conduct disorder and substance use disorders may be present in as many as a quarter of this population [16].

Depressive Disorder Not Otherwise Specified

Many of the descriptive criteria in the DSM-IV-TR were derived from adult studies. It is not surprising, then, that many children and adolescents are diagnosed with depressive disorder not otherwise specified, since they typically do not clearly fall into one of the DSM-IV-TR categories for affective disturbances. Nevertheless, this type of mood disorder does result in significant distress and impairment in daily functioning that is sufficient to warrant a diagnosis and formal treatment.

CASE STUDY

A.J. was a 13-year-old eighth grader when she was referred for outpatient treatment after being assessed at but not admitted to an inpatient adolescent unit. Her parents were initially alerted to come to school by her school counselor and have her evaluated at the hospital. The school counselor had learned from one of A.J.'s girlfriends that she had cut her wrists superficially last evening at home. The parents reported that A.J. had always been a rather shy child experiencing separation anxiety when she first started school. She was typically a compliant child who did well academically. Her parents reported they often had to push A.J. to be more active socially or with extracurricular activities. This past year A.J. had significant difficulty transitioning to junior high feeling no one liked her. This was precipitated in large part by her best friend moving away before the start of the school year. She had quit her school dance team that she previously seemed to enjoy and her parents were concerned about the steady decline in her grades. A.J. appeared sad, listless with a very constricted affect. She wore no make-up and dressed in bland clothing. A.J. related life no longer seemed worth living and she wished she were dead. She disliked everything about her appearance and especially being overweight although she had lost 12 pounds over the past six months. A.J. spent increasing amounts of time in her room and would often sleep after school which likely contributed to her inability to fall asleep at night and making it difficult to awake in the morning. While her motivation for school and academics had declined markedly she also admitted she could no longer concentrate in school and found it increasingly difficult to complete her work even when she tried. A.J. feared she was losing her mind as she was

occasionally hearing her voice being whispered for the past two weeks. Her parents were concerned about the changes in A.J.'s behavior but wondered if this was somewhat normal behavior for a socially struggling teenager who had entered puberty. Additionally, A.J.'s father was a junior executive who was frequently away from home on business and her mother reported being lonely and dysthymic for years. Family history was notable for several maternal aunts being described as chronic worriers and on medication. A.J. was referred for individual and family therapy. Individual therapy addressed her low self-concept and negative thought patterns to initially reduce her self-abusive behavior and suicidal ideation. Family therapy addressed the distant relationships in the family and eventually sought to have the parents engage in marital therapy. Concurrently with this counseling A.J. was started on fluoxetine after discussing the risks, benefits and side effects of antidepressant medications including the need to be vigilant for signs of suicidality or activation. A.J's progress was slow but after six months of treatment she reported being back to 80% of her prior functioning without further suicidal ideation.

Bipolar Disorders

Just as depression in children was only officially recognized as recently as the 1970s, serious investigation into and acceptance of bipolar disorder's existence in children and adolescence has only belatedly occurred. Bipolar affective disorder (BAD), once known as manic depression, was previously thought to rarely occur in pediatric populations. We now believe pediatric bipolar disorder (PBD) may occur in as much as 1% of the pediatric population. Over the past decade there has been a substantial increase in the number of children and adolescents diagnosed with bipolar disorder. Previously, these youth would have been assessed as suffering from conduct disorder (CD), ODD, ADHD, borderline personality disorder, schizophrenia or simply undersocialization due to poor parenting. However, some clinicians remain skeptical of the frequency with which PBD is now diagnosed and question if this diagnostic shift and inherent change in somatic treatment has gone too far given the lack of diagnostic accuracy and certainty in many cases.

Case reports of mania in early childhood were made as far back as the mid-nineteenth century by Esquirol [17]. There are multiple contributors to the difficulty in diagnosing bipolar disorder in childhood, such as the fact that adolescent turmoil ('sturm und drang') is often seen incorrectly as an expected developmental occurrence and therefore not deemed significant. Additionally, while developmental variations have been accepted in previous DSM manuals for major depression, no comparable developmental concessions have been made for childhood bipolar disorder and there is considerable overlap with symptoms of other childhood diagnoses.

There are many difficulties in diagnosing manic disorders in children and adolescents due to the low base rate 1.0% [18], overlap with other disorders (ADHD) and atypical symptoms of the prodromal state (lack of clear distinct episodes and chronic, mixed symptoms) compared to the better described adult condition. Indeed, many child and adolescent patients are diagnosed as atypical BPD or bipolar disorder N.O.S. per DSM-IVr criteria. Another complicating variable is that depression is frequently the first manifestation of BPD in this pediatric population [19]. Twenty to 40 percent of adolescents with major depression develop bipolar disorder within five years after depression onset [20].

It is only now being accepted that bipolar illness may have a developmentally different presentation in young children and adolescents than in adults. Variable clinical presentations, which reflect the differing developmental levels of children, as well the symptomatic overlap with other more common disorders as discussed later, create an obstacle to the accurate diagnosis of PBD. Pavuluri *et al.* [21] contends empirical evidence indicates that there are two variants of PBD: prepubertal and early adolescent-onset bipolar disorder (PEA-BD) – children usually under the age of 12 years; and adolescent-onset bipolar disorder (AO-BD) – postpubertal adolescents.

Findings from phenomenological studies in both of these age groups indicate that PEA-BD and AO-BD have distinguishing presentations. PEA-BD children seem to exhibit more irritability, rapid cycling (ultradian), emotional lability, little interepisode recovery, and high comorbidity with ADHD and ODD. A distinct cycling is often difficult to elicit, and there is a greater chronicity to the symptoms.

Due to the lability of the affective state of many children and adolescents with bipolar illness, one might assume that it is often a very 'rapid cycling' (four or more episodes a year) form. However, it appears that rapid cycling bipolar disorders by definition are actually less common in children and adolescents than adults. This phenomenon may be more clearly understood if one accepts the premise that the juvenile presentation more often consists of chronic episodes with incomplete recoveries and rapidly fluctuating affective states. Geller [22] found using specific definitions of cycling that of the 60 bipolar patients she studied aged 7–16 years old, 83% were some form of rapid cycling with 8% classified as 'ultra-rapid' (episodes lasting a few days to a few weeks) and 75% classified as 'ultradian' (variation occurring within a 24-hour period). She also identified 87% of the pediatric bipolar cases as suffering from mixed mania when mania occurred.

Often bipolar children exhibit marked disruptive behaviors, extreme moodiness, difficulty falling asleep at night, explosive anger that may take 1–2 hours to de-escalate, and dysphoric mood. Poor academic performance is frequently present, related to their high impulsivity, hyperactivity, low frustration tolerance and inability to concentrate and attend. At times the clinician will be able to detect more overt symptomatology such as increased sexual activity, pressured speech, racing thoughts, increased talkativeness, and flight of ideas. Even visual or auditory hallucinations with delusional thinking of both persecutory and grandiose themes may be present. Clinicians may receive reports from parents describing very severe aggressive behaviors directed at siblings, peers, parents or animals.

Despite an increased awareness of bipolar disorder, it appears many children are still misdiagnosed. It is not uncommon to find children with ADHD syndromes diagnosed as BPD. This may be attributed, in part, to the definitional change that occurred in the diagnosis of ADHD when DSM-III was released. The symptoms of emotional lability were removed from the ADHD diagnostic criteria, as they were not deemed to be specific enough for ADHD given that they occur in many other pediatric illnesses such as autism, for example. Many clinicians, however, believe it to have been a mistake to do so, as emotional lability is a well-known symptom of many pediatric and adult ADHD patients. It has resulted in some clinicians diagnosing the oppositional emotional type of ADHD patient with the diagnosis of BAD. Occasionally, children with marked psychotic symptoms likely secondary to a schizophrenic process are diagnosed with BPD despite the lack of symptoms of bipolar illness. Conversely, it is probably beneficial to consider the diagnosis of bipolar disorder in the differential diagnosis of psychotic children, especially those with affective symptoms since these two populations require

Table 12.2 Mania items significantly and substantially more frequent among bipolar vs. ADHD cases.

	Bipolar disorder	ADHD
Elated mood	86.7%	5.0%
Grandiosity	85.0%	6.7%
Decreased need for sleep	43.3%	5.0%
Racing thoughts	48.3%	0.0%
Hypersexuality	45.0%	8.3%

different pharmacologic treatment approaches and have distinctly different long-term prognoses.

As stated above, there may be significant symptomatic overlap with ADHD and comorbidity with CD making the diagnosis difficult in this juvenile population. Geller *et al.* [23] found that mania symptoms are useful to differentiate prepubertal and early adolescent bipolar patients from ADHD patients (Table 12.2).

It is becoming more generally accepted that childhood bipolar disorder typically presents in children with a dysphoric rather than a euphoric mood disturbance, a chronic rather than episodic course, and a mixed presentation with simultaneous symptoms of depression and mania. This broad spectrum of behaviorally and affectively dysregulated states is unidentifiable as bipolar disorder conventionally seen in adults. This alternative phenotype may include behavioral dyscontrol and extreme explosive tantrums that escalate very rapidly and de-escalate very slowly, often occurring in conjunction with behavioral problems of the type seen in ADHD. Emily L. Fergus, M.D. [24], of the National Institute of Mental Health, proposes a model of five symptoms that when they occur together predicts bipolar disorder in 91% of cases:

• grandiosity;
• suicidal gesture;
• irritability;
• decreased attention span;
• racing thoughts.

Typically at the point of adolescence there appears to be a change in the phenomenology where the disorder exhibits more of the classic cycling of manic and depressive states. Postpubertal adolescent-onset bipolar disorder (AO-BD) children may demonstrate more classic symptoms of adult euphoria, elation, paranoia and grandiose delusions. This can be misdiagnosed as schizophrenia or other related psychotic disorders. The irritable insomnia and agitation characteristic of childhood depression may change to lethargic hypersomnia and retardation postpubertally. AO-BD is also characterized by high rates of substance abuse, anxiety symptoms, and an episodic nature in at least a quarter of the subjects [25–29].

A current debate exists as to whether there is comorbidity between bipolar disorder and other disorders such as ADHD, or rather whether these diagnoses represent the early expression of distinct nosological entities. Kutcher [30] reported that in US studies 29%–98% of the PBD population is also diagnosed with comorbid ADHD. However, he notes that in studies outside the US, the frequency of comorbidity between PBD and ADHD is less than 10%. He further contends longitudinal studies of ADHD cohorts indicate an infrequent comorbidity between the two disorders.

Geller *et al.* [31] found a mean age of onset of 7.3 years and a mean episode duration of 3.6 years. Unfortunately, this age of onset is only slightly later than when ADHD may be diagnosed and due to system overlap with ADHD may cause diagnostic confusion to a clinician. Unfortunately this is no small matter as a misdiagnosis of ADHD with subsequent placement on a stimulant or a misdiagnosis of unipolar depression with placement on an antidepressant could lead to a disastrous exacerbation of affective symptoms in a BAD patient.

Geller *et al.* [32] believe the frequent ADHD observed in pediatric bipolar disorder is an issue of 'phenocopy ADHD' i.e., prepubertal bipolar children may fit ADHD criteria, but will *not* continue to fit these criteria as they age. She notes that this 'phenocopy' hypothesis is supported by an earlier study she completed in which she found a decrease in ADHD from a prevalence of approximately 100% during prepuberty to 70% during young adolescence to 30% among older adolescents [33]. This conflicting data is evidence of the confusion and controversy that currently exists surrounding PBD. Whether childhood bipolar disorder with its atypical presentation is indeed a unique clinical entity, separate from adult bipolar disorder and demonstrating symptom overlap with other disorders such as ADHD or CD is an issue that requires further study.

Cyclothymia

This disorder may be on the spectrum of BPDs; however, the fluctuation of affective states, both depressed and elevated, is less intense and causes less impairment than with BPD proper. Numerous episodes of hypomanic and depressed symptoms must occur over a period of at least one year period with no more than a two months without symptoms.

Bipolar II Disorder

This disorder stipulates a history of at least one major depressive episode and at least one hypomanic episode in the absence of a full manic episode.

Bipolar Disorder Not Otherwise Specified

This category is used when the clinician concludes that a bipolar spectrum disorder is present whose features do not meet the criteria for a specific disorder (e.g., very rapidly – within hours or days – fluctuating mood states or hypomanic episodes without intercurrent depression). The only well-established criteria are for bipolar I disorder.

Although Kraepelin [34] described subtypes such as mixed mania or rapid cycling over 70 years ago, true systematic research into this area has only occurred within the past 10 years. Bowden [35] contended that the term 'classic mania' is misleading and made a key distinction between this subgroup and the so-called 'mixed mania' patients, whom he described as having all the symptoms of mania but lacking elation. He recommended classifying these symptoms as 'elated mania' and not using the terms classic or 'pure mania', since these have a different illness courses and responses to pharmacotherapy approaches. Bowden estimated that 40%–50% of all patients with manic episodes experience elated mania.

CASE STUDY

P.J. was a 10-year-old male who initially presented due to academic and behavioral difficulties at school that threatened his removal from the classroom. P.J. was described as out of control in the classroom due to his hyperactivity, lack of willingness to complete tasks and his lack of respect for teacher authority. He was disliked by his classmates and frequently engaged in fights, especially during unstructured times such as recess. His single mother felt overwhelmed by the situation as she also had several other children who were not well behaved. P.J.'s mother feared she would lose her job if she had to leave work one more time to pick P.J. up from school because of his misbehavior. She too felt unable to make P.J. listen at home. He would frequently instigate fights with his older brothers and despite receiving physical retaliation from them never seemed to learn from these altercations. His mother would frequently awake in the middle of the night to find P.J. making a mess in the kitchen, watching TV, or playing video games. A referral was made to his pediatrician and based on the available data started treatment for ADHD with stimulants. Initially, P.J. demonstrated a significant improvement in his school performance and was moderately more controlled at home. Despite receiving school services, therapy, and ongoing medical management by his pediatrician, P.J.'s improvement began to decline after four months. His defiance at school and aggression increased dramatically resulting in P.J. being suspended after he hit his teacher and kicked the police officer that was called to remove him. His mother noted an increase in sexualized behavior as P.J. was repeatedly caught attempting to watch his sisters undress and viewing adult channels on cable TV. P.J.'s dysphoric mood swings were more apparent during the initial beneficial period with stimulant treatment when his disruptive and hyperkinetic behaviors subsided somewhat. A consult was subsequently initiated with a child psychiatrist to assess for bipolar disorder. A more complete family history inquiry revealed that P.J.'s biological father was incarcerated and had a history of violent mood swings and substance abuse as did his father who also committed suicide. Several paternal aunts were believed to have been treated for depression. A diagnosis of pediatric bipolar was made, his stimulant discontinued, and a mood stabilizer was initiated while he was in a partial hospital program for two weeks. P.J.'s mood stability, anger, and sleep improved markedly over the ensuing month. P.J. was returned to school but continued to demonstrate difficulties with focus, concentration, task completion and hyperactivity. After a period of observation without improvement in these ADHD symptoms his stimulant was gradually restarted with good benefit. Eventually P.J. required the addition of a second mood stabilizer when his mood stability and anger began to worsen. Subsequently, P.J. has been able to attend school with a modified school plan and with family services in place has functioned in the home setting in a much more appropriate manner.

Outcome and Follow-Up Data

Depressive Disorders

It appears that the clinical course of depression may be affected by the age of the patient and an early onset is a harbinger of a more virulent course and prognosis [36]. Kovacs [37] found that among clinically referred youth the average length of a depressive episode is about 7–9 months with approximately 90% of these major depressive episodes remitting 1–2 years after onset. She noted that about 50% of previously clinically referred children and adolescents have a recurrent MDD when followed up for 1–2 years and 70% have a recurrence within five or more years, highlighting the need for ongoing treatment. Depression in adolescents confers an increased risk for substance abuse and suicidal behavior. The suicide risk is particularly high in adolescent males if depression is comorbid with conduct disorder and alcohol or other substance abuse [38].

There is an increased risk of development of bipolar disorders in early-onset depressive disorders as described below in the discussion of BPD. In general 30% of depressed children can be expected to evolve into bipolar illness by their teens or early twenties [39,40].

Bipolar Disorders

Akiskal and colleagues [41] proposed in 1983 that an early age of onset of depressive disorder is a prognosticator of bipolar outcome. Bipolarity seems to be predicted by a depressive symptom cluster comprising an early-pubertal age at onset with rapid symptom development, hypersomnic/psychomotor retardation and mood-congruent psychotic features; a loading of affective disorders in the family pedigree; a family history of bipolar illness and a presence of illness in three successive generations of the pedigree; and pharmacologically induced tricyclic hypomania [42,43].

The overall conversion rate of childhood depression to bipolar I or bipolar II disorder may be over 30% [44,45].

Akiskal et al. [46] reported the risk of bipolar outcome is up to threefold higher in childhood-onset depression versus later-onset depression. He found the time from the onset of unipolar depression to the conversion to a bipolar course appears to have decreased. In a comparison of patients he reviewed whose first onset of clinical depression was several decades ago and patients recently diagnosed with BPD, the 'switch' in polarity to a manic episode occurred after more than 10 years and less than five years, respectively. In addi-tion, Akiskal found the number of intervening depressive episodes between the onset of the illness and the switch in polarity has decreased from about seven to two or three. When a switch in polarity does occur, it does so only 4–8 months after the onset of the illness in most patients. Strober and Carlson [47] found that severe melancholic and delusional depressions were associated with increased rates of manic switching in teenagers from 13 to 17 years of age.

Kovacs and Pollock [48] originally found that comorbid CD in bipolar youths appears to be associated with a worse clinical course and may identify a severe subtype of very early-onset BPD. The CD in and of itself does not appear to confer any risk for the development of a manic episode.

Epidemiology

Depressive Disorders

The prevalence of depression in children and adolescents varies widely among the different populations sampled. Epidemiological studies using a community sample have estimated the incidence of depression to be about 1% in preschoolers, 2% in school-age children and close to 5% in adolescents [49]. Carlson and Cantwell [50] found that 28% of patients in a child psychiatric clinic were depressed. Robbins et al. [51] found 27% of adolescent inpatients and Petti [52] reported 59% of psychiatric inpatients were diagnosable as depressed. Hankin et al. [53] indicates that depression is more common in boys than girls, with the ratio as high as 5:1 before the age of 10 years. By adolescence, they found a reversal in the gender ratio, which becomes consistent with the adult male-to-female ratio of approximately 1:2. Since this switch in the gender ratio occurs before the onset of puberty, it is speculated that a presently unknown neurophysiologic or hormonal change predates the onset of puberty and is responsible for this switch.

For years, clinicians have anecdotally reported increasing numbers of children and adolescents presenting with depression in clinical practice. Indeed, several recent studies in the US and abroad have demonstrated that there is an increased prevalence of major depression in the cohorts born since World War II as well as a period effect, shown as an increase in rates between 1960 and 1980 (Figure 12.1) [54]. The rate of depression in females consistently surpasses that in males across all birth cohorts in these studies. Growing evidence indicates that these data reflect a real change worldwide in the clinical rates of depression, rather than an artifact such as increased psychi-

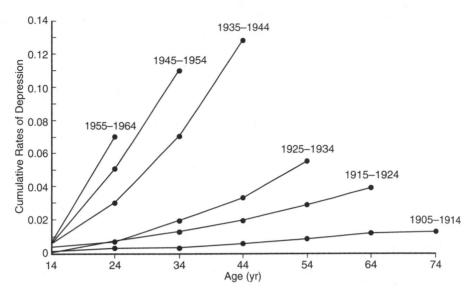

Figure 12.1 The temporal trends (period-cohort effects) and lifetime prevalence of major depression, from the National Institute of Mental Health and the US Epidemiologic Area Catchment study at five sites. Includes both sexes, white only. (From Klerman GL, Weissman MM: Increasing rates of depression. *JAMA* 1989; **261**:2229–2235. Copyright 1989, American Medical Association. All rights reserved.)

atric care. Some researchers believe that this may be an example of 'genetic anticipation' where a condition becomes more virulent and prevalent with each subsequent generation. The age of onset for depression appears to be occurring earlier as well (Figure 12.2) [55].

Bipolar Disorders

Only one epidemiological study has attempted to determine the incidence or prevalence of diagnosable bipolar illness in juvenile samples. Lewinsohn and colleagues administered structured diagnostic interviews to a community sample of 1709 older adolescents (age 14–18 years) and found a lifetime prevalence of BPDs (primarily bipolar II disorder and cyclothymia) of approximately 1% [56]. In retrospective studies that examined the onset of BPD in adult patients, 0.5% reported their onset to be between the ages of five and nine years, and 7.5% reported their onset between the age of 10 and 14 years [57]. Although as many as 20%–30% of bipolar adults are felt to have experienced the onset of their illness before the age of 20 years, fewer than half of these individuals were so impaired at the time that their symptoms necessitated psychiatric intervention. Although BPD disorder is less common than depression, prevalence rates within

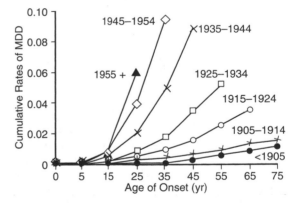

Figure 12.2 Cumulative life-time rates of major depression by birth cohort and age of onset – North America, from The US Epidemiologic Catchment Area study at five sites (N = 18,244). MDD, major depressive disorder. (Adapted from Cross-National Collaborative Group: The changing rate of major depression – Cross-National Comparisons. *JAMA* 1992; **268**:3098–3105. Copyright 1992, American Medical Association. All rights reserved.)

restricted samples such as inpatient populations or other psychiatrically referred groups challenge the common belief that mania is rare or nonexistent in children. Weller et al. [58] estimated the rate of mania at 22% among severely disturbed children. Wozniak et al. [59] identified 43 children (16%) aged 12 years or younger who were referred to their outpatient psychopharmacology clinic and who met diagnostic criteria for mania using the Schedule for Affective Disorders and Schizophrenia for School-Age Children – Epidemiologic Version structured interview. The data available indicates that in psychiatrically referred children and adolescents, BAD may not be uncommon at all.

Etiology and Pathogenesis

Although significant progress has been made in the diagnosis and treatment of affective disturbances in children and adolescents, a thorough understanding of the cause or causes of these early-onset affective disturbances remains elusive. As with other areas of psychiatry, many of the explanatory models have been adapted from studies of depressive disorders in adults. At present, no single model or even combination of models satisfactorily provides a causal mechanism that can consistently explain the production of an affective disturbance in childhood. Several models do address the biopsychosocial factors as etiologic agents in an affective disturbance, however; owing to the prevalence of such models, each will be discussed in brief detail.

Familial and Care Giver Influences

Multiple studies have indicated that major depressive disorders – and to an even greater degree, BPDs – do aggregate in families [60,61]. It appears there are genetic components (discussed later) as well as environmental influences that contribute to the development of depression. The trend in most studies poses a higher degree of genetic loading in affective disorders; however, the fact that about one half of all depressed children do *not* demonstrate a family history of depression indicates that variables other than genetic factors are at play. One theory that has received much attention is that dysfunctional intrafamilial interactions may lead to depression in the child and/or parent. Descriptions of family interactions support the clinical impression that an affectively disturbed child often has an affectively ill parent. Concurrent with this are observations of poor child–parent relations, a lack of caring in these interactions, and conflictual interactions with siblings and peers. Associated parental dis-

orders such as alcoholism may also increase the role of depression in offspring [62]. A history of physical abuse is more common among all adolescents with psychiatric disorders, and not just those with mood disorders. Parental impairment and specifically parental mood disorders are risk factors, but they appear to be independent, nonspecific risk factors that contribute to the production of major depression in their children. It appears the degree of parental impairment – regardless of the cause – may be more important than the specific psychiatric disorder exhibited by the parent. Surprisingly, clinical lore would contend severe depression in mothers may have a more detrimental effect on the development of a child than schizophrenia in the mother. This pattern may result from differing behaviors between the mother and the child. The stimulation and interactions – however altered they may be – that occur between the child and schizophrenic mother may result in the development of an emotional bond, whereas the depressed mother's interactions may be so emotionally retarded that a bond is never formed.

Psychodynamic tradition has held that following the loss of an imaginary or real love object, the individual experiences feelings of anger toward the lost loved one. In theory, these aggressive drives can be directed inward toward (toward the self) or outward (towards the environment). If directed inward, this anger may lead to depression; if directed outward, these aggressive drives may result in more conduct-disordered behaviors. This dichotomy in part explains the concept of 'masked depression', in which children and adolescents with varying diagnoses ranging from ODD to ADHD to encopresis are felt to demonstrate a clinical picture of depression unique to children.

The work of Bowlby [63] and Ainsworth and colleagues [64] expanded the concept of object loss and separation and its relation to depression. This concept appears to have some intrinsic validity, although the subjective experience of loss seems to be of critical importance as well. Tenant [65] found that loss of a parent by death actually appeared to have less pathogenic developmental effects later in life than did severe parental discord with subsequent divorce.

The conception of a 'normal' grief reaction to loss is now being reevaluated and, as Freud espoused in *Mourning and Melancholia* [66], is considered at times to be a pathologic condition warranting treatment.

Bipolar Disorders

It is interesting to contemplate what factors might predispose one to the onset of bipolar illness, especially when one is a young child. The illness becomes apparent early in the lives of children who demonstrate disruptive behavioral problems and marked affective dysregulation, compared with children who do not demonstrate these early life problems. Akiskal [67] argues that temperamental dysregulation or subaffective temperaments are the developmental substrates from which affective episodes arise, and are possibly genetically linked to manic depressive illness. This model of manic depressive illness is based on a model that sees these disorders as a 'bipolar spectrum' ranging from temperamental dysregulation to extreme affective dysregulation with psychosis in the most extreme cases. Looking at bipolar disorders as a spectrum of disorders is consistent with the finding that more patients meet the criteria for bipolar II or cyclothymia than bipolar I, due to the less frequent occurrence of frank mania symptoms in children. This is consistent with the view that differences from adult-onset mania are often one of degree rather than quality, which can be adjusted for by considering the developmental stage. Thus one may see the cycling of extreme emotional storms with mood lability and irritability as well as explosive outbursts which abruptly switch to more dysphoria and self-devaluation. If one accepts that this temperamental dysregulation is on the continuum of bipolar spectrum disorders, it would seem likely that certain developmental considerations such as a dysfunctional, overstimulating family and environment could predispose to the development of bipolar affective illness. Whether a more nurturing supportive and less stimulating environment could prevent the developments of such a disorder or just delay its onset is debatable. Additionally, the comorbid development of severe behavior problems, such as externalizing disorders or substance abuse, are likely to increase the likelihood of a conflictual atmosphere developing during childhood which could exacerbate ` or accelerate the onset of the bipolar illness. Akiskal believes the temperamental excesses and dysregulation generate the very life events such as stormy relationships and biological precipitants such as substance use and sleep dysregulation and such a causal fashion of temperament leads to the stressors, which bring about the affective disorder. He proposes such a model as summarized in Figure 12.3 [68].

One of the risks of expanding bipolar disorder into such a spectrum of disorders is that the criteria can be expanded or adjusted to become meaningless. One worries that undersocialized behavior with poor self-control and self-modulation due to parental psychopathology or inconsistent parenting will lead to an overdiagnosis of bipolar spectrum disorders. The

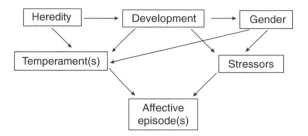

Figure 12.3 Affective temperaments – cyclothymia and its variants – as an intermediary between predisposing factors and full-blown clinical expressions of recurrent mood disorders. (From Akiskal HS: Developmental pathways to bipolarity: Are juvenile-onset depressions pre-bipolar? *J Am Acad Child Adolesc Psychiatry* 1995; **34**:754–763. © Hagop S Akiskal.)

bipolar condition could become overdiagnosed if psychiatrists expand the criteria for bipolar disorder excessively and assume the dysphoric labile mood states found in many juveniles with externalizing disorders to always represent a precursor of bipolar disorder. It may be prudent to adopt a more conservative approach as prescribed by Strober [69], and delineate only those with an uncomplicated bipolar history (without such confounding diagnoses as substance abuse and ADHD) as reliably predictive of who will later develop adult bipolar disorder. The debate is far from over.

Genetic Model

Depressive Disorders

In treating children and adolescents, it is very common to find other close family members who also suffer from an affective disturbance. One of the best ways to study heredity is via twin studies. Akiskal and Weller [70] reported that the concordance rate for mood disorders in monozygotic twins is 76% declining to 19% in dizygotic twins. Monozygotic twins reared apart in this study showed a concordance rate of 67% indicating an environmental factor as well. Family studies [71] of depression in adults have shown that a positive family history for depression increases the likelihood of depression occurring in relatives. This genetic loading and predisposition seem to be increased even further for relatives of children and adolescents with major depression. The earlier the age of onset of depression in children, the greater the degree of genetic loading for the affective disorder: first-degree relatives of prepubertal children with depression have the greatest risk, and the first-degree relatives of adolescents with depression have a somewhat lesser risk [72,73].

Conversely, a study [74] involving children and adolescents indicated that having a single parent with a unipolar or bipolar affective disorder imparts to the offspring a 25% risk and having two parents affected imparts a 75% risk of developing an affective disturbance.

Bipolar Disorder

In treating children and adolescents, it is very common to find other close family members who also suffer from an affective disturbance. Akiskal [75] states that genetic studies have shown that if one parent has bipolar disorder the risk to the offspring of developing BPD is 30%–40% and when both parents are diagnosed with bipolar disorder the risk is 50%–70%.

One of the best ways to study heredity is via twin or adoption studies. Twin studies show the concordance rate of mania in monozygotic twins to be 65%, versus 14% in dizygotic twins [76]. An adoption study by Mendlewicz and Rainer [77] found that 31% of the biological parents of adopted children who developed mania suffered from BPD, whereas only 2% of the adoptive parents did so. Klein and colleagues [78] found an association of cyclothymia among the adolescent offspring of bipolar adults. Among the children or siblings of bipolar adults, however, depressive spectrum disorders (major depression, dysthymia, and melancholic) are actually the most common finding.

Pedigree studies [79] involving the chromosomal mapping of identified families with a high incidence of affective disorders including BPD (such as those found within the Amish community) initially led to the hope that a 'bipolar gene' could be identified. Akiskal [80] reported that molecular genetic studies have focused on 'hot spots' on chromosomes 18 and 22 as the most promising leads for bipolar-related genes. He indicates there is evidence that panic attacks associated with BPD have been strongly linked with genes on chromosome 18 and some genetic overlap with schizophrenia on both chromosomes 18 and 22. There also appears to be some association with obsessive–compulsive disorder (OCD) and migraine headaches as these conditions are comorbid at higher prevalence rates than one would predict based on their individual prevalence rates in the population. The specific genetic etiology remains elusive, but should be more fully elucidated within the next decade.

Biological Factors

It is believed that affective disorders may result from or produce biological changes of a brief or lasting duration. Biological inquiry and tests have sought to elucidate these biological changes in the hopes of developing a laboratory test that could confirm or rule out an affective disorder. Biological markers are differentiated either as 'state markers' which are detectable only during the episode and eventually revert to normal, or 'trait markers' which are detectable prior to the onset of the illness in question. Several tests or studies such as the dexamethasone suppression test (DST), growth hormone release to an insulin challenge, and sleep studies have been used rather extensively in adults. These tests have been applied to children and adolescents as well to aid in diagnosis but are only state markers of depression and should only be interpreted in the broader range of clinical findings. The overall sensitivity of the DST is reported at 70% in prepubertal children and 47% in adolescents. Thus, the test seems to have limited utility in the juvenile population as given the sensitivity it is unlikely that a clinician would withhold treatment if the patient met full clinical criteria for an affective disorder regardless of the results of the DST. Given the lack of conclusive data regarding these tests and their costs (often several hundreds of dollars), these studies have limited use, especially in the present medical environment of cost containment as they may help to confirm a diagnosis of depression but not diagnose it. Thus these studies are likely to be increasingly relegated to patients in specific research protocols or studies.

Numerous conditions are known to mimic depressive disorders but there is no consensus as to what should constitute a routine screening battery of bloodwork and tests to rule out many of these potentially treatable disorders. A chemistry panel may indicate an electrolyte disturbance or alteration in calcium, which could effect one's mental state. A complete blood count (CBC) with differential may help to identify a central nervous system (CNS) infection or anemia which would prompt the physician to pursue a B12 or folate deficiency as such disorders are well known to have psychiatric manifestations. A thyroid stimulating hormone (TSH) and a free thyroid (T4 free) serum level will typically screen for most thyroid disorders. Testing for sexually transmitted diseases that affect the CNS, such as syphilis or AIDS, is increasingly relevant in an age when so many adolescents are sexually active. An elevation of one's liver enzymes could signal alcohol abuse or mononucleosis. If accompanying mental or neurological symptoms are present these liver abnormalities may also indicate Wilson's disease or a porphyria which can be further evaluated via a ceruloplasmin level or 24-hour quantitative urine screen for porphyrins respectively. Other mental or neurological symptoms may indicate the need for an electroencephalogram (EEG) or brain imaging with computerized axial tomography (CT) or magnetic resonance imaging (MRI).

Assessment and Formulation

The symptomology exhibited by children and adolescents must be accurately and comprehensively evaluated so that a formulation and appropriate treatment plan can be instituted. The assessment process in children and adolescents is more complex than in adults. The evaluation process should include diagnostic interviews with the child and parents individually and together. As well, collaboration with teachers and school counsellors is prerequisite as children spend a significant portion of their awake hours in school or related functions. Additional areas to be addressed include the physical well-being of the child with a possible referral for more specific laboratory, genetic and neurological testing if indicated. Also, psychological or neuropsychological testing may help to provide missing pieces of a diagnostic puzzle.

The younger the child, the more the emphasis is often placed upon parents' report and descriptions in obtaining a useful history and diagnostic picture. Some of the earlier studies show that an interview with the parents was the single best technique for detecting psychiatric disorders in children [81]. One must remember, however, that parental perceptions may be altered by their own personal psychological make-up and possible pathology.

Traditionally, child psychiatrists used play therapy to assess the unconscious functioning of patients by eliciting their fantasies and observing the symbolic meanings of their play. This type of therapeutic interaction can provide information related to the dynamic and cognitive functioning of the child, and additionally may provide a window into the environment in which the child interacts. While it may be true that only certain aspects of a clinical evaluation could be ascertained in this setting, a limiting factor in this type of assessment is the number of sessions that may be needed before a full diagnostic picture is completed. Given the short length of treatment demanded by most insurance companies today, the use of traditional long-term dynamic therapy techniques such as play therapy is becoming increasingly difficult. In an age when descriptive phenomenology drives the diagnostic basis for DSM-IV-TR criteria, play therapy alone may limit the therapist in arriving at comprehensive diagnostic assessment and diagnosis(es). Such interactions

however, may be utilized for the young child who is demonstrating marked social anxiety and who would provide little information in a more direct clinical interview. In these young or anxious children the parent's input is essential. The young child may have difficulty recognizing or relating their feelings and use words not typically associated with classic depression. Often one must use several different terms or phrases to describe a mood state before the young child will comprehend. Poznanski [82] and Puig-Antich and colleagues [83] suggest questions that could be used when interviewing younger children to help solicit information regarding their mood states, social functioning, academic functioning and physical state. From middle childhood onward, children are able to describe their internal mood states fairly clearly to adults. Indeed as discussed above, children are typically better reporters of their subjective feelings related to internal mood states such as with depressive disorders than are their parents or teachers. It is not uncommon for parents to be unaware of their child's suicidal thoughts or even prior suicide attempts. Parents and teachers, however, tend to be better reporters and identifiers of externalizing disorders such as ODD or CD.

When trying to index the onset or duration of psychiatric symptoms in children, it is often necessary to use or relate the occurrence to significant events in their life such as the onset of school, holidays, birthdays and the different seasons. The clinician must also keep in mind the sociocultural background of the child and family being interviewed. Often different ethnic groups or races may use terminology in describing symptoms or mood states that is foreign to the interviewing clinician and his cultural background (and thus not fully or clearly understood) which can result in miscommunication and misunderstandings. One must learn to speak the language of the patient, so to speak, if they are to be fully successful in understanding their psychological or mood states.

Previously, structured and semistructured interviews were considered the domain of research psychiatrists. Increasingly, however, these types of assessment tools are finding their way into clinical practice, especially among adult psychiatrists. At first many clinicians feel that they put an artificial element into the diagnostic process and at times can be time consuming; but as one becomes rather proficient in their use, they may not in actuality extend the diagnostic process significantly and should provide a more objective outcome measure. These types of assessments or instruments are now available and being used for children and adolescents. They all use the children and primary caretaker as informants. Gould and Shaffer [84] describe diagnos-

Table 12.3 Structured or semistructured interviews for assessing mood disorders in children and adolescents.

	K-SADS	DICA	DISC	CAPA	CAS	ISC
Type	Semistructured	Structured	Structured	Semistructured	Semi-structured	Semi-structured
Ages (years)	6–17	6–17	8–17	7–17	7–17	8–17
Period assessed	Present or lifetime	Lifetime	Past year	Present	Present	Present
Administrator	Clinician	Clinician	Lay	Clinician or trained lay (4–5 weeks of training)	Clinician	Clinician

K-SADS, Affective Disorders and Schizophrenia for School-Age Children; DICA, Diagnostic Interview for Children and Adolescents; DISC, Diagnostic Interview Schedule for Children; CAPA, Child and Adolescent Psychiatric Assessment; CAS, Child Assessment Schedule; ISC, Interview Schedule for Children.

tic interviews as generally either respondent or investigator-based. Respondent-based or 'structured' interviews consist of a series of questions that are asked verbatim. Investigator-based or 'semistructured' interviews allow the more clinically trained interviewer to inquire about specific behaviors and mood states via the use of any questions they deem appropriate. The handful of structured or semistructured interviews for assessing mood disorders in children and adolescents are summarized in Table 12.3.

They use information gathered from both the primary caretaker and the child informant to derive the diagnoses therein. It was the use of such instruments that helped to elucidate the phenomenon alluded to above: that children and adolescents in comparison to their parents sometimes showed major discrepancies in their reports of current functioning especially in terms of describing internalizing versus externalizing disorders. Some of these structured diagnostic interviews are more applicable for use in clinical practice while others are primarily designed as instruments for use in large-scale epidemiological research. Typically they require some training, but can be used by either clinicians or trained lay interviewers.

Behavioral rating scales can be utilized to assess the severity of a particular mood disorder such as depression or bipolar disorder. These scales can be completed by patients in a self-report questionnaire format or be completed by external evaluators such as parents or school teachers. They can be useful in *screening* for patients demonstrating symptoms that may indicate an affective disturbance, to assess the degree of disturbance, or to obtain a baseline by which further treatment can be assessed by repeating the instrument. The

Childhood Depression Inventory (CDI) [85] developed by Kovacs is a self-report questionnaire that helps to assess the severity of depression and assess for suicidality but not diagnose it. Other parent and self-report assessments can be purchased from suppliers of psychometric test materials but unfortunately there is no conclusive data as to which tests are the most clinically useful. One must remember these are not diagnostic instruments but can be helpful when used in conjunction with more formal diagnostic assessment tools, i.e., a thorough clinical interview. A mood lifetime chart or mood diary describing a child's mood state over the school years with reference to life stressors can be useful in diagnosing a mood disorder, especially a bipolar spectrum disorder. Several of these mood charts can be downloaded from the internet at www.bpkids.org.

Fristad, Weller, and Weller [86] modified the Mania Rating Scale of Young *et al.* [87] and found it helpful in teasing out the difficult differential between prepubertal manic and hyperactive children.

More recently Geller [88] modified the Kiddie Schedule for Affective Disorders and Schizophrenia (K-SADS) [89] to develop the WASH-U-KSADS. She made the 16 mania items more prepubertal-specific; added items to assess even ultradian cycling; and added specific items on onset and offset of each symptom and syndrome. Geller developed the WASH-U K-SADS Mania Scale to include developmentally appropriate items i.e., grandiosity – a child may truly believe they could teach the class better than their instructor or run their sports team better than their coach – to better assist in studying, diagnosing and treating pediatric BPD patients. Geller proposes, however, that while there is significant overlap between BPD and ADHD (60%–98% in some studies), certain criteria (Table 12.2) may help to separate the two.

Youngstrom *et al.* compared the diagnostic accuracy of six screening instruments for predicting juvenile bipolar disorder in two outpatient youth groups aged 5–10 years or youths aged 11–17 years. This study also looked at the comparative diagnostic value of parent, teacher, and youth reports. The six screeners included the Parent Young Mania Rating Scale (P-YMRS) [90], an 11-item questionnaire adapted from the Young Mania Rating Scale, the General Behavior Inventory (A-GBI) [91], a 73-item self-report questionnaire measuring depressive, hypomanic, manic, and mixed mood symptoms in adolescents as young as 11 years, the Parent General Behavior Inventory (P-GBI) [92], an adaptation of the GBI that allows parents to rate the mood symptoms of their children aged 5–17 years, the Child Behavior Checklist (CBCL) [93], a parent report which includes 118 problem behavior items, the Youth Self Report (YSR) [94], which allows youths ages 11–17 years to assess the same behavior problems as does the CBCL, and the Teacher Report Form (TRM) [95], the teacher report version of the CBCL. While none of these measures are sufficient alone to make a diagnosis of bipolar disorder they can prove useful in the decision process. Some of the clinical implications and recommendations from the study include:

- parent report provided the most powerful information for the recognition and diagnosis of bipolar disorder in youths aged 5–17 years;
- for the older sample, the P-GBI performed significantly better than the CBCL externalizing score;
- for the younger cohort, the three parent measures did not show significant differences in diagnostic performance, but all three parent measures did substantially better than did the TRF;
- the CBCL, P-GBI, and P-YMRS are roughly equal in their global diagnostic efficiency and combining tests does not help clinically.
- If one suspects juvenile bipolar disorder from risk factors or clinical concerns the P-GBI or P-YMRS are the best candidates to provide information to change the likelihood of a bipolar diagnosis to a meaningful degree.

Treatment

The comprehensive diagnostic assessment and subsequent formulation serves as the basis or foundation for an effective treatment plan. The assessment ideally identifies the strengths and deficiencies of the identified patient and his/her environment as they pertain to their intrapsychic make-up, family, peers, school and religious affiliations. Treatment should then address the precipitators of the condition as well as those factors maintaining the maladjustment and then attempt to initiate a multimodal treatment intervention that utilizes and optimizes those curative factors that will promote a return to a normal developmental track. One must guard against utilizing a treatment approach solely because it aligns with the therapist's theoretical orientation when other approaches may better serve the patient and family.

Developmental practicalities of children and adolescents such as their emotional and economic dependency on their caregivers necessitates that treatment address family system dynamics along with other environmental interventions. A nonjudgmental attitude that doesn't overemphasize blame and highlights the positive healthy functioning of the child and family will serve the treatment well. The therapist or treatment team must strive to align with the patient and family to hopefully be seen as an advocate or resource for positive change. These principles are well addressed by those therapists who practice brief-solution focused therapy [96]. The range of therapeutic interventions open to the therapist(s) are varied and include individual therapy, family therapy, parent education, school collaboration and out of home placement as some examples. An in-depth discussion of each of these modalities is beyond the scope of this chapter but is summarized Table 12.4.

Bipolar Disorders

Psychosocial Therapies
Pharmacologic intervention alone is seldom sufficient in treating patients with bipolar disorder in large part due to the finding that over 50% of adult patients are noncompliant with their medication regimen [97].

Psychotherapy may prove invaluable and enhance outcomes by facilitating understanding and acceptance of one's illness and thereby improving medication compliance. Additionally, psychotherapy can be used to educate the patient and family to monitor the patient's affective state, to hopefully identify early the symptoms of a budding depressive or manic episode so that appropriate treatments can be initiated promptly. Difficulty sleeping or reduced need for sleep can be both a symptom and a precipitator of a manic episode. Treatment can focus on insuring good sleep habits and a healthy lifestyle as individuals with bipolar disorder are often at risk for substance abuse.

Table 12.4 The range of therapeutic interventions available for treatment of children and adolescents with bipolar disorder.

Individual therapies	Theory	Appropriate populations	Goals	Interventions	Length
Interpersonal	Depression determined by the interpersonal relationships between person and environment: abnormal grief interpersonal role conflicts difficult role transitions interpersonal deficits	Adolescents	Relieve symptoms through resolution of interpersonal problems Improved social adaptation	Role playing	Short-term Focused
Analytic	Aggression turned inward Object loss Loss of self-esteem Negative cognitive set	Cognitively mature child/adolescents	Sustained improvement: personality reorganization adoption of mature defenses realistic sense of self resolve past traumas	Development of transference relationship which is interpreted to gain insight	Long-term six months to years
Play	Use of play as therapeutic communication to understand wishes, fantasies, traumas Discharging feelings via physical activity	School-age children immature	Corrective emotional experience Reworking and mastery of trauma	Encourage verbalization of repetitive themes while staying in the metaphor Connect past experiences with present feelings of sadness, low self-esteem, anger	Long-term
Cognitive	Irrational negative beliefs about self/world promote sadness and their correction promotes euthymia	Average IQ	Clarify links between thoughts and feelings foster rational self-talk	Logs of daily negative thought processes (self- critical, irrational) for review in session in an A-	

	Negative schemata or automatic thoughts			B-C format (antecedent events → incorrect beliefs → emotional consequences) Prescriptions to engage in activities that will disprove irrational beliefs about self (see Lewinsohn manual)	
Behavioral	Reduced positive reinforcement from environment produces depression (stimulus → response)	All ages Low IQ and above	Enhance social skills Modify behaviors via use of external reinforcers	Modeling/shaping appropriate prosocial behaviors Role playing specific problem situations	
Social learning	Learned helplessness Loss of reinforcement	All ages	Changing negative expectations Relinquish nonattainable goals Teach social skills and decision making		
Family	Family is a system which functions to maintain homeostasis	All ages	Determine what homeostatic role the identified patient serves in the family system 'Joining' with family to restructure and reorganize dysfunctional family dynamics	Positive reframing decrease blaming and scapegoating, altering unhealthy family rules, recognizing cross-generational dynamics	
Group	Varied orientations (psychodynamic, cognitive, behavioral etc.) Diagnostically homogeneous vs. heterogeneous groups	Children (activities and play) Adolescents (more verbally expressive)	Group leader(s) develop(s) a safe and supportive environment in which a therapeutic process can	Yalom's 11 curative factors: installation of hope universality imparting of information altruism	Open ended vs. time limited Group moves through early →

Table 12.4 *Continued*

Individual therapies	Theory	Appropriate populations	Goals	Interventions	Length
	Provide a social forum in which family dynamics, interpersonal issues, and developmental issues can be immediately explored and corrected		evolve	corrective recapitulation of the primary family group development of socialization techniques imitative behavior interpersonal learning catharsis existential factors	middle→ termination phases
School intervention	School serves as the primary social system and is the childhood equivalent of work (a vocation of the developing child) thus able to directly effect their emotional state	All ages	Facilitate participation and motivation for the learning process thereby increasing likelihood of positive reinforcement Optimize learning and preparation for life	Diagnose and address special needs in regards language or learning disabilities, social inadequacies, etc., by altering classroom environment or mode of teaching (tutors or aides) Identify and treat biological conditions such as ADHD which may contribute to depression	As appropriate
Out-of-home placement respite care foster home group home residential	Home environment is not conducive to normal development either because of parental pathology or child's behavior is unmanageable in this setting	All ages	Stabilize the child's or parent's condition Destabilize maladaptive systems Restore a therapeutic parent/child relationship	Milieu therapy Establish a holding environment while other interventions are implemented Supervised visitation leading to a gradual transition back to home	As indicated

Unfortunately, there are no proven psychosocial therapies for PBD children and their families. The National Institute of Mental Health is funding two studies by Fristad [98] and Miklowitz *et al.* [99] to test psychoeducational models. Greene [100] has developed a model that teaches parents when to intervene and utilize collaborative problem-solving with their PBD children after a rage attack has subsided. Additionally, Basco has written a book detailing a cognitive-behavioral approach that can be used in therapy with the chronic bipolar patient to enhance outcomes [101].

Community involvement is often vital as a family member or friend who is educated about the disorder may be the first one to identify the presence of symptoms indicating the reemergence of the disorder and thus, could support the patient in seeking needed treatment. Reports are that 25% of patients with PBD [102] will eventually attempt suicide and unfortunately many manic episodes are characterized by overt acts of physical violence. These alarming percentages indicate that indeed this is a severe disorder that requires chronic treatment.

Pharmacotherapy and Other Somatic Treatments

Over the past decade the emphasis or attention paid to biological therapies has increased significantly. The hope of finding somatic treatments that will quickly and significantly improve affective dysregulation is very compelling.

Depressive Disorders

Tricyclic antidepressants (TCAs) have been available for many years and were previously the most commonly used medications to treat depressive disturbances in children and adolescents. While no TCA antidepressant has been approved by the FDA for use in depressed children, these medications do have a rather long track record and a good safety profile when administered and monitored appropriately. While TCAs have been shown in a number of adult studies to have an overall response rate around 75%, it appears that these medications are not as effective in children and adolescents. Indeed, most double-blind placebo-controlled studies typically using imipramine in depressed children, have shown that these medications are not significantly better than placebo. One notable sideline of the studies is that the placebo rate has approached almost 70% in some studies and thus, it would be very difficult to show a positive response rate versus placebo given this finding. Nevertheless, most clinicians would contend that for a *given* patient, TCAs

might be beneficial. The present difficulty appears to be the inability to predict which patients will respond to medication therapy. Despite the lack of supportive data from studies, some clinicians continue to treat a child or adolescent with severe depression with TCAs, especially if they have failed trials on serotonin reuptake inhibitor antidepressants (SSRIs).

If one is going to use TCA antidepressant therapy, several guidelines should be followed to insure their utmost safety and minimize possible adverse side effects – in the most extreme cases, sudden death. A sound approach is to obtain an ECG to assess baseline parameters such as PR, QRS and QTC intervals before starting a TCA. As most studies do show that patients receive the greatest benefit when these medications are at a therapeutic serum level, one may gradually increase a patient to approximately 3 mg/kg for most TCAs such as amitriptyline, doxepin, imipramine and desipramine. Nortriptyline and protriptyline typically require a significantly lower mg/kg dose. At 3 mg/kg of amitriptyline, doxepin, imipramine and desipramine, clinicians should recheck the EKG to assess the cardiac function via monitoring conduction parameters such as the QTC interval. If the QTC interval is greater than 440–450 milliseconds, it may be inadvisable to increase the dosage further if the patient has not yet responded. If the QTC and other parameters (resting heart rate not over 130 b.p.m., P-R interval length not over 0.21 seconds, and a QRS width not over 130% of baseline) are within normal limits, one may gradually increase up to 5 mg/kg and then recheck the EKG and serum level. Several of the TCAs have specified serum levels that are felt to be their 'therapeutic range' and theoretically one has the best odds of obtaining a response when within these parameters. One must be cautious in 'treating by the lab values,' however, as is illustrated in interesting case studies where patients with treatment resistant depression only responded to extraordinarily high doses of medication and supranormal serum levels. Additionally, in these cases, the depressive symptoms reemerged whenever the dosage was decreased. Despite the alarming high dosages and serum levels in these cases, the EKGs were found to be normal and the patient without adverse side effects. From such reports one can make a case that as long as the EKG is acceptable and the patient is tolerating the medication in regards to side effects there is no definitive standard upper dosage (except possibly for nortriptyline which has a reported 'therapeutic window').

After Quitkin's [103] now landmark article most clinicians adopted the common lore that TCAs require 4–6 weeks to work. Interestingly, the article in fact, demonstrates that some individuals actually respond within two weeks while others may take longer than 6–8 weeks before achieving beneficial response. Thus, if one changes medications too abruptly, some patients may miss out on a treatment which would have eventually been effective for them. These examples and points are cited to help bring home the point that as with most other treatments, if one tries to become too 'cookbookish' some patients may actually be denied beneficial treatment.

Since the introduction of selective serotonin reuptake inhibitors (SSRIs) there has been a move by many clinicians to use these medications preferentially in place of TCAs due to their perceived efficacy, more benign side effect profile, low lethality in overdose, ease of administration (often once a day dosing), and lack of EKG and serum level monitoring required. This initially seemed very reasonable in view of the lack of impressive double-blind placebo-controlled studies conducted with TCAs and the safer side effect profile with SSRIs. However, while open studies have reported a 70%–90% response rate to fluoxetine in adolescents with MDD, subsequent double-blind, placebo-controlled studies were initially unable to show clinical efficacy. This was probably due to several factors. While response rates in pediatric studies often approach 70%, similar to that in adult studies, the placebo response rate has been over 50% in some of the studies making it very difficult to show a statistically significant response. Eventually, fluoxetine was shown to be effective and now has FDA approval for treatment of depression in adolescents. SSRIs as a class appear to work very well for pediatric anxiety disorders. Indeed, fluvoxamine and sertraline have been granted FDA approval for OCD in children and adolescents.

FDA Warnings on Antidepressants for Children

During some of these pediatric studies utilizing SSRIs however, there were possible indicators that study subjects on medication demonstrated an increased frequency of suicidal ideation (no completed suicides occurred in these studies). While these studies were never designed to look at these issues, it did appear that some subjects demonstrated an increase in emotionality and others actual suicidal ideation or acts. A syndrome of behavioral 'activation' or 'disinhibition' has been noted by clinicians occasionally in the pediatric population since the initiation of treatment with SSRIs. In the author's opinion this can at times be correlated with too rapid a titration or too high a final dosage of the SSRI in question and can often be corrected by lowering the dose of SSRI. This activation or disinhibition period may account for some of the impulsive, out of character or even self-abusive/suicidal behavior that has been observed in a small number of these study subjects.

The FDA in 2004 commissioned two expert panels, the Psychopharmacologic Drugs and Pediatric Advisory Committees, to look at this issue and hopefully provide direction to this important but controversial issue. A commissioned FDA analysis of 24 clinical trials concluded that 4% of young people treated with antidepressants run the risk of suicidal thoughts or actions, which was twice the placebo risk of 2%. While there were 4400 patients in these studies, there were no completed suicides. Most of the trials were scientifically flawed and not designed to address the issue of suicidality and so causality could not be scientifically assigned to the medications.

The American Academy of Child and Adolescent Psychiatry reports that the rate of depression in children and adolescents is approximately 5%. Five hundred thousand children and adolescents experience suicidal ideation or acts each year and 2000 of these youth commit suicide each year. Unfortunately, at least 7% will eventually commit suicide [105]. While the 2% increase in suicidality associated with these medications is a concern, the finding that the underlying illness carries a 15% increase in suicide if left untreated is also clearly relevant and must be considered in a risk–benefit analysis. However, in September of 2004, the panels in a split vote of 15 to 8 urged the FDA to require 'black box' warnings on *all* antidepressants related to the possible link between antidepressants and an increased risk of suicidality, defined as suicidal ideation or acts, in pediatric patients. The labels advise close monitoring of patients particularly in the early stages of treatment or when dosage changes are made.

Some of the panelists were understandably concerned that such a black box warning could impede access to treatment. There is a shortage of child psychiatrists and many primary care physicians and pediatricians would now be unwilling to prescribe these medications and parents more reluctant to seek medical treatment. Many clinicians would also contend that the decrease in the suicide rate over the past decade could, in part, be attributed to the earlier recognition and medical treatment of depression in the pediatric age group. Most clinicians support the tenet that the benefits of medication still outweigh the risks. It would be unfortunate if clinicians and parents become unduly alarmed and discontinue the appropriate application of these medications in the comprehensive treatment of a markedly depressed pediatric patient in the absence of further data.

One of the benefits of the FDA review of these pediatric studies is that some summary data is now available regarding these trials. There were 15 short-term 4–16-week MDD studies in children aged 7–18 years. Only three studies – two fluoxetine studies and one citalopram study – were positive. The overall success rate was only 20%, which is below the 50% failure rate seen in adult studies. The other trials consisted of five OCD trials, one social anxiety disorder trial, and two ADHD trials.

March *et al.* [105] in 2004 completed an NIMH-sponsored Treatment for Adolescents with Depression Study (TADS) which included more than 400 children aged 12–17 years with MDD. In this multicenter, randomized, controlled, 12-week study with four treatment arms, adolescents receiving fluoxetine alone did nearly as well as those patients receiving both fluoxetine and cognitive behavioral therapy (CBT). Both of these treatment arms did significantly better than those adolescents receiving either CBT alone or placebo (see Figure 12.4). CBT did demonstrate an important benefit by reducing suicidal thoughts and behaviors whether used alone or in conjunction with fluoxetine treatment. Thus combination treatment may be the best therapy for teenagers with major depression, especially when there is a history of past or present suicidal ideation.

Unfortunately, there are no head-to-head studies comparing these SSRI compounds in children, but experience seems to indicate that for a given patient one antidepressant may be better tolerated and provide better efficacy than another. This is often only determined by trial and error. In regards to initial selection however, a specific SSRI may have an advantage for a select patient, often based on its pharmacologic or side effect profile. For instance, fluoxetine with its long half-life may be a good option for the patient who is often noncompliant.

In addition to SSRIs clinicians could also use serotonin norepinephrine reuptake inhibitors (SNRIs) such as venlafaxine and duloxetine. These compounds may be more efficacious for select patients as they modulate both noradrenergic and serotoninergic activity, with even some dopaminergic effect possible for venlafaxine at higher dosages. Once again, however, these compounds are not FDA approved for children yet.

As children and adolescents with affective disturbances typically have multiple comorbid diagnoses this often becomes the determining factor as to which medication should be used. For instance, a child with depression or dysthymia and concomitant ADHD may lead the clinician to use a TCA, bupropion, atomoxetine, or duloxetine as these medications – because of their noradrenergic effects – should have benefit in both of these comorbid conditions. Unfortunately, more controlled studies are needed to confirm these clinical assumptions. If a patient has a depressive dis-

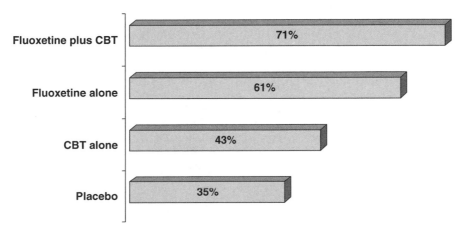

Figure 12.4 Adolescents exhibiting improvement on clinical global impressions score. (Adapted from March J: Fluoxetine, cognitive-behavioral therapy, and their combination for adolescents with depression. *JAMA* 2004; **292**(7): 807–820.

turbance and prominent anxiety symptoms or OCD, use of an SSRI compound, which may be helpful for both disorders, would be indicated. In short, one should adhere to the principle of pharmacologic parsimony whenever feasible.

Antidepressants and the Cytochrome P450 System

When the SSRI antidepressants were initially made available for patient use it was felt that their implementation would be much easier and safer due to their side effect profile. While overall they still appear medically to be a fairly safe class of medications, there is potential for severe drug–drug interactions in selected patients. As polypharmacy may be more the rule than the exception these days, it is imperative that the clinician be aware of the specific cytochrome P450 enzyme systems involved when prescribing SSRIs or TCAs together with other medications such as antipsychotics, benzodiazepines, warfarin, antiarrhythmics and even allergy medications. There are differences in the cytochrome P450 characteristics of each of the SSRIs and thus the modern prescriber must be aware of the potential drug–drug interactions for a given patient and choose the appropriate medication based on a risk–benefit analysis of all the relevant clinical variables. Unfortunately medicine is never simple!

Other Pharmacologic Treatments

Numerous other somatic agents have been found to be useful in the treatment of unipolar and bipolar mood disorders. Lithium, thyroid hormones, psychostimulants, and light therapy are some of the more common augmenting strategies used to supplement conventional monotherapy agents in treatment resistant unipolar and bipolar mood disorders. Lithium and psychostimulants can often have a rather rapid potentiating effect to antidepressants and mood stabilizers. Thyroid hormone dysregulation is felt to be an important and yet often overlooked contributing factor related to mood disorders. Thyroid function testing and thyroid hormone dosing is often perceived by many clinicians as too complicated which may in part explain the likely underutilization of this augmentation strategy. For the interested reader Bowers (1998) [106] described briefly the role of thyroid function testing and thyroid hormone treatment in an effort to clarify this issue.

Bipolar Disorder

As previously discussed, a diagnosis of bipolar disorder is not always easily made, especially if the 'index episode' was one of severe agitated depression. Often an initial manic episode will require an inpatient hospitalization to stabilize the patient and implement treatment. If one is fortunate enough to appreciate the budding emergence of a manic episode early enough, however, the development into a full blown manic episode at times can be prevented by aggressive and rapid pharmacologic treatment. The most common mood stabilizers are lithium, the anti-seizure medications, and the atypical antipsychotics, which now have FDA approval as mood stabilizers in adults. All the mood stabilizers except lamotrigine appear to have better antimanic properties than antidepressant effects.

Lithium

Lithium has been the standard therapy for bipolar disorder for a quarter of a century and has the unique distinction of being approved by the FDA for the treatment of bipolar disorder in adolescents who are 12 years of age or older. Despite this FDA approval there are few controlled studies utilizing lithium. Geller [107] published a double-blind randomized controlled trial of lithium in the pediatric age group. By the end of the six-week study, lithium treated subjects showed a significant improvement in their global assessment of functioning and also showed a significant decrease in their substance abuse. Kafantaris et al. [108] published the first placebo-controlled study of lithium for treatment of acute mania in children and adolescents. In this discontinuation study 40 adolescents aged 12–18 years, who initially responded to lithium treatment over 4–8 weeks, were then randomized to continue lithium or to be placed on placebo. After two weeks 53% of the lithium group and 62% of the placebo group relapsed clinically. Lithium appeared to decrease manic symptoms initially but the subsequent relapse rates did not appear to support long-term treatment or at least indicated that 4–8 weeks of treatment with a mood stabilizer may not be adequate to stabilize this condition.

Lithium may be most effective when the first episode is representative of mania since it has an 80% response rate in adults and an 80% nonresponse when the first episode is a depression [109].

Before lithium therapy is initiated several baseline laboratory studies are completed. Typically, a CBC with a differential (due to lithium's potential to cause neutrophilia) is obtained. Electrolytes, blood urea nitrogen, creatinine, creatinine clearance, urine osmolality, urinalysis and fasting blood sugar should be obtained for baseline measures and repeated every 6–12 months due to lithium's possible effects on kidney function and association with nephrogenic diabetes insipidus. It is known that lithium does cause morphologic changes in the kidney but the significance of these changes are not yet fully known. Overall, this young population typically does not experience significant renal dysfunction. Baseline thyroid function tests (TSH, T4, T3 uptake) should be obtained and repeated annually due to lithium's potential to cause hypothyroidism. There is some evidence that obtaining baseline thyroid antibodies may help to predict who will later develop hypothyroidism as this is likely an autoimmune related disorder. Lithium does have the disadvantage that many of its side effects are not acceptable to children or adolescents. It is not uncommon for this pediatric population to complain of thirst, polyuria (including enuresis), sedation, gastrointestinal upset, tremor (even at therapeutic dosages), cognitive/short-term memory impairment and as the dreaded facial acne and weight gain. These side effects and the need for blood monitoring are the major reasons for the high noncompliance rate with the use of lithium. Strober [110] has found that as many as 50% of adolescent bipolar patients are noncompliant with lithium treatment. Noncompliance with lithium treatment occurs even when the high potential for relapse is stressed to the patient and family.

The two types of lithium on the market (lithium carbonate and lithium citrate) have no major clinical differences. If one is not using a lithium dosing protocol [111], it is often started at 300 mg p.o. b.i.d. and increased 300 mg every 3–4 days. Lithium can be given in a b.i.d. dosage but a single bedtime dosage may produce less polyuria and chronic renal complications. Lithium levels of 0.6–1.2 mEq/L are typically cited as therapeutic ranges. Emerging data seems to indicate that serum lithium levels from 0.8 to 1.2 mEq/L are more effective in treating bipolar disorder than lower serum levels. In fact, the risk of relapse may be as much as 2.5 times higher in those who are in the low lithium dosage range than among those in the standard ranges. It has been cautioned that when treating organic or retarded children one should use lower dosages to avoid cognitive impairment. Some clinicians feel that the sustained release forms of lithium may lower side effects such as tremor and nausea at peak levels, but they may increase diarrhea. As with the other mood stabilizers, serum levels are usually checked 4–5 days after a change or increase in dosage and serum levels drawn 12 hours after the last ingested dose by standard. While lithium levels may be checked initially weekly during the titration phase, the frequency may be decreased to every 6–12 months once a stable therapeutic level has been achieved.

Lithium has been associated with Ebstein's Anomaly, a rare cardiac birth defect, found in 0.10% of exposed individuals. Despite this, many clinicians still believe lithium to be the safest choice for a mood stabilizer in pregnancy, but its dosage must often be adjusted upward during pregnancy and reduced by 25%–30% just before delivery to allow for the rapid shifts in fluid balance that occur following delivery.

Valproic Acid (Depakene) and Divalproex Sodium (Depakote)

The terms valproic acid and divalproex sodium are often used interchangeably. While lithium has been the standard of therapy for a quarter of a century, divalproex sodium is also FDA approved for bipolar disorder in adults and believed by many clinicians to be at least equally efficacious and better tolerated in this younger age group. Divalproex and carbamazepine (CBZ) may be even more efficacious for rapid cycling, dysphoric or mixed mania patients and those with comorbid substance abuse, all of which are common subgroups in adolescents [112]. Kowatch et al. [113] found valproate to be an effective treatment in adolescents. These agents are fairly well tolerated and can be administered in a loading dose of 20 mg/kg [114]; this dosage allows one to reach therapeutic plasma concentrations within 24 hours of treatment, compared to several days for lithium. Clinical dosages for mood stabilization range from 25 to 60 mg/kg/day with desired serum levels between 80 and 120 mg/L to achieve efficacy and avoid side effects [115]. The most common side effect consists of weight gain, sedation and nausea. Very rarely, valproic acid has been implicated in fatal hepatotoxicity/liver failure (one in 45 000 cases on monotherapy), although this occurs predominantly in children less than 2–3 years of age. In adults, the rate of liver failure is only one in 118 000. Pancreatitis can also be a very rare complication. Due to these issues, valproic acid requires initial blood monitoring to follow serum levels and then subsequent blood monitoring that can be as infrequently as every 6–12 months to monitor for these adverse events. Divalproex sodium, valproic acid, and CBZ may all temporarily raise liver function tests during the first three months of therapy and are not a health concern unless they elevate 2.5 to 3 times the upper limit of the normal values.

In 1993, Isojarvi et al. [116] raised questions about valproate's relationship to polycystic ovary syndrome in women with epilepsy. Two recent studies [117,118] appear to suggest that this is related more to the epilepsy than to the anticonvulsant exposure; however, it is probably prudent to monitor menstrual abnormalities, infertility, weight gain, and hair growth changes in female patients and obtain an endocrine consultation if concern arises.

Carbamazepine

Carbamazepine (CBZ), a tricyclic compound, is usually initiated during inpatient therapy at 200 mg twice a day and can be increased 200 mg/day with a targeted range of 15–30 mg/kg in divided dosages to minimize peak levels and side effects. Dosing can be weighted towards bedtime or even given solely at bedtime if daytime sedation or insomnia is problematic. Recently a long acting form of CBZ received FDA approval for the treatment of bipolar disorder in adults. This long acting preparation allows less frequent dosing and a more beneficial side effect profile. Serum levels should be checked five days after a change in dosage. Therapeutic plasma levels vary between labs but are typically between 6 and 12 mEq/L. Due to hepatic autoinduction of its own metabolism, after 2–4 weeks of treatment the CBZ plasma half-life decreases from 24 to 12 hours and thus the dosage may have to be increased. Carbamazepine's most serious potential side effect is that of bone marrow suppression with neutropenia, which can lead to life-threatening infections. Because of this risk of bone marrow suppression and even aplastic anemia (in adults about six per one million usually during the first three months of therapy) the use of CBZ typically requires laboratory monitoring similar to that suggested for divalproex. If the white blood count should drop below 2500 to 3000/mm^3 or the absolute neutrophil count below 1000 to 1500/mm^3, the medication should usually be discontinued promptly. Clinicians should instruct the family to be alert for signs of an infection, such as fever, sore throat, or easy bruising, which could be an indication of neutropenia. Rashes are fairly common in 10%–15% of patients and generally warrant discontinuation of CBZ. The hypersensitivity reaction can progress to more severe conditions such as exfoliative dermatitis or Stevens–Johnson syndrome, which can be fatal.

Both CBZ and valproate can cause teratogenic neural tube defects (spina bifida) at rates of 1.0% and 1.0 to 5.0%, respectively, in addition to possible facial clefts; they are therefore relatively contraindicated for use during pregnancy.

Lamotrigine

Lamotrigine is a new anticonvulsant that in 2003 received FDA approval for treatment of bipolar disorder in adults. Lamotrigine seems to be one of the few mood stabilizers that have good antidepressant prop-

erties despite being a mood stabilizer. Lamotrigine appears to have better antidepressant properties than antimanic properties but is approved in the long-term prevention of both manic and depressive affective states. The antidepressant effect may be due to its known inhibitory effects on glutamate, which is consistent with NMDA-receptor downregulation seen with other antidepressants. Lamotrigine may allow patients to discontinue adjunctive therapy with antidepressants, which are known to increase the risk of cycling and mania. Lamotrigine has a very favorable side effect profile, which is reflected in its common usage in pediatric seizure disorders. When prescribing lamotrigine there is no requirement for blood work and serum levels are not typically useful. Unlike most other mood stabilizers, lamotrigine does not have significant side effects such as weight gain or cognitive impairment, which makes it very useful as an augmenting agent as well. Lamotrigine does have a well-described relationship to Stevens–Johnson syndrome if the dosage is increased at too rapid a rate. Strict guidelines are in place for the gradual titration of lamotrigine, but when followed it has a Stevens–Johnson's risk comparable to that of divalproex sodium.

Comparative Studies of Mood Stabilizers in Pediatrics

Kowatch et al. [119] conducted an open study in children and adolescents comparing effect-sizes of valproate, lithium and CBZ over an eight-week period. All three medications showed a large effect-size (a medium effect-size is one that a trained observer will recognize in a clinical situation), and response rates for both lithium and valproate were in the same range as other reports in adults and adolescents (less than 50%). More than half of the study patients did not respond to monotherapy with any of these medications. Clinical experience with these patients indicates that they frequently require combination treatment with either: (a) two (or more) mood stabilizers; (b) a mood stabilizer plus an atypical antipsychotic agent; or (c) addition of a stimulant. This study also examined time-to-response data for each of the three study medications and found that subjects treated with lithium continued to respond until week eight, whereas no new subjects responded after week five of CBZ and week six of valproate.

Atypical Antipsychotics Approved as Mood Stabilizers

Bipolar patients, especially severely manic patients, may require the addition of an antipsychotic medication, particularly during the acute treatment phase. Although traditional neuroleptics (such as haloperidol) have been shown to be effective, atypical antipsychotics such as olanzapine, risperidone, quetiapine, ziprasidone, and aripiprazole are increasingly being used due to their perceived better tolerability and efficacy. All of these atypical antipsychotics now have FDA approval for bipolar disorder in adults and thus should be considered as true mood stabilizers although large-scale pediatric studies are lacking.

There are however several open label studies in children and adolescents that suggest effectiveness of these medications in the pediatric population. Frazier *et al.* [120] in 1999 completed a retrospective chart review of risperidone as an adjunctive treatment in an outpatient 'bipolar disorder' population (mean age 10 years) with 82% reporting symptoms much improved. There is one open-label trial of olanzapine as monotherapy in children (mean age of 10 years) with bipolar I, treated as outpatients for eight weeks, by Frazier *et al.* [121] in 2001 that showed a 74% response rate (>50% improvement). In the one double-blind, placebo-controlled combination study, Delbello *et al.* [122] in 2002 found valproate plus quetiapine to be more efficacious than valproate monotherapy in a group of hospitalized adolescents with bipolar I disorder. Several more studies are currently in press.

These mood stabilizers have been proven to provide clear benefit for manic and to some degree depressive symptoms in bipolar patients. These agents cause less extrapyramidal (EPS) and tardive dyskinesia symptoms. Risperidone, for example, has a reported tardive dyskinesia risk of 0.034% per year, which is significantly lower than that of traditional neuroleptics [123]. These agents also typically cause less prolactin elevation, except for risperidone. Prolactin elevation may cause unwanted breast enlargement in males and lactation in females, which in and of itself is not a serious medical issue. However, if a female has an elevated prolactin level and experiences cessation of her periods there does appear to be an associated risk of osteoporosis and thus a medication change may be indicated if clinically appropriate. Traditionally, as many as 25% or more of bipolar patients will require chronic treatment with antipsychotic medication and thus these agents with their more tolerant side effects seem to have an advantage over older neuroleptics. Unfortunately, significant weight gain is a typical side effect of these agents except for ziprasidone and aripiprazole. Additionally, diabetes mellitus, hypercholesterolemia, and hypertriglyceridemia have been associated with these agents and occasionally even in patients who do not gain extreme amounts of weight. These disorders

are now being described as part of a syndrome referred to as Metabolic Syndrome or Syndrome X, which is occurring in epidemic proportions in children and adults. Metabolic Syndrome includes insulin resistance and one or more related health problems such as obesity, high cholesterol, high blood pressure, and high triglycerides. The FDA now recommends screening and treating adult patients who are on these medications for diabetes and hyperlipidemia. The American Diabetes Association/American Psychiatric Association Consensus Conference on Antipsychotic Drugs and Obesity and Diabetes in 2003 made recommendations for monitoring (Table 12.5).

One change that may occur in the future will be the recommendation for yearly lipid screening in patients. The American Diabetes Association Clinical Practice Recommendations [124] state that all children and adolescents aged 10 years or older should be screened for diabetes every two years if they are overweight (body mass index >85th percentile for age and sex, weight for height >85th percentile, or weight >120% of ideal weight) plus any two of the following risk factors:

- family history of Type 2 diabetes in first- or second-degree relative;
- race/ethnicity (Native American, African–American, Latino, Asian–American, Pacific Islander);
- signs of insulin resistance or conditions associated with insulin resistance (acanthosis nigrans, hypertension, dyslipidemia, or polycystic ovary syndrome.)

Children and adolescents with these risk factors may be candidates for another class of mood stabilizer or at least preferentially tried on ziprasidone or aripiprazole.

Other Potential Mood Stabilizers

A search for new medications is always ongoing, as a substantial percentage of patients exhibit bipolar disorder, which is not adequately controlled with the currently available mood stabilizers.

Some other anticonvulsants, such as oxcarbazepine and topiramate appear to be beneficial for some patients. Oxcarbazepine is often used in place of CBZ because it does not require bloodwork as has a much lower potential for blood dyscrasias. Topiramate has a unique and desirable property of weight loss in dosages of 200–400 mg/day, but is also associated with cognitive blunting. Nevertheless, it is often used in conjunction with other bipolar agents to minimize their all too common side effect of weight gain. Other anti-seizure medications, such as gabapentin and tiagabine may be beneficial for some bipolar patients, but studies

Table 12.5 ADA/APA Consensus Conference on Antipsychotic Drugs and Obesity and Diabetes Monitoring Recommendations. Copyright © 2004 American Diabetes Association. From Diabetes Care, Vol. 27, 2004; 596–601. Reprinted with permission from The American Diabetes Association.

	Baseline	4 weeks	8 weeks	12 weeks	Quarterly	Annually	Every 5 years
Personal/family history	X					X	
Weight (BMI)	X	X	X	X	X		
Waist circumference	X					X	
Blood pressure	X			X		X	
FPG	X			X		X	
Fasting lipid profile	X			X			X

FPG, Fast Plasma Glucose.
Data from: *J Clin Psychiatry* 2004; **65**:267–272; *Diabetes Care* 2004; **27**:596–601.

Table 12.6 Pharmacotherapies for bipolar disorder.

	Typical antipsychotics	Anticonvulsants	Atypical antipsychotics
Lithium 1973[a]	Chlorpromazine 1973[a]	Divalproex sodium 1995[a]	Clozapine
		Lamotrigine 2003[a]	Olanzapine 2000[a]
		Carbamazepine 2005[a]	Risperidone 2003[a]
		Oxcarbazepine	Olanzapine/fluoxetine 2004[a]
			Quetiapine 2004[a]
			Ziprasidone 2004[a]
			Aripiprazole 2004[a]

[a] FDA approval for bipolar disorder.

seem to indicate they have better anti-anxiety properties than antimanic properties. Thus these agents are typically used in treatment resistant or treatment intolerant patients (Table 12.6).

The benzodiazepine clonazepam is sometimes used as an augmenting strategy in the treatment of manic patients. It is felt to have some mood stabilizing qualities and anxiolytic effects that may be particularly helpful in the agitated manic patient. Also, clonazepam can be quite sedating and is often successfully used at bedtime to restore sleep/awake cycles that appear to be very important in the treatment of bipolar patients. Some patients, during the developing early phase of a manic episode, may receive benefit from using clonazepam 1–2 mg/hour until one falls asleep. The total dosage that is required for sleep induction is then divided into a t.i.d. dosing schedule to be given daily over the next couple of days to aid in averting a full-blown manic episode. The severe bipolar patient may require a combination of mood stabilizers such as valproic acid and CBZ or lithium plus a neuroleptic. This type of polypharmacy is inherently more complicated due to the number of possible drug–drug interactions. For instance, valproic acid displaces CBZ from plasma proteins resulting in an increase in free CBZ and possible toxicity, which may be heralded by diplopia and truncal ataxia. CBZ induces the metabolism of TCAs and bupropion lowering their serum levels. Fluoxetine, fluvoxamine, and nefazodone reportedly inhibit CBZ metabolism, resulting in elevated CBZ levels and potential toxicity. To minimize these potential complications the eventual goal is to maintain the patient on the fewest medications and at the lowest dosages that prove efficacious in bringing about a reduction in the rate of the patient's cycling or number of episodes. Due to unwanted side effects and risk of tardive dyskinesia with neuroleptics these medications should be weaned when clinically appropriate. Clonazepam should be reduced gradually to minimize withdrawal and seizure activity. As a rule, slow weaning should probably be performed with any mood stabilizer as abrupt discontinuation may bring about dysregulation in the patient's affective state. For all bipolar patients the mood stabilizers are better at maintaining the manic symptoms than improving the depressive symptoms as they have only moderate antidepressant effects. This poses a dilemma when a patient's depressive periods are severe to the point of suicidal ideation and specific antidepressant pharmacotherapy is needed, as there is clinical concern that antidepressants can, with differing propensity (TCAs > SSRIs > bupropion), induce mania or permanently increase the frequency of affective cycling. Sachs et al. [125] found that with bupropion the risk of mania is one-fifth that of desipramine. In treating bipolar depression one approach is to initiate one of the mood stabilizers and if the patient does not respond to add a second mood stabilizer. If the patient is still not improved with two mood stabilizers one may add an antidepressant slowly and then consider tapering the antidepressant in three months to minimize the risk of rapid cycling.

It remains unclear if one type of antidepressant is better than another in reducing the risk of possible mania precipitation in children and adolescents. Longitudinal studies addressing the course of depression over the life span [126] seem to indicate that unipolar depression converts to bipolar illness more frequently in childhood than in adulthood, and thus raises another consideration in initial treatment, since some antidepressants may pose a slightly less risk of precipitating 'switching' than others (see below).

A careful risk–benefit analysis should be discussed with the patient before antidepressant therapy is initiated.

Adolescents of Childbearing Age and Considerations in Pregnancy

Many teenagers are at risk for becoming pregnant, but this is even more of a concern in the bipolar female. Therefore, it may be advisable to have bipolar female of childbearing age to consider the use of birth control measures, especially if CBZ or valproate is implemented. Due to the fact that medication noncompliance is so prominent in this age group, long acting contraceptives such as intramuscular progesterone or Norplant may have considerable advantages over oral birth control pills, although their side effect profile may be unacceptable to some teenagers. It is not advisable to suddenly stop a mood stabilizer if a patient reports she is pregnant. Rapid discontinuation of mood stabilizers may precipitate bipolar relapse and adult studies indicate 30% relapse rates even in medication compliant patients. Typically, by the time the adolescent is aware she is pregnant and then notifies someone, she is several months pregnant and any effect on the fetus is complete. For this reason, some clinicians advocate

placing all female bipolar patients of childbearing age on birth control and or at least using supplemental folic acid 4 mg/day. Additionally, if a patient desires pregnancy and uninterrupted administration of CBZ or valproate is clinically necessary, the use of supplemental folic acid four weeks before conception and continuing through the first trimester to reduce the risk of spina bifida is recommended.

In the depressed adolescent female a similar argument can be made for continuing antidepressant therapy. While somewhat controversial, this recommendation follows the growing body of evidence in adult pregnant females that the pre- and postnatal period is unfortunately a high risk period for serious relapse in depressed and bipolar females. Women on medication participate in better prenatal care, which is a high predictor of postnatal outcome. Maternal depression is now known to be a significant risk factor for poor postnatal outcomes, poor mother–child bonding and higher risk for depression and delinquency later in the offspring. Decisions regarding these issues must be made on a case-by-case basis in close consultation with the patient, her family and physicians.

Electroconvulsive Therapy in Adolescents

Given the high rates of relapse and treatment resistance among children and adolescents with mood disorders, it seems surprising that more attention has not been given to electroconvulsive therapy (ECT). Although controversial with the lay public, ECT has been shown through numerous studies in adults to be safe and effective when standardized methods of administering it are used. Medical opinion about its appropriateness in treating children and adolescents, however, is more polarized and only a few practitioners and medical centers have utilized ECT with any frequency. No controlled studies have been conducted in children and adolescents, and as was learned with antidepressants, results obtained with adults are not necessarily applicable to younger populations. Nevertheless, one must question carefully whether this attitude protects children from a procedure that would be ineffective and stigmatizing or whether the current reluctance to use ECT in children and adolescents is in fact overly conservative and is depriving this population from receiving an effective treatment.

Historical Perspectives

It was not until the 1940s that many children and adolescents were administered ECT; the first child reported to receive ECT was a three-year-old with epilepsy in 1941 [127]. With few effective somatic treatments available for children and adolescents in the 1940s, ECT was used more liberally by such psychiatrists as Lauretta Bender at Bellevue Hospital in New York. In 1947, Dr. Bender reported on the efficacy of ECT in 98 children [128]; the encompassing diagnosis of 'childhood schizophrenia' was applied to many of these children who received ECT but who probably suffered from oppositional or developmental disorders by today's classifications. The early case reports generally cited favorable results from ECT; with the advent of psychotropic drugs in the following decades, however, the use of ECT fell out of favor. Today, ECT for children and adolescents is outlawed in some countries and in some states in the US.

In 1997 Rey and Walter [129] published a retrospective analysis of all studies worldwide on the use of ECT in persons 18 years of age or younger. They identified 60 reports describing ECT in 396 patients; most (63%) were case reports and none were controlled trials. The quality of the reports was found to be poor overall in the following respects: the absence of controlled studies; the lack of reported symptoms to make a diagnosis or the complete lack of a diagnosis; the failure to list previous and concurrent treatments; the omission of adverse effects data; and in many instances failure to specify the position of electrode placement and the number and frequency of ECT treatments.

Given the shortcomings of these studies, conclusions must be drawn cautiously; overall, however, it appeared that one-half to two-thirds of the patients showed benefit after completing their course of ECT. This parallels the response rate found in adults. ECT appeared to be effective for patients with major depression unless they exhibited psychotic features; patients with bipolar disorders responded favorably, especially those with manic states. Subjects diagnosed as schizophrenic responded rather poorly, however. Electrode placement (unilateral vs. bilateral), age, and comorbidity did not appear to affect response rates. No fatalities were reported in the 60 studies and, long-term sequelae attributable to the ECT were not noted. The most common acute adverse events were headache, confusion, agitation, the development of hypomania/mania, subjective memory loss, and vomiting. Overall, adverse events appeared to be similar in type and frequency to those experienced by adults.

Presently, ECT is seldom if ever used in prepubertal children and only rarely in adolescents as a treatment of last resort. Given the refractory nature of some juvenile mood disorders to current psychotherapy or psychopharmacologic approaches as well as the fact that probably less than 1% of patients who receive ECT are less than 18 years of age, ECT is likely underused in this population. Relatively few clinicians have any knowledge of ECT usage in the juvenile population, and even fewer clinicians have first-hand experience with it. In carefully selected cases of mood disorders, ECT can have a beneficial, dramatic, or even lifesaving effect. Dramatic responses to ECT have been described repeatedly in psychiatric case reports where all prior therapy and somatic treatments had failed miserably. In this era of health care cost containment, health–economic issues may spur more research on ECT. With the addition of controlled studies of ECT in this population, this treatment could then be judged by its merits (or lack thereof), rather than by the current stigma still associated with it by laypersons and professionals alike.

Conclusion

The present field of child and adolescent psychiatry may best be described by a quote from Dickens' *Tale of Two Cities*, 'It was the best of times. It was the worst of times.' The *best* is the exciting research currently underway in the form of controlled studies investigating efficacy of both traditional and new cognitive therapy approaches as well as the development of numerous pharmacologic agents that hold the prospect of being better tolerated, safer, and more effective. Our understanding of the complexities of brain functioning is progressing at an astonishing rate, owing to research in neurotransmitters, receptors, and neuroimaging. The predicted outcome of this research – improved and *proven* treatments available to child and adolescent psychiatrists – may hold great promise for both clinicians and patients.

The *worst* of current-day psychiatry is the loss of autonomy that many psychiatrists feel in their treatment of patients. Shortened hospital stays of less than a week, the lack of residential treatment options, abbreviated outpatient therapy, and restrictive formularies often do not allow the modern psychiatrist to function as they see most fitting for their patients. The unfortunate practice of defensive medicine due to fears of civil liability perceived by clinicians and its associated health care costs are issues that will hopefully be addressed in the near future if our health care system is to remain of high quality, efficient and cost effective.

Child and adolescent psychiatrists have always been strong advocates for the welfare of this underserved population. Given the current flux of the rapidly changing health care delivery system in this country, in the future, psychiatrists will need to champion their causes with renewed vigor.

References

1. Schulterbrandt JG, Raskin A, eds: *Depression in Childhood: Diagnosis, Treatment, and Conceptual Models.* Rockville, MD: National Institute of Mental Health, 1977: 168, DHEW publ. No. (ADM) 77–476.
2. Kraepelin E: *Manic Depressive Insanity and Paranoia.* Edinburgh: Livingstone, 1921.
3. American Psychiatric Association: *Diagnostic and Statistical Manual of Mental Disorders*, 4th ed, Text Revision. Washington, DC: American Psychiatric Association, 2000.
4. Weller EB, Weller RA: Depressive disorders in children and adolescents. In: Garfinkel B, Carlson G, Weller EB, eds. *Psychiatric Disorders in Children and Adolescents.* Philadelphia, WB Saunders, 1990:3–20.
5. Weller EB, Weller RA: Depressive disorders in children and adolescents. In: Garfinkel B, Carlson G, Weller EB, eds. *Psychiatric Disorders in Children and Adolescents.* Philadelphia, WB Saunders, 1990:37–47.
6. Weller EB, Weller RA, Fristad MA: Assessment and treatment of childhood depression. In: Weller EB, Weller RA, eds. *Current Perspectives on Major Depressive Disorders in Children.* Washington, DC: American Psychiatric Press, 1984:1–18.
7. Weller EB, Weller RA, Fristad MA: Historical and theoretical perspectives on childhood depression. In: Weller EB, Weller RA, eds. *Current Perspectives on Major Depressive Disorders in Children.* Washington, DC: American Psychiatric Press, 1984:1–18.
8. Youngstrom EA, Findling RL, Calabrese JR, *et al.*: Comparing the diagnostic accuracy of six potential screening instruments for bipolar disorder in youths aged 5 to 17 years. *J Am Acad Child Adolesc Psychiatry* 2004; **43**(7):847–858.
9. American Psychiatric Association: *Diagnostic and Statistical Manual of Mental Disorders*, Fourth Edition, Text Revision. Washington, DC: American Psychiatric Association, 2000.
10. WebMD Medical reference. Depression in children, edited by Charlotte E. Grayson, MD, October. 2004.
11. Chambers WJ, Puig-Antich J, Tabrizi MA, Davies M: Psychotic symptoms in prepubertal major depressive disorder. *Arch Gen Psychiatry* 1982; **39**:921–927.
12. WebMD Medical reference, Depression in children, edited by Charlotte E. Grayson, MD, October. 2004.
13. Blackman MB: You asked about . . . adolescent depression. *Can J CME* May 1995.
14. Klein DN, Schwartz JE, Rose S, *et al.*: Five-year course and outcome of dysthymic disorder: A prospective, naturalistic follow-up study. *Am J Psychiatry* 2000; **157**(6):931–939.
15. Kovacs M, Feinberg TL, Crouse-Novak M, *et al.*: Depressive disorders in childhood ii: Longitudinal study of the risk for a subsequent major depression. *Arch Gen Psychiatry* 1984; **41**:643–649.
16. Angold A, Costello EJ: Depressive comorbidity in children and adolescents: Empirical, theoretical, and methodological issues. *Am J Psychiatry* 1993; **150**(12):1779–1791.
17. Esquirol E: *Mental Maladies.* (Hunt EK, trans.) Philadelphia: Lea and Blanehard, 1845:33.
18. Lewinsohn PM, Klein DL, Seeley JR: Bipolar disorders in a community sample of older adolescents: Prevalence, phenomenology, comorbidity, and course. *J Am Acad Child Adolesc Psychiatry* 1995; **34**:454–463.
19. Lish JD, Dime-Meenan S, Whybrow PC, *et al.*: The National Depressive and Manic-Depressive Association (DMDA) survey of bipolar members. *J Affect Disord* 1994; **31**:281–294.
20. Birmaher B, Ryan ND, Williamson DE, *et al.*: Childhood and adolescent depression: A review of the past 10 years. Part I. *J Am Acad Child Adolesc Psychiatry* 1996; **35**(11):1427–1439.
21. Pavuluri M, Naylor M, Janicak P: Recognition and treatment of pediatric bipolar disorder. *Contemporary Psychiatry* 2002; April:1–9.
22. Geller B: Prepubertal and early adolescent bipolarity differentiate from ADHD by manic symptoms, grandiose delusions, ultra-rapid or ultradian cycling. *J Affect Disord* 1998; **51**:81–91.
23. Geller B, Williams M, Zimmerman B, Frazier J, Beringer L, Warner K: Prepubertal and early adolescent bipolarity differentiate from ADHD by manic symptoms, grandiose delusions, ultra-rapid or ultradian cycling. *J Affect Disord* 1998; **51**:81–91.
24. Fergus E: How can we differentiate between ADHD, bipolar disorder in children? *The Brown University Child and Adolescent Psychopharmacology Update* 1999; **1**(5):4–5.
25. Lewinsohn PM, Klein DL, Seeley JR: Bipolar disorders in a community sample of older adolescents: Prevalence, phenomenology, comorbidity, and course. *J Am Acad Child Adolesc Psychiatry* 1995; **34**:454–463.
26. Werry JS, McClellan JM, Chard L: Childhood and adolescent schizophrenic, bipolar, and schizoaffective disorders: A clinical and outcome study. *J Am Acad Child Adolesc Psychiatry* 1991; **30**:457–465.
27. Strober M, Schmidt-Lackner S, Freeman R, *et al.*: Recovery and relapse in adolescents with bipolar affective illness: A five-year naturalistic, prospective follow-up. *J Am Acad Child Adolesc Psychiatry* 1995; **34**:724–731.
28. McClellan J, McCurry C, Snell J, *et al.*: Early-onset psychotic disorders; course and outcome over a 2-year period. *J Am Acad Child Adolesc Psychiatry* 1999; **38**: 1380–1388.
29. Carlson GA, Bromet EJ, Sievers S: Phenomenology and outcome of subjects with early- and adult-onset psychotic mania. *Am J Psychiatry* 2000; **157**:213–219.
30. Kutcher S: Bipolar disorder in children and adolescents: Identification, diagnosis, and treatment. Presented at the World Assembly for Mental Health. Vancouver, Canada, July 24, 2001.
31. Geller B, Zimmerman B, Williams M, Bolhofner K, Craney JL, Delbello MP, Soutullo CA: Diagnostic characteristics of 93 cases of a prepubertal and early adolescent bipolar disorder phenotype by gender, puberty and comorbid attention deficit hyperactivity disorder. *J Child Adolesc Psychopharmacol* 2000; **10**(3):157–164.
32. Geller B, Williams M, Zimmerman B, Frazier J, Beringer L, Warner K: Prepubertal and early adolescent bipolarity differentiate from ADHD by manic symptoms, grandiose delusions, ultra-rapid or ultradian cycling. *J Affect Disord* 1998: **51**:81–91.
33. Geller B, Luby J: Child and adolescent bipolar disorder: A review of the past 10 years. *J Am Acad Child Adolesc Psychiatry* 1997; **36**:1168–1176.

34. Kraepelin E: *Manic Depressive Insanity and Paranoia.* Edinburgh: Livingstone, 1921.

35. Bowden C: Pharmacotherapy for classic euphoric mania. *Psychiatric Times' Bipolar Disorders Letter*, May 1997.

36. Weissman MM, Wolk S, Goldstein RB, *et al.*: Depressed adolescents grown up. *JAMA* 1999; **281**: 1701–1713.

37. Kovacs M: Presentation and course of major depressive disorder during childhood and later years of the life span. *J Am Acad Child Adolesc Psychiatry* 1996; **35**:710.

38. Shaffer D, Craft L: Methods of adolescent suicide prevention. Methods of adolescent suicide prevention. *J Clin Psychiatry* 1999; **60**(Suppl 2):70–74.

39. Akiskal HS, Walker T, Puzantian VR, King D, Rosenthal TL, Dranon M: Bipolar outcome in the course of depressive illness. Phenomenologic, familial, and pharmacologic predictors. *J Affect Disord* 1983; **5**:115–128.

40. Geller B, Fox LW, Clark KA: Rate and predictors of prepubertal bipolarity during follow-up of 6- to 12-year-old depressed children. *J Am Acad Child Adolesc Psychiatry* 1994; **33**:461–468.

41. Akiskal HS, Walker T, Puzantian VR, King D, Rosenthal TL, Dranon M: Bipolar outcome in the course of depressive illness. Phenomenologic, familial, and pharmacologic predictors. *J Affect Disord* 1983; **5**:115–128.

42. Akiskal HS, Walker T, Puzantian VR, King D, Rosenthal TL, Dranon M: Bipolar outcome in the course of depressive illness. Phenomenologic, familial, and pharmacologic predictors. *J Affect Disord* 1983; **5**:115–128.

43. Strober M, Carlson G: Bipolar illness in adolescents with major depression: Clinical, genetic and psychopharmacologic predictors in a three-to-four year perspective follow-up. *Arch Gen Psychiatry* 1982; **39**:549–555.

44. Geller B, Fox LW, Clark KA: Rate and predictors of prepubertal bipolarity during follow-up of 6- to 12-year-old depressed children. *J Am Acad Child Adolesc Psychiatry* 1994; **33**:461–468.

45. Akiskal HS, Walker P, Puzantian VR, King D, Rosenthal TL, Dranon M: Bipolar outcome in the course of depressive illness: Phenomenological, familial, and pharmacological predictors. *J Affect Disord* 1983; **5**:115–128.

46. Akiskal HS, Walker P, Puzantian VR, King D, Rosenthal TL, Dranon M: Bipolar outcome in the course of depressive illness: Phenomenological, familial, and pharmacological predictors. *J Affect Disord* 1983; **5**:115–128.

47. Strober M, Carlson G: Bipolar illness in adolescents with major depression: Clinical, genetic and psychopharmacologic predictors in a three-to-four year perspective follow-up. *Arch Gen Psychiatry* 1982; **39**:549–555.

48. Kovacs-M, Pollock M: Bipolar disorder and comorbid conduct disorder in childhood and adolescents. *J Am Acad Child Adolesc Psychiatry* 1995; **34**:715–723.

49. Kashani JH, Sherman DD: Childhood depression: Epidemiology, etiological models and treatment implications. *Integrative Psychiatry* 1988; **6**:1–8.

50. Carlson GA, Cantwell DP: A survey of depressive symptoms, syndrome and disorder in a child psychiatric population. *J Child Psychol Psychiatry* 1980; **1**:19–25.

51. Robbins DR, Alessi NE, Cook SC, *et al.*: The use of the research diagnostic criteria (RDC) for depression in adolescent psychiatric inpatients. *J Am Acad Child Psychiatry* 1982; **21**:251–255.

52. Petti TA: Depression in hospitalized child psychiatry patients: Approaches to measuring depression. *J AM Acad Child Psychiatry* 1978; **17**:49–59.

53. Hankin BL, Abramson LY, Moffitt TE, *et al.*: Development of depression from preadolescence to young adulthood: Emerging gender differences in a 10-year longitudinal study. *J Abnorm Psychol* 1998; **107**:128–140.

54. Klerman GL, Weissman MM: Increasing rates of depression. *JAMA* 1989; **261**:2229–2235.

55. Cross-National Collaborative Group: The changing rate of major depression – Cross-National comparisons. *JAMA* 1992; **268**:3098–3105.

56. Lewinsohn PM, Klein DL, Seeley JR: Bipolar disorders in a community sample of older adolescents: Prevalence, phenomenology, comorbidity, and course. *J Am Acad Child Adolesc Psychiatry* 1995; **34**:454–463.

57. Loranger A, Leivene P: Age and onset of bipolar affective illness. *Arch Gen Psychiatry* 1978; **35**:1345–1348.

58. Weller RA, Weller EB, Tucker SG, Fristad MA: Mania in prepubertal children: Has it been underdiagnosed? *J Affect Disorder* 1986; **11**:151–154.

59. Wozniak J, Biederman J, Mundy E, *et al.*: A pilot family study of childhood onset mania. *J Am Acad Child Adolesc Psychiatry* 1995; **34**(12):1577–1583.

60. Weissman MM, Gershon ES, Kidd KK: Psychiatric disorders in the relatives of probands with affective disorders: The Yale-NIMH collaborative family study. *Arch Gen Psychiatry* 1984; **41**:13.

61. Fergus EL: Offspring study of pediatric bipolar disorder. Poster presented at AACAP; 1999.

62. Mitchell J, McCauley E, Burke P, *et al.*: Psychopathology in parents of depressed children and adolescents. *J Am Acad Child Adolesc Psychiatry* 1989; **28**:352–357.

63. Bowlby J: Grief and mourning in infancy and early childhood. *Psychoanal Study Child* 1960; **15**:9–52.

64. Ainsworth MDS, Blehar MC, Waters E, *et al.*: *Patterns of Attachment.* Hillsdale NJ: Lawrence Erlbaum, 1978.

65. Tenant C: Parental loss of childhood. *Arch Gen Psychiatry* 1988; **45**:1045–1050.

66. Freud S: Mourning and melancholia. In: Strachey J, ed. *The Standard Edition of the Complete Psychological Works of Sigmund Freud (Vol. 14).* London: Hogarth Press, 1966.

67. Akiskal HS: Developmental pathways to bipolarity: Are juvenile-onset depressions pre-bipolar? *J Am Acad Child Adolesc Psychiatry* 1995; **34**:754–763.

68. Akiskal HS: Developmental pathways to bipolarity: Are juvenile-onset depressions pre-bipolar? *J Am Acad Child Adolesc Psychiatry* 1995; **34**:754–763.

69. Strober M: Childhood onset of bipolar disorder: Identification and treatment. *Psychiatric times bipolar disorders letter*, June, 1996.

70. Akiskal HS, Weller EB: Mood disorders and suicide in children and adolescents. In: Kaplan HI, Sadock BJ, eds. *Comprehensive Textbook of Psychiatry*, Volume II, 5th ed. Baltimore: Williams and Wilkins, 1989.

71. Weissman MM, Gershon ES, Kidd KK: Psychiatric disorders in the relatives of probands with affective disorders: The Yale-NIMH collaborative family study. *Arch Gen Psychiatry* 1984; **41**:13.

72. Puig-Antich J, Goetz D, Davies M, *et al.*: A controlled family history study of prepubertal major depressive disorder. *Arch Gen Psychiatry* 1988; **46**:406–420.

73. Strober M, Carlson G, Ryan N, *et al.*: Advances in the psychopharmacology of childhood and adolescent affective disorders. Paper presented at the Scientific Proceedings of the Annual Meeting of the American Academy of Child and Adolescent Psychiatry, Washington, DC, 1987.

74. Gershon ES, Hamovit J, Guroff JJ, *et al.*: A family study of schizoaffective, bipolar I, bipolar II, unipolar, and normal control probands. *Arch Gen Psychiat* 1982; **39**:1157.

75. Akiskal H: Recent progress in genetic studies of bipolar disorder. Presented at the World Assembly for Mental Health. Vancouver, Canada, July 24, 2001.

76. Nurnberger JI, Gershon E: Genetics. In: Paykel ES, ed. *Handbook of Affective Disorders.* Edinburgh: Church-Livingstone, 1982.

77. Mendlewicz J, Rainer JD: Adoption study supporting genetic transmission in manic depressive illness. *Nature* 1977; **265**:327–329.

78. Klein DN, Depue RA, Slater JF: Cyclothymia in the adolescent offspring of parents with bipolar affective disorder. *J Abnorm Psychol* 1985; **94**:115–127.

79. Egeland J, Sussex J: Suicide and family loading for affective disorders. *JAMA* 1985; **254**:915.

80. Akiskal H: Recent progress in genetic studies of bipolar disorder. Presented at the World Assembly for Mental Health. Vancouver, Canada, July 24, 2001.

81. Reinherz HC, Stewart-Berghaue G, Pakiz B, *et al.*: The relationship of early risk in current mediators to depressive symptomatology in adolescents. *J Am Acad Child Adolesc Psychiatry* 1989; **28**:942–947.

82. Poznanski EO: The clinical phenomenology of childhood depression. *Am J Orthopsychiatry* 1982; **52**: 308–313.

83. Puig-Antich J, Chambers WJ, Tabrizi MA: The clinical assessment of current episodes in children and adolescents: Interviews with parents and children. In: Cantwell DP, Carlson GA, eds. *Affective Disorders in Childhood and Adolescence.* New York: Spectrum, 1983.

84. Gould M, Shaffer D: *Psychiatry, Vol II.* Philadelphia: J.B. Lippincott Co., 1991:11.7.

85. Kovacs M: Rating scales to assess depression in school-aged children. *Acta Paedopsychiatr* 1981; **46**:305–315.

86. Fristad M, Weller E, Weller RA: The mania rating scale: Can it be used in children? A preliminary report. *J Am Acad Child Adolesc Psychiatry* 1992; **31**:252–257.

87. Young RC, Biggs JT, Ziegler VE, *et al.*: A rating scale for mania: Reliability, validity and sensitivity. *Br J Psychiatry* 1978; **133**:429–435.

88. Geller B, Warner K, Williams M, *et al.*: Prepubertal and early adolescent bipolarity differentiate from ADHD: Assessment and validity using the WASH-U-KSADS, CBCL, and TRF. *J Affect Disord* 1998; **51**:93–100.

89. Puig-Antich J, Chambers W: *The Schedule for Affective Disorders and Schizophrenia for School-age Children (Kiddie SADS).* New York: New York State Psychiatric Institute, 1978.

90. Gracious BL, Youngstrom EA, Findling RL, Calabrese JR: Discriminative validity of a parent version of the Young Mania Rating Scale. *J Am Acad Adolesc Psychiatry* 2002; **41**:1350–1359.

91. Depue RA, Krauss S, Spoont MR, Arbisi P: General Behavioral Inventory identification of unipolar and bipolar affective conditions in a nonclinical university population. *J Abnorm Psychol* 1989; **98**:117–126.

92. Youngstrom EA, Findling RL, Danielson CK, Calabrese JR: Discriminative validity of parent report of hypomanic and depressive symptoms on the General Behavior Inventory. *Psychol Assess* 2001; **13**:267–276.

93. Achenbach TM: *Manual for the Child Behavior Checklist/4–18 and 1991 Profile.* Burlington: University of Vermont, 1991.

94. Achenbach TM: *Manual for the Youth Self-Report Form and 1991 Profile.* Burlington: University of Vermont, 1991.

95. Achenbach TM: *Manual for the Teacher's Report Form and 1991 Profile.* Burlington: University of Vermont, 1991.

96. Insoo Kim Berg: Pretend a miracle happened: A brief therapy task. In: Nelson T, Trepper T, eds. *101 Interventions in Family Therapy.* New York: Haworth Press, 1993.

97. Basco MR, Rush AJ: Compliance with pharmacotherapy in mood disorders. *Psych Ann* 1995; **25**:78–82.

98. Fristad MA, Gavazzi SM, Soldano KW: Multi-family psychoeducation groups for childhood mood disorders: A program description and preliminary efficacy data. *Contemp Fam Ther* 1998; **20**:385–402.

99. Miklowitz DJ: Coping with bipolar disorder during the transition to young adulthood. Presented at the Jean Paul Ohadi Conference on Children and Adolescents with Bipolar Disorders: November 30, 2001.

100. Greene RW: *The Explosive Child: A New Approach for Understanding and Parenting Easily Frustrated, 'Chronically Inflexible' Children,* 2nd ed. New York: Harper Collins, 2001.

101. Basco M: *Cognitive-Behavioral Therapy for Bipolar Disorder.* Guilford Press, 1996.

102. Geller B, Zimerman B, Williams M, *et al.*: DSM-IV mania symptoms in a prepubertal and early adolescent bipolar disorder phenotype compared to attention-deficit hyperactive and normal controls. *J Child Adolesc Psychopharmacol* 2002; **12**(1):11–25.

103. Quitkin, Frederic M, *et al.*: Duration of antidepressant drug treatment. *Arch Gen Psychiatry* 1984; **41**:242.

104. March J: Antidepressants for children and adolescents: Dangerous medicine? *DukeMed Magazine* 2004; **4**(2):53.

105. March J: Fluoxetine, cognitive-behavioral therapy, and their combination for adolescents with depression. *JAMA* 2004; **292**(7):807–820.

106. Bowers R: A primer in thyroid function and guidelines for thyroid augmentation in affective disorders. In: Klykylo W, Kay J, Rube D, eds. *Clinical Child Psychiatry.* Philadelphia, PA: WB Saunders Co, 1998: 202.

107. Geller B, Cooper TB, Sun K, Zimmerman B, Frazier J, Williams M, Heath J: Double-blind and conceivable controlled study of lithium for adolescent bipolar disorders the secondary substance dependency. *J Am Acad Child Adolesc Psychiatry* 1998; **37**:171–178.

108. Kafantaris V, Coletti DJ, Dicker R, Padula G, Pleak RR, Alvir JM. Lithium treatment of acute mania in adolescents: A placebo-controlled discontinuation study. *J Am Acad Child Adolesc Psychiatry* 2004 **43**(8):984–993.

109. Baastrup TC, Shou M: Lithium as a prophylactic agent: Its effects against recurrent depression and manic-

depressive psychosis. *Arch Gen Psychiatry* 1967; **16**:162–172.

110. Strober M, Morrell W, Lambert C, *et al.*: Relapse following discontinuation of lithium maintenance therapy in adolescents with bipolar I illness: A naturalistic study. *Am J Psychiatry* 1990; **147**:457–461.

111. Weller EB, Weller RA, Fristad MA: Lithium dosage guide for prepubertal children: A preliminary report. *J Am Acad Child Psychiatry* 1986; **25**:92–95.

112. Keck PE Jr, Bennett JA, Stanton S: Health-economic aspects of the treatment of manic-depressive illness with divalproex. *Rev Contemp Pharmacother* 1995; **6**:597–604.

113. Kowatch R, Suppes T, Carmody TJ, Bucci JP, Hume JH, Kromelis M, Emsilie GJ, Weinberg W, Rush AJ: Effect size of lithium, divalproex sodium, and carbamazepine in children and adolescents with bipolar disorder. *J Am Acad Child Adolesc Psychiatry* 2000; **39**(6):713–720.

114. Hirschfield RM, Allen MH, McEnvoy JP, Keck PE Jr, Russell JM: Safety and tolerability of oral loading divalproex sodium in acutely manic bipolar patients. *J Clin Psychiatry* 1999; **60**:815–818.

115. Bowden CL, Janicak PG, Orsulak P, *et al.*: Relation of serum valproate concentration to response in mania. *Am J Psychiatry* 1996; **153**:765–770.

116. Isojarvi JI: Polycystic ovaries and hyperandrogenism in women taking valproate for epilepsy. *New England Journal of Medicine* 1993; **329**(19):1383–1388.

117. Bowden CL, Lecrubier Y, Bauer M: Maintenance therapies for classic and other forms of bipolar disorder. *Journal of Affective Disorders* 2000; **59**(Suppl. 1):S57–S67.

118. Rasgon NL, Altshuler LL, Gudeman D: Medication status and polycystic ovary syndrome in women with bipolar disorder: A preliminary report. *J Clinl Psychiatry* 2000; **61**(3):173–178.

119. Kowatch R, Suppes T, Carmody TJ, Bucci JP, Hume JH, Kromelis M, Emsilie GJ, Weinberg W, Rush AJ: Effect size of lithium, divalproex sodium, and carbamazepine in children and adolescents with bipolar dis-

120. Frazier JA, Meyer MC, Biederman J, Wozniak J, Wilens TE, Spencer TJ, Kim GS, Shapiro S: Risperidone treatment for juvenile bipolar disorder: A retrospective chart review. *J Am Acad Child Adolesc Psychiatry* 1999; **38**(8):960–965.

121. Frazier JA, Biederman J, Tohen M, Feldman PD, Jacobs TG, Toma V, Rater MA, Tarazi RA, Kim GS, Garfield SB, Sohma M, Gonzalez-Heydrich J, Risser RC, Nowlin ZM: A prospective open-label treatment of olanzapine monotherapy in children and adolescents with bipolar disorder. *J Child Adolesc Psychopharmacol* 2001; **11**(3):239–250.

122. Delbello MP, Schwiers ML, Rosenberg HL, Strakowski SM: A double-blind, randomized, placebo-controlled study of quetiapine as adjunctive treatment for adolescent mania. *J Am Acad Child Adolesc Psychiatry* 2002; **41**(10):1216–1223.

123. Ghaemi SN: Antidepressants overused in bipolar treatment. *Psychiatric Times' Bipolar Disorders Letter* 1997; **May**:3–4.

124. American Diabetes Association: Clinical Practice Recommendations 2004. *Diabetes Care* 2004; **27**(Suppl.):S1–142.

125. Sachs GS, Lafer B, Stoll AL, *et al.*: A double-blind trial of bupropion versus desipramine for bipolar depression. *J Clin Psychiatry* 1994; **55**(9):391–393.

126. Kovacs M: Presentation and course of major depressive disorder during childhood and later years of the life span. *J Am Acad Child Adolesc Psychiatry* 1996; **35**:705–715.

127. Hemphill RE, Walter WG: The treatment of mental disorders by electrically induced convulsions. *J Ment Sci* 1941; **87**:256–275.

128. Bender L: One hundred cases of childhood schizophrenia treated with electric shock. *Trans Am Neurol Soc* 1947, **72**:165–169.

129. Rey JM, Walter G: Half a century of ECT use in young people. *Am J Psychiatry* 1997; **154**:595–602.

13

Anxiety Disorders in Childhood and Adolescence

Craig L. Donnelly, Debra V. McQuade

Introduction

Fear and anxiety are common experiences across childhood and adolescence. It is in the adaptive management and development of coping strategies for these affective states that the processes of mastery, autonomy, skill acquisition and cognitive maturation unfold. The clinician evaluating childhood anxiety disorders faces the task of differentiating the normal, transient and developmentally appropriate expressions of anxiety from pathological anxiety.

Anxiety disorders are characterized as 'internalizing' disorders, along with depression and dysthymia, and stand in distinction to the 'externalizing' disorders of childhood such as oppositional defiant disorder (ODD), conduct disorder (CD) and attention deficit hyperactivity disorder (ADHD). Anxiety disorders are among the most common psychiatric disorders in children and adolescents affecting from 7% to 15% of individuals under 18 years of age [1]. The latest version of the *Diagnostic and Statistical Manual of Mental Disorders-IV* (*Text Revision*) has refined the diagnostic nomenclature of childhood anxiety disorders to attain greater consistency with the adult anxiety disorders. In assessing the criteria for diagnostic threshold, the clinician is expected to exercise clinical judgment in terms of the severity, the degree of distress, and the relative dysfunction manifested by the individual child.

The developmental course of anxiety, its appropriateness and boundaries with psychiatric disorder are areas of intense research interest in child psychiatry, and yet surprisingly little empirical data exists in these areas. To effectively engage the assessment process a wide and thorough clinical perspective is necessary.

First, clinicians need to maintain a high level of suspicion for anxiety disorders when evaluating children.

Anxiety disorders are not rare and often mimic or are comorbid with other childhood disorders. Symptoms such as school refusal, tantrums, or irritability may be less reflective of oppositional behavior than an underlying social phobia or generalized anxiety disorder (GAD). Second, children need to be evaluated within a biopsychosocial framework. Genetic vulnerability, biological etiologies, life experience, social and family contexts, and developmental phase are interwoven to a greater or lesser extent in the expression of pathological anxiety and their roles need to be clarified. The clinician must understand the inner experiential context and the external behavioral contingencies in which the anxious child is operating. Third, given the uniqueness of each child and the complex interplay among the internal and external variables that drive anxiety, a multimodal approach to diagnosis and treatment is warranted.

This chapter will provide the basics for evaluating and treating each of the recognized childhood anxiety disorders. In using this chapter the clinician should bear in mind that the assessment and treatment of childhood anxiety is often quite complex and time consuming. The clinician undertaking this task should not hesitate to consult an expert in childhood anxiety if time constraints, lack of experience or the intricacies of a particular child's presentation prove problematic.

Separation Anxiety

Definition

Separation anxiety disorder (SAD) is the sole childhood anxiety disorder classified in DSM-IV-TR as one of the 'disorders usually diagnosed in infancy, child-

Clinical Child Psychiatry, Second Edition. Edited by W.M. Klykylo and J.L. Kay
© 2005 John Wiley & Sons Ltd.

hood or adolescence.' Its cardinal feature is excessive anxiety engendered by separation from major attachment figures or the home environment. Four weeks' duration and clinically significant or subjectively distressful impairment in social, academic or occupational functioning are necessary to make this diagnosis.

Sometime past their first birthday, normal children begin to exhibit signs of distress when confronted with possible separation from their caretakers. Called separation protest, this behavior peaks at about 15 months of age, after which it continues on a course of resolution. This is qualitatively different from the experience of children with SAD, who, at a later age, exhibit excessive distress and abnormal reactivity at the thought of, or at the time of, separation from a parent. Children with SAD may be burdened with unrelenting worries about losing or possible harm befalling a parent or loved one. Getting lost or kidnapped are frequent fears. They may be reluctant to attend school, go to bed at night or be alone in the house without their major attachment figure present. These children often suffer nightmares with themes of separation and will complain of multiple somatic symptoms, such as headaches, stomach aches or nausea. They are often fretful, whiny and pester their parents with reassurance seeking. Children with separation anxiety are typically unable to do sleepovers at friend's houses or endure overnight summer camps. Commonly, children and their parents seek treatment in the context of school refusal or excessive somatic complaints.

Incidence and Prevalence

The estimated prevalence of SAD is 4%–5% [2], making it one of the most common childhood psychiatric disorders. About half of all anxious children seeking psychiatric attention have separation anxiety [3]. Most studies report a higher rate of SAD for girls than boys [4], however, the symptom presentation does not differ between them [4]. It can be diagnosed up until age 18 years, but it is primarily a disorder of prepubertal children with an average age of onset of 7.5 years [5], making SAD the earliest of all anxiety disorders to be diagnosed in children. Two age related trends are worth noting: younger children report more symptoms and experience more distress than older children; and, as children age, prevalence rates go down [6]. Interestingly, while most children with anxiety disorders come from middle to upper-middle classes, children with SAD more frequently come from lower socioeconomic homes [2], which may relate to an interaction between an otherwise 'hidden' biological propensity that is more likely to be expressed owing to

the cumulative stress burden that is likely to be higher among children in these settings.

Etiology and Natural History

Attempts have been made to attribute the onset of separation anxiety to inadequately resolved separation/individuation conflict [7], vulnerability determined by temperament [8] or behavioral contingencies. Genetic and familial/environmental factors have also been advanced as causes. Decisive empirical or epidemiological proof supporting any of these theories is lacking. Multiple and interactive etiologies appear most likely.

The fact that SAD is a risk factor for panic disorder (PD) has led some investigators to posit a developmental link between them [9,10]. Evidence in support of a specific SAD–PD link is mixed, given that SAD is a risk factor for other anxiety disorders. A more recent formulation is that SAD may persist into adulthood as part of the same 'panic diathesis'' or panic spectrum [11,12]. These ideas continue to be investigated.

Separation anxiety is typically a disorder of middle childhood (ages 7–9 years), although it has also been described in adolescents. If the disorder develops acutely, a precipitating stressor can often be identified. Common precipitating factors include a move, change of school, loss of a loved one, illness in the family or prolonged absence from school. Sometimes the symptoms develop more insidiously, worsening over 3–6 months before a clinical referral is necessitated. Separation anxiety waxes and wanes, with exacerbations in times of stress. While some children recover fully after a single episode, others may experience a more protracted and chronic course. Later age of onset, comorbidities, familial pathology and missing more than one year of school seem to be associated with a greater risk of chronicity [13].

Comorbidities with separation anxiety are common. As many as 60% of the children diagnosed with separation anxiety have at least one comorbid anxiety disorder, and 30% have two [14], the most likely being GAD and specific phobias. Separation anxiety is also closely associated with depression; one third of the children diagnosed with SAD have comorbid depression [5]. Conversely, SAD is the most commonly diagnosed anxiety disorder for prepubertal children with depression. [15]. Typically, separation anxiety precedes depression, raising the question of whether the mood disorder is a consequence of enduring functional impairment. Finally, when children are diagnosed with separation anxiety, they are at risk for developing not only PD, but also social phobia (SP) and depression as adults [14,16].

Diagnosis

Children suffering from SAD often come to the clinician's attention when problems with school attendance develop. Presentation may range from great reluctance to refusal and temper tantrums if parents insist on taking the child to school. Separation from loved ones is often an issue around sleep time and the separation-anxious child often winds up in the parents' bed. Increasing anxiety interferes with spending the night at a friend's house or going to camp. Once separation takes place, these children may worry incessantly about the misfortunes that might befall their loved ones. Nightmares with prominent themes of separation are sometimes reported. Fears of being lost and never reunited with their families often beset these children. Typically the 'storm' is resolved once the child is returned to home. Somatic complaints such as morning stomach aches, headaches, nausea and vomiting, are more often seen in younger children, while older ones may also complain of palpitations and feeling faint.

A detailed history is the most helpful diagnostic resource. As is true for most of the internalizing disorders (i.e., anxiety, depression), accounts from the child are usually more telling than parents' and teachers' reports. Descriptions of the events preceding the separation, response to parents' departure, ensuing behavior (usually in school) and the consequences of separation are helpful in understanding the pattern of distress and precipitants. Gathering a comprehensive family history of psychiatric disorders is important, given the notable family patterns involving SAD. Clinicians should be sensitive to hearing the family's expressed and unexpressed feelings about the child as well as separation from the child, as these may be precipitating and maintaining factors. For example, as is typical with many childhood anxiety disorders, parents initial and well intended attempts to reassure the child may be inadvertently supporting the child's anxiety and, or escape/avoidance responses. Cooperation with a pediatrician is valuable, especially when somatic complaints are prominent.

Anxiety rating scales such as the Screen for Child Anxiety Related Emotional Disorders (SCARED) [17] or the Multidimensional Anxiety Scale for Children (MASC) [18] may be used diagnostically and as measures of treatment outcome. General psychiatric symptom rating scales, such as the Connors Parent and Teacher Questionnaires [19] may assist in the diagnosis of comorbid disorders, which are common for these children. Routinely available laboratory studies do not increase the accuracy of the diagnosis.

Differential Diagnosis

The clinician must differentiate separation anxiety from developmentally appropriate fears accompanying separation from loved ones. These developmentally normal separation fears occur earlier in childhood, have milder presentations, and tend to be transient and self-limiting. Functional impairment is not a typical feature of fears accompanying normal development (See Table 13.1 for a list of normal developmental fears).

Delineation of SAD from other disorders sharing 'school refusal' as a symptom is sometimes a challenging task. After CD and ODD (i.e., truancy) have been ruled out, one should carefully evaluate evidence for other anxiety disorders. School refusal may be based in a specific phobia (e.g., test taking and, or fear of humiliation), in situationally bound panic disorder or in social phobia, as well as SAD.

Generalized anxiety disorder (GAD) has a more varied presentation and the fears involved tend to stem from matters other than separation. Although children with separation anxiety can experience panic attacks,

Table 13.1 Normal developmental fears.

Birth–6 months	Loud noises, loss of physical support, rapid position changes, rapidly approaching unfamiliar objects
7–12 months	Strangers, looming objects, sudden confrontation by unexpected objects or unfamiliar people
1–5 years	Strangers, storms, animals, the dark, separation from parents, objects, machines, loud noises, the toilet, monsters, ghosts, insects, bodily harm
6–12 years	Supernatural beings, bodily injury, disease (AIDS, cancer), burglars, staying alone, failure, criticism, punishment
12–18 years	Tests and exams in school, school performance, bodily injury, appearance, peer scrutiny, athletic performance, social embarrassment

in panic disorder, attacks will occur in other unrelated situations. Relative comfort in social settings will differentiate separation anxiety from social phobia. Specific phobias are characterized by well defined and usually singular phobic objects; distress can occur even in the presence of an attachment figure. Pervasiveness of a mood disorder, especially if it precedes onset of separation anxiety, demands a separate diagnosis. Teasing apart major depression from separation anxiety is not always easy as they often occur together, but both diagnoses should be given, when appropriate, as treatment interventions differ for the two disorders.

Psychotic disorders, post-traumatic stress disorder (PTSD), pervasive developmental disorders and learning disorders should also be addressed.

Familial dysfunction, substance abuse, medical problems (especially ones causing abdominal distress) and iatrogenically caused syndromes (e.g., neuroleptic induced anxieties) need to be ruled out.

Several additional points bear emphasizing. First, children with SAD commonly have parents with an anxiety or depressive disorder. Careful assessment and, if necessary, treatment of the parent may be called for. This may entail simple psychoeducation of the parents regarding their inadvertent support of the child's anxiety versus frank treatment for an anxiety disorder in the parent. Second, a complete evaluation is important as over half of children with SAD have a second comorbid anxiety diagnosis which can unnecessarily complicate treatment if it is missed.

Treatment

If the child presents with school refusal, this needs addressing. Treatment of school refusal is discussed in a subsequent section. For separation difficulties which do not involve school, use of psychoeducational, behavioral and cognitive techniques is recommended.

Psychoeducational interventions targeting the family members should focus on explaining the diagnoses given to the child, how these relate to the child's current maladaptive behaviors, and how behavioral, cognitive and emotional changes made by members of the family may help the child. Educating parents about age-appropriate developmental tasks, informing them how they might encourage and support their child's attainment of these and instructions on how to deal with negative family dynamics should also be undertaken, where required. The essential and core feature of this approach is to assist parents in helping their child confront the separation experience and avoid the typical escape/avoidance response that reinforces the anxiety. Gradual mastery of minor separations, with parents modeling coping and nondistress and reinforcing the child's successes, supports children in facing and overcoming separation fears. Note that for mild cases of separation anxiety, this may be sufficient treatment.

Behavioral techniques have been demonstrated to be successful in SAD related behaviors. Shaping the desired behavior through contingency management by positively reinforcing nonfearful behavior and withdrawing rewards for anxious behaviors may yield results. Modeling and exposure based treatments have also been reported as effective. In these, children are rewarded for practicing 'being brave' and are taught new skills for managing old anxious behaviors. Success in this endeavor depends upon identification of manageable target behaviors, practicing new behaviors and appropriate reinforcement strategies.

Cognitive interventions focusing on the maladaptiveness of 'catastrophic' thoughts and their replacement with more adaptive cognitions, in combination with self-instruction and teaching realistic appraisal of fear producing circumstances, can be fruitful. Generally referred to as CBT (cognitive behavioral therapy), this type of treatment is now widely used with children, and some manualized protocols are becoming available [20].

Some somatic complaints can be countered by instruction in deep muscle relaxation or tension-relaxation exercises that can serve as anxiety counter-responses. Group and family therapies can be valuable adjunct treatments and may be more efficient venues for skill teaching, modeling and generalization.

Psychopharmacologic approaches may be useful in selected cases, especially when combined with psychosocial interventions. The reader is referred to recent summaries of the psychopharmacological literature for comprehensive assessment of current options [21–23]. Psychotropic agents should be reserved for more refractory and complicated cases, or when anxiety is so severe that it limits therapy based exposure practice [24]. Although there is no currently approved medication for the treatment of SAD, standard of care consensus suggests that the selective serotonin uptake inhibitors (SSRIs) are first-line pharmacotherapy. Adjunctive medications may include clonazepam, particularly while awaiting benefit of the SSRI, although this strategy might best be reserved for older children. Tricyclic antidepressants (TCA; e.g., clomipramine, imipramine) have been used successfully in the past, although use of these agents is currently limited due to their side effect profile and potential for cardiac toxicity. It should be borne in mind that CBT is likely to be the most powerful and enduring treatment. Studies of combined CBT and medication therapies in children are currently underway [25].

School Refusal

Definition

School refusal is not an anxiety disorder diagnosis, per se, but it bears mentioning as it often presents in relation to other psychiatric diagnoses. School refusal is defined as difficulty attending school, associated with emotional distress, especially anxiety and depression [26]. It is distinguished from truancy and conduct disorder because the child is home from school with the parent's knowledge, and the child does not have any associated antisocial behaviors, such as lying, stealing or destructiveness. As noted, school refusal is not a separate diagnostic entity, but rather a symptom of other diagnoses. It is most commonly thought to be a behavioral manifestation of SAD, however, accumulating evidence supports significant heterogeneity in its presentation. Not all children with separation anxiety become school refusers and not all children who refuse to go to school meet criteria for separation anxiety [13].

Incidence and Prevalence

Between 1% and 2% of all school aged children and 5% of all clinic referred children become school refusers. Boys and girls are equally affected. There is an unequal distribution of cases of school refusers across the age span, with certain ages and school grades reflecting a greater vulnerability to the behavior. Peak expression of school refusal tends to come at ages 5–6, 10–11 and 13–15 years [27]. These ages represent the times that children typically face transition entry into elementary, middle and high school, respectively.

Etiology and Natural History

There is a wide variation in the presentation of school refusal, suggesting multiple etiologies. Some children go to school, but spend much of their day in distress in the nurse's office, making multiple phone contacts with parents. Others refuse to leave home. Some make partial progress towards school, but become anxious while en route. Some miss weeks and months of school, others manage to attend school on an intermittent basis. When school refusers are confronted with going to school, they manifest true physiological distress with increased muscle tension and breathing irregularities [28]. Many complain of feeling ill, most frequently complaining of headaches or stomach distress. When fear is involved, it is directed differentially, depending on the age of the child. Younger children fear separation from their parent(s), older children fear their teachers or other children. Social-evaluative fears dominate the presentation of adolescents.

School refusers meet criteria for other psychiatric disorders more often than not. Frequently associated diagnoses are SAD, social phobia, GAD (overanxious disorder), specific phobia for school; less frequently PD and PTSD are part of their presentation [28]. Some family patterns are identifiable; school refusers with SAD have an increased likelihood of having a parent with PD, with or without agoraphobia. School refusers diagnosed with specific phobias have an increased likelihood of having a parent who also has specific phobias or social phobia. Several types of problematic family function have been identified, such as the enmeshed family, the conflictive family, the isolated family and the detached family [29]. However, many school refusing children have healthy families [29]. Single parent families are overrepresented in this group of children [30].

Diagnosis

Because of the variability in the clinical presentations of school refusal, evaluations prior to treatment should engage multiple informants. The child and the family should undergo clinical interviews. Members of the school, daycare and the family doctor are all potentially important sources of collateral information. Patterns of family dynamics need to be explored for potential weaknesses, e.g., inadequate parental oversight, conflicting parental tactics. Psychoeducational reports and discussion with teachers should be requested from the school, if these are available. Developmental patterns need to be reviewed, especially language, academic and social skills development. A thorough medical exam should be undertaken to rule out any organic cause for the child's somatic complaints, if these are part of the presentation. Once the primary diagnosis is made, search should continue for associated comorbid disorders, as comorbidities are common [31].

Differential Diagnosis

Because school refusal is not a diagnostic entity, the goal of a clinical evaluation will be to identify the primary disorder, of which the school refusal is a

Table 13.2 Differential diagnosis of school refusal.

Diagnosis	Features
Separation anxiety disorder	Fears separation from parent or attachment figure Spends out-of-school time in presence of parent
Generalized anxiety disorder	Anxiety in multiple domains, not limited to school setting, fretful, overly conscientious/fearful
Specific phobia	Exhibits anxiety toward teacher, other student, activity, test taking or other specific object or circumstance
Social phobia	Social setting per se is the primary fear May fear scrutiny in test taking, being observed in bathroom etc.
Panic disorder	May have situationally bound or predisposed panic attacks Some panic attacks have occurred out of school or unexpectedly, anticipatory anxiety, agoraphobia
Post-traumatic stress disorder	Multiple symptoms in addition to school refusal: irritability, depression, reexperiencing, all related to a specified trauma
Obsessive–compulsive disorder	Presence of obsessive thoughts/compulsive rituals that may be a source of embarrassment or result in phobic avoidance
Conduct/Oppositional defiant disorder (truancy)	Multiple oppositional/disruptive behavior symptoms in addition to school refusal, 'hangs out' with friends when not in school, often complicated by substance abuse or antisocial behavior

symptom (see Table 13.2). Consideration needs to be given to SAD, GAD, specific phobias, including school and social phobia, and depression. Other anxiety disorders, such as PTSD and PD need to be considered. Competing explanations for school attendance failure are uncomplicated truancy versus truancy as part of CD. Both are distinguished from school refusal because truant and/or conduct disordered children do not suffer significant emotional distress as part of their attempts to attend school. Additionally, unlike parents of school refusers, parents of truant children are typically not aware of their children's failure to be in school. The potential for learning disabilities or developmental disabilities needs to be ruled out and a more straightforward fear of failure needs to be identified, when present.

Treatment

In uncomplicated cases where school refusal has not lasted more than two weeks, treatment is fairly straightforward. After informing the parents about the nature of the disorder and eliciting their cooperation as well as that of school authorities, the child is encouraged to return to school as soon as possible. Parents are instructed to show empathy and understanding for the child's distress but to insist in a firm and consistent manner on regular school attendance. The child is

supported and provided skills to master the fears and worries incumbent in the separation. This may involve the parent being present in the classroom for a brief period and then fading out their presence. Reward and praise should accompany desired behavior.

If school refusal has become entrenched, especially in older adolescents, therapy is much more difficult. Under these circumstances, CBT is considered first-line treatment for school refusal. King and Bernstein [26] recommend the use of the School Refusal Assessment Scale (SRAS) [32,33] as an aid to identification of the negative and positive reinforcers which maintain the school refusal behavior. Associated with the SRAS are manuals that prescribe treatments for each of the functional conditions identified [34,35] and involves school as well as family. Whether this or other protocols are used, success will likely be dependent upon successful identification of the positive reinforcers at home and the negative reinforcers at school, and some combination of relaxation therapy, systematic desensitization, modeling, shaping and contingency management [35,36] and involves school as well as family. A gradual return to school is the typical goal. Identifying the common negative perceptions, such as 'the kids think I'm stupid,' and replacing them with more positive and realistic perceptions are frequently part of the plan. Teaching self-monitoring skills and counter anxiety responses is common. Extended treatment to family and the teacher helps to make the behavioral plan consistent throughout the course of the child's day. The best treatments span the home and school domains.

Several reports of successful CBT treatments of school refusal are in the literature. [26]. Interestingly, there is also one report [37] of a successful 'placebo' treatment group which underwent 'educational therapy' to be compared with an experimental CBT-based therapy. Educational therapy consisted of a combination of educational presentations, supportive psychotherapy, and a daily diary for the recording of thoughts and fears. No treatment for modifying thoughts or encouragement for confronting fears was given. On all measures of success, the 'educational therapy' matched the CBT for success. While it is not clear what elements of the educational therapy made it successful, and perhaps a common element of exposure was at work in both groups, the possibility is open for alternative types of therapy as potential remedial tools.

The use of medications has been addressed in several studies. While most reports involve the use of TCAs (with or without CBT), the general feeling of clinicians is that these medications should not be considered first line, given new reports of the effectiveness of the safer SSRIs, such as fluoxetine in treating anxiety disorders in children [38]. Additionally, it is general clinical opinion that medication should not be added to treatment until a trial of CBT based therapy has been undertake, or in particularly entrenched cases [27].

Finally, prognosis of school refusal behaviors is better for younger children and for children with a higher baseline of school attendance prior to the initiation of treatment. Older children, and those with longer periods of failed school attendance, fare worse [28].

Generalized Anxiety Disorder

Definition

In 1994 with the publication of DSM-IV [29], the American Psychiatric Association replaced the diagnostic category 'overanxious disorder' (OAD) with 'generalized anxiety disorder' (GAD) for use with the pediatric population. Diagnostic modification of the criteria for adult GAD included the reduction in the number of physical/somatic complaints required, from three to one (of six alternatives), as well as a replacement of the former descriptor 'unrealistic worries,' with 'excessive anxiety and worry that is difficult to control.' These changes, first articulated in DSM-IV, have been maintained in the current diagnostic nosology system, DSM-IV-TR. To be diagnosed with GAD, the child or adolescent must additionally experience excessive worry that impairs daily function and continues for at least six months.

Several challenges complicate the diagnosis of GAD in this population. Due to the significant overlap of anxiety with depressive symptoms in children – such as concentrating, irritability and sleep disturbance – clinicians face the task of differentiating GAD from depressive disorders. This is complicated by the high comorbidity of GAD with depressive disorders that is found in children and adolescents [32,39] as well as adults [40]. In order to better discriminate between the disorders, work is continuing to identify those symptoms of GAD which are most common in the pediatric populations. In her report of 58 children, Masi et al. (2004) [39] reported that the most common symptoms of GAD are tension, apprehension, need for reassurance, irritability, negative self-image and physical complaints. Less common symptoms were psychomotor agitation, fear of sleeping alone and fear of being alone.

Additionally, some amount of anxiety is typical of normal development [41]. Fears, worries and scary dreams are experienced by the majority of children, at one time or another [42]. This leaves the distinction between pathological and developmentally appropriate anxiety to be made by the clinician (see Table 13.1). Pathological worries of children with GAD tend to encompass more domains of concerns (such as health of family members, school performance, social relationships), be associated with greater distress, cause stronger daily interference, are more difficult to control [41,42] and, to a lesser extent, occur more frequently [43] than those of healthy children.

Incidence and Prevalence

Current understanding of the epidemiology of GAD in children and adolescents continues to rely heavily on data collected using the older diagnostic entity OAD [39]. Using the older criteria, youth prevalence rates for GAD are estimated to be from 2.7% to 5.7% [44,45]; prevalence rates increase with age [46]. The mean age of onset of GAD/OAD is reported to be 8.8 years [47]. Younger females and males are equally likely to receive the diagnosis, although this changes in adolescence when it becomes more common in girls [48]. Muris and colleagues reports 3.8% of boys and 9.0% of girls meet diagnostic criteria in their sample of 8–13-year-olds [41]. Comorbidities with GAD are high; Masi et al. [49] reported 87% of their 7–13-year-old group to have comorbid diagnoses, most frequently a depressive disorder (62%). SAD was a common comorbidity for younger children (42%).

Etiology and Natural History

Freud postulated that anxiety is a byproduct of suppression of unacceptable libidinous or aggressive drives. In a later revision of this theory, he postulated 'signal anxiety' as a warning to the approach of highly conflictual and potentially devastating repressed material [50].

Behavioral theories conceptualize anxiety as an arousal response inadvertently rewarded and perpetuated. Recent cognitive theories tend to view maladaptive cognitions associated with arousal as precipitants, which are subsequently reinforced through escape or avoidance. Familial factors, such as high levels of parental expectation and an emphasis on achievement, or conversely, excessive permissiveness, may facilitate the development of anxiety.

Data indicate that behavioral inhibition (BI), a temperamental profile described as a stable tendency to be avoidant, quiet and behaviorally restrained in unfamiliar situations, seen in about 20% of Caucasian children, may constitute a substantial risk for the development of GAD (OAD) [51]. Increasing evidence supports BI as a distinct physiological profile [52], with a substantial heritability index, as documented in twin studies [53].

Efforts to track the neurodevelopmental trajectory of pediatric GAD have only recently begun. Neurobiological theories suggest disturbance in the hypothalamic–pituitary–adrenal axis, and regulation of thyroid and growth hormone secretion as possible causes of anxiety. GABA, noraderenalin, serotonin and adenosine dysfunction have all been implicated as contributing to anxiety [54].

Recently, DeBellis and colleagues identified structural differences in both the amygdala and the superior temporal gyrus (STG) associated with pediatric GAD. In two separate reports, they initially described significantly larger right and total amygdala volumes [55], and later identified STG increases in both total and white matter volume which were more pronounced on the right side [56]. Further, their index of this asymmetry correlated with child reports on the SCARED (Screen for Child Anxiety Related Emotional Disorders Scale). Although a theoretical accounting of these findings would be premature, the data are intriguing in that they link regions of the brain known to be involved with fear responses (amygdale) and social intelligence (STG) to GAD in a clinically meaningful way. Additionally, the right/left structural asymmetry fits nicely with demonstrations of right-sided prefrontal activation in behaviorally inhibited children as well as increased responses to angry faces and novel situations that have recently been reported [51].

Diagnosis

The differential diagnosis of GAD can be complicated, as it frequently involves symptom overlap with other anxiety disorders. Children and adolescents with GAD tend to worry excessively about their performance and competence, even in the absence of external scrutiny. Ruminating about past mistakes and worrying about future adversities (i.e., 'what if' concerns) may cause a decline in academic function and precipitate a referral. Parents will often report children's apprehension about 'adult issues:' illness, old age, death, financial matters, wars and natural disasters. Children with GAD are often seen as perfectionistic and self-cautious, frequently seeking reassurance. Because they 'cannot stop worrying' these youths often appear de-concentrated, restless, fragile, tense and irritable. Where there is a discrepancy between their high expectations and the level of achievement, depression often ensues, especially in teenagers. Comorbid phobias, panic attacks or PD are not uncommon [49,57]. Younger children sometimes have concomitant symptoms of SAD and ADHD [58]. Somatic complaints such as stomach aches and headaches are often reported by youngsters suffering from GAD [59] and can precipitate frequent visits to pediatricians.

An extensive and detailed history, including family history of psychiatric disorders, is important in establishing a correct diagnosis and differentiating GAD from other anxiety disorders. Multiple sources of information are preferable. Formal or informal reports from teachers, day care providers and past or present mental health providers can be invaluable. Assessment of family dynamics can reveal stressors to the child which are not easy for the patient or family members to share without encouragement. As with all childhood anxiety disorders, gathering history from both child and parents is essential. Cooperation with the family doctor or pediatrician and school authorities assures better evaluation and more effective treatment.

Several anxiety scales are available for use. These include: the Revised Children's Manifest Anxiety Scale (RCMAS) [60], the Multidimensional Anxiety Scale for Children (MASC) [18] the Child Behavior Checklist (CBCL) [61] and the Pediatric Anxiety Rating Scale (PARS) [62]. These scales have potential value both in identifying anxiety disorders as well as monitoring treatment progress. Detailed descriptions of useful psychometric instruments are available [63,64].

Differential Diagnosis

GAD can be differentiated from separation anxiety by its pervasive nature and presence across different contexts (e.g., school, home and peer relations). Panic disorder is more 'phasic' in comparison to the more 'tonic' GAD. The content of anxiety in panic disorder is usually focused on future panic attacks. In specific phobia, fears center on the phobic object. Obsessive thoughts can be distinguished from GAD by their intrusive nature and concomitant compulsive rituals used to alleviate anxiety. In PTSD, anxiety is usually related to a past traumatic event or reexperiencing of the event. Prevalence of depressed mood, anhedonia and vegetative signs set depressive episodes apart from GAD, in spite of significant symptom overlap.

Finally, medical conditions often present with symptoms that may mimic GAD. Caution is warranted not to overlook hyperthyroidism, diabetes mellitus, and the more rare syndromes such as pheochromocytoma or systemic lupus erythematosis. Excessive stimulant use, alcohol withdrawal or drug dependence can also mimic GAD. The recreational use of steroids, primarily by adolescent boys, bears monitoring as this practice has been associated with anxiety [65].

Treatment

Traditionally, psychodynamic therapy focused on the expanding awareness of the defensive and maladaptive nature of the anxiety. Empirical validation is lacking for this approach in the treatment of children. Neither does empirical support exist for the use of play therapy or supportive psychotherapy for pediatric GAD.

In contrast, a growing number of studies demonstrate the efficacy of CBT. Common treatment components include desensitization, prolonged exposure, modeling, contingency management, and self-management/cognitive strategies [66]. Relaxation, visual imagery, self-affirmative statements, self-instruction, identifying faulty cognitions and replacing them with adaptive thoughts have been combined in various ways in different cognitive behavioral approaches.

There is some evidence that CBT which has a family therapy component improves treatment outcome [67], although this benefit may disappear with time [68]. If a child has at least one parent with anxiety, parental anxiety management combined with child-focused CBT is superior to the CBT component alone [69].

Several reports have been made of the successful use of The Coping Cat, a manualized treatment protocol developed by Kendall [70]. In two separate studies, 50% [71] and 64% [72] of participating children no longer met criteria for OAD after undergoing this manualized treatment approach. Long-term maintenance of improvement was documented in each of these randomized trials. More recently, comparisons have been made of the efficacy of The Coping Cat protocol, when presented in either individual versus group format. Significant improvement was reported with both formats, with nonsignificant differences between them [73].

Increasingly, practitioners are turning to psychopharmacological therapy for treatment of pediatric GAD. Many now consider the use of SSRIs as first-line agents for pediatric GAD. The RUPP (Research Unit on Pediatric Psychopharmacology) Anxiety Subgroup has presented compelling evidence that these medications [specifically, fluvoxamine (Luvox)] are both effective for anxiety disorders (including GAD) and tolerated well [74,75]. Other controlled studies support the efficacy and tolerability of sertraline [76], fluoxetine [77], and citalopram [78] for pediatric GAD.

Limited information exists concerning the efficacy of benzodiazepine use in pediatric GAD. An early study of alprazolam failed to demonstrate significant improvement over placebo [79]. Concerns for previously demonstrated behavioral disinhibition [80], as well as theoretical concerns for dependence and abuse are limiting clinical use of benzodiazepines in this context. Short-term use for highly anxious children, especially while awaiting onset of the action of an SSRI remains a potential treatment choice.

Specific Phobia

Definition

A specific phobia is a marked and persistent fear of a specific object or situation whose exposure invariably provokes intense anxiety, much like a situationally bound or predisposed panic attack. Children with specific phobias will avoid the object or situation; if they cannot, they react with distress, often crying, exhibiting tantrums, freezing or clinging. Although their fearful responses are excessive or unreasonable for the event, children may not recognize them as such. The DSM-IV-TR currently recognizes five types of phobias: animal, natural environment, blood-injection-injury, situational and other types. To meet DSM-IV-TR criteria for specific phobia, the child must be in significant distress or suffer clinical impairment for at least six months.

Incidence and Prevalence

Specific phobia is a relatively common anxiety disorder for children. Prevalence is estimated to be at 3%–4% and is somewhat higher for girls than for boys [81]. It peaks in prevalence between 10 and 13 years of age [82,83]. Some fears are common to normal development: preschoolers are often afraid of strangers, the dark, animals and imaginary creatures; elementary children may fear animals, the dark, threats to safety and thunder/lightening; adolescents may be agoraphobic or have fears with sexual or failure themes [84]. Normally, these fears decrease with age [85,86]. Normal fears are distinguished from true phobias by their intensity and degree of impairment. Specific phobias may parallel age related fears for content, or they may be unique.

Etiology and Natural History

Psychoanalytical theory viewed phobias as attempts to master anxiety and fear stemming from repressed conflictual libidinal and aggressive urges. Thus, fear disconnected from repressed material is displaced onto a phobic object, allowing the child a degree of control through the act of phobic avoidance.

Current theories emphasize the role of learned experiences in the generation and maintenance of phobias. Strong empirical evidence supports each of the three mechanisms touted in Rachman's (1977) three-pathway theory [87]: aversive classical conditioning, modeling, and negative information transmission [88]. Stated differently, children may learn phobias by having one (or more) frightening experiences with an object/situation (e.g., developing a phobia of dogs after having been bitten by one), by witnessing the behavior of somebody who has an established phobia (e.g., seeing an older sibling respond fearfully to dogs) or by direct instruction (e.g., hearing from a parent, 'Don't go near dogs, they are dangerous and can hurt you.') Once developed, phobic fears are maintained by the positive consequences of avoidance.

There are some fears, shared by many children, which have been described as occurring spontaneously, without identifiable experiences of prior learning (e.g., fear of water, thunder). This has led to the intriguing notion of evolutionary-dependent or 'instrinsic' fears that are hard-wired, and which become phobias either because the child's experiences fail to habituate them properly, or due to some flaw in the child's internal 'danger detection' system [82]. While acceptance of this nonassociative theory of fear is mixed, evidence does suggest that genetic factors play a substantial role in propagating specific phobias [89].

Phobic symptoms tend to vacillate over time, and in the majority of children they will gradually subside without treatment. However, clinicians are cautioned against hasty dismissal of a child's fears. A portion of children will not get over their phobias, which may eventually hamper their normal development and functioning. Specific phobias have been reported to be highly cormorbid with SP and SAD [90].

Diagnosis

Children usually present with excessive fear related to some well circumscribed situation or object. Often parents will complain that the child is preoccupied with the object, causing the fear or the attempts to avoid it to interfere with family life. The child's play, relationship with peers and family members as well as school performance can be negatively influenced by avoidance of a feared situation or even by incapacitating anticipatory anxiety.

Exposure to the phobic object elicits a response that has cognitive, emotional, behavioral, motoric and physiologic components. Each of these components presents the clinician with the opportunity for assessment by observation and clinical history, increasing diagnostic accuracy.

The path to correct diagnosis lies in a detailed history containing an accurate description of the sequence of events, fear producing situation, consequences and the intensity of fear. The behavioral component is usually measured indirectly by distance from the phobic object at which one experiences distress. Heart rate is a quantifiable correlate of physiologic response. A comprehensive description of psychometric instruments may be found in King et al. [91].

Differential Diagnosis

The initial task is to differentiate developmentally appropriate fears from a specific phobia. Specific phobia is not diagnosed if the child's anxiety is better accounted for by another disorder. In social phobia, fears are confined to social situations, especially if one's performance is subject to scrutiny. Fears in PD are related to anticipation of reexperience of an attack. Anxiety peaks during separation from loved ones in SAD. In GAD, fears and worries tend not to be confined to a specific object or situation. Post-traumatic stress disorder is characterized by fear and avoidance of memories related to past traumatic experiences. In anorexia nervosa, obsessions with food and its avoidance can be suggestive of a phobia although the eating disorder symptoms are pervasive and dominate the clinical picture. Bizarre fears are often a part of a psychotic disorder, but here, the presence of a thought disorder in an obvious differentiating feature.

Treatment

Both exclusively behavioral as well as CBT are widely used to treat children with specific phobias. In their comprehensive review, Ollendick and King [92] identify participant modeling and contingency management techniques as the most efficacious. Thus, a combination of exposure, reinforced practice with shaping, positive reinforcement and extinction techniques best predisposes to symptom control. They identify other therapeutic techniques, including variants of systematic desensitization, live or filmed modeling, and CBT, as good choices for treatment. Self-control strategies (which use the cognitive tools of self-evaluation and self-reward) used in combination with contingency management and *in vivo* exposure (a variant of systematic desensitization) has been touted as a successful treatment combination [93].

Flooding, or implosive therapy, is not a recommended modality for the treatment of children. Psychodynamic therapy, described in numerous case studies, has had scarce empirical support.

Family therapy is a useful adjunct. It can be fruitful in dealing with disturbed family relationships, especially where they cause the child's phobia of serve to support it. Psychoeducation of parents about the basics of anxiety reinforcement and extinction are necessary features of treatment. Often, providing them with a 'rule of thumb' that avoidance increases anxiety and exposure decreases it, can be helpful.

Anecdotal reports of benzodiazepine or antidepressant use for treatment of phobias should not encourage the clinician to pursue medication intervention. Psychosocial treatments are efficacious and are the standard of care.

Social Phobia (Social Anxiety Disorder)

Definition

Sociability is the preference for companionship and affiliation with others, and shyness is a form of social withdrawal accompanied by distress and inhibited behaviors. Both are enduring personality features, detectable at an early age and stable across development [94]. Children who indicate a desire for affiliation with other children but who experience significant distress in social setting may meet criteria for social phobia.

Social phobia and social anxiety disorder are interchangeable terms, with a trend towards preferred use of the latter in the adult literature. Social phobia is characterized by a marked and persistent fear of one or more social or performance situations in which the individual is exposed to unfamiliar people or possible scrutiny. In children, there must be the capacity for age appropriate social relationships and the anxiety must occur in peer settings, not just in adult interactions. Youngsters may express the anxiety in the form of crying, tantrums, freezing, avoidance or may exhibit a full blown panic attack. Children may not recognize that their fears are excessive, although adolescents typically do.

Incidence and Prevalence

Social phobia has the distinction of being the most common adult anxiety disorder, and is the third most common psychiatric disorder overall, with a lifetime prevalence of nearly 15%. Only depression and alcohol abuse occur more frequently. In children and adolescents, prevalence is frequently cited to be 1%, with the caveat that it is generally underdiagnosed in childhood and adolescence. Reasons for this include widespread failure of both parents and school personnel to identify the disorder, partially because they may not understand it be anything other than 'shyness' [95], and partially because these children, in their efforts to reduce their anxiety, do not draw attention to themselves and can be 'invisible' to inattentive or misinformed adults.

Etiology and Natural History

Symptoms of SP begin to appear in adolescence, with diagnosis around age 15 years. Its typical course is chronic and unremitting, with lifelong symptoms which can lead to multiple, significant social impairments. Adults with SP are less likely to be married, more likely to be underemployed, less likely to attain a high educational level [96]. From 70% to 80% of adults with SP have at least one other psychiatric disorder, most frequently panic with agoraphobia, GAD or simple phobia. In adults, the illness is now recognized for its pervasive and severely disabling nature.

Much less is known about pediatric SP. It has been diagnosed as young as eight years of age, but is more commonly identified in early- to mid-adolescence. Its presentation varies with age. Younger children may cry, cling to their parents or have temper tantrums when faced with a feared social situation. School-aged children may become oppositional and resist going to school. When in school, they may avoid class presentations, discussions and physical education classes. Adolescents have an increased risk of alcohol abuse, school drop-out, suicide ideation and suicide attempts. Conduct problems may appear [93]. Like adults with SP, children and adolescents are thought to have impaired social skills, although it has been suggested that it is less the absence of social skills and more the presence of anxiety which limits their use. Across all ages, somatic symptoms of distress, such as racing heart, sweating, tremulousness, lightheadedness and gastrointestinal discomfort, are common [97].

Both concordance data [89] and proband studies [98] suggest a genetic predisposition to SP. Behavioral inhibition, the predisposition to withdraw from novel circumstances, may be developmentally linked to SP [99]. High levels of parental criticism and overcontrol may be predisposing experiences [100], as may peer rejection and victimization experiences [101]. Once manifested, SP is maintained by negative perceptions and affect, social skill deficits and the positive reinforcement of avoidance [102].

Diagnosis

Children with SP typically do not spontaneously report nor seek treatment for their disorder. Symptoms such as school refusal, test anxiety, shyness, poor peer relationships, difficulty using public restrooms, problems using the telephone, eating in front of others and shrinking from social settings should alert the clinician to the need for a more systematic evaluation for SP. A thorough clinical evaluation should include interviews with both the child and the parents or primary caretakers with a focus on physical symptoms, specific worries and distressful situations characteristic of SP. Clinicians will often have to 'pin down' the specific fears and situations with the child, as children are less adept at articulating their symptoms and will often report complaints in vague terms, e.g., stomach aches, hating school, and 'not liking' situations.

To date, there are no laboratory tests nor physiological probes that have been demonstrated to be pathognomonic for SP. The Social Phobia and Anxiety Inventory for Children (SPAI-C) and the Social Phobia and Anxiety Inventory (SPAI) are empirically derived inventories meant to be used with children ages 8–14 years of age and over 14 years of age, respectively [103]

for diagnostic assessment and clinical monitoring of treatment.

Differential Diagnosis

Panic disorder with agoraphobia, SAD, GAD and specific phobia are chief considerations in the differential diagnosis of SP.

Classically, SP is characterized by the avoidance of social situations in the absence of panic attacks. Although social avoidance may occur in PD with agoraphobia, it is the specific fear of having a panic attack or being seen while having a panic attack that discriminates the two disorders. Fears in individuals with agoraphobia may or may not include the fear of scrutiny by others. Also, unlike SP, agoraphobic individuals may be reassured in social situations by the presence of a companion.

In SAD, the primary fear is one of separation from the primary caretaker. These individuals are usually comfortable in social settings in the home, whereas socially phobic individuals are distressed in social situations, even in the home.

In children with GAD and specific phobia, fear of embarrassment or humiliation in social settings may occur but it is not the main focus of their anxiety. These individuals experience fear and anxiety apart from social contexts.

Social anxiety and avoidance are common in many disorders, e.g., major depressive disorder, general medical disorders, personality disorders, and the diagnosis of SP should not be made if another disorder better accounts for the social anxiety or if its occurrence is limited to the occurrence of the other disorder.

Finally, school refusal is a descriptive term for behavior which may indicate the presence of a specific phobia, separation anxiety, truancy or SP, among other causes but does not imply a specific psychiatric diagnosis.

Treatment

Rigorous treatment outcome data for children with SP are limited. While published support for the efficacy of CBT are available, most studies do not focus on children with SP, but instead include them in the larger category of children with anxiety disorders [104]. Nonetheless, some SP-specific data are slowly becoming available. Beidel and colleagues [97] report considerable success with preadolescent children with SP symptoms, using a multifaceted behavioral treatment that combines social skills training with individual and group exposure sessions (but does not include cognitive restructuring) which she calls Social Effectiveness Therapy for Children (SET-C). Albano and colleagues [105] have treated adolescents with a version of Cognitive Behavioral Group Therapy for Adolescents (CBGT-A) adapted for SP, consisting of psychoeducation, cognitive restructuring, exposure and skills building. Both short- and long-term control of symptoms were evidenced. Other reports have demonstrated the additional benefit of including parents in CBT based treatment [106] and the potential for school based CBT for adolescents [107]. The reports of successful interventions with CBT all share four treatment components: psychoeducation, exposure, skill building (relaxation training, cognitive restructuring, social skills, problem-solving skills) and homework [93].

Following the lead of investigators of adult SP, preliminary reports on the utility of pharmacotherapy for children and adolescents with the disorder are beginning to appear. Both fluoxetine [108] and fluvoxamine [92] have been described as effective and well tolerated by children with anxiety disorders, including SP.

Cognitive and behavioral based strategies are the preferred treatment approach for social phobia in children and adolescents. Where medications are indicated, despite the absence of a Food and Drugs Administration (FDA) label indication in childhood, SSRIs are considered the pharmacological treatment of choice. Empirical evidence and downward extrapolation from adult studies supports the use of medication in treating SP.

Panic Disorder

Definition

Panic attacks are discrete, intense periods of fear and discomfort with cognitive and somatic symptoms that escalate in a crescendo fashion. Attacks may last minutes to, rarely, several hours. The attacks may be unexpected or 'out of the blue' or they may be situationally predisposed (more likely but not always occurring in a specific context), or situationally bound (almost always occurring in a specific situation). Panic attacks, but not necessarily the disorder itself, may occur in association with specific phobias, PTSD, SP, but by definition, in panic disorder at least some of the panic attacks are unexpected.

Panic disorder is diagnosed when the attacks are recurrent, and at least one of the attacks is followed by

a month or more period of worried anticipation for additional attacks and/or concern for negative consequences of an attack, to the point where it may change behavior. Agoraphobia (fear and avoidance of situation in which a panic attack may occur or in which escape may be difficult) may or may not complicate the disorder.

Incidence and Prevalence

Studies of adolescents in community samples report that between 2% and 18% of adolescents have experienced at least one four-symptom panic attack, when these are identified via a structured psychiatric interview. Higher prevalence reports of 43%–60% are found with adolescent self-report questionnaires. Prevalence of PD is reported to be between 0.5% and 5%, with greater representation in pediatric psychiatric clinic populations, e.g., up to 10% of referrals [109]. Females are more frequently afflicted than males [110]. Reliable epidemiological data are not available for pre-adolescents.

An earlier and well accepted model of PD [111] posited that panic attacks were the result of 'catastrophic misinterpretation' of ongoing somatic sensations. Because young children are considered lacking in the cognitive skills necessary to make these cognitive evaluations, it was long believed that children could not be diagnosed with PD [112]. Subsequent reports of clear panic attacks in children have challenged this theory, although it has remained useful for treatment.

Etiology and Natural History

Panic disorder may have a bimodal onset, the first peak occurring from ages 15 to 19 years, and the second, smaller peak in the mid-30s. Development of PD in early childhood or after the mid-40s, while possible, is considered a rarity. Panic attacks, as well as PD, are more likely in older children and adolescents than in younger children [113]. In adolescence, boys and girls are equally likely to experience panic attacks, but a diagnosis of PD is made more frequently with girls [114].

Following a lively debate in the literature which eventually acknowledged the existence or pre-pubertal panic attacks, some investigators still maintain that pre-adolescent 'panic' is not a genuine disorder, but rather an associated feature of another disorder, such as SP [81]. A more common position is that SP is linked to PD, via genetics, experience or in some other indirect way, such as a shared relation to major depressive disorder (MDD). While this issue remains open, recent evidence disputes a direct developmental link [109,115].

The symptoms most frequently reported by children and adolescents during panic attacks change with age [116]. For the youngest children, the most common somatic complaints are palpitations, shortness of breath, sweating, fainting and weakness. In adolescence, new somatic symptoms emerge, including chest pain, flushing, trembling, headache and vertigo. Cognitive symptoms are a delayed manifestation, relative to somatic symptoms, with the earliest reports of children and early adolescents being typically limited to fear of dying. Fear of going crazy and depersonalization–derealization tend to follow.

Risk factors for PD include female sex, MDD, high anxiety sensitivity (an increased tendency to respond fearfully to anxiety symptoms) negative affectivity (a temperamental tendency towards fear, sadness, self-dissatisfaction, hostility and worry in the face of negative stimuli) and a family history of MDD and PD [109,114]. Up to 90% of children and adolescents with PD have comorbities, most frequently MDD and other anxiety disorders (GAD, SAD, social phobia, agoraphobia). Up to 50% report somatoform disorders, substance use disorders, CD, ODD, ADHD and bipolar disorder [109].

Diagnosis

A somewhat intricate relationship between PD, other anxiety disorders and depression calls for a thorough clinical assessment. A detailed history should be obtained from the patient, family members, teachers and other professionals acquainted with the child, as with the child. Discerning whether the child can predict the onset of the attack is important for differential diagnosis. Pediatric and neurological exams can be helpful in some instances to elucidate the origin of somatic complaints or unusual sensations. Anxiety symptom scales may provide useful diagnostic information and later assist in evaluating treatment progress.

Differential Diagnosis

It is essential to differentiate PD from medical conditions such as hyperthyroidism, hyperparathyroidism, pheochromocytoma, diabetes, asthma, seizures, vestibular dysfunction or cardiac problems. Intoxica-

tion with stimulants or withdrawal from sedatives can produce symptoms which mimic panic attacks.

Differentiating PD from other anxiety disorders can be challenging. Fear and panic occurring only when a child is separated from an attachment figure points to SAD rather than PD. If the discomfort is experienced only in situations when one is subjected to scrutiny, SP is a more likely diagnosis. In specific phobia, fear and anxiety are an expected response to confrontation of the phobic object. Recollection of past trauma usually precedes emotional and autonomic distress in PTSD sufferers. Obsessions and compulsive rituals will help differentiate PD from obsessive–compulsive disorder (OCD). The generic descriptor 'school phobia' needs to be precisely defined symptomatically and operationally in order to differentiate its etiology as anxiety related (panic, phobic or separation) or due to another cause (e.g., truancy).

The absence of panic-like symptoms will distinguish PD from dissociative disorders manifested by depersonalization/derealization. Although some psychotic disorders may have panic as an associated feature, PD patients do not have thought disorders.

Treatment

Behavioral, cognitive and pharmacologic treatments of PD in children have for the most part been extrapolated from the adult literature, with some necessary modifications. Ollendick [117] and Hoffman and Mattis [118] report success using modified CBT programs with adolescents diagnosed with PD. Diler [109] recommends that such therapies focus on modifying patient's interpretation of their bodily processes, as well as changing the behaviors which maintain their previous 'catastrophic' interpretations.

While no controlled trials to evaluate the efficacy of behavioral and cognitive approaches in children have been undertaken, anecdotal data suggest that systematic desensitization may be helpful in the treatment of agoraphobia. Exposure techniques may be particularly helpful in situationally bound and predisposed panic attacks.

Masi and colleagues [119] reported considerable success in their open label treatment of adolescent PD with paroxetine. Diler [109] reviews small scale studies describing success with imipramine, alprazolam, clonazepam and other SSRIs. More systematic studies are necessary before a recommendation regarding pharmacotherapy can be made. However, clinical wisdom is leaning heavily in favor of the use of SSRIs, when there is significant debility.

Obsessive–Compulsive Disorder

Definition

The essential features of OCD include the recurrence of obsessions and, or compulsions severe enough to be time consuming (i.e., more than one hour per day), cause marked impairment or significant distress. Obsessions are recurrent and persistent thoughts, urges, impulses or images that are experienced as intrusive and inappropriate and which cause anxiety or distress. Compulsions are repetitive behaviors (e.g., hand washing, ordering, checking) or mental acts (e.g., praying, counting, repeating words silently) that the person feels driven to perform in response to an obsession. The behaviors or mental acts are aimed at preventing some dreaded event or situation, or in order to get something 'just so.' Children may or may not recognize that the obsessions or compulsions are unreasonable or excessive, and this criterion is not necessary in order to make a pediatric diagnosis.

Incidence and Prevalence

Obsessive–compulsive disorder is more common in children and adolescents than was once thought. Prevalence estimates, which have been widely discrepant in the past due to varied collection and diagnostic techniques [120], are now reported to be around 2% [121]. Cases of clinically significant OCD need to be distinguished from the subclinical obsessions and compulsions experienced by large numbers of children and adolescents in the course of normal development [86,122].

Etiology and Natural History

Like adults, children with OCD tend to present with both obsessions and compulsions, although independent presentations of compulsions and (less likely) obsessions are possible. Young children particularly, may present with ritualistic behaviors unassociated with compulsions and may not experience anxiety or feel distressed while performing them [123]. Symptoms tend to follow adult patterns: at some time during the course of the illness, washing rituals affecting more than 85% of children with OCD, repeating rituals 51% and checking rituals 46% [124]. Ordering, arranging, counting, collecting, ensuring symmetry and a preoccupation with having said or done the right thing are all common.

The mean age of onset is 10.3 years, with males outnumbering females by a 3:2 ratio [121]. Surprisingly, symptoms are present for 5–8 years before they come to clinical attention [122]. The disproportionate representation of male to female cases in childhood OCD is different from the adult disorder (where males and females are equally affected) and likely due to the earlier age of onset for boys [125]. Early-onset OCD has been posited as a special subtype of OCD, perhaps genetically related to tic disorders, which are more prevalent for males [126].

OCD is characterized by a waxing and waning course, with symptoms often worsened by stress, although this is not invariant. Males are more likely than females to have a chronic rather than episodic course [127,128]. In the vast majority of patients, specific symptoms are numerous, appear and disappear, vary in intensity and change in content over the course of the illness.

Childhood-onset OCD is a chronic and debilitating illness. It is complicated by high comorbidity rates with other disorders, including mood disorders (8%–73%), other anxiety disorders (13% 70%), disruptive behavior disorders (3%–57%), tic disorders/Tourette's syndrome (13%–26%), speech/developmental disorders (13%–27%), enuresis (7%–37%) and pervasive developmental disorders (3%–7%) [121]. Studies indicate that the majority of children with OCD will require long-term medication treatment and that although as many as 80% will experience improvement, a significant proportion (43%–68%) will continue to meet diagnostic criteria for OCD [124]).

Since the presentation and initial support for the serotonin hypothesis [129], much new information has come to light with respect to the pathogenesis of OCD. While support for the major role played by serotonin has continued, other neurotransmitters, such as dopamine and glutamate, have been suggested as important mediators of the disorder. The cortico-striato-thalamo-cortical circuit (CSTC) has been identified, with dysfunction in this circuit tied to OCD symptoms in ways consistent with our understanding of mediating neurotransmitters [130]. Structural and functional imaging studies of children and adolescents with OCD are currently being undertaken, although they lag behind information obtained with adult patients, but so far support the accumulating data and developing theory of functional deficits in the CSTC [131,132].

Current clinical research focuses on the heterogeneity of OCD. Several factor analytic studies have consistently identified at least four stable dimensions: contamination/washing, aggressive/checking, hoarding and asymmetry/ordering, each posited to represent a potential subtype, with different presumed genetic features, comorbidities and responses to treatment.

How these subtypes converge upon shared cortical and subcortical circuitry remains to be illuminated, although presumably it will involve a model of different phenotypes, different or overlapping etiologies, but a shared common pathway of expression.

Diagnosis

Accurate diagnosis of pediatric OCD is complicated by comorbid disorders, a waxing and waning course, changes in favored obsessions and compulsions, and potential confusion with developmentally appropriate expression of fearful preoccupations and rituals. Additionally, many children feel shameful about their obsessions and compulsions, making disclosure difficult. Consequently, careful history taking from the parents or primary caregiver and the use of semi-stuctured interview scales are useful in making the diagnosis. Input from siblings, teachers and day care providers can be helpful.

The primary instrument for assessing OCD in children and adolescents is the Children's version of the Yale-Brown Obsessive–Compulsive Scale (CY-BOCS) which can be useful to rate the severity of the disorder as well as to monitor its treatment progress [133]. A companion instrument, the CY-BOCS Symptom Checklist, is an extremely useful paper and pencil checklist for parents and children to identify current and past obsessions and compulsions. It is a time efficient way to survey a vast array of symptoms and is helpful in mapping treatment target symptoms. The Leyton Obsessional Inventory-Child Version (LOI-CV) [134] is an acceptable self-report assessment instrument. Recently, a shorter version of the LOI-CV became available, purporting to have similar psychometric soundness [135].

Differential Diagnosis

Because of the comorbity of OCD and Tourette's syndrome, a disorder of chronic motor and vocal tics, it is necessary to distinguish complex motor tics from a true ritual. Tics are usually not heralded by a preceding thought or obsession.

The stereotypies and repetitive movements seen in mental retardation and pervasive developmental disorder tend to be more fixed than the broader symptom picture of OCD.

Obsessive ruminations in depressed or dysthymic individuals can often mimic OCD symptoms although in the former case mood symptoms predominate. Similarly, although obsessions or compulsions can occur in psychotic disorders, there is by definition no disor-der in reality testing in OCD. The individual with OCD is often aware of the ridiculous or unreasonable nature of the cognition or behavior, although in younger children this is not a required feature of the diagnosis.

Obsessive–compulsive disorder symptoms associated with PANDAS (pediatric autoimmune neuropsychiatric disorders associated with streptococcal infections) have a temporal relationship with Group A beta-hemolytic streptococcal infections and are sometimes associated with choreiform movements [136].

The eating rituals of anorexic or bulimic patients and the rigid personality traits characteristic of obsessive–compulsive personality disorder need to be considered in the differential diagnosis of OCD. OCPD is present in a minority of cases and often improves with successful treatment of OCD. Curiously, individuals with OCPD may not find their 'symptoms' debilitating and may in fact believe their rigidity and obsessiveness are means to success.

Treatment

The American Academy of Child and Adolescent Psychiatry has established practice parameters for the treatment of OCD for pediatric patients [137]. Here, recommendation is made that CBT, with or without medication, be considered first-line treatment. Graduated exposure and response prevention (E/RP) has been demonstrated to have a respectable success rate with durability of effect [138]. In this technique, identification of all obsessions and compulsions is followed by assignment of a stimulus hierarchy, ranked by 'subjective units of discomfort' (SUDS). Exposure tasks are then undertaken with concurrent prevention of the usual obsessive or compulsive behavior. Repeated presentation of the anxiety invoking stimulus ensues, based on least to greatest SUDS, in the absence of the avoidance response, until they evoke minimal anxiety. This treatment approach is based on the principle that anxiety responses will habituate and eventually extinguish in the presence of repeated presentations of the anxiety stimulus, in the absence of an escape or avoidance response (i.e., performing the compulsive ritual). The specifics of the treatment have been described elsewhere [139] and a manualized treatment program of E/RP is available [140]. Mild cases of OCD are likely best treated initially with behavioral techniques exclusively, with adjunctive pharmacological treatment reserved for moderate-to-severe cases.

Pharmacotherapy with serotonergic agents such as clomipramine (at 3–5 mg/kg/day) [141] and various SSRIs (fluoxetine up to 60 mg/day/, sertraline up to

200 mg/day, fluvoxamine up to 200 mg/day) has demonstrated effectiveness in the treatment of children with OCD [142–144]. Three SSRIs, fluvoxamine (Luvox), sertraline (Zoloft) and fluoxetine (Prozac) have FDA label indications for the treatment of OCD in childhood and adolescence. Because side effects with the SSRIs tend to be fewer, these agents are typically preferred, with a 12-week trial of an adequate dose recommended before the trial is considered a failure. Following failure of a second SSRI, a course of clomipramine should be considered. Augmentation with a neuroleptic, such as risperidone [145] is an alternative strategy for those with a limited response to SSRIs. In general, published studies reveal that 40%–50% of patients will experience a 25%–40% reduction in symptoms with their first trial of medication. Medication treatment may be particularly indicated in cases of OCD where primary obsessional OCD is present (e.g., primary obsessional slowness) and target compulsions amenable to CBT are lacking. Treatment reports of PANDAS related OCD with immunoglobulin and plasma pheresis therapies have been primarily limited to specialty or research settings [136].

Selective Mutism

Definition

The term elective mutism was coined by Tramer in 1934 [146] to describe a population of children who speak only in certain situations or to certain people. Historically, a variety of etiologies for this disorder have been presented, with support for a particular etiology frequently limited to a single case study. In this manner, the disorder has variously been attributed to early psychological trauma [147], dysfunctional family dynamics involving mother–child enmeshment [148], a learned behavior reinforced by the child's environment [149], a manifestation of unresolved conflict [150], or the defiant refusal to speak [151]. The heterogeneous nature of these proposed etiologies has been cited as one justification for the disorder's current classification as a disorder usually first diagnosed in infancy [152].

In 1994, DSM-IV renamed the disorder selective mutism. Consistent with that change has since come theoretical consideration of selective mutism as a symptom of an anxiety disorder, or a variant of a specific anxiety disorder, such as SP, which would address the 'selective' nature of the mutism [153].

Selective mutism is characterized by the consistent failure to speak in specific social situations in which there is the expectancy for speech, despite speaking in other situations, such as the home. The failure to speak is not due to a lack of knowledge or comfort with social communication or a specific language (such as might occur for immigrants), and is debilitating to the individual. It is not diagnosed when better accounted for by embarrassment related to speech or language abilities, or by another psychiatric disorder.

Incidence and Prevalence

Prevalence estimates of selective mutism range from 0.03% to 2% [93]. While it has widely been assumed to be rare, some investigators are now calling this into question [154], as estimates are increasing with accumulating data. Most cases do not come to medical attention and resolve with age.

Etiology and Natural History

The age of onset is usually between three and six years [155]. Seventy percent of referrals occur during kindergarten years, with boys being referred an average of 2.3 years earlier than girls. The disorder is more common in girls than boys, with a ratio of about 3:1. Symptoms may be present several years before a referral is made, which typically occurs through the school in the early school age years [156].

A wide variety of psychiatric symptoms have been reported to be associated with selective mutism. Premorbid speech and language difficulties [157], developmental disorders [158], and Asperger's disorder [159] have all been reported to occur at elevated rates for this group. Higher rates of enuresis, encopresis, depression and separation anxiety have been suggested [160] although demonstrations of these are not consistent [161].

Remarkably consistent are associations between selective mutism and anxiety disorders. Black and Uhde described a population of children with selective mutism, nearly all of whom (97%) also met criteria for social phobia or avoidant behavior, and most of them (70%) had a parent who met the same criteria [161]. Dummit and colleagues [162] reported 100% of their sample of 50 to be comorbid for either social anxiety or avoidant disorder, and 48% of them had additional anxiety disorders. Kristensen [158] found selective mutism to have 74% comorbidity with anxiety disorders. In general, there is increasing evidence for a high association of selective mutism with anxiety disorders.

The majority of children with selective mutism appear to outgrow their disorder although it is not uncommon for the disorder to persist for several years in elementary school. There is some evidence to indicate that children who do not improve by the age of 10 years have an intractable form of the disorder [157].

Diagnosis

Diagnosis is based on clinical history. Children with selective autism should receive a complete medical history and physical examination. Neurological examination and developmental history should focus on motor, cognitive, language and social milestones. Quality of temperament, social interactions and the precise contexts in which speech occurs should be assessed. Formal hearing, speech and language assessment (sometimes utilizing the child's audio-recorded speech) may be necessary.

Differential Diagnosis

Shyness, unfamiliarity with the language or the presence of a communication disorder may be mistaken for selective mutism. Children with disorders such as schizophrenia, mental retardation or PDD may be unable to speak in social situations. However, selective mutism should only be diagnosed in a child with an established capacity to speak in some social situations, such as at home. The presence of a comorbid anxiety (e.g., social phobia), communication (e.g., stuttering) or other disorder should be diagnosed when present. It is worth noting that the presence of selective mutism *does not* imply that a child has been abused. Finally, rare cases of mutism can occur following operations on the posterior fossa, usually to remove large tumors, or on the corpus callosum, usually to improve intractable epilepsy [163].

Treatment

Historically, treatments for selective mutism have included a range of individual, family, behavioral and psychodynamic modalities. Evidence-based treatment literature is limited. Psychodynamic treatments, in isolation, have generally fared poorly, though they may provide a supportive role, facilitate social interactions and understanding of family issues unique to the child.

A multimodal approach with or without pharmacotherapy is the treatment of choice. The child should not be removed from the classroom for initiation of treatment. Cognitive behavioral therapy is the primary intervention aimed at reducing the child's anxiety inhibiting speech and positively reinforcing the child

for speaking. An attitude of expectation for normal speech and reinforcement for efforts to speak are important. Behavioral treatments are time consuming, requiring persistence and the cooperation of parents, teachers and other professionals. The child should not be removed from the classroom setting during treatment.

Psychosocial interventions utilizing modeling and peer pressure may be used to reinforce incremental or successive approximations of speech (e.g., hand raising, whispering) in the context of small groups of adults or peers. Family therapy may provide a powerful context for support, understanding the dynamics of the mutism and an opportunity for application of cognitive and behavioral interventions.

Pharmacotherapy for selective mutism includes the use of SSRIs, such as fluoxetine and sertraline [161,164] and the monoamine oxidase inhibitor phenelzine (at doses up to 2 mg/kg/day) [165]. Evidence is preliminary at best, but a trial of an SSRI, or phenelzine failing that, should be considered when the symptoms of selective mutism are debilitating, of long duration or refractory to other interventions (Table 13.3).

Summary

Anxiety symptoms are ubiquitous in youth. Clinicians need to be familiar with the normal developmental course of anxieties in youth and their consequent mastery by children in order to differentiate normative versus pathological anxiety and in order to discriminate between the anxiety disorders themselves (Table 13.4). Anxiety symptoms do not necessarily constitute an anxiety disorder. Adept assessment and management of anxiety symptoms through reassurance, anticipatory guidance and psychoeducation of parents may forestall the development of full blown anxiety syndromes.

Owing to their being among the most common psychiatric disorders in youth, clinicians need to maintain a high index of suspicion for anxiety disorders. A biopsychosocial approach to assessment utilizing multiple informants as well as paper and pencil assessment instruments will assist in the accurate screening and diagnosis of these disorders. The hallmark of all anxiety disorders is debility in life functioning that is attributable to fear or distress that is inappropriate in its intensity, frequency or context.

Empirically driven theories and treatment strategies, often in manualized form, are emerging for children and adolescents with anxiety disorders. Data is beginning to emerge regarding the effectiveness of

Table 13.3 Child and adolescent anxiety disorders: pearls and perils.

DSM-IV-TR diagnosis	Discriminating features	Associated features	Pharmacologic treatments	
			Primary	Secondary
Generalized anxiety disorder	Anxiety in multiple settings Common anxiety disorder in 12–19-year-olds	SAD, specific phobia	SSRI	Benzodiazepine Buspirone
Obsessive–compulsive disorder	Ruminations and rituals Washing, repeating, checking, 'just so' concerns, counting	Motor/vocal tics, second anxiety disorder	SSRI Clomipramine	Atypical Neuroleptic
Panic disorder	Rare in children Unexpected panic attacks, crescendo anxiety	Agoraphobia, anticipatory anxiety, somatic symptoms	SSRI	Benzodiazepine
Separation anxiety disorder	Middle childhood (7–10 years) Fears specific to separation from primary attachment figure	Phobia Depression GAD	SSRI	Buspirone Benzodiazepine
Selective mutism	Refusal to speak socially, despite ability Early childhood onset (3–6 years)	Social phobia	SSRI	
Social phobia	Relatively common, typically mid-teen onset, fear of social or performance setting	School refusal Shyness Somatic complaints	SSRI	Buspirone Benzodiazepine
Specific phobia	Specific phobic object or circumstance		Not indicated	

Table 13.4 Child and adolescent anxiety disorders: discriminating features.

DSM IV-TR diagnosis	Discriminating features	Associated features
Generalized anxiety disorder	Anxiety in multiple settings	SAD, specific phobia
	Common anxiety disorder in 12–19-year-olds	
	Often overlooked/underdiagnosed	
	Fretful, reassurrance seeking	
	Multiple sources of worry	
	'Achey-painy'/somatic/stomach pain	
	Worries about inconsequential items	
Obsessive–compulsive disorder	Ruminations and rituals	Motor/vocal tics
	Washing, repeating, checking, 'just so'	Second anxiety disorder
	concerns, counting, getting stuck, rigid	
	routines	ADHD
Panic disorder	Rare in children	Agoraphobia
	Unexpected panic attacks	
	Sudden/crescendo, disaster/impending	
	doom, discrete episodes of extreme	
	anxiety	
	Anticipatory anxiety 'fear of fear'	
	Somatic anxiety, feelings of symptoms	
	(tachycardia, tachypnea, chest tightness)	
Separation anxiety disorder	Middle childhood (7–10 years)	Phobia, depression, GAD
	Fears specific to separation from primary	
	attachment figure	
	Frequent reassurance seeking, bedtime	
	anxiety	
	Cannot do overnights at friends'	
	Crying/whining	
Selective	Refusal to speak	Social

pharmacologic strategies for treating childhood anxiety, especially in regard to the SSRIs. Despite the current controversy regarding potential suicidal ideation in youth related to these agents, they can be used safely and effectively with judicious selection and appropriate symptom monitoring by clinicians. The most successful treatments are typically multimodal, involving interventions that are educational, skills based, with a focus on exposure and mastery, and which involve both the child and important adults in the child's environment. The two case vignettes at the end of the chapter illustrate some of the complexities involved in assessment and treatment of rather typical anxiety disorder presentations in youth.

The field of child and adolescent anxiety disorder research is rapidly evolving, offering new insights into the etiology, developmental course and outcome of childhood anxiety disorders as well as the promise for ever more effective treatment interventions.

Vignette 1: Anxiety Comorbid with ADHD in an Adolescent Female

HISTORY AND CHIEF COMPLAINT

Sheila, a 13-year-old 8th grader, presented for evaluation of depression on referral from her school guidance counselor. Sheila's history was significant for shyness noted in kindergarten and elementary school. She struggled academically throughout her early school years to attain average grades despite special education accommodations in the classroom. Her elementary school teachers described Sheila as being 'spacey and disconnected.' Psychoeducational testing revealed that Sheila had a full-scale IQ of 102 (Verbal = 104, Performance = 98) and did not meet criteria for a specific learning disability.

Sheila's parents described her as a shy and immature girl who was somewhat overdependent, disorganized and unsure of herself. Socially she had few friends and tended to avoid group activities or sports. At home, Sheila exhibited a low tolerance for frustration and was known to be 'prickly' and bossy, often becoming irritable and frequently whining when her needs were not immediately met. She also engaged in frequent reassurance seeking from her parents and tended to have multiple somatic complaints including stomach aches, which contributed to her frequent absences from school.

The 8th grade represented a transition to a new school for Sheila. She started out the year without apparent problems but over the course of the first quarter, her academic performance began to decline. She had increasing trouble completing her homework without hours of prompting and assistance from her parents. She had frequent absences and tended to withdraw and isolate herself from peers while in school. Sensing that Sheila was depressed, her guidance counselor advised Sheila's parents to pursue an evaluation for possible depression.

PSYCHIATRIC EVALUATION

Sheila presented as a thin, quiet, early adolescent female who was appropriately, if plainly, dressed and groomed. She had difficulty maintaining eye contact, spoke in a quiet voice and gave only brief answers to interviewer questions. There was no evidence of psychosis, suicidal ideation or suicidal intent. Sheila's mood was self-described as 'OK,' but she appeared mildly dysphoric. Sheila denied frank depressed mood. She did, however, endorse multiple symptoms of anxiety as well as anxious cognitions. Sheila stated that she had great difficulty keeping focused on her teacher's lectures in the classroom setting and was often easily distracted by sounds in or outside the classroom as well as getting lost in her own thoughts. She reported that she was always anxious that she would be called on in class and that she would say something stupid and be laughed at by her peers. She was highly anxious of both peer criticism as well as performance situations such as test taking and in-class oral presentations. In these situa-

tions her heart would pound, her palms and underarms would sweat, her mouth would become dry and she would feel short of breath. In several oral classroom presentations Sheila reported that she became so paralyzed by her anxiety symptoms that she froze and subsequently fled the classroom. She reported that she had begun to anticipate these highly distressing anxiety episodes and that she feared entering the school building in the morning. Sheila's difficulties were compounded by a social scene that had intimidating cliques of seemingly confident and outgoing girls who were more physically mature than Sheila.

Family history was positive for a presumptive history of ADHD in Sheila's father. Sheila's mother had been treated as a late adolescent for depression.

PSYCHIATRIC ASSESSMENT

Assessment revealed that Sheila met DSM-IV diagnostic criteria for attention deficit hyperactivity, inattentive subtype as well as for generalized anxiety disorder. In addition, although Sheila did not meet criteria for panic disorder, she did experience isolated situationally bound panic attacks in performance situations.

TREATMENT

Sheila was referred for cognitive behavioral therapy to target her anxiety symptoms with a focus on skills based training. Special emphasis was given to targeting performance based situations in which Sheila could practice exposure and response prevention as well as anxiety management training skills. Pharmacotherapy trials resulted in several medications being evaluated before arriving at a successful combination of a long-acting stimulant plus a selective serotonin reuptake inhibitor.

DISCUSSION

Sheila's case highlights several important features of anxiety disorder presentations in adolescence. First, anxiety can often mimic other psychiatric disorders. Sheila's counselor mistakenly attributed her isolation, withdrawal, school absences and academic struggles as

signs of depression rather than the consequences of anxiety and ADHD. Second,
anxiety disorders frequently occur comorbidly
with other diagnoses. In this case Sheila's
comorbid condition was ADHD, inattentive
type, a diagnosis frequently overlooked in
girls who present without disruptive behavioral problems. Comorbid psychiatric conditions can often display a complex array of
symptoms that, taken together, may mimic
other psychiatric disorders such as depression. In Sheila's case, a thorough and detailed
psychiatric evaluation was able to pinpoint
the presence of attention and concentration
problems along with significant anxiety symptoms. The two disorders acted synergistically
to exacerbate one another leading to a progressive downward spiral of performance
across all important domains of Sheila's functioning. Finally, Sheila's treatment involved a
multiple modality approach with combination
CBT and pharmacotherapy. Because the combination of ADHD and anxiety can be difficult
to treat pharmacologically, several medication
trials were necessary before arriving at a successful combination.

Vignette 2: ADHD with Comorbid Anxiety in a School-Age Boy

HISTORY AND CHIEF COMPLAINT

Tommy, a six-year-old first grader, was
referred for psychiatric evaluation for attention deficit hyperactivity disorder. Tommy's
mother reported that he had been anxious and
a 'worry wort' since the age of two years.
Tommy's parents had divorced when he was
three years old and he currently lived with his
mother. Mother noted that Tommy had
become increasingly irritable and clingy over
the past year, subsequent to the death of his
grandmother, with whom he was particularly
close. Tommy had experienced academic and
behavioral difficulties since kindergarten.
Always an active and rambunctious youngster, Tommy was seen as disruptive and somewhat aggressive toward peers in kindergarten.
He would often throw temper tantrums in the
morning and refuse to allow his mother to
leave him in the kindergarten classroom. In

first grade, Tommy's teacher noted that he
appeared de-concentrated, had difficulty settling down to complete his work, and was
often oppositional, argumentative and disruptive with peers in class. Reading was difficult
owing to Tommy's impatience and he was
seen as a highly impulsive youngster with low
frustration tolerance. Transitions were particularly difficult.

At home mother reported that Tommy was
a high need youngster who was very busy. He
demanded constant attention and could not
engage in independent activities, even for
short periods of time. Mother noted that she
could not be in the bathroom by herself and
that Tommy insisted on being there with her,
although he would turn away from her in
order to 'give her privacy.' Bedtime was difficult. Typically, it would take several hours for
Tommy to get to sleep. He would cry out,
leave his room for the company of his mother,
and make repeated demands for a drink, a
story or trips to the bathroom. At the time of
psychiatric evaluation, Tommy's mother
reported that she was exhausted and despite
the seemingly endless time commitment to
Tommy, the situation was worsening.

PSYCHIATRIC EVALUATION

Tommy presented as a healthy appearing six-
year-old male who was noted to be fidgety
and who continuously interrupted his mother
during the psychiatric interview. Tommy was
seen as a highly distractible youngster who
had difficulty sustaining his focus in either
play activities or in direct conversation with
the examiner. His mood was noted to be
mildly irritable but he denied frank sadness,
tearfulness or depression. There was no evidence of psychosis, hypomanic or manic
symptoms. Tommy endorsed multiple fears
and worries. Since the death of his grandmother, Tommy had been having nightmares
that his mother was killed in an automobile
accident. He had intrusive thoughts during
the day that his mother would become ill or
would die, and that he would be left alone in
the world. He reported that these fears were
especially strong in the morning, when his
mother would drop him off at school, and in
the evening prior to bedtime.

History was negative for abuse or trauma exposure. Family history was significant for probable ADHD, anger problems and substance abuse in Tommy's father.

The Child Behavior Checklist, filled out by mother and teacher, indicated that Tommy had clinically significant scores on both internalizing and externalizing symptom domains. His Connors ADHD rating scale, which his mother and teacher completed, indicated highly significant core symptoms of ADHD including concentration problems, impulsivity and hyperactivity.

ASSESSMENT

Tommy was diagnosed with attention deficit hyperactivity disorder, combined type; oppositional defiant disorder; and separation anxiety disorder and generalized anxiety disorder.

TREATMENT

Treatment was initiated involving parent guided behavioral management training to target Tommy's oppositional and defiant symptoms, along with individual skills based CBT to give Tommy tactics that he could use to identify and combat his anxious thoughts. Tommy and his mother 'rehearsed being brave' in progressively longer and longer separations, after which Tommy was reinforced with access to his game boy. Pharmacotherapy was initiated with a long acting stimulant medication in the morning supplemented by clonidine at bedtime for sleep initiation. However, Tommy exhibited an increase in daytime anxiety symptoms and irritability in response to stimulant medication. Ultimately, Tommy was switched to a nonstimulant ADHD treatment and his stimulant and clonidine were tapered to discontinuation. Improvement was noted in core ADHD symptoms as well as anxiety. Tommy was able to separate from his mother without undue distress and sleep latency was less than 30 minutes.

DISCUSSION

Owing to the disruptive nature of Tommy's behaviors, Tommy's teacher failed to see the significant anxiety component in Tommy's symptom picture. Much of Tommy's seemingly disruptive, oppositional and hyperactive behaviors were in fact being driven, or at least exacerbated, by the significant anxiety that Tommy was experiencing. Treatment involved multiple modalities. Pharmacotherapy targeted Tommy's core ADHD and anxiety symptoms; CBT provided Tommy anxiety management skills; and, parent behavioral management training provided his mother skills for dealing with Tommy's anxious and oppositional behaviors.

References

1. Costello J, Angold A: A test–retest reliability study of child-reported psychiatric symptoms and diagnoses using the Child and Adolescent Psychiatric Assessment (CAPA-C). *Psychol Med* 1995; **25**(4):755–762.
2. Masi G, Mucci M, Millepiedi S: Separation anxiety disorder in children and adolescents: epidemiology, diagnosis and management. *CNS Drugs* 2001; **15**(2):93–104.
3. Bell-Dolan D, Brazeal TJ: Separation anxiety disorder, overanxious disorder and school refusal, *Child Adolesc Psychiatr Clin North Am* 1993; **2**(1):563–580.
4. Compton SN, Nelson AH, March JS: Social phobia and separation anxiety symptoms in community and clinical samples of children and adolescents, *J Am Acad Child Adolesc Psychiatry* 2000; **39**(8):1040–1046.
5. Last CG, Hersen M, Kazdin AE, Finkelstein R, Strauss CC: Comparison of DSM-III separation anxiety and overanxious disorders: Demographic characteristics and patterns of comorbidity. *J Am Acad Child Adolesc Psychiatry* 1987; **26**(4):527–531.
6. Francis G, Last CG, Strauss CC: Expression of separation anxiety disorder: The roles of age and gender. *Child Psychiatry Hum Dev* 1987; **18**(2):82–89.
7. Mahler MS, Pine F, Bergman A: *The Psychological Birth of the Human Infant: Symbiosis and Individualtion.* New York: Basic Books, 1975.
8. Kagan J, Snidman N, Arcus D: Childhood derivatives of high and low reactivity in infancy. *Child Dev* 1998; **69**(6):1483–1493.
9. Silove D, Harris M, Morgan A, Boyce P, Manicavasagar V, Hadzi-Pavlovic D, Wilhlm K: Is early separation anxiety a specific precursor of panic disorder-agoraphobia? A community study. *Psychol Med* 1995; **25**(2):405–411.
10. Silove D, Manicasagar V: Adults who feared school: Is early separation anxiety specific to the pathogenesis of panic disorder? *Acta Psychiatr Scand* 1993; **88**(6):385–390.
11. Fagiolinia, Shear MK, Cassano GB: Is lifetime separation anxiety a manifestation of a panic spectrum? *CNS Spectrums* 1992; **33**(4):249–279.
12. Manicavasagar V, Silove D: Is there an adult form of separation anxiety disorder? A clinical report. *Aust N Z J Psychiatry* 1997; **31**(2):299–303.

13. Black B: Separation anxiety disorder and panic disorder. In: March JS. ed. *Anxiety Disorders in Children and Adolescents*. New York: Guilford Press, 1995.

14. Kashani JH, Orvaschel H: A community study of anxiety in children and adolescents. *Am J Psychiatry* 1990; **147**(3):313–318.

15. Keller MB, Lavori PW, Wunder J, Beardslee WR, Schwartz CE, Roth J: Chronic course of anxiety disorders in children and adolescents. *J Am Acad Child Adolesc Pscychiatry* 1992; **331**:595–599.

16. Battaglia M, Bertella S, Politi E, Bernardeschi L, Perna G, Gabriele A, Bellodi L: Age at onset of panic disorder: Influence of familial liability to the disease and of childhood separation anxiety disorder. *Am J Psychiatry* 1995; **52**(9):1362–1364.

17. Birmaher B, Brent DA, Chiapetta L, Bridge J, Monga S, Baugher M: Psychometric properties of the Screen for Anxiety Related Emotional Disorders (SCARED): a replication study. *J Am Acad Child Adoles Psychiatry* 1999; **38**(10):1230–1236.

18. March JS, Parker JD, Sullivan K, Stallings P, Connors CK: The Multidimensional Anxiety Scale for Children (MASC): Factor structure, reliability and validity. *J Am Acad Child Adolesc Psychiatry* 1997; **36**(4):333–341.

19. Connors CK: 1997, *Connors Rating Scales-Revised Technical Manual*. North Tonawanda NY: Multi-Health Systems, 1978.

20. Barrett PM, Lowrey-Webster D, Turner SM: *FRIENDS Program for Children*. Brisbane Australia: Academic Press, 2000.

21. Kratochvil CJ, Harrington MJ, Burke WJ, March JS: Pharmacotherapy of childhood anxiety disorders. *Curr Psychiatry Rep* 2002; **4**(4):264–269.

22. Murphy TK, Bengston MA, Tan JY, Carbonell E, Levin GM: Selective serotonin reuptake inhibitors in the treatment of paediatric anxiety disorders: A review. *Int Clin Psychopharmacol* 2000; **15**(Suppl 2):S47–S63.

23. Velosa JF, Riddle MA: Pharmacologic treatment of anxiety disorders in children and adolescents. *Child Adolesc Psychiatr Clin N Am* 2000; **9**(1):119–133.

24. Bernstein GA, Shaw K: Practice parameters for the assessment and treatment of children and adolescents with anxiety disorders: American Academy of Child and Adolescent Psychiatry. *J Am Acad Child Adolesc Psychiatry* 1997; **36**(10 Suppl):69S–84S.

25. Bernstein GA, Layne A: Separation anxiety disorder and generalized anxiety disorder, In: Weiner JM, Dulcan MK, eds. *Textbook of Child and Adolescent Psychiatry*, Washington DC: APA Publishing, 2004.

26. King NJ, Bernstein GA: School refusal in children and adolescents: A review of the past 10 years. *J Am Acad Child Adolesc Psychiatry* 2001; **40**(2):197–205.

27. Heyne D, King NJ, Tonge BJ, Cooper H: School refusal: Epidemiology and management. *Paediatr Drugs* 2001; **3**(10):719–732.

28. King NJ, Ollendick TH, Tonge BJ: *School Refusal: Assessment and Treatment*. Boston MA: Allyn and Bacon, 1995.

29. American Psychiatric Association. *Diagnostic and Statistical Manual of Mental Disorders-Fourth Edition (DSM-IV)*. Washington, DC: American Psychiatric Association, 1994.

30. Kearney CA, Silverman WK: Family environments of youngsters with school refusal behavior: A synopsis with implications for assessment and treatment, *Am J Fam Ther* 1995; **23**(1):59–72.

31. Bernstein GA, Borchardt CM: School refusal: Family constellation and family functioning. *J Anxiety Disord* 1996; **10**(1):1–19.

32. Kendall PC, Brady EU, Verduin TL: Comorbidity in childhood anxiety disorders and treatment outcome. *J Am Acad Child Adolesc Psychiatry* 2001; **40**(7): 787–794.

33. Kearney CA, Silverman WK: A preliminary analysis of a functional model of assessment and treatment for school refusal behavior. *Behav Modif* 1990; **14**(3):340–366.

34. SilvermanWK, Kearney CA: Listening to our clinical partners: Informing researchers about children's fears and phobias. *J Behav Ther Exp Psychiatry* 1992; **23**(2):71–76.

35. Kearney CA: *School Refusal Behavior in Youth: A Functional Approach to Assessment and Treatment*. Washington DC: American Psychological Association, 2001.

36. Kearney CA, Albano AM: *When Children Refuse School: A Cognitive Therapy Approach*. San Antonio TX: Psychological Corporation, 2000.

37. Last CG, Hansen C, Franco N: Cognitive-behavioral treatment of school phobia. *J Am Acad Child Adolesc Psychiatry* 1998; **37**(4):404–411.

38. Labellarte MJ, Ginsburg GS, Walkup JT, Riddle MA: The treatment of anxiety disorders in children and adolescents. *Biol Psychiatry* 1999; **46**(11):1567–1578.

39. Masi G, Millepiedi S, Mucci M, Poli P, Bertini N, Milantoni L: Generalized anxiety disorder in referred children and adolescents. *J Am Acad Child Adolesc Psychiatry* 2004; **43**(6):752–760.

40. Judd LL, Kessler RC, Paulus MP, Zeller PV, Wittchen HU, Kunovac JL: Comorbidity as a fundamental feature of generalized anxiety disorders: Results from the National Comorbidity Study (NCS). *Acta Psychiatr Scand* 1998; **393**:6–11.

41. Muris P, Merckelback H, Schmidt H, Tierney S: Disgust sensitivity, trait anxiety, and anxiety disorders symptoms in normal children. *Behav Res Ther* 1999; **37**(10):953–961.

42. Weems CF, Silverman WK, LaGreca AM: What do youth referred for anxiety problems worry about? Worry and its relation to anxiety and anxiety disorders in children and adolescents. *J Abnorm Child Psychol* 2000; **28**(1):63–72.

43. Perrin S, Last CG: Worrisome thoughts in children clinically referred for anxiety disorder. *J Clin Child Psychol* 1997; **26**(2):181–189.

44. Costello EJ: Developments in child psychiatric epidemiology. *J Am Acad Child Adolesc Psychiatry* 1989; **28**(6):836–841.

45. Schaffer D, Fisher P, Dulcan MD, Davies M, Piacentini J, Schwab-Stone MjE, Lahey BB, Bourdon K, Jensen PS, Bird HR, Canino G, Regier DA: The NIMH Diagnostic Interview Schedule for Children Version 2.3 (DISC-2.3): Description, acceptability, prevalence rates, and performance in the MECA study-Methods for the Epidemiology of Child and Adolescent Mental Disorders Study. *J Am Acad Child Adolesc Psychiatry* 1996; **35**(7):865–877.

46. McGee R, Feehan M, Williams S, Partridge F, Silva PA, Kelly J: DSM-III disorders in a large sample of ado-

lescents. *J Am Acad Child Adolesc Psychiatry* 1990; **29**(4):611–619.

47. Last CG, Perrin S, Hersen M, Kazdin AE: DSM-III-R anxiety disorders in children: Sociodemographic and clinical characteristics. *J Am Acad Child Adolesc Psychiatry* 1992; **31**(6):1070–1076.

48. Werry JS: Overanxious disorder: A review of its taxonomic properties. *J Am Acad Child Adolesc Psychiatry* 1991; **30**(4):533–544.

49. Masi G, Mucci M, Favilla L, Romano R, Poli P: Symptomatology and comorbidity of generalized anxiety disorder in children and adolescents. *Compr Psychiatry* 1999; 3:210–205.

50. Freud S: *Inhibitions, Symptoms and Anxiety*. New York: WW Norton and Co., 1959.

51. Biederman J, Rosenbaum JF, Bolduc-Murphy EA, Faraone SV, Chaloff J, Hirshfeld DR, Kagan J: A 3-year follow-up of children with and without behavioral inhibition. *J Am Acad Child Adolesc Psychiatry*, 1993; **32**(4):814–821.

52. Kagan J, Snidman N: Early childhood predictors of adult anxiety disorders. *Biol Psychiatry* 1999; **46**(11):1536–1541.

53. Carey G, DiLalla DL: Personality and psychopathology: genetic perspectives. *J Abnorm Psychol* 1994; **103**(1):32–43.

54. Millan MJ: The neurobiology and control of anxious states. *Prog Neurobiol* 2003; **70**(2):83–244.

55. DeBellis D, Casey BJ, Dahl RE, Birmaher B, Williamson DE, Thomas KM, Axelson DA, Frustaci K, Boring AM, Hall J, Ryan ND: A pilot study of amygdale volumes in pediatric generalized anxiety disorder. *Biol Psychiatry* 2000; **48**(1):51–57.

56. DeBellis MD, Keshaven MS, Shifflett H, Iyengar S, Dahl RE, Axelson DA, Birmaher B, Hall J, Moritz G, Ryan ND: Superior temporal gyrus volumes in pediatric generalized anxiety disorder. *Biol Psychiatry* 2002; **51**(7):553–562.

57. Verduin TL, Kendall PC: Differential occurrence of comorbidity within childhood anxiety disorders. *J Clin Child Adolesc Psychol* 2003; **32**(2):290–295.

58. Wilens TE, Biederman J, Brown S, Tanguay S, Monuteaux MC, Blake C, Spencer TJ: Psychiatric comorbidity and functioning in clinically referred preschool children and school-age youths with ADHD. *J Am Acad Child Adolesc Psychiatry* 2002; **41**(3): 262–268.

59. Kendall PC, Pimental SS: On the physiological symptom constellation in youth with Generalized Anxiety Disorder (GAS). *J Anxiety Disord* 2003; **17**(2):211–221.

60. Reynolds CR, Richmond BO: What I think and feel: A revised measure of children''s manifest anxiety. *J Abnorm Child Psychol* 1978; **6**(2):271–280.

61. Achenbach TM, Rescoral LA: *Manual for the ASEBA School Age Forms and Profiles*. Burlington, VT: University of VT Research Center for Children, Youth and Families, 2001.

62. Silverman WK, La Greca AM, Wasserstein S: What do children worry about? Worries and their relation to anxiety. *Child Dev* 1995; **66**(3):671–686.

63. Walkup J, Labellarte M, Riddle MA, Pine DS, Greenhill L, Fairbanks J, Klein R, Davies M, Sweeney M, Abikoff H, Hack S, Klee B, Bergman RL, Lynn D,

McCracken J, March J, Gammon P, Vitiello B, Ritz L, Roper M: Research Units on Pediatric Psychopharmacology Anxiety Study Group: Treatment of pediatric anxiety disorders: an open-label extension of the research units on pediatric psychopharmacology anxiety study. *J Child Adolesc Psychopharmacol* 2002 **12**(3):175–188.

64. Brooks SJ, Kutcher S: Diagnosis and measurement of anxiety disorder in adolescents: A review of commonly used instruments, *J Child Adolesc Psychopharmacol* 2003; **13**(3):351–400.

65. Clark AS, Henderson LP: Behavioral and physiological responses to anabolic-androgenic steroids, *Neurosci Biobehav Rev*, 2003; **27**(5):413–436.

66. Compton SN, March JS, Brent D, Albano AM, Weersing R, Curry J: Cognitive-behavioral psychotherapy for anxiety and depressive disorders in children and adolescents: An evidence-based medicine review. *J Am Acad Child Adolesc Psychiatry* 2004; **43**(80): 930–959.

67. Mendlowitz SL, Manassis K, Bradley S, Scapillato D, Miezitis S, Shaw BF: Cogniitive-behavioral group treatments in childhood anxiety disorders: The role of parental involvement. *J Am Acad Child Adolesc Psychiatry* 1999; **38**(10):1223–1229.

68. Barrett PM, Duffy AL, Dadds MR, Rapee RM: Cognitive-behavioral treatment of anxiety disorders in children: Long-term (6 year) follow-up. *J Consult Clin Psychol* 2001; **69**(1):135–141.

69. Cobham VE, Dadds MR, Spence SH: The role of parental anxiety in the treatment of childhood anxiety. *J Consult Clin Psychol* 1998; **66**(6):893–905.

70. Kendall PC: *Coping Cat Workbook*, Ardmore PA: Workbook Publishing, 1990.

71. Kendall PC, Southam-Gerow MA: Long-term follow-up of a cognitive-behavioral therapy for anxiety-disordered youth. *J Consult Clin Psychol* 1996; **64**(4):724–730.

72. Kendall PC: Treating anxiety disorders in children: results of a randomized clinical trial. *J Consult Clin Psychol* 1994; **62**(1):100–110.

73. Flannery-Schroeder EC, Kendall PC: Group and individual cognitive-behavioral treatments for youth with anxiety disorders: A randomized clinical trial. *Cognit Ther Res* 2000; **24** (3):251–278.

74. Research Units on Pediatric Psychopharmacology Anxiety Study Group (RUPP): Fluvoxamine for the treatment of anxiety disorders in children and adolescents. *N Engl J Med* 2001; **344**(17):1279–1285.

75. Research Units on Pediatric Psychopharmacology Anxiety Study Group (RUPP): Pediatric anxiety disorders: An open-label extension of the research units on pediatric psychopharmacology anxiety study. *J Child Adolesc Psychopharmacol* 2002; **12**(3): 175–188.

76. Rynn MA, Siqueland L, and Rickels K: Placebo-controlled trial of sertraline in the treatment of children with generalized anxiety disorder. *Am J Psychiatry* 2001; **158**(12):2008–2014.

77. Birmaher B, Axelson DA, Monk K, Kalas C, Clark DB, Ehmann M, Bridge J, Heo J, Brent DA: Fluoxetine for the treatment of childhood anxiety disorders, *J Am Acad Child Adolesc Psychiatry* 2003; **42**(4): 415–423.

78. Baumgartner JL, Emslei GJ, Crismon ML: Citalopram in children and adolescents with depression or anxiety. *Ann Pharmacother* 2002; **36**(11):1692–1697.

79. Simeaon JG, Ferfuson HB, Knott V, Roberts N, Gauthier B, Dubois C, Wiggins D: Clinical, cognitive and neurophysiological effects of alprazolam in children and adolescents with overanxious and avoidant disorders. *J Am Acad Child Adolesc Psychiatry* 1992; **31**(1):29–33.

80. Graae F, Milner J, Rizzotto L, Klein RG: Clonazepam in childhood anxiety disorders. *J Am Acad Child Adolesc Psychiatry* 1994; **33**(3):372–376.

81. Freeman JB, Garcia AM, Leonard HL: Anxiety disorders. In: Lewis M, ed. *Child and Adolescent Psychiatry: A Comprehensive Textbook*. New York: LW&W, 2002.

82. Fyer AJ: Current approaches to etiology and pathophysiology of specific phobia. *Biol Psychiatry* 1998; **44**(12):1295–1304.

83. Essau CA, Conradt J, Petermann F: Frequency, comorbidity and psychosocial impairment of specific phobia in adolescents. *J Clin Child Psychol* 2000; **29**(2):221–231.

84. Marks IM: *Fears, Phobias and Rituals*. New York: Oxford University Press, 1987.

85. Gullone E: The development of normal fear: a century of research. *Clin Psychol Rev* 2000; **20**(4):429–451.

86. Evans DW, Leckman JF, Carter A, Reznick JS, Henshaw D, King RA, Pauls D: Ritual, habit and perfectionism: The prevalence and development of compulsive-like behavior in normal young children. *Child Dev* 1997; **68**(1):58–68.

87. Rachman S: The conditioning theory of fear acquisition: A critical examination. *Behav Res Ther* 1977; **15**(5):375–387.

88. Muris P, Merckelbach H, deJong P, Ollendick TH: The etiology of specific fears and phobias in children: A critique of the non-associative account. *Behav Res Ther* 2002; **40**(2):185–195.

89. Kendler KS, Neale MC, Kessler RC, Heath AC, Eaves LJ: The genetic epidemiology of phobias in women: The interrelationship of agoraphobia, social phobia, situational phobia and simple phobia. *Arch Gen Psychiatry* 1992; **49**(4):273–281.

90. Lewinsohn PM, Zinbarg R, Seeley JR, Lewinsohn M, Sach WH: Lifetime comorbidity among anxiety disorders and between anxiety disorders and other mental disorders in adolescents. *J Anxiety Disord* 1997; **11**(4):377–394.

91. King NJ, Ollendick TH, Murphy GC: Assessment of childhood phobias. *Clin Psychol Rev* 1997; **17**(7):667–687.

92. Ollendick TH, King NJ: Empirically supported treatments for children with phobic and anxiety disorders: current status. *J Clin Child Psychol* 1998; **27**(2):156–167.

93. Black B, Garcia AM, Freeman JB: Specific phobia, panic disorder, social phobia and selelctive mutism. In: Weiner JM, Dulcan MK, eds. *Textbook of Child and Adolescent Psychiatry*. Washington DC: APA Publishing, 2004.

94. Thomas A, Chess S: *Temperament and Development*, New York: Brunner/Mazel, 1977.

95. Albano AM, Chorpita BF, Barlow DH: Childhood anxiety disorders, In: Mash EJ, Barkeley RA, eds. *Child Psychopathology*, Guilford Press, New York, 1996.

96. Keller MB: The lifelong course of social anxiety disorder: A clinical perspective. *Acta Psychiatry Scand Suppl* 2003; **417**:85–94.

97. Beidel DC, Turner SM, Morris TL: Behavioral treatment of childhood social phobia. *J Consult Clin Psychol* 2000; **68**(6):1072–1080.

98. Stein MB, Chartier MJ, Kozak MV, King N, Kennedy JL: Genetic linkage to the serotonin transporter protein and 5HT2A receptor genes excluded in social phobia. *Psychiatry Res* 1998; **81**(3):283–291.

99. Schwartz CE, Snidman N, Kagan J: Adolescent social anxiety as an outcome of inhibited temperament in childhood. *J Am Acad Child Adolesc Psychiatry* 1999; **38**(8):1008–1015.

100. Whaley SE, Pinto A, Sigman M: Characterizing interactions between anxious mothers and their children. *J Consult Clin Psychol* 1999; **67**, (6):826–836.

101. LaGreca AM, Lopez N: Social anxiety among adolescents: Linkages with peer relationships and friendships. *J Abnorm Child Psychol* 1998; **26**(2):83–94.

102. Kashdan TB, Herbert JD: Social anxiety disorder in childhood and adolescence: Current status and future directions. *Clin Child Fam Psychol Rev* 2001; **4**(1):37–61.

103. Storch EA, Masia-Warner C, Dent HC, Roberti JW, Fisher PH: Psychometric evaluation of the Social Anxiety Scale for Adolescents and the Social Phobia and Anxiety Inventory for Children: Construct validity and normative data. *J Anxiety Disord* 2004; **18**(5):665–679.

104. Zaider TI, Heimberg RG: Non-pharmacologic treatments for social anxiety disorder. *Acta Psychiatr Scand Suppl* 2003; **417**:72–84.

105. Albano AM, Marten PA, Holt CS, Heimberg RG, Barlow DH: Cognitive-behavioral group treatment for social phobia in adolescents. *J Nerv Ment Dis* 1995; **183**(10):649–656.

106. Spence SH, Donovan C, Brechman-Toussaint M: The treatment of childhood social phobia: The effectiveness of a social skills training based, cognitive behavioral intervention, with and without parental involvement. *J Child Psychol Psychiatry* 2000; **41**(6):713–726.

107. Masia CL, Klein RG, Storch EA, Corda B: School-based behavioral treatment for social anxiety disorder in adolescents: Results of a pilot study. *J Am Acad Child Adolesc Psychiatry* 2001; **40**(7):780–786.

108. Birmaher B, Waterman CGS, Ryan N, Cully M, Balach L, Ingram J, Brodsky M: Fluoxetine for childhood anxiety disorders, *J Am Acad Child Adoles Psychiatry* 1994; **33**(7):993–999.

109. Diler RS: Panic disorder in children and adolescents, *Yonsei Medical Journal*, 2003; **44**(1):174–179.

110. Whitaker A, Johnson J, Shaffer D, Rapoport JL, Kalikow K, Walsh BT, Davies M, Braiman S, Dolinsky A: Uncommon troubles in young people: Prevalence estimates of selected psychiatric disorders in a non-referred adolescent population. *Arch Gen Psychiatry* 1990; **47**(5):487–496.

111. Clark DM: A cognitive approach to panic. *Behav Res Ther* 1986; **24**(4):461–470.

112. Nelles WB, Barlow DH: Why do children panic? *Clin Psychol Rev* 1998; **8**(4):359–372.

113. Hayward C, Killen JD, Hammer LD, Litt IF, Wilson DM, Simmonds B, Taylor CB: Pubertal stage and panic attack history in sixth and seventh grade girls. *Am J Psychiatry* 1992; **9**(9):1239–1243.

114. Hayward C, Killen JD, Kraemer HC, Taylor CB: Predictors of panic attacks in adolescents. *J Am Acad Child Adolesc Psychiatry* 2000; **39**(2):207–214.

115. Aschenbrand SG, Kendall PC, Webb A, Safford SM and Flannery-Schroeder E: Is childhood separation anxiety disorder a predictor of adult panic disorder and agoraphobia? A seven year longitudinal study. *J Am Acad Child Adolesc Psychiatry* 2003; **42**(12):1478–1485

116. Masi G, Favilla L, Mucci M, Millepiedi S: Panic disorder in clinically referred children and adolescents. *Child Psychiatry Hum Dev* 2000; **31**(2):139–151.

117. Ollendick TH: Cognitive behavioral treatment of panic disorder with agoraphobia in adolescents: A multiple baseline design analysis. *Behav Ther* 1995; **26**(3): 517–531.

118. Hoffman EC, Mattis SG: A developmental adaptation of panic control treatment for panic disorder in adolescents. *Cogn Behav Pract* 2000; **7**(3):253–261.

119. Masi G, Toni C, Mucci M, Millepiedi S, Mata B, Perugi G: Paroxetine in child and adolescent outpatients with panic disorder. *J Child Adolesc Psychopharmacol* 2001; **11**(2):151–157.

120. Towbin KE, Riddle MA: Obsessive-compulsive disorder. In: Lewis M, ed. *Child and Adolescent Psychiatry: A Comprehensive Textbook*. New York: LW&W, 2002.

121. Geller DA, Spencer T: Obsessive-compulsive disorder. In: Martin A, Scahill L, Charney D, Leckman J, eds. *Pediatric Psychopharmacology: Principles and Practice*. New York: Oxford University Press, 2003.

122. Zohaan AH, Bruno R: Normative and pathological obsessive-compulsive behavior and ideation in childhood: A question of timing. *J Child Psychol Psychiatry* 1997; **38**(8):99309.

123. Geller D, Biederman J, Jones J, Park K, Schwartz S, Shapiro S, Coffey B: Is juvenile obsessive-compulsive disorder a developmental subtype of the disorder? A review of the pediatric literature, *J Am Acad Child Adolesc Psychiatry* 1998; **37**(4):420–427.

124. Leonard HL, Swedo SE, Lenane MC, Hamburger SD, Bartko JJ, Rapoport JL: A 2- to 7-year follow-up study of 54 obsessive-compulsive children and adolescents. *Arch Gen Psychiatry* 1993; **50**(6):429–439.

125. Eichstadt JA, Arnold SL: Childhood-onset obsessive-compulsive disorder: A tic-related subtype of OCD? *Clin Psychol Rev* 2001; **21**(1):137–157.

126. Lochner C, Stein DJ: Heterogeneity of obsessive-compulsive disorder: A literature review. *Harv Rev Psychiatry* 2003; **11**(3):113–132.

127. Rettew DC, Swedo SE, Leonard HL, Lenane MC, Rapoport JL: Obsessions and compulsions across time in 79 children and adolescents with obsessive-compulsive disorder. *J Am Acad Child Adolesc Psychiatry* 1992; **31**(6):1050–1056.

128. Lensi P, Cassano GB, Correddu G, Ravagli S, Kunovac JL, Akiskal HS: Obsessive-compulsive disorder: Familial-developmental history, symptomatology, comorbidity and course with special reference to gender-related differences. *Br J Psychiatry* 1996; **169**(1):101–107.

129. Thoren P, Asberg M, Berilsson L, Mellstrom B, Sjoqvist F, Traskman L: Clomipramine treatment of obsessive-compulsive disorder. II Biochemical aspects. *Arch Gen Psychiatry* 1980; **37**(11):1289–1294.

130. Baxter L: Functional imaging of brain systems mediating obsessive compulsive disorder, In: Charney DL, Nessler E, Bunney BS, eds. *Neurobiology of Mental Illness*. New York: Oxford University Press, 1999.

131. Fitzgerald KD, Moore GJ, Paulson LA, Steward CM, Rosenberg DR: Proton spectroscopic imaging of the thalamus in treatment-naïve pediatric obsessive-compulsive disorder. *Biol Psychiatry* 2000; **47**(3): 174–182.

132. Rosenberg DR, MacMaster FP, Keshavean MS, Fitzgerald KD, Stewart CM, Moore GJ: Decrease in caudate glutamatergic concentrations in pediatric obsessive-compulsive disorder patients taking paroxetine. *J Am Acad Child Adolesc Psychiatry* 2000; **39**(9):1096–1103.

133. Scahill L, Riddle MA, McSwiggin-Hardin M, Ort SI, King RA, Goodman WK, Cicchetti D, Leckman JF: Children''s Yale-Brown Obsessive Compulsive Scale: Reliability and validity. *J Am Acad Child Adolesc Psychiatry* 1997; **36**(6):844–852.

134. Berg CJ, Rapoport JL, Flament M: The Leyton Obsessional Inventory-Child Version. *J Am Acad Child Psychiatry* 1986; **25**(1):84–91.

135. Bamber D, Tamplin A, Park RJ, Kyte ZA, Goodyer IM: *J Am Acad Child Adolesc Psychiatry* 2002; **41**(10):1246–1252.

136. Swedo SE, Leonard HL, Garvey M, Mittleman B, Allen AJ, Perlmutter S, Lougee L, Dow S, Zamkoff J, Dubbert BK: Pediatric autoimmune neuropsychiatric disorders associated with streptococcal infections: Clinical description of the first 50 cases. *Am J Psychiatry* 1998; **155**(2):264–271.

137. King RA, Leonard H, March JS: Summary of the practice parameters for the assessment and treatment of children with obsessive-compulsive disorder: American Academy of Child and Adolescent Psychiatry. *J Am Acad Child Adolesc Psychiatry* 1998; **37**(10 Suppl): 27S–45S.

138. March JS, Mulle K, Herbel B: Behavioral psychotherapy for children and adolescents with obsessive-compulsive disorder: An open trial of a new protocol-driven treatment package. *J Am Acad Child Adolesc Psychiatry* 1994; **36**(4):554–565.

139. Berg CZ, Rapoport JL, Whitaker A, Davies M, Leonard H, Swedo SE, Braiman S, Lenane M: Childhood obsessive compulsive disorder: A two-year prospective follow-up of a community sample. *J Am Acad Child Adolesc Psychiatry* 1989; **28**(4):528–533.

140. March JS, Mulle K: *OCD in Children and Adolescents: A Cognitive-Behavioral Treatment Manual*. New York: Guilford Press, 1998.

141. DeVeaugh-Geiss J, Moroz G, Biederman J, Cantwell D, Fontaine R, Greist JH, Reichler R, Katz R, Landau P: Clomipramine hydrochloride in childhood and adolescent obsessive-compulsive disorder – a multicenter trial. *J Am Acad Child Adolesc Psychiatry* 1992; **31**(1):45–49.

142. March JS, Biederman J, Wolkow R, Safferman A, Mardekian J, Cook EH, Cutler NR, Dominguiez R, Ferguson J, Muller B, Riesenberg R, Rosenthal M, Salle FR, Wagner KD, Steiner H: Sertraline in children and adolescents with obsessive-compulsive disorder: A multicenter randomized controlled trial. *JAMA* 1998; **280**(20):1752–1756.

143. Riddle MA, Reeve EA, Yaryura-Tobias JA, Yang HM, Claghorn JL, Gaffney G, Greist JH, Holland K, McConville BJ, Pigott T, Walkup JT: Fluvoxamine for children and adolescents with obsessive-compulsive disorder: A randomized, controlled, multicenter trial. *J Am Acad Child Adolesc Psychiatry* 2001; **40**(2): 222–229.

144. Geller DA, Hoog SL, Heilegenstein JH, Ricardi RK, Tamura R, Kluszynski S, Jacobson JG: Fluoxetine treatment for obsessive-compulsive disorder in children and adolescents: A placebo-controlled clinical trial. *J Am Acad Child Adolesc Psychiatry* 2001; **40**(7):773–779.

145. Fitzgerald KD, Steward CM, Tawile V, Rosenberg DR: Risperidone augmentation of serotonin reuptake inhibitor treatment of pediatric obsessive compulsive disorder. *J Child Adolesc Psychopharmacol* 1999; **9**(2):115–123.

146. Tramer M: *Electiver mutismus bei kindern*, Kinderpsychiatrie. 1934.

147. Hayden TL: Classification of elective mutism. *J Am Acad Child Adolesc Psychiatry* 1980; **19**(1):118–133.

148. Meyers S: Elective mutism in children: A family systems approach. *American Journal of Family Therapy* 1984; **12**(4):39–45.

149. Porjes M: Intervention with the selectively mute child. *Psychol Schools* 1992; **29**(4):367–376.

150. Valner J, Nemiroff M: Silent eulogy. Elective mutism in a six-year-old Hispanic girl. *Psychoanal Study Child* 1995; **50**(1):327–340.

151. Hoffman S, Lamb B: Paradoxical intervention using a polarized model of cotherapy in the treatment of elective mutism: A case study. *Contemporary Family Therapy* 1986; **8**(2):136–143.

152. Astendig KD: Is selective mutism an anxiety disorder: rethinking its DSM-IV classification, *J Anxiety Disord* 1999; **13**(4):417–434.

153. Dow SP, Sonies BC, Scheib D, Moss SE, Leonard HL: Practical guidelines for the assessment and treatment of selective mutism. *J Am Acad Child Adolesc Psychiatry* 1995; **34**(7):836–846.

154. Bergman RL, Piacentini J, McCracken JT: Prevalence and description of selective mutism in a school-based sample, *J Am Acad Child Adolesc Psychiatry*, 2002; **41**(8):938–946.

155. Wright HH, Miller MD, Cook MA, Littman JR: Early identification and intervention with children who refuse to speak. *J Am Acad Child Adolesc Psychiatry* 1985; **24**(6):739–746.

156. Kumpulainen K: Phenomenology and treatment of selective mutism. *CNS Drugs*, 2002; **16**(3):175–180.

157. Kolvin I, Fundudis T: Elective mute children: Psychological development and background factors. *J Child Psychol Psychiatry* 1981; **22**(3):219–232.

158. Kristensen H: Selective mutism and comorbidity with developmental disorder/delay, anxiety disorder and elimination disorder. *J Am Acad Child Adolesc Psychiatry* 2000; **39**(2):249–256.

159. Gillberg C: *Clinical Child Neuropsychiatry*. Cambridge England: Cambridge University Press, 1995.

160. Tancer NK: Elective mutism: A review of the literature. In: Lahey BB, Kazdin AE, eds. *Advances in Clinical Child Psychology*. New York: Plenum Press, New York, 1992.

161. Black B, Uhde TW: Treatment of elective mutism with fluoxetine: A double-blind, placebo-controlled study. *J Am Acad Child Adolesc Psychiatry* 1994; **33**(7): 1000–1006.

162. Dummit ES, Klein RG, Tancer NK, Asche B, Martin J, Fairbanks JA: Systematic assessment of 50 children with selective mutism. *J Am Acad Child Adoles Psychiatry* 1997; **36**(5):653–660.

163. Gordon N: Mutism: elective or selective and acquired. *Brain Dev*, 2001; **23**(2):83–87.

164. Carlson JS, Kratochwill TR, Johnston HF: Sertraline treatment of 5 children diagnosed with selective mutism: A single-case research trial. *J Child Adolesc Psychopharmacol*, 1999; **9**(4):293–306.

165. Golwyn DH, Sevlie CP: Phenelzine treatment of selective mutism in four prepubertal children. *J Child Adolesc Psychopharmacol* 1999; **9**(2):109–113.

14

Substance Use in Adolescents

Jacqueline Countryman

Introduction

Despite some evidence indicating that adolescent substance use is a normal part of development it is one of the strongest predictors of later adult substance abuse disorders [1]. Over 90% of adult addicts started substance use in adolescence [2]. Substance use among the adolescent population is increasing and is responsible for multiple problems including an increase in mortality among this age group [3]. The three leading causes of death in young people between the ages of 15 and 24 years in the US in descending order are accidents, homicides, and suicide. Alcohol and other drugs have contributed to each of these causes [4].

Most adolescents have not obtained a mature level of cognitive, emotional, social or physical growth and will experiment with a range of attitudes and behaviors. This experimentation also includes use of substances. Typically adolescents start experimenting with 'gateway' drugs including tobacco and alcohol. The use of substances in the preteen population has not been researched as well as the adolescent population and therefore, this chapter concentrates on the use of substances in adolescents.

Epidemiology

The number of adolescents using drugs and alcohol has been falling in the recent past but numbers overall continue to be worrisome. In 2003 the National Institute on Drug Abuse, Monitoring the Future found the following:

- 51% of 12th graders had used illicit drugs during their lifetimes;
- 58% of 12th graders reported having been intoxicated;
- 46% reported use of marijuana;
- 14% reported use of amphetamines;

- 11% reported use of hallucinogens;
- 9% reported use of barbiturates;
- 8% reported use of cocaine;
- 1.5% reported use of heroin;
- 8% reported use of MDMA (ecstasy).

Positive findings from were reported in this study include:

- use of any illicit drug in the past 30 days (current use) was down 11%. As a result of this decline approximately 400 000 fewer youth in 2003 were using illicit drugs than in 2001;
- Current use of marijuana declined 11%;
- lifetime use of LSD declined 43%;
- lifetime use of ecstasy declined 32%;
- lifetime use of inhalants declined 12%;
- lifetime use of amphetamines declined 15%;
- current use of alcohol declined 7% [5].

Risk Factors

Family/Parent Factors

Parents and siblings are role models for adolescents. Their attitudes toward drinking and their drinking habits correlate with adolescents' drinking patterns [6]. The influence of siblings has been a stronger correlate on adolescent drug-taking behaviors than parents' influence. The gender of the parent also has shown to be an influence on substance use. Mothers' drinking habits have been shown to be more relevant for adolescents' drinking than is the fathers' [7]. Family bonding has been shown to decrease the risk of alcohol and other drug use among adolescents [8].

Family environmental risk factors that stem from substance use include: excessively high family conflict, low parent–child attachment, poor parenting skills, lax or excessive punishment, physical or sexual abuse,

Clinical Child Psychiatry, Second Edition. Edited by W.M. Klykylo and J.L. Kay
© 2005 John Wiley & Sons Ltd.

ineffective communication, lack of sharing of proso-cial family values, little time spent supervising and monitoring children's activities and friends, and no sharing of positive leisure time activities and ways to reduce stress [9]. The discipline style of the parent influences substance use. Inconsistent and unpre-dictable parental discipline and parental permissive-ness have been shown to increase the risk of substance use in adolescents [10].

Family protective factors include supportive parent–child relationships, positive discipline methods, monitoring and supervision, family advocacy for their children, and seeking information and support for the benefit of children [11].

Open communication with parents and feeling sup-ported by parents are protective factors. Even when parents use substances there can be protective factors. Seeing the ramifications of substance use in their parents can deter adolescents from using [12]. Anti-drug parental attitudes are reasons why adolescents do not use drugs and alcohol [13]. Parental attitudes con-cerning drug use play a greater role for girls than boys. In contrast the community and neighborhood envi-ronment has a greater influence on boys than girls [14].

Peer Factors

Peer tolerance or approval of drug use, and whether friends have asked, encouraged, or pressured an ado-lescent all influence an adolescents' drug usage [15]. Parental norms have been found to be more important for early adolescents (mean age 13 years) and peer norms more important for middle adolescents (mean age 15 years). During mid-adolescence peer influence may peek as children spend more time with their peers than with family [16]. The single strongest predictor of adolescent substance use is having friends who use drugs. Eighty-eight percent of substance users stated that they had friends who also use [13].

Community Factors

Social environmental norms, role models, social support, and opportunities for nonuse of drugs have been shown to be related to adolescent drug use [17]. Other factors that have shown an influence include low socioeconomic status, high population density, physi-cal deterioration of the neighborhood, and high crime [18]. With children an important component is the school environment. Those adolescents who feel con-nected to the school are at a lower risk for using and abusing substances [19]. Adolescents expected to have high academic achievement by their parents are also

at lower risk [20]. Adolescents with poor academic achievement and low commitment to education are more likely to engage in substance use [12]. Work is also included in community factors and those adoles-cents who work more than 20 hours per week are at a greater risk for use and abuse [21].

Genetic Factors

The role of genetics in alcoholism has been studied with adoption and twin studies. Studies done in the 1930s and 1940s in Denmark showed an association between alcoholic biological fathers and male adoptees developing alcoholism [21]. More recent research has implicated the A1 allele of the dopamine D2 receptor being associated with alcoholism [22]. Sons of alco-holics have a higher tolerance to the effects of alcohol and therefore may not notice the effects that alcohol can have until they drink larger quantities [23].

Cloninger has concluded that risk factors for alco-holism are mediated in large part by inborn, heritable differences in temperament and learning styles [24]. Cloninger type 2 alcoholics demonstrate interpersonal risk factors that lead to continued use. These risk factors are a high-level of novelty seeking, a low-level of harm avoidance, and a low-level of reward depend-ence. They also show other risk factors including: early onset of spontaneous alcohol-seeking behavior; diag-nosis during adolescence; rapid course of onset; possible genetic precursors that put them at risk for substance use; and severe symptoms of deviant behav-ior, including fighting and arrests while drinking.

Individual Factors

Traits that are associated with substance use are aggression, depression, impulsivity, sensation-seeking behavior, and positive attitudes toward substance use [13]. Gender and age are also risk factors. Males have higher rates of alcoholism than females. The age of greatest risk to initiate alcohol and marijuana use is between the ages of 16 and 18 years [25]. Use of sub-stances before the age of 15 years increases the risk of future substance use/abuse. Table 14.1 lists risk factors associated with drug use.

Comorbidity

Studies of treatment seeking adolescents with sub-stance use disorders have documented that 50%–90% also have nonsubstance use comorbid psychiatric dis-orders [27]. Although a high prevalence of comorbid-ity has been reported among adolescent inpatients with

Table 14.1 Risk Factors Associated with Drug Use

I.   Family/Parent Factors
     Family conflict
     Low parent-child attachment
     Poor parenting
     Lax/excessive punishment
     Physical/sexual abuse
     Ineffective communication
     Little time supervising/monitoring children's
          activities
     Parental drug attitudes

II. Peer Factors
     Peer tolerance/approval of drug use
     Peer rejection

III. Community Factors
     Low socioeconomic status
     High population density
     Physical deterioration of neighborhood
     High crime
     Availability of drugs in community

IV. School Factors
     No connection with school
     Poor academic achievement

V.   Genetic Factors
     Inherited susceptibility to drug abuse

VI. Individual Factors
     Age
     Gender
     Aggression, especially early onset
     Depression
     Impulsivity
     Sensation-seeking behavior
     Positive attitudes towards substance use

Newcomb MD: Psychosocial predictors and consequences of drug use: a development perspective within a prospective study. J Addict Dis 1997; 16:57–89. Reproduced by permission of The Haworth Press.

drug use disorders, it is unclear how many of them exhibit psychiatric symptoms secondary to the substance abuse disorder and how many have a primary or coexisting psychiatric diagnosis. Some researchers have felt that methodological considerations, including the length of abstinence required before the diagnosis is made, the population studied, and the perspective of the examiner, affect prevalence rates for psychiatric dis-

orders in persons who abuse substances and account for the variability. They see the prevalence rates artificially elevated by the tendency to make a diagnosis before abatement of some of the psychiatric symptomatology secondary to substance use [28].

Depression

Depression is thought to be the primary component of substance dependence in women [29]. The question of which came first is an ongoing one with depressive disorders. One study of inpatient adolescent substance abusers with major depression showed that 60% had a secondary depression and 16% had a primary diagnosis [30]. Another study showed that 53% of inpatients with substance use disorders had dysthymia prior to the substance problems [31].

Bipolar Disorder

In teens, the diagnosis of bipolar disorder is a difficult diagnosis to make and even more difficult when there is possible substance abuse. Studies have shown an increased risk of substance use disorders in adolescents diagnosed with bipolar disorder. Children who are treated at a younger age for bipolar disorder have a decreased risk of substance use. It is important to make the diagnosis of bipolar disorder during a period of abstinence from substance use because there is an overlap of manic symptoms with substance intoxication [32].

Anxiety Disorders

Anxiety disorders are among the most common psychiatric conditions in adolescents and often can be missed if there is a coexisting substance abuse disorder. Many patients first use substances to help reduce or relieve anxiety. The onset of anxiety disorders is more likely to precede a substance use disorder in all countries [33]. Adolescents with anxiety often do not come to the attention of teachers and clinicians because they don't usually exhibit behavioral problems. The combination of shyness and aggressiveness has been shown to be a valid predictor of future cocaine use in boys [34]. Adolescents who have experienced trauma may use substances to help relieve symptoms of post-traumatic stress disorder [35].

Schizophrenia

The onset of schizophrenia typically is in the late teenage years. The use of substances may precipitate an incipient psychosis [28]. Young persons with schizophrenia may abuse substances in an attempt to manage or deny their symptoms. Their use of substances often interferes with treatment for their psychotic disorder [36].

Attention Deficit Hyperactivity Disorder

Attention deficit hyperactivity disorder (ADHD) is a common comorbid diagnosis with adolescents who have substance abuse problems. There has been debate whether ADHD is directly connected with the increased risk for substance abuse or if the presence of conduct disorder in addition to the ADHD is the true risk factor. Children with ADHD with conduct disorder have a much greater risk for substance abuse than do children with ADHD alone. [37] Studies have shown that individuals with ADHD began drug use at an earlier age, had more severe substance abuse, and had a more negative self-image before drug use [38].

The issue of medicating adolescents with psychostimulants and increasing their risk of substance abuse has been studied. Studies have been consistent in showing that successful treatment of adolescents with stimulants actually lowers their probability of developing a substance use disorder [37]. In fact one study showed that if an adolescent has ADHD and is treated, the risk for a substance use disorder is reduced by 85% [39].

Conduct Disorder

Conduct disorder is one of the most common comorbid diagnoses with substance abuse, especially in boys [40]. Reebye *et al.* have found that 52% of pre-adolescents and adolescents they studied with conduct disorder also met criteria for a substance use disorder [41]. In the younger age group the probability of comorbidity was greater. The prognosis of adolescents who develop conduct disorder prior to a substance abuse disorder is poorer than for those who develop conduct disorder during the substance abuse disorder [42].

Eating Disorders

One fourth of patients with an eating disorder have a history of substance abuse or are currently abusing substances [43]. Persons with eating disorders may abuse amphetamines to lose weight. The use of substances is more prevalent in bulimia nervosa than in anorexia nervosa.

Suicidality

In a study done by Shafii *et al.* postmortem analysis of adolescents who committed suicide demonstrated that 70% were drug and alcohol users [44].

Assessment

The first part of assessment should be a clinical interview with the patient and collateral sources. Part of substance abuse is deception and denial and thus collateral sources are extremely important. Areas to explore include substance use behaviors; psychiatric and behavior problems; school functioning; family functioning; peer relationships; and leisure activities. In the area of substance use behavior it is important to ask about the quantity, frequency, onset, type of substance used, negative consequences, context of use, and control of use. These questions need to be asked with each substance identified. As part of the clinical interview risk factors should be evaluated. Of particular importance is the parent's own history of substance use, attitudes about drug use, the type and level of discipline used within the home, and the level of attachment between the child and parent.

Laboratory measures are often used to detect use. Urinalysis is the most widely used test but is limited to the short and variable detection period for substances. Stimulants are detected up to 1–2 days after use. Cocaine is detected for several days after use. Sedative hypnotic drugs are variable ranging from one day to one week or more for the long acting benzodiazepines, to about two weeks for long acting barbiturates. Opiates are detected for up to two days. Cannabis can be detected up to 30 days especially with chronic use. A positive drug screening test does not confirm a diagnosis of abuse or dependence but does confirm use.

Self report instruments can be used as an adjunct to the clinical interview but should not be relied upon as the only source to make a diagnosis. Table 14.2 lists several examples of self-report screening and diagnostic instruments that can be used with adolescents. Most can be self or clinician administered and take a short time to take and score.

The diagnosis of Substance Abuse and Dependence are defined by the DSM-IV-TR as a maladaptive pattern of substance abuse leading to clinically significant impairment. Other criteria are listed in Table 14.3 that distinguish between the two.

Medical Concerns

Alcohol and other Central Nervous System Depressants

Clinicians who work with adolescents should be familiar with the presentation of alcohol intoxication, alcohol withdrawal, and symptoms of abuse and dependence especially in the emergency room setting. The CAGE questionnaire can be used as a screening

Table 14.2 Self-help and diagnostic instruments.

Measure	Type
Adolescent Drug Abuse Diagnosis ADAD (Friedman and Ueada 1989)	Structured interview, comprehensive assessment drug/alcohol use
Adolescent Diagnostic Interview ADI (Winters and Henly 1993)	Structured interview, diagnostic assessment
Adolescent Problem Severity Index APSI (Metzger *et al.* 1991)	Semistructured interview; comprehensive assessment, identifies drug use patterns
Diagnostic Interview Schedule for Children DISC (Shaffer *et al.* 1996)	Structured interview; diagnostic assessment
Minnesota Multiphasic Personality Inventory – Adolescent MMPI-A (Wood *et al.* 1994)	Self-administered screen, identifies and describes drug/alcohol related problems
Personal Experience Inventory PEI (Winters and Henly, 1989)	Self-administered, comprehensive assessment; identifies drug/alcohol use patterns
Personal Experience Screening Questionnaire PESQ (Winters 1993)	Self-administered screen; identifies drug/alcohol use
Problem Oriented Screening Instrument for Teenagers POSIT (Rahden 1991)	Self-administered screen; identifies potential drug/alcohol use
Substance Abuse Subtle Screening Inventory SASSI (Miller 1990)	Self-administered screen; identifies drug/alcohol use and tendency to deny use
Teen Addiction Severity Index TASI (Kaminer *et al.* 1991)	Structured interview; comprehensive assessment

tool though it is used more in adults than in adolescents [45]. The CAGE consists of four questions with two or more positive answers suggestive of alcoholism.

1. Have you ever felt the need to **C**ut down on your drinking?
2. Have you ever felt **A**nnoyed that others criticized your drinking?
3. Have you ever felt bad or **G**uilty about your drinking?
4. Have you ever felt the need for an **E**ye-Opener first thing in the morning?

A more developmentally appropriate questionnaire is the CRAFFT [46]. It consists of six questions with two or more yes answers suggestive of a significant problem.

1. Have you ever ridden in a **C**ar driven by someone (including yourself) who was 'high' or had been using alcohol or drugs?
2. Do you ever use alcohol or drugs to **R**elax, feel better about yourself, or fit in?
3. Have you ever used alcohol or drugs while you are **A**lone?
4. Do any of your **F**amily or **F**riends ever tell you that you should cut down on your drinking or drug use?
5. Do you ever **F**orget things you did while using alcohol or drugs?
6. Have you gotten in **T**rouble while you were using alcohol or drugs?

Alcohol intoxication in adolescents is identical to that in adults. This can be broken down into three stages. The initial stage consists of low-levels of blood alcohol concentration (BAC) leading to an increase in disinhibition, increased feelings of self-confidence, impaired judgment, and a loss of fine-motor tasks. The next stage, the excitement stage begins with a BAC of 100 mg/dL and leads to impaired memory, increased distractibility, and impaired concentration. Above a

Table 14.3 DSM-IV TR diagnosis. Reprinted with permission from the Diagnostic and Statistical Manual of Mental Disorders, Copyright 2000. American Psychiatric Association.

Substance Abuse
A maladaptive pattern of substance use leading to clinically significant impairment or distress, as manifested by one (or more) of the following, occurring within a 12-month period:

- recurrent substance use resulting in a failure to fulfill major role obligations at work, school, or home;
- recurrent substance use in situations in which it is physically hazardous;
- recurrent substance-related legal problems;
- continued substance use despite having persistent or recurrent social or interpersonal problems caused or exacerbated by the effects of the substance;
- the symptoms have never met the criteria for substance dependence for this class of substance.

Substance Dependence
A maladaptive pattern of substance use, leading to clinically significant impairment or distress, as manifested by three (or more) of the following, occurring at any time in the same 12-month period.

(1) Tolerance, as defined by either of the following:
    (a) a need for markedly increased amounts of the substance to achieve intoxication or desired effect;
    (b) markedly diminished effect with continued use of the same amount of the substance.
(2) Withdrawal, as manifested by either of the following:
    (a) the characteristic withdrawal syndrome for the substance;
    (b) the same substance is taken to relieve or avoid withdrawal symptoms.
(3) The substance is often taken in larger amounts or over a longer period than was intended.
(4) There is a persistent desire or unsuccessful efforts to cut down or control substance use.
(5) A great deal of time is spent in activities necessary to obtain the substance, use the substance, or recover from its effects.
(6) Important social, occupational, or recreational activities are given up or reduced because of substance use.
(7) The substance use is continued despite knowledge of having a persistent or recurrent physical or psychological problem that is likely to have been caused or exacerbated by the substance.

From: American Psychiatric Association: *Diagnostic and Statistical Manual, Fourth Edition, Text Revision (DSM-IV-TR)*. Washington DC: American Psychiatric Press, 2000.

BAC of 200 mg/dL persons exhibit confusion, disorientation, dizziness, ataxia, diplopia, and slurred speech.

Alcohol withdrawal for adolescents is usually not as severe as it is with adults possibly due to adolescents being in better health and using substances for less time than adults. The symptoms of alcohol withdrawal generally begin 24 hours after cessation of use and will resolve within several days. The treatment of uncomplicated alcohol withdrawal is generally the same in adolescents as in adults though the literature is sparse on this topic. Long-acting benzodiazepines are typically used and administered on a fixed or symptom triggered schedule. Alcohol withdrawal seizures are typically seen 24–48 hours after last use. Delirium tremens is a medical emergency and are seen 48–120 hours after last use. Symptoms are autonomic instability, severe tremors, and mental status changes. They are rare in adolescents but require intensive care unit monitoring if seen.

Marijuana

Intoxication symptoms include impaired motor coordination, anxiety, impaired judgment, conjunctival injection, increased appetite, dry mouth, and tachycardia. Withdrawal with marijuana is a controversial subject. The DSM-IV does not recognize cannabis withdrawal though it has been described in the literature [47]. Its symptoms are insomnia, irritability, restlessness, drug craving, depression, and nervousness. Pharmacologic treatment for intoxication and withdrawal are rarely indicated.

Cocaine

During cocaine intoxication agitation and anxiety may occur. A person may also present with psychotic symptoms including formication. Other symptoms include hypertension, arrhythmias, or seizures. Withdrawal symptoms include mild depression, anxiety, and fatigue. Treatment for intoxication and withdrawal is typically supportive. Complications can arise from the method of use including nasal perforation, HIV, Hepatitis C and infections at the injection site.

Opiates

Intoxication symptoms include initial euphoria followed by apathy, dysphoria, psychomotor agitation or retardation, impaired judgment, or impaired social or occupational functioning. Physical symptoms include papillary constriction, drowsiness, slurred speech, and impaired attention. Naloxone use causes opiate withdrawal and can be life saving. Withdrawal symptoms include dysphoric mood, nausea, muscle aches, lacrimation, piloerection, diarrhea, yawning. Methadone or clonidine have been used for treatment [48].

Phencyclidine (PCP)

Intoxication symptoms include nystagmus, hypertension, numbness, ataxia, dysarthria, seizures. Agitation and psychotic symptoms can result. Treatment is typically supportive. Severe intoxication may require medical or psychiatric monitoring. The DSM-IV does not recognize PCP withdrawal though in animal models symptoms include tremor, lethargy, piloerection, and seizures [49].

Ecstasy

Intoxication consists of disorientation, increased sociability, increased mental clarity, a feeling of closeness to others, and a general sense of well-being. Other physical symptoms noted with intoxication include hyperthermia, tachycardia, hypertension, agitation and confusion. A 'hang-over' feeling is often noted 24–48 hours after last use consisting of confusion, depression, restlessness, insomnia and paranoia. Treatment is supportive [50].

Ketamine

Ketamine is a noncompetitive NMDA receptor antagonist and is considered a psychotmimetic or schizophrenomimetic drug. In large doses it produces reactions similar to PCP. At lower doses it results in impaired attention and memory. At higher doses it can result in delirium, amnesia, hypertension or depression [51]. Treatment is supportive [52].

Gamma Hydrxybutyrate (GHB)

GHB is a naturally occurring inhibitory neurotransmitter. It is used for its intoxicating, sedating and euphoria-producing effects or for its growth hormone-releasing effects. Withdrawal from GHB has been described and looks similar to alcohol withdrawal [53].

Treatment

The goals of treatment for substance use disorders with adolescents are first achieving and maintaining abstinence from substance use. These goals are difficult to achieve and practitioners need to keep in mind that because of the chronicity of the problem in some adolescents, and the self-limiting nature of substance use in other adolescents, a reduction of harm may be a more achievable goal.

Many adolescents with substance use disorders have comorbid psychiatric diagnosis or have social/family/educational problems that should also be addressed in the treatment plan.

Characteristics of treatment that have been shown to be related to improved abstinence and lower relapse rates are [54,55]:

- Treatment that is intensive and of needed duration to achieve change. The intensity and duration should depend on the level of substance involvement, level of motivation of the adolescent and the family, the quality of social supports, the presence of comorbid psychiatric diagnosis, and the existence of deficits in other psychosocial areas.
- Treatment should be comprehensive and target all areas that are noted to be dysfunctional in the adolescent's life.
- Treatment should encourage family involvement. Working with the parents to provide appropriate and effective limits should be a focus. Also any addiction noted in the parents should be addressed.
- Treatment should address the adolescent and the family developing a drug-free lifestyle.
- Treatment should include self-help groups for both the adolescent and the family.
- Treatment should be sensitive to the culture and socioeconomic limitations of the family.
- Treatment programs should work with social service agencies, juvenile justice and the school system.
- Treatment should include an after-care component.
- Treatment should be multimodal to achieve the above goals.

Treatment Settings

As with any care rendered to patients the least restrictive setting that is safe and effective should be sought for adolescents with substance use disorders. The treatment settings that are available include: inpatient, residential, partial hospitalization and outpatients treatment with or without community treatment (self-help groups). Factors that providers should look at to determine the appropriate level of care include:

- motivation and willingness to cooperate;
- need for structure and limit-setting;
- need for a safe environment;
- adolescent's ability to care for him/her self;
- comorbid conditions;
- availability of treatment settings;
- adolescent/families preference for treatment;
- past treatment failure in a less restrictive setting.

Listed in Table 14.4 are each treatment setting and when to utilize the setting for a specific patient.

Treatment Modalities

Cognitive Behavioral Therapy (CBT)
CBT is used to identify negative thinking patterns and cognitive distortions and then modify these to reduce negative feelings and behavior. Adolescents in a CBT program have demonstrated a reduction in the severity of substance use [56,57].

Table 14.4 Treatment settings.

Inpatient
Severe psychiatric disorders, treatment failure in less restrictive setting, patients with withdrawal risk/history

Residential
Severe personality disorders, inadequate psychosocial supports, history of treatment failure after inpatient care

Partial hospitalization
Twenty-four hour supervision not necessary, step-down from inpatient; stable social supports

Outpatient
Highly motivated, stable social supports, limited comorbid psychopathology, following successful treatment in higher level of care

---

Behavioral Therapy
Inpatient, residential, and partial hospitalization programs often use the operant conditioning methods that are part of behavioral therapy. This includes rewarding and punishing the adolescent for appropriate and inappropriate behaviors. Parent management training is also included in behavioral therapy. Behavioral contingency contracting pairs a specific behavior to a positive reinforcer after a certain goal is obtained. Parents are then trained on how to continue this method when the adolescent returns home.

Dynamic and Interpersonal Therapy
These methods are used often in clinical practice with adolescents with substance use disorders. However, there are no controlled studies in this population.

Self-Help Groups
Participation in self-help groups is a part of many treatment programs. Adolescents receive support from other recovering peers. Role models for recovery and abstinence are available. The 12-step approach is the most widely used to treat adolescents with substance use disorders. The philosophy of the 12-step approach is that recovery from addiction is possible only if the person recognizes his/her problem with drugs/alcohol and admits that he/she is unable to use substances in moderation without significant consequences. Spiritual growth is seen as critical to this process. There has been little published research on the use of 12-step approaches with adolescents. Studies that have been done show a lower substance use rate in those who attend Alcoholics Anonymous (AA) or Narcotics Anonymous (NA) groups than those who do not (Table 14.5) [58].

Family Therapy
Family approaches have been found to be critical for good outcomes in adolescent substance use. This makes sense when looking at the number of risk factors for substance use that involve the family or parents. Goals of family therapy include psychoeducation, assisting the family on getting the adolescent into treatment, assisting the family in establishing structure with consistent limit-setting and monitoring, and improving communication within the family. There are many approaches to family therapy. Cognitive behavioral family focused programs have the largest evidence of effectiveness, the largest effect size, and the most lasting effects [59,60]. In contrast parent education programs have not been found to be effective. Structural–strategic family therapy has been

Table 14.5 The 12 steps of Alcoholics Anonymous and Narcotics Anonymous.

(1) We admitted we were powerless over alcohol (our addiction) – that our lives had become unmanageable.

(2) We came to believe that a Power greater than ourselves could restore us to sanity.

(3) We made a decision to turn our will and our lives over to the care of God, as we understood Him.

(4) We made a searching and fearless moral inventory of ourselves.

(5) We admitted to God, to ourselves, and to another human being the exact nature of our wrongs.

(6) We were entirely ready to have God remove all these defects of character.

(7) We humbly asked Him to remove our shortcomings.

(8) We made a list of persons we had harmed and became willing to make amends to them all.

(9) We made direct amends to such people wherever possible, except when to do so would injure them or others.

(10) We continued to take a personal inventory and when we were wrong promptly admitted it.

(11) We sought through prayer and medication to improve our conscious contact with God, as we understood Him, praying only for knowledge of His will for us and the power to carry that out.

(12) Having had a spiritual awakening as the result of these steps, we tried to carry this message to alcoholics (addicts) and to practice these principles in all our affairs.

shown to improve the parent–adolescent relationship and in turn reduces the adolescent's drug use [61]. Structural–strategic family therapy involves the whole family and focuses on the dysfunctional family structure and interactional patterns.

Community Based Interventions

Multisystemic therapy (MST) has been shown to be an effective model for community based alternatives for violent chronic juvenile offenders with substance use disorders. MST targets individual, family, peer, school, and community factors. Studies have shown that it reduces substance use and deviant behaviors in subjects [62,63].

Medication Management

Few clinical trials have been conducted on pharmacotherapuetic agents for treating adolescent substance use disorders. Data from adult studies should be extrapolated to adolescents with caution. Treatment of withdrawal symptoms in adolescents is rare [64]. Treatment should proceed as would the treatment of withdrawal in adults. The use of pharmacologic agents to decrease the subjective reinforcing effects of a substance is limited to case reports in the literature. The use of such agents should be reserved for treatment after other proven methods have been utilized. The use of aversive agents, such as disulfiram, should also be limited in use in adolescents due to concerns with safety and compliance.

The treatment of comorbid psychiatric disorders with psychopharmacologic agents is critical in the overall treatment plan. A period of abstinence is recommended so that a definitive assessment can be made. Few studies have been done in this population. A placebo controlled study has examined lithium use in children and adolescents with comorbid bipolar disorder and substance use disorders. Twenty-six subjects aged 7–18 years were treated with lithium or placebo for six weeks. Positive urine toxicology screens decreased significantly, and global assessment of functioning improved in 46% of those receiving lithium versus 8% of those receiving placebo [65].

An assessment of the risk of abuse of a therapeutic agent by the adolescent or family should be done. All medications should be monitored under adult supervision. Also the choice of agent should be considered with agents with lower abuse potential being chosen first.

Prevention

Clinicians need to be aware of the risk factors for substance use disorders in youth. These risk factors need to be targeted and appropriate intervention made. School-based interventions are the mainstay of prevention research. Research by Botvin et al. showed significant reductions in drug use with long-term positive results after implementation of a classroom-based intervention [66]. Interactive as opposed to didactic programs have been shown to have greater effect [67]. Another preventive target is parent training. Parents who included consistent limit-setting and discipline combined with love, warmth, and involvement raise children who are engaged in fewer high-risk behaviors [68].

Conclusion

Substance abuse and dependence is a major problem facing the adolescent population today. Research on this topic has made many advances over the past 10 years but much still needs to be discovered. We know a great deal about the risk and preventive factors involved in substance use disorders. We know that in treatment the involvement of the family is critical and we know what treatments are the most effective. Further studies on the cause and on definitive treatments are needed to continue to help this population with this widespread problem.

References

1. Shedler J, Block J: Adolescent drug use and psychological health. *Am Psychol* 1990; **45**:612–630.
2. Sheehan M, Oppenheimer E, Taylor C: Who comes for treatment: Drug misusers at three London agencies. *Br J Addict* 1988, **83**:311–320.
3. Johnston L, Bachman JG, O'Malley PM: National trends in Drug Use and Related Factors Among American High School Students and Young Adults, 1975–1987. National Institute on Drug Abuse Publ. no. ADM-87-1587. Washington, DC: US Department of Health and Human Services, 1987.
4. Kaplan HI, Sadock BJ: Synopsis of Psychiatry. 8th ed. Baltimore: Williams & Wilkins, 1998.
5. Johnston L, O'Malley P, Bachman J: *Monitoring the Future. National Results on Adolescent Drug Use: Overview of Key Findings, 2003.* Bethesda, MD: National Institute on Drug Abuse, 2004.
6. D'Amico EJ, Fromme K: Health risk behaviors of adolescent and young adult siblings. *Health Psychol* 1997; **16**(5):426–432.
7. White HR, Johnson V, Buyske S: Parental modeling and parenting behavior effects on offspring alcohol and cigarette use. A growth curve analysis. *J Substance Abuse* 2000; **12**(3):287–310.
8. Bahr SJ, Marcos AC, Maughan SL: Family, educational and peer influences on the alcohol use of female and male adolescents. *J Stud Alcohol* 1995; **56**(4):457–469.
9. Kumpfer KL: Special populations: Etiology and prevention of vulnerability to chemical dependency in children of substance abusers. In: Brown BS, Mills AR, eds. *Youth at High Risk for Substance Abuse.* Rockville, MD: NIDA Monograph, 1987:1–71.
10. Dielman TE, Butchart AT, Shope JT, Miller M: Environmental correlates of adolescent substance use and misuse: Implications for prevention programs. *Int J Addict* 1990/1991; **25**:855–880.
11. Bry BH, Catalano RF, Kumpfer KL, Lochman JE, Szapocznik J: Scientific findings from family prevention intervention research. In: Ashery RS, Robertson E, Kumpfer KL, eds. Family focused prevention of drug abuse: Research and interventions. NIDA Research Monograph, Washington, DC: Superintendent of Documents, US Government Printing Office, 1998:103–129.
12. Patton LH: Adolescent substance abuse: Risk factors and protective factors. *Pediatr Clin North Am* 1995; **42**: 283–293.
13. Dembo R, Wothke W, Shemwell M, Pacheco K, Seeberger W, Rollie M, Schmeidler J: A structural model of the influence of family problems and child abuse factors on serious delinquency among youths processed at a juvenile assessment center. *J Child and Adolesc Substance Abuse* 2000; **10**:17–31.
14. Center for Substance Abuse Prevention. Preventing Substance Abuse Among Children and Adolescents: Family-Centered Approaches. Prevention enhancement protocols system. DHHS Publication No. 3223-FY'98. Washington DC: Supt. Of Docs. US Government Printing Office.
15. Graham JW, Marks G, Hansen WB: Social influences processes affecting adolescent substance use. *J Appl Psychol* 1991; **76**(2):291–298.
16. Biddle BJ, Bank BJ, Marlin MM: Parental and peer influences on adolescence. *Social Forces* 1980; **58**(4):1057–1080.
17. Roski J, Perry CL, McGovern PG, Williams CL, Farbakhsh K, Veblen-Mortenson S: School and community influences on adolescent alcohol and drug use. *Health Educ Res* 1997; **12**(2):255–266.
18. Brook JS, Whiteman M, Gordon AS, Brook DW: The psychosocial etiology of adolescent drug use: A family interactional approach. *Gen Social Psychol Monogr* 1990; **116**, entire issue.
19. Resnick MD, Harris LJ, Blum RW: The impact of caring and connectedness on adolescent health and well-being. *J Paediatr Child Health* 1993; **29**(Suppl 1): 3–9.
20. Resnick MD, Bearman PS, Blum RW, *et al.*: Protecting adolescents from harm: Findings from the national longitudinal study on adolescent health. *JAMA* 1997; **278**:823–832.
21. Goodwin DW, Schulsinger F, Hermansen L, *et al.*: Alcohol problems in adoptees raised apart from alcoholic biological parents. *Arch Gen Psychiatry* 1973; **28**: 238–443.
22. Blum K, Noble EP, Sheridan PJ, *et al.* Alleic association of human dopamine D2 receptor gene in alcoholism. *JAMA* 1990; **263**:2055–2060.
23. Schukit MA: A 10 year study of sons of alcoholics: Preliminary results. *Alcohol* 1999(Suppl 1):147–149.
24. Cloninger CR: Neurogenetic adoptive mechanisms in alcoholism. *Science* 1987; **236**:410–416.
25. Beman DS: Risk factors leading to adolescent substance abuse. *Adolescence* 1995; **30**:201–208.
26. Newcomb MD: Psychosocial predictors and consequences of drug use: A development perspective within a prospective study. *J Addict Dis* 1997; **16**:57–89.
27. Clark DB, Bukstein OG: Psychopathology in adolescent alcohol abuse and dependence. *Alcohol Health Res World* 1998; **22**:117–126.
28. Miller NS, Fine J: Current epidemiology of comorbidity of psychiatric and addictive disorders. *Psychiatr Clin N Am* 1993; **16**:1–10.
29. Whitmore EA, Milulick SK, Thompson LL, *et al.*: Influences on adolescent substance dependence, conduct disorders, depression, attention deficit hyperactivity disorder, and gender. *Drug Alcohol Depend* 1997; **47**: 87–97.
30. Bukstein OG, Glancy LJ, Kaminer Y: Patterns of affective comorbidity in a clinical population of dually diagnosed adolescent substance abusers. *J Am Acad Child Adolesc Psychiatry* 1992; **31**:1041–105.

31. Hovens JG, Cantwell DP, Kiriakos R: Psychiatric comorbidity in hospitalized adolescent substance abusers. *J Am Acad Child Adolesc Psychiatry* 1994; 33: 476–483.

32. Wilens TE, Biederman J, Millstein RB, et al. Risk for substance use disorders in youths with child and adolescent-onset bipolar disorder. *J Am Acad Child Adolesc Psychiatry* 1999; 38:680–685.

33. Merikangas KR, Mehta RL, Molnar BE, et al.: Comorbidity of substance use disorders with mood and anxiety disorders: Results of international consortium in psychiatric epidemiology. *Addict Behav* 1998; 23: 893–907.

34. Swan N: Early childhood behavior and temperament predict later substance abuse. *National Institute on Drug Abuse Notes* 1995; 10:1–6.

35. Clark DB, Lesnick L, Hegedus AM: Traumas and other adverse life events in adolescents with alcohol use and dependence. *J Am Acad Child Adolesc Psychiatry* 1997; 36:1744–1751.

36. Buckley PF: Substance abuse in schizophrenia; a review. *J Clin Psychiatry* 1999; 59(Supp 3):26–30.

37. Wilens TE, Biederman J, Spencer TJ: Attention deficit hyperactivity disorder and psychoactive substance use disorders. *Child Adolesc Psychiatr Clin N Am* 1996; 5:73–91.

38. Horner B, Scheibe K: Prevalence and implications of attention-deficit hyperactivity disorder among adolescents in treatment for substance abuse. *J Am Acad Child Adolesc Psychiatry* 1997; 36:30–36.

39. Biederman J, Wilens T, Mick E, et al. Pharmacotherapy of ADHD reduces risk of substance use disorder. *Pediatrics* 1999; 104:e20.

40. American Academy of Child and Adolescent Psychiatry. Practice parameters for the assessment and treatment of children and adolescents with substance abuse disorders. *J Am Acad Child Adolesc Psychiatry* 1998; 37: 122–126.

41. Reebye P, Moretti M, Lessard J: Conduct disorder and substance use disorders: Comorbidity in a clinical sample of preadolescents and adolescents. *Can J Psychiatry* 1995; 40;313–319.

42. Myers MG, Stewart DG, Brown SA: Progression of conduct disorder to antisocial personality disorder following treatment for adolescent substance abuse. *Am J Psychiatry* 1998; 155:479–485.

43. Katz JL: Eating disorders: A primer for the substance abuse specialist. I: Clinical features. *J Subst Abuse Treat* 1990; 7:143–149.

44. Shafii M, Stelz-Linarsky J, Derrick AM, et al.: Comorbidity of mental disorders in the post mortem diagnosis of completed suicides in children and adolescents. *J Affect Disord* 1998; 15:227–233.

45. Issacson JH, Schorling JB: Screening for alcohol problems in primary care. *Med Clin N Am* 1999; 83:1547–1563.

46. Knight JR, Shrier LA, Bravender TD, et al.: A new brief screen for adolescent substance abuse. *Arch Pediatr Adolesc Med* 1999; 153:591–596.

47. Duffy A, Millin R: Case study: Withdrawal syndrome in adolescent chronic cannabis users. *J Am Acad Child Adolesc Psychiatry* 1996; 35:1618–1621.

48. Jaffe SL, Estroff TW: Use of medications with substance-abusing adolescents. In: Estroff TW, ed. *Manual of Adolescent Substance Abuse Treatment.*

Washington, DC: American Psychiatric Publishing; 2001:187–203.

49. Baldridge EB, Besson HA: Phencyclidine. *Emerg Med Clin N Am* 1990; 8:541–550.

50. Schwartz RH, Miller NS: MDMA (ecstasy) and the rave: A review. *Pediatrics* 1997; 100:705–708.

51. Krystat JH, Karper LP, Siebyl JP, et al.: Subanesthetic effects of the noncompetitive NMDA antagonist, ketamine, in humans: Psychotmimetic, perceptual, cognitive, and neuroendocrine responses. *Arch Gen Psychiatry* 1994; 51:199–214.

52. Koesters SC, Rogers PD, Rajasingham CR: MDMA (ecstasy) and other club drugs: The new epidemic. *Pediatr Clin N Am* 2002; 49:415–433.

53. Galloway GP, Frederick SL, Staggers FE, et al.: Gamma-hydroxybutyrate: An emerging drug of abuse that causes physical dependence. *Addiction* 1997; 92:89–96.

54. Friedman AS, Beschner GM (eds): *Treatment Services for Adolescent Substance Abusers.* DHSS Pub No. (ADM) 85–1342, 1985; Washington DC: US Government Printing Office.

55. Fleisch B: *Approaches in the Treatment of Adolescents with Emotional and Substance Abuse Problems.* DHSS Pub. No. (ADM) 91–1744. 1991; Washington DC: US Government Printing Office.

56. Kaminer Y: Alcohol and drug abuse: Adolescent substance abuse treatment: Where do we go from here? *Psychiatr Serv* 2001; 52:147–149.

57. Kaminer Y, Burleson JA: Psychotherapies for adolescent substance abusers: 15 month follow-up of a pilot study. *Am J Addict* 1999; 8:114–119.

58. Alford GS, Koehler RA, Leonard J: Alcoholics anonymous-narcotics anonymous model inpatient treatment of chemically dependent adolescents: A 2-year outcome study. *J Studies Alcohol* 1991; 52:118–126.

59. Taylor TK, Biglan A: Behavioral family interventions for improving child-rearing: A review for clinicians and policy makers. *Clin Child Fam Psychol Rev* 1998; 1:41–60.

60. Webster-Stratton C, Taylor T: Nipping early risk factors in the bud: Preventing substance abuse, delinquency, and violence in adolescence through interventions targeted at young children-8 years. *Prev Science* 2000; 2: 165–192.

61. Joanning H, Quinn TF, Mullen R: Treating adolescent drug abuse: A comparison of family systems therapy, group therapy, and family drug education. *J Marital Fam Ther* 1992; 18:345–356.

62. Henggeler SW, Melton GB, Smith LA, et al.: Family preservation using multi-systemic treatment: Long term follow-up to a clinical trial with serious juvenile offenders. *J Child Fam Studies* 1993; 2:283–293.

63. Henggeler SW, Schoenwald SK, Pickrel SG, et al.: *Treatment Manual for Family Preservation Using Multisystemic Therapy.* Charleston: Medical University of South Carolina, 1994.

64. Martin CS, Kaczynski NA, Maiston SA, et al.: Patterns of alcohol abuse and dependence symptoms in adolescent drinkers. *J Studies on Alcohol* 1995; 56:672–680.

65. Geller B, Cooper TB, Watts HE, et al.: Early findings from a pharmacokinetically designed double-blind and placebo-controlled study of lithium for adolescents comorbid with bipolar and substance dependency disorders. *Prog Neuropsychopharmacol Biol Psychiatry* 1992; 16:281–299.

66. Botvin GJ, Baker E, Dusenbury L, *et al.*: Long-term follow-up results of a randomized drug abuse prevention trial in a white middle-class population. *JAMA* 1995; **273**;1106–1112.

67. Tobler NS, Stratton HS: Effectiveness of school-based drug prevention programs: A meta-analysis of the research. *J Prim Prevent* 1997; **18**:71–128.

68. Brook JS, Brook DW, Gordon AS, *et al.*: The psychological etiology of adolescent drug use: A family interactional approach. *Gen Soc Gen Psychol Monogr* 1990; **116**:111–267.

15

Childhood Trauma

Sidney Edsall, Niranjan S. Karnik, Hans Steiner

Introduction

Childhood trauma is a common presenting issue for the practicing clinician. The range of phenomena that bring about these issues can range from pediatric acute and chronic illness, to sexual abuse, and even entail mass trauma as the events surrounding the destruction of the World Trade Center in New York City highlight. Clinicians working with these varied populations of children need to be cognizant of current advances in the neurobiological underpinnings of trauma and post-traumatic stress, and its implications on treatment, as well as being sensitive to the social and family milieu that can help form the basis of good therapeutic interventions.

History of Trauma-Related Diagnosis

The diagnosis and treatment of psychological sequelae associated with traumatic events have changed greatly over the years and have only recently expanded to include children. Initially, the definition of traumatic events and the research that ensued were limited to war duty. The experiences of soldiers in World Wars I and II led to terms such as 'shell shock' and 'combat fatigue' and established a relationship between traumatic events and the resulting behavior and affect. It was not until the Vietnam War and the 1970s that the diagnosis of post-traumatic stress disorder (PTSD) was formally introduced into the mental health nomenclature. Although the early conceptualizations of the effects of trauma were significant in shaping our current understanding, the research in this area was largely based on adult men. Only in the last 20 years has the conceptualization of trauma and the incidents that induce trauma-related psychopathology been broadened to include the experiences of the general population, women, specific ethnic groups, and most

recently, those of children [1–3]. The association between the range of traumatic events and the resulting psychological and biological effects continues to challenge researchers and clinicians in the mental health community.

Traumatic Events

Traumatic events can be described as impacting children on at least one of the following three levels: the self, the community, and environment. Depending on their developmental stage, children may be particularly susceptible to the adverse effects of trauma because of their dependency on adults for care and safety, their limited ability to influence the events and surroundings in which they live, and their cognitive and emotional level of development. Over the past decade, there has been a considerable amount of research examining the impact of trauma on children. Studies to date suggest the psychiatric consequences of trauma are influenced by several variables, such as the level of exposure and duration of trauma [4,5], pre-existing psychopathology prior to trauma exposure [6–8], the impact of trauma on a child's social structure [9], and biological factors contributing to a child's predisposition to trauma-related pathology as well as resilience in the development of pathology [10]. In addition, a child's subjective experience of potential harm during trauma has been found to be associated with trauma-related symptoms as opposed to more objective accounts of traumatic events [11–13]. It is also apparent that different types of trauma impact children to varying degrees. For example, exposure to natural disasters results in a lower rate of PTSD development compared to more chronic, war-related traumas [14]. Interpersonal-related traumas, such as physical or sexual abuse, seem to be associated with the highest rates of PTSD [14–17].

Clinical Child Psychiatry, Second Edition. Edited by W.M. Klykylo and J.L. Kay
© 2005 John Wiley & Sons Ltd.

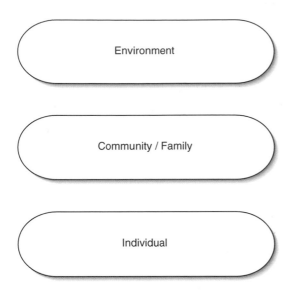

Figure 15.1 Levels of trauma experience.

Studies assessing the psychological sequelae of physical and sexual abuse in children have revealed the presence of significant trauma-related pathology [18–21]. The duration of abuse, the closeness of the perpetrator, and the use of violence all influence the severity of psychological symptoms that present during and following abuse [20]. Sexual abuse in children is associated with the development of depression, anxiety, behavioral problems, sexualized behaviors, and PTSD [19,21]. Victims of sexual abuse as children are at higher risk for having psychiatric problems in adulthood as well, including substance use disorders, social anxiety, and depression, and are at higher risk for attempting suicide [22,23]. Children who experience significant accidents, such as those involving motor vehicles and fires, or who suffer life-threatening illness and invasive medical procedures are at risk for developing psychological symptoms [24–26]. Additionally, children who are victims of violent crimes such as robbery, assault, and attempted murder are at high risk for developing PTSD, anxiety, and depressive disorders [27], and may demonstrate increased rates of internalizing and externalizing behavioral problems [28].

Children who witness violence in their immediate environment may develop trauma-related pathology. Violence within the family, such as abuse between parents or abuse between a parent and sibling, can create an environment of fear resulting in psychologi-cal distress and symptomatology [29–31]. Children who witness the assault or murder of a parent exhibit trauma-related symptoms such as anxiety, hypervigilance, and decreased concentration [32].

Trauma within the community can cause psychiatric disturbance in children, as reflected by research of violence in US inner cities [12,27,33–35]. US inner-city environments can parallel the environments of combat zones, as violence and aggression creates an atmosphere of potential danger and fear for personal safety and security. Ninety-two percent of 90 female adolescents living within a US urban environment and presenting for routine medical care endorsed at least one trauma, including witnessing community violence (86%) and hearing about a homicide (68%) [36]. Other community-based studies have reported more than 80% of inner-city adolescents have seen someone physically assaulted, 40% have seen someone shot or stabbed, and almost 25% have witnessed a homicide [34,37,38]. Mazza *et al.* reported a significant relationship between violence exposure and PTSD symptomatology, suicidal ideation, and depression in 94 young adolescents from an inner-city school within the US [39].

Terrorism-induced trauma imposes unique stress on the community and the individual. Due to its unpredictability and devastating effects, terrorism can create an environment of fear and intimidation within society persisting for prolonged periods of time. Few studies have been conducted to determine the effects on children in the aftermath of terrorist events such as the September 11, 2001 terrorist attacks, the 1995 bombing of the Alfred P. Murrah Building in Oklahoma City, the Scud missile attacks in Israel, state terrorism attacks in Guatemala between 1981 and 1983, and terrorist activity in Northern Ireland [40]. The rates of PTSD in children exposed to terrorism activity ranges from 28% to 50% [41–43]. Other psychiatric problems have been associated with terrorism, such as depression, anxiety, separation problems, mood changes, sleep difficulties, behavioral problems and regressive symptoms [40,41,43].

The terrorist attacks of September 11, 2001 have increased concerns for personal safety and security in both adults and children. Schuster *et al.* surveyed 560 adults throughout the USA 3–5 days after September 11. Thirty-five percent of adults surveyed noted their children were experiencing one or more stress symptoms. Parents experiencing stress reactions were more likely to report symptoms in their children [44]. Pfefferbaum *et al.* examined the impact of peri-traumatic responses in over 2000 middle school children seven weeks after the 1995 Oklahoma City bombing, finding that peri-traumatic responses such as nervousness, fear, or fear that a family member or friend would be hurt, were the strongest predictors of PTSD reactions [11].

Research addressing the effects of war on children in Cambodia [45,46], South Africa [47], Kuwait [48], Rwanda [49], and the Israeli–Palestinian conflict [50] have documented the psychological sequelae resulting from wartime experiences. As expected, traumatic events and development of pathology varies between populations due to multiple psychosocial factors. Of note, 3000 Rwandan children interviewed 13 months after the genocide in April 1994 described exposure to extreme levels of violence in the form of witnessing the deaths of close family members and others in massacres. The majority of these children (90%) had believed they would die and 61% had severe levels of PTSD symptoms, predominantly presenting as avoidance and intrusive thoughts [49]. Eighty-seven percent of Palestinian children living the areas of bombardment were found to have moderate to severe levels of PTSD [50].

War also creates significant numbers of child refugees who are uniquely at risk for developing trauma-related pathology due to the multiple and compounding stressors experienced before escape from their country of origin, during their flight from home, and during resettlement [51]. An estimated 300 000 children under the age of 18 years have fought in armed conflicts, with approximately 10 million refugee children in the world [52]. In addition, traumatic events often occur during detainment in refugee camps. For example, among Cuban refugees detained in a refugee camp prior to arrival in the USA, 80% witnessed acts of violence and 37% saw someone attempt or commit suicide, and 19% were separated from family members [53]. Yet refugee children have also been reported to have significant levels of resiliency. Ideological commitment to issues of war, peace, patriotism and the political enemy were found to be associated with less anxiety, insecurity and depression in Israeli Jewish young adolescents faced with low-levels of war exposure [54]. Social support, parental well-being and maintaining connections to one's culture of origin have also been found to be protective in refugee children [55,56].

Indirect exposure to violence, such as television viewing of traumatic events, has been shown to increase children's risk for trauma-related symptoms, in particular PTSD-related symptoms [11,48,57,58]. For example, PTSD symptoms in Kuwaiti children following the Gulf War were found to be positively cor-

related with television coverage exposure of combat-related events [48]. Terr *et al.* studied children's reactions to the Challenger space shuttle explosion, describing their experience as 'distant trauma' being they had witnessed the disaster at the time of its occurrence, but indirectly via television and from a safe distance from the disaster. Children's symptom patterns were similar to PTSD, in addition to trauma-specific fear, fear of being alone, clinging to others, and event-specific fears [57]. Following the September 11 terrorist attacks, the number of hours of television viewing by children was correlated with the number of reported stress symptoms [59]. Also, children who have experienced direct loss are more likely to watch television coverage of a traumatic event [42,58], thereby exacerbating their trauma-related symptoms.

Natural disasters such as flash floods, hurricanes, and earthquakes have all been found to produce trauma-related pathology in children [60–63]. Anxiety, depression, PTSD symptoms and diagnosis, as well as behavior problems such as aggression and enuresis, have been found in children who survive these types of trauma. The perceived severity of the disaster, level of injury, and level of predisaster functioning are all moderating factors that can contribute to the extent of psychological distress [61,63,64]. Physical proximity to a trauma has also been associated with increased PTSD symptomatology [5,65]. Vernberg *et al.* described children's level of exposure to Hurricane Andrew, including their perceived life threat, was highly predictive of later development of PTSD symptoms [63].

Displacement and relocation may have varying effects on children. Children whose families are displaced because of political violence have higher levels of psychiatric symptoms compared to families who are not displaced [66]. Relocation due to nonwar situations, as may occur during natural disasters, has been shown to have comparatively fewer negative psychological effects on children [67].

It is also important to recognize children's responses to traumatic events can be influenced by their parents' response. Positive correlations have been found between children's and parents' symptomatology following trauma [50,55,68,69]. In addition, having a parent who models appropriate coping mechanisms, as well as having a stable and secure emotional relationship with at least one parent, has been shown to increase resiliency in children experiencing trauma-related stress [55,69,70]. Other psychosocial factors which have been associated with children's resiliency during and after traumatic events include social support and community educational, political and religious support [55,71]. It is apparent further under-standing of resilient factors will help to better identify children's optimal coping strategies, and differentiate these strategies from their parents'.

Epidemiology

The pattern in which trauma-related pathology occurs in the general population is an issue of ongoing study. Studies involving children are scarce, due in part to dif-ficulties in reporting traumatic events and in the diag-nostic process, both of which will be discussed later. Although literature is lacking in this area, several studies have generated a fairly complete picture.

A person in the general population has an approxi-mately 69% chance of experiencing an extraordinary event during his or her lifetime [72]. Of the individuals that do experience such an event, about 20% become traumatized. Tragic deaths are the most frequent form of trauma experienced, and sexual assault yields the highest rates of trauma-related pathology. Motor vehicle crashes present the most adverse combination of frequency and impact but low socioeconomic status also puts individuals at risk [73,74]. Approximately one-fifth of all psychiatric outpatients show symptoms of PTSD [72].

In an urban population study, Breslau and col-leagues [7,75] reported that over one-third of a sample of young adults experienced some type of trauma in their lifetime, as defined in DSM-III-R. Approximately 24% of these individuals (9% of the total sample) also exhibited symptoms consistent with a diagnosis of PTSD. A separate assessment of the general adolescent population reported that 40% of the adolescents eval-uated experienced some type of traumatic event during their teen years [8,76]. Of those adolescents, approxi-mately 14% (6% of the sample population) later devel-oped PTSD. No differences across gender were identified for the occurrence of trauma, but females were six times as likely as males to develop PTSD. A study of urban school-age children found that 57% of the students sampled had been the victim of a violent act or knew someone who had been a victim [33]. More recently, Cuffe and colleagues found a rate of 3% for females and 1% for males in a community sample of older adolescents met DSM-IV criteria for PTSD [77].

Rates of trauma-related symptoms are often higher in those populations whose risk of exposure to trau-matic events is greater than that of the general popu-lation. Incarcerated delinquent males, for example, present with high rates of active PTSD and dissocia-tive symptoms [78,79]. Approximately 32% of these males meet the full criteria for a trauma-related diag-nosis, and 15% fulfill partial criteria. Many of these youths come from communities in which they are exposed to community violence, which thus places them at greater risk for trauma-related pathology. In addition, many of these individuals are traumatized by the circumstances and events of their crime.

Among the children who experience specific traumas the rates of PTSD vary depending on the methods used for data collection and the criteria used. For example, PTSD has been reported as high as 44% for sexual abuse and 20% for physical abuse, with an even larger percentage for partial criteria [18,80–82]. The variability reported is due in part to differences in abuse circumstances. The closeness of the relationship between the child and the perpetrator (i.e., parent versus stranger), the duration of the abuse, and the level of violence all contribute to the presence of a PTSD diagnosis. Females and young children appear to be more susceptible to the disorder [20]. Method-ological design and length of time posttrauma vary among the studies and likely account for some differ-ences in rates; few studies use longitudinal designs with adequate follow-up time.

As many as 38% of children exposed to violence in the community show symptoms of PTSD. A study conducted by Fitzpatrick and Boldizar found that 27% of African–American youths between the ages of 7 and 18 years exhibited PTSD symptoms as a result of community violence [27]. Studies of the effects of natural disasters vary greatly in their method of reporting PTSD, owing to the length of time post trauma at which the children are evaluated and to the type of disaster. Rates of PTSD and PTSD symptoms range from as high as 54% immediately following a disaster such as an earthquake to 37% two years fol-lowing a flood to 7% six months following a hurricane [62,65,83–85]. The more intense a child's experience during and following a disaster, the more likely the child is to develop PTSD symptoms. Factors influenc-ing the development of symptoms include the severity of the disaster, the extent of injury, the degree of mate-rial and personal loss, and the level of trait anxiety [60,61].

The picture that emerges is incomplete but useful. Only a fraction of people going through extraordinary situations become ill and this varies depending on the intensity of experience and nature of trauma. Although a substantial amount of information is known about the factors that contribute to the pres-ence of trauma-related symptoms for specific types of trauma, less is known about what factors protect chil-dren from developing symptoms or, conversely, place them at risk. Emerging research discussed later in this chapter suggests that personality and coping styles play a part in a child's response to events [78,86,87]. Further information is needed on the clinical profiles and prevalence of PTSD and trauma-related symptoms in the clinical child and adolescent population. Future studies should also obtain profiles of the general population and examine the influence of protective factors that insulate those who do not develop psychopathology [88].

Developmental Traumatology

The field of developmental traumatology is a relatively new focus of child psychiatric study. It is defined as a systematic investigation of biological, psychological and sociological impacts on children who have experienced maltreatment and/or trauma, in an attempt to identify varying biopsychosocial effects throughout the developmental stages of a child into adulthood [1]. This area of study attempts to clarify the interactions between biological and environmental variables in the developing child, such as genetic constitution, psychosocial stressors, and identification of critical periods of vulnerability and resilience for traumatic experiences. Information regarding psychosocial stressors, such as low socioeconomic status, parental mental illnesses, and poor social support, can be integrated with research from developmental psychopathology, developmental neuroscience, and stress and trauma research. Developmental traumatology is the study of these complex interactions, as stressful life experiences can affect biological systems leading to a variety of psychiatric and psychological consequences.

Recent advances in neuroimaging and neurochemical research has shed considerable light onto the biological effects of trauma in children. These effects can have significant and ongoing developmental impact on children. Neurobiological systems provide the structural framework not only for physical and cognitive development, but emotional and behavioral development as well. Acute and chronic stress causes significant alterations in these neurobiological pathways [10,89]. Stress also impacts the regulation and expression of genes, which in effect impacts the development of brain and its processes [90,91].

Neurobiological Processes Involved in the Stress Response

Research regarding the neurobiological aspects of PTSD and its development from single and/or multiple traumatic event(s) in childhood is limited to date.

Initial findings appear to reflect PTSD in childhood as a different developmental process compared to PTSD in adults. These differences may be reflected in the finding that children appear to be less resilient to trauma than adults. Results of a meta-analysis demonstrated children and adolescents who have experienced trauma are approximately 1.5 times more likely to be diagnosed with PTSD compared to adults [92].

Traumatic stress activates the catecholamine system, i.e., the sympathetic nervous system, leading to increases in heart rate, blood pressure, metabolic rate, and alertness. In addition, during a stress response, corticotropin-releasing hormone (CRH) is released from the hypothalamus, thereby activating the hypothalamic–pituitary–adrenal (HPA) axis by stimulating secretion of adrenocorticotropin (ACTH) from the pituitary. Cortisol is then released from the adrenal glands, further stimulating the sympathetic nervous system during stress. These biological processes are consistent with the 'fight-or-flight' response evolutionarily adapted to protect the individual from danger and potential harm but in chronic experience may become counterproductive. HPA regulation eventually leads to restoration of basal cortisol levels via negative feedback inhibition. It is hypothesized that dysregulation of the catecholamine system and HPA axis in response to stress and trauma may significantly contribute to the negative symptoms of PTSD.

It has generally been hypothesized that early stress on brain development could exert only deleterious effects on neural development. An alternative hypothesis has been proposed, suggesting that early stressors can create new developmental pathways, allowing the brain to adapt itself for continued survival and reproduction, despite existence in a stressful environment [89,91]. Nonetheless, elevated levels of catecholamines and dysregulation of the HPA axis associated with stress and trauma appears to lead to adverse neuronal development through a variety of mechanisms. There is evidence of accelerated loss of neurons [93–95], delays in myelination [96], decreased number and length of dendritic processes [97], disruptions in neural pruning [98], inhibition of neurogenesis [99,100], and decreases in brain-derived neurotrophic factor expression [101]. Early stressful experiences have also been shown to have neurobiological structural consequences, such as reduced corpus callosum size, attenuated development of the left neocortex, hippocampus and amygdala, enhanced electrical irritability in limbic structures, and reduced functional activity of the cerebellar vermis [89]. Loss of the corpus callosum volume can lead to reduced communication between the hemispheres, and has been shown to produce lateralization that can lead to catecholamine dysregulation. The brain regions effected during stressful experiences appear to have one or more of the following features: (a) a prolonged postnatal development; (b) a high density of glucocorticoid receptors; and (c) some degree of postnatal neurogenesis [89]. While the picture at this point is still preliminary, there appears to be increasing evidence that collectively damage to these areas of the brain can lead to difficulties in social integration, attachment and bonding, as well as mood and anxiety disorders. These features suggest there are potential on-going, developmental consequences to traumatic stress. In order to better understand the neurobiological and psychological sequelae of trauma, it is worthwhile to review neurobiological findings in children at varying developmental stages into adulthood.

The Catecholamine System and Trauma

There has been significant evidence to suggest maltreated children and adolescents with mood and anxiety symptoms have altered catecholamine levels. Maltreated children with PTSD have been shown to have elevated concentrations of urinary norepinephrine and dopamine over 24 hours compared to nontraumatized children diagnosed with overanxious disorder and healthy controls, with a significant positive correlation between urinary catecholamine levels and duration of trauma and severity of PTSD symptoms [102]. Increased 24-hour urinary norepinephrine concentrations in neglected depressed male children has been reported [103], as well as greater 24-hour urinary catecholamine and catecholamine metabolite concentrations in dysthymic, sexually abused girls [104]. This is a consistent finding in adult populations, as adult patients with chronic PTSD have been shown to have increased circulating levels of norepinephrine [105] and increased reactivity of α2-adrenergic receptors [106].

The HPA Axis and Trauma

The HPA axis has also been implicated in the pathophysiology of PTSD, although current PTSD research reflects conflicting theories regarding the regulation of the HPA axis in PTSD, both in child and adult populations. Still, it appears some trends in HPA axis research have been identified. For example, most studies of traumatized pediatric populations have found increased basal levels of cortisol, whereas cortisol levels in adult populations with PTSD are generally decreased.

The theory that adults with PTSD have low basal cortisol levels is supported by evidence of lower plasma cortisol levels in adult combat veteran populations with PTSD compared to controls without PTSD [107], and findings of low urinary cortisol excretion in adult holocaust survivor with PTSD compared to holocaust survivors without PTSD [108]. It is hypothesized that cortisol levels in adults with chronic PTSD are decreased compared to nontraumatized control subjects due to a down-regulation of anterior pituitary CRH receptors secondary to chronic elevations in CRH levels and also due to an enhanced negative feedback inhibition of cortisol at the level of the pituitary [109]. This down-regulation may be an adaptive response, as chronically elevated cortisol levels are potentially neurotoxic. This theory is supported by studies by Yehuda et al. demonstrating combat veterans with PTSD have an exaggerated cortisol suppression following the administration of low dose dexamethasone (an analog of cortisol) and an exaggerated decline of cytosolic lymphocyte glucocorticoid receptors compared to those without PTSD [110]. Also compatible with this hypothesis are the findings that individuals with PTSD have high levels of corticotropin-releasing factor (CRF) in their cerebrospinal fluid (CSF) [111], a blunted ACTH response to CRH [112], and an enhanced ACTH response to doses of metyrapone suppressing cortisol production [113].

Other studies have not been compatible with the above-mentioned theory regarding PTSD in adults. Specifically, three studies reported elevated 24-hour urinary cortisol excretion in adult patients with PTSD [114–116]. In addition, a greater ACTH response to CRF in PTSD compared to control subjects has been reported [117], as well as greater ACTH responses to current psychosocial stress among women with histories of childhood physical and sexual abuse compared to women with no such histories [118]. These studies postulate an alternative theory explaining baseline low cortisol levels; such being a chronically low adrenal output of cortisol, or rather, adrenal insufficiency [119]. These discrepant findings may be associated with the confounding effects of assay methodology as well as potential current life stressors influencing the regulation of the HPA axis.

Studies of the HPA axis and its regulation following trauma in children have generally demonstrated elevated cortisol levels, suggesting different biological consequences to traumatic stress compared to adult populations. De Bellis et al. reported maltreated prepubertal children diagnosed with PTSD have increased 24-hour urinary cortisol levels compared to matched control subjects [102]. Carrion *et al.* demonstrated significantly elevated salivary cortisol levels in children with trauma exposure histories and PTSD symptoms when compared with control groups [120]. Gunnar *et al.* demonstrated elevated salivary cortisol levels in 6–12-year-old children raised in Romanian orphanages for eight months of their lives compared with early adopted and Canadian born children tested at 6.5 years after adoption [121]. In a relatively large study, Hart *et al.* demonstrated depressed maltreated children had elevated afternoon salivary cortisol levels compared to depressed nonmaltreated children [122].

In contrast, Goenjian *et al.* studied adolescents five years after the 1988 Armenian earthquake and reported reduced levels of cortisol in children in closest proximity to the disaster [123]. Also King *et al.* found that girls with a history of sexual abuse within the last two months had lower cortisol in comparison to control subjects [124]. Comparing and interpreting the results of these studies in children, as well as in adult PTSD studies, is limited by varying methodological approaches and differing population samples. While there is no absolute consensus on whether cortisol levels in children with PTSD are elevated or decreased, most studies show an elevation in cortisol levels in children diagnosed with PTSD.

It is possible that some variations in study results could also be explained by examining the developmental stage when trauma occurred as well as the duration of time elapsed since exposure to trauma in children as well as adults. One could postulate CRH and cortisol levels are elevated acutely after a trauma. Long-term, or rather, developmental effects of trauma could eventually lead to decreased levels of cortisol due to chronic elevations in CRH and the enhanced negative feedback on the HPA axis. This hypothesis is supported by a study comparing pituitary volume differences using magnetic resonance imaging (MRI) in children of varying ages with PTSD and nontraumatized healthy comparison subjects [125]. Although there were no differences seen in pituitary volumes between PTSD and control subjects, there was a significant age-by-group effect for PTSD subjects showing greater differences in pituitary volume with age compared to control subjects. *Post hoc* analyses revealed pituitary volumes were significantly larger in pubertal and postpubertal maltreated subjects with PTSD compared to control subjects, but were similar in prepubertal maltreated subjects with PTSD and control subjects. Pituitary volumes changes in response to stress and dysregulation of the HPA axis have already been demonstrated in various research models. Chronically administrating CRH to rats shows an increase in the number and size of pituitary corticotroph cells [126,127]. Also, suicide victims have been shown to have larger pituitary corticotroph cells [128].

Clearly, neurobiological research regarding PTSD in children is only beginning to elucidate the biological effects of trauma. While preliminary data and developing theory regarding HPA regulation in children with PTSD is provocative, it is still with incomplete evidence to date. Further research is needed to clarify HPA regulation in PTSD in children at varying developmental stages.

Neuroanatomical Findings Associated with Traumatic Stress

A growing body of evidence is reflecting significant involvement of glucocorticoids (cortisol) and their impact on the hippocampus in a stress response [129]. There is significant evidence for hippocampal atrophy in adult populations with PTSD [130–133], Cushing syndrome (characterized by a pathologic oversecretion of glucocorticoids) [134,135], and recurrent major depressive disorder [136,137] also frequently associated with oversecretion of glucocorticoids. There is also significant evidence that glucocorticoid toxicity may, in part, be mediated by prolonged elevations in excitatory amino acids such as glutamate [138].

With the use of high-resolution MRI, significant hippocampal atrophy has been demonstrated in adult combat veterans with the diagnosis of PTSD compared to control subjects [130,131]. In addition, studies have reported significant left hippocampal volume reduction in adult populations with histories of childhood trauma and a current diagnosis of PTSD [132,133].

In contrast, studies of children with PTSD have not demonstrated any significant differences in hippocampal volumes compared to normal controls. Carrion *et al.* did not observe any significant differences in hippocampal volumes between abused children with the diagnosis of PTSD and subthreshold diagnosis of PTSD compared to normal control subjects [139]. De Bellis *et al.* [140] and in a subsequent study [141] studied hippocampal volumes by MRI in maltreated children with PTSD and healthy controls, finding no significant differences in volume. Rather, it was reported that subjects with PTSD had smaller intracranial, cerebral, and prefrontal cortex, prefrontal cortical white matter, right temporal lobe volumes, and smaller areas of the corpus callosum. Teicher *et al.* found a marked reduction in the middle portions of the corpus callosum in child psychiatric inpatients with a

Table 15.1 Recent HPA studies of PTSD and trauma in children.

Study	N	Location	Population	DSM diagnosis	Findings
Goenjian *et al.* 1996	37 Trauma exposed from 1988 Armenia earthquake (five years after event)	Armenia	Adolescents	PTSD symptoms	Lower morning salivary cortisol, and greater suppression with dexmethasone challenge
De Bellis *et al.* 1999	18 PTSD 10 Overanxious disorder (OAD) 24 Control	USA	Ages 8–12 mixed gender	PTSD diagnosis	Urine catecholamines PTSD > OAD = Control
Gunnar *et al.* 2001	18 Romanian orphans (adopted at eight months) 15 Early adopted (prior to four months) 27 Canadian born	Canada/Romania	Ages 6–12	None	Salivary cortisol greater in eight-month institutionalized infants
King *et al.* 2001	10 girls with sexual abuse histories 10 Control	USA	Ages 5–7 girls	None	Lower basal cortisol levels than controls
Carrion *et al.* 2002	51 PTSD symptoms 31 Control	USA	Ages 7–14 mixed gender	PTSD symptoms	Salivary cortisol elevated in PTSD > control

substantiated history of abuse or neglect verses control subjects [142]. De Bellis *et al* [140] also reported reduced corpus callosum size in children with a history of abuse and PTSD with more notable volume changes in males versus females. This neurobiological finding may be associated with decreased communication between the cortical hemispheres, which may be related to memories difficulties and dissociative disorders, both of which are often found to be comorbid with PTSD.

There are several possible explanations for the differences in neuroanatomical findings between adult and child populations with diagnoses of PTSD. One possibility may be associated with the fact that many adults with PTSD have comorbid substance use disorders and reduced hippocampal volumes may be associated with this alcohol and/or drug use. De Bellis *et al.* has demonstrated a decrease in hippocampal volumes in adolescent-onset alcohol abuse [143]. Yet neuroimaging studies described in adults have continued to reflect significant hippocampal volume changes even after matching controls for years of substance use [131,143] or adjusting volume changes for cumulative alcohol exposure [130,133].

Another possible cause of these discrepancies could be that neurobiological findings may take time to present, suggesting the stress response is gradual and progressive in nature. The hippocampus, as well as other brain structures, is known to have continued neurogenesis postnatally. In addition, the hippocampus has been shown to have an overproduction of axonal and dendritic arborization, as well as synapses and receptors, which are not pruned and eliminated until the postpubertal period [144–146]. Animal models suggest that psychological and physical stress produce measurable changes in brain-derived neurotrophic factor (BDNF) which has effects on neurogenesis and prevention of apoptosis [147]. Cumulatively, these findings suggest that the effects of childhood trauma could have ongoing developmental implications on brain structure and function. Traumatic injury could therefore be partially dependent on the individual's stage of postnatal neural development.

A third possibility may be that the neurobiological finding of a smaller hippocampal volume is actually not a result of chronic stress, but rather is a predisposition for the development of PTSD. This is supported by a study comparing monozygotic twin veterans and normal control subjects. It was found that combat veterans with PTSD, as well as their identical twin without exposure to trauma, both had smaller hippocampi compared to normal, nontraumatized

controls. In addition, veterans with PTSD had significantly smaller hippocampal volumes compared to their nontraumatized twins [148]. This may suggest smaller hippocampal volumes may be a both predisposition to the development of PTSD as well as an effect of trauma in adults.

The majority of research involving metabolic activity of the brain in PTSD has been conducted in adult populations although there are a few recent studies in children as well. Positron-emission tomography and functional MRI have shown increased reactivity in the amygdala and anterior paralimbic region [149,150] and decreased reactivity in the anterior cingulate and orbitofrontal areas in adults who have experienced childhood sexual abuse while reading trauma-related scripts [151]. Preliminary studies in child populations with PTSD have reported some similar metabolic activity, implicating specific brain areas as metabolically affected in PTSD. Using proton MRI spectroscopy, De Bellis *et al.* found a decreased ratio of N-acetylaspartate to creatine in the anterior cingulate in 11 maltreated children and adolescents with PTSD compared to control subjects, suggesting the anterior cingulate's metabolism is altered in childhood PTSD [152]. Of note, these brain areas described have been implicated in the fear response.

One caveat to these studies must be noted. Functional imaging studies are labor intensive to produce, and have yield interesting preliminary data, but to this point the sample sizes are generally small, number less than 20 in the best studies. The data emerging must therefore be interpreted with caution, and clinicians are strongly discouraged at this point from using imaging techniques as the sole or primary basis for diagnosis. Expense, expertise and the need to interpret images very carefully are cautionary flags for the practicing clinician. In contrast, these cautions need not extend to the endocrine literature that is much better established, and represent a long history of research with some degree of clinical correlation. But here again, the diagnostic value of this information still remains in doubt and only further studies will shed light on these complex pathways and their utility in practice.

Research on the neurobiological and neuroanatomical effects of PTSD from single and/or multiple traumatic event(s) in childhood is limited to date. Initial findings may appear to demonstrate PTSD in childhood as a different developmental process compared to PTSD in adults with potentially evolving neurobiological consequences during the course of an individual's early life. It is important to consider the likelihood of prolonged effects from childhood trauma, not only impacting the development of coping strategies, impact on interpersonal relationships and academic performance, but also the neurobiological effects in children and adolescent populations. These neurobiological effects may indeed demonstrate significant impact on behavior and cognition, and may in part be influenced by the neurobiological developmental stages in children and adolescents. Further research is needed to clarify these complexities in PTSD development in childhood through adolescence and into young adulthood.

The Workup

The Interview

When making a trauma-related diagnosis in children, the clinician should recognize that the necessary information is often not forthcoming. Since most of the symptoms of PTSD and acute stress disorder (ASD) [153] are of an internalizing kind, the younger the child, the worse he or she is as a self-observer and reporter. Much information about internal states is provided by the parents of young children and is displayed by the children in play. As children reach school age, they develop some psychological structures to report complex internal states; these reports can nevertheless involve fairly simple reports and misunderstanding.

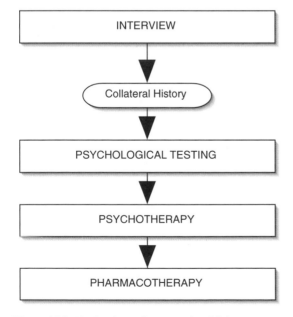

Figure 15.2 Evaluation of trauma in children.

Children, in particular young children, often do not associate the emotional repercussions with the traumatic events that caused them; as a result, they are not likely to volunteer information regarding events that may seem far in the past. Children who are sexually abused are often sworn to secrecy by the abuser and are therefore less likely to reveal the occurrence of the trauma. Parents often bring their children to treatment with recognition of problematic behavior but without specific knowledge of the trauma from which it originated. The situation is further complicated in adolescence. Although most adolescents have the capacity to self-observe, many do not have the motivation to collaborate in their own treatment. Adolescents as well as children often presume personal responsibility and guilt and may experience threats from the perpetrator, all of which decrease the likelihood of reporting.

When assessing for traumatic events, it is crucial that the clinician administer interviews with the child as well as the parents or primary caregiver to establish as accurate a history as possible. This is especially important, because many trauma victims deny or minimize the factors surrounding the event, depending on the stage of trauma recovery. In addition, contact with teachers, school counselors, and school psychologists should be conducted to form a more objective assessment of the child's behavior in structured settings. The absence of a thorough assessment from different parties can lead to misdiagnosis, ineffective treatment, and a continuation of symptoms as well as the appearance of new symptoms.

Trauma can often be the hidden cause of psychopathology in the absence of significant reported life events. This does not mean, however, that one should assume trauma as fallback diagnosis. Rather, when a child presents with difficulties in attention and concentration or mood changes, the clinician should explore possible experiences with traumatic events and the reactions that ensued. In the absence of an explained cause of behavior difficulties, traumatic events should be investigated but not assumed. It is becoming increasingly apparent that memory is a complex experience, and that the mind is capable of repressing trauma [154,155]. Nevertheless, care must be taken when interviewing children if the clinical data is to be used for judicial or investigative purposes. Children and adolescents are suggestible, and thus leading questions (for example, the type of questions that are usually part of a structured interview), although never a good strategy in clinical practice, are especially problematic in this context. Combining structured techniques with skilled clinical exploration is likely the best method for conducting interviews where trauma is suspected. We advocate that clinicians initially prepare and the child and family or guardians in an unstructured format to allow open-ended exploration of leads that may arise, and then proceed in a more structured and thorough way to obtain details of the history. While we believe this combination approach represents a good set of practices, there may be circumstances where alternative approaches are needed and therefore clinical judgment is always necessary.

The differentiation of false from true traumatic memories is complex and inconsistent. Williams in her study of victims of sexual abuse 17 years after the event found that younger age at the time of abuse and closeness of relationship with the abuser correlated with the inability to recall the event [156]. A recent functional MRI study by John Gabrieli and colleagues has demonstrated that prefrontal cortical and right hippocampal regions of the brain exhibit higher degrees of activation in individuals who repressed unwanted memories [157]. Their study, while limited to adults in nontraumatic situations, sheds light on the ways that the brain may produce traumatic forgetting and also leads to the realization that memories might indeed emerge at a later time in the event that these pathways normalize at a neurochemical level.

It is clear that memories are reconstructed and not simply laid down, and thus not simply recalled as a photographic image or 100% accurate event. Memories are narrated and constantly being reconstructed, and individuals can therefore be induced to believe that certain events happened when in fact they did not; however, it is not yet clear whether complex events typically reported by trauma victims can also be implanted. In clinical practice, we have helped several patients with this kind of problem and were impressed with several features of the emergence of long-forgotten material:

(1) the emergence occurred in the context of a long-established and trusted therapeutic relationship after many months of treatment for other related problems;
(2) the emergence was triggered by a current event in the patient's life that in some form was reminiscent of the original event;
(3) the traumatic event did not come as a total surprise, since the patient usually assessed the victimizer to be a problematic person in his or her life;
(4) the memories were disjointed and fragmented at first and were accompanied by appropriate emo-

tions such as anxiety and rage, but there was a general hesitancy to draw the appropriate inferences;
(5) nightmares at times reemerged that had been present a long time ago;
(6) our own clinical conduct during the time of the emergence of these traumatic events was at all times receptive and facilitative but never pressuring and prescriptive.

As further research is conducted to help deal with these complex issues, clinicians can be helpful to patients but still not 'muddy the waters.'

Assessment

Psychological and neuropsychological testing can be beneficial in assessing a trauma-related diagnosis, particularly when there is a question of differential diagnosis or comorbidity or when children are reluctant or unable to discuss the trauma or their feelings: the Child Trauma Inventory (CTI) and the Child Trauma Questionnaire (CTQ) [158]. In addition to the standard psychological assessment measures, more specific measures have been designed to assess problematic behavior of children who have been sexually abused [159,160]. The presence of commonly occurring traumas that often lead to psychopathology can also be investigated with specific measures such as the Impact of Event Scale and the Response Evaluation Measure (REM-71) [161,162]. Other measures, such as the Child Behavior Checklist and the Schedule for Affective Disorders and Schizophrenia, can help assess the presence of certain target symptoms such as depression, anxiety, and dissociation.

Treatment

PTSD and trauma-related psychopathology have been treated for many decades. Numerous studies have reported many different kinds of interventions, for example, eye roll movements, hypnosis, psychoanalysis, cognitive therapy, and psychopharmacology.

Only a handful of studies, however, were conducted to allow the formation of firm conclusions about treatment efficacy, and none of those studies involved children and adolescents. The present literature concludes (after much extrapolation from adult studies – which is itself problematic as demonstrated in the depression literature) that psychopharmacology and various forms of psychotherapy are all moderately effective, that many interventions show promise (none of them being superior to others *a priori*), and that most interventions are not rigorously tested in children and adolescents. It also appears that various treatments target different aspects of the syndrome. Medications seem to reduce intrusion and 'startle response' problems, as do behavioral treatments. Psychodynamic treatments seem to work better on avoidance symptoms, although this result is variable across studies and has not been adequately studied in children. There are likely to be differences across ages, given the different nature of child PTSD.

Factors that Influence Treatment

As in the treatment of any disorder, the culture of the patient should be considered. The race, ethnicity, and religion of a patient can influence his or her willingness to present symptoms that may be considered taboo or embarrassing. In cases of sexual abuse, patients may be embarrassed about what took place and attribute blame to themselves. Family and communities may also blame, ostracize, and distance themselves from the victim. If a family member has perpetrated the abuse, some cultures may dictate that the perpetrator be taken care of within the family (e.g., moved to another location) and resent the interference of 'outsiders.' Behaviors such as hitting or alienating a child for unacceptable behavior may be the standard form of punishment in certain countries and cultures. Although this behavior should be understood within its cultural framework, it should not be sanctioned as acceptable in this country. Behaviors that occur because of cultural differences and a lack of knowledge regarding the laws in this country can often be resolved in family therapy.

The limits of confidentiality can significantly affect therapy with trauma victims. Although the specific laws vary slightly among states, clinicians are legally and ethically obligated to report suspected abuse and in most cases are legally protected in making reports that turn out to be without merit. Parents, children, and adolescents should all be informed about the limits of confidentiality. In cases in which abuse is the presenting problem, the issue of confidentiality can be addressed at the beginning of therapy in relation to the trauma; patients should be made aware, however, that these limits also apply to other instances of abuse that might be revealed during the course of therapy. This is an important point to stress, since traumatized or abused patients have often experienced more than one significant trauma.

Clearly defining the limits of confidentiality does not preclude difficulties from arising later in therapy,

should confidentiality be broken. Reporting information revealed during therapy to the police and to child protection agencies can bring up issues of trust, security, and betrayal for patients, particularly if they are not in agreement with the reporting. One fourth of families drop out of therapy after a report is made. The integrity of the therapeutic relationship is influenced by the manner in which the need to report is presented, the identity and relationship of the perpetrator to the patient, and the ability of the patient to cope with the effect of such reporting on his or her relationships, both in and out of therapy.

Psychotherapy

Individual treatment is the mainstay of intervention. In our clinic, we usually prescribe a mixture of behavioral interventions that are delivered in the context of a psychodynamic treatment package. The psychodynamic elements are intended to help develop a treatment alliance with children, help the clinician manage the therapeutic relationship, and possibly target memories in order to uncover important details of the original trauma. The typical course progresses in three stages. Phase one is exploratory (two to five sessions): the nature and extent of the traumatic event is established while a solid working alliance is built. This phase is completed when the patient and clinician agree on a scenario of the events that traumatized the patient and on a course of exposure or desensitization (depending on the comorbidity), the familial resources, and the patient's ego strengths and defense profile. More resilient patients with many resources usually receive some form of exposure, in which the traumatic event is reworked and the patient rapidly works up to flooding therapy. These patients, however, are still cognizant of some of the severe side effects this method may produce. More complicated cases should be approached gradually, with a model based on the prevention of relapse.

In phase two (6–15 sessions), the behavioral program is carried out and is supplemented by further exploratory sessions as needed to work through patient resistance. In the first two phases, ongoing treatment is provided every week. After these phases, regular clinic contact is terminated. In the third phase of treatment (up to 2–3 years as necessary, with very intermittent contacts), the patient is encouraged to practice on his or her own and to return when progress stops or symptoms reoccur. Such relapses are then handled in the course of one to three sessions. Play therapy and drawings are productive with younger children, and more traditional forms of therapy benefit older adolescents. At all phases of treatment, the patient's need for psychopharmacology is assessed.

Cognitive behavioral therapy (CBT) has shown effectiveness in treating children who are victims of sexual abuse [163]. Judith Cohen and colleagues in a recent study have shown specific benefit to children experience PTSD as a result of sexual abuse by using trauma-focused cognitive behavioral therapy (TF-CBT) over a child centered therapeutic approach for both children and their parents [21]. TF-CBT develops skills in expressing feelings, coping, and developing a sense of the connections between emotion, behavior and feeling. It also includes some exposure by using narrative, processing, parenting skills and psychoeducation. Along a similar line, Barry Nurcombe and colleagues in a review of the limited published studies for the treatment of sexual abuse likewise found benefit from CBT, as well as from group therapy and play therapy [164]. Ramchandani and Jones in their recent review of the literature on treatment of sexually abused children, likewise conclude that CBT has the most evidence in randomized clinical trials for its efficaciousness [165].

Additional Forms of Therapy

Psychoeducation can be extremely beneficial for parents of children who have experienced a trauma. Often parents are scared, confused, and uncertain about the origins of their child's behavior and the prevalence of symptoms. They often need to learn new strategies and parenting skills to deal with problematic behavior such as anger outbursts and flashbacks. In addition, children and especially adolescents can gain security in knowing that their symptoms are valid and within the normal range of experiences for individuals affected by a traumatic event.

Group therapy often helps children and adolescents understand that their symptoms are experienced by others and allow them to learn coping strategies from those who have been through similar circumstances. Group therapy should begin following an initial assessment of the trauma and related symptoms. It is not recommended as the initial form of therapy in the case of severe trauma, since children are likely to experience symptoms during the initial telling of their traumas that may be better managed in initial individual sessions. An initial assessment should differentiate between those patients who can present their experience in a group and withstand the exposure to others' traumas and those who require individual work prior

to sharing with others. For the latter patients, once individual therapy has started, group therapy can be used as a means of continued support.

Particularly in the instance of abuse, family therapy can be beneficial for the patient as well as the individual family members. These approaches have been manualized and tested in community settings [164]. When one member of a family experiences a trauma, everyone in the family is affected. Feelings of insecurity, fear, guilt, and shame can all be present in family members as a result of the trauma. These feelings along with changes in the family routine because of care for the identified patient can upset the previously held dynamics of the family. When the perpetrator of abuse is within the family, family therapy is essential for assessing family structure and relationships within the family, as well as the development of new roles within the family. Decisions about whether to include the perpetrator in therapy should be decided on a case-by-case basis and should take into consideration the stage of recovery of the victim, the perpetrator's understanding of the abuse and his or her involvement in treatment, and reunification issues.

Psychopharmacology

If the evidence for the efficacy of drugs is not strong in adults, it is quite weak for the treatment of children and adolescents with PTSD. At present, one can only extrapolate from studies of adults, which is of course problematic. Psychotherapeutic interventions should be tried first; only if patients fail to progress or if symptoms are so overwhelming as to incapacitate the patient should the clinician consider medications. A trial of medicine should be started if symptoms do not begin to recede after about four weeks of adequate intervention or when symptoms are so incapacitating to make management impossible and there is pronounced interference with developmental tasks.

What are the appropriate targets for treatment? Based on what can be gleaned from the adult literature, predominantly the intrusion and hyperactivity-related symptoms of PTSD respond to intervention. Post and colleagues propose a kindling model for the development of PTSD [166,167]. Three general stages can be discerned. First there are the traumatic events that serve to prime the system and can result in acute stress disorder. Second there is the development of PTSD with the presence of flashbacks, nightmares, hyperarousal, avoidance and numbing. In the third phase, chronic PTSD develops whereby explosiveness, irritability, panics, generalized anxiety, depression, social phobia and somatization can occur. Pharmacologically, these stages can be approached with different sets of medications but will likely require multiple interventions including psychotherapy and family therapy. The kindling theory of PTSD holds that prompt intervention to address core symptoms is necessary in order to prevent further progression of the disease, and medications may play one significant role in this process.

Selective serotonin reuptake inhibitors (SSRIs) have been the mainstay of PTSD treatment for the past decade. The evidence for their utility in children is supported by limited studies, and most practitioners draw from the adult literature on this point. Seedat and colleagues studied eight adolescents with a 20-mg fixed dose of citalopram and found improvements in arousal level and startle response [168]. The use of SSRIs in children has become a point of controversy in recent years, and all drugs in this class now have a block box warning for the possible development of suicidal ideation with the initiation of SSRI therapy. Clinicians need to monitor all children for this potential effect, and caution should be exercised when starting any new medication.

Limited data is available on the use of mood stabilizers like divalproex sodium for populations with high levels of PTSD and comorbid conduct disorder [169]. Further recent studies by our group have shown that divalproex sodium can significantly reduce intrusion, avoidance and arousal in children with PTSD [170]. The efficacy of mood stabilizers seems consistent with Post's kindling theory of PTSD, in that this medication can reduce arousal, irritability, and explosiveness, and thereby theoretically blunt the transition from PTSD to chronic PTSD.

Should SSRIs and mood stabilizers fail, then consideration can be given to using beta-blockers [171], alpha-blockers [172] and atypicals. Each of these classes of medications has had some limited success in treating PTSD symptoms in children. Minor tranquilizers are apparently not useful on an ongoing basis, changing little of the core pathology of PTSD, but can be used for brief symptomatic relief. One has to be mindful of the potential abuse of these drugs, especially in teenagers or in chaotic families in which parents might avail themselves of medications prescribed for their children.

Drugs should never be considered the primary mode of treating PTSD in this age group, and all patients, given the current state of knowledge, should receive a carefully reviewed and comprehensive psychotherapy package.

Conclusion

It is evident that knowledge about childhood trauma is rapidly changing. The field of developmental traumatology is newly emerging and evolving, and the results will likely be to change our understanding of the mind and the effects of early trauma. In addition, as the neuroscience behind childhood trauma becomes clearer, the resulting changes in interventions from pharmacological, psychotherapeutic, and sociotherapeutic perspectives [173] will have to alter and progress. It is incumbent on practitioners to be vigilant about these coming changes in order to provide the highest level of care for this population of children.

References

1. Ohmi H, Kojima S, Awai Y, Kamata S, Sasaki K, Tanaka Y, *et al.*: Post-traumatic stress disorder in preschool aged children after a gas explosion. *Eur J Pediatr* 2002; **161**:643–648.
2. Scheeringa MS, Zeanah CH, Drell MJ, Larrieu JA: Two approaches to the diagnosis of posttraumatic stress disorder in infancy and early childhood. *J Am Acad Child Adolesc Psychiatry* 1995; **34**:191–200.
3. Shaw JA, Applegate B, Schorr C: Twenty-one-month follow-up study of school-age children exposed to Hurricane Andrew. *J Am Acad Child Adolesc Psychiatry* 1996; **35**:359–364.
4. Allwood MA, Bell-Dolan D, Husain SA: Children's trauma and adjustment reactions to violent and nonviolent war experiences. *J Am Acad Child Adolesc Psychiatry* 2002; **41**:450–457.
5. March JS, Amaya-Jackson L, Terry R, Costanzo P: Posttraumatic symptomatology in children and adolescents after an industrial fire. *J Am Acad Child Adolesc Psychiatry* 1997; **36**:1080–1088.
6. Breslau N, Chilcoat HD, Kessler RC, Davis GC: Previous exposure to trauma and PTSD effects of subsequent trauma: Results from the Detroit Area Survey of Trauma. *Am J Psychiatry* 1999; **156**:902–907.
7. Breslau N, Davis GC: Posttraumatic stress disorder in an urban population of young adults: Risk factors for chronicity. *Am J Psychiatry* 1992; **149**:671–675.
8. Giaconia RM, Reinherz HZ, Silverman AB, Pakiz B, Frost AK, Cohen E: Traumas and posttraumatic stress disorder in a community population of older adolescents. *J Am Acad Child Adolesc Psychiatry* 1995; **34**: 1369–1380.
9. Pine DS, Cohen JA: Trauma in children and adolescents: Risk and treatment of psychiatric sequelae. *Biol Psychiatry* 2002; **51**(7):519–531.
10. De Bellis MD: Developmental traumatology: The psychobiological development of maltreated children and its implications for research, treatment and policy. *Dev Psychopathol* 2001; **13**:539–564.
11. Pfefferbaum B, Doughty DE, Reddy C, Patel N, Gurwitch RH, Nixon SJ, *et al.*: Exposure and peritraumatic response as predictors of posttraumatic stress in children following the 1995 Oklahoma City bombing. *J Urban Health* 2002; **79**(3):354–363.

12. Schwarz ED, Kowalski JM: Malignant memories: PTSD in children and adults after a school shooting. *J Am Acad Child Adolesc Psychiatry* 1991; **30**(6):936–944.

13. Aaron J, Zaglul H, Emery RE: Posttraumatic stress in children following acute physical injury. *J Pediatr Psychol* 1999; **24**(4):335–343.

14. Yehuda R: Post-traumatic stress disorder. *N Engl J Med* 2002; **346**(2):108–114.

15. Fergusson DM, Lynskey MT, Horwood LJ: Childhood sexual abuse and psychiatric disorder in young adulthood: I. Prevalence of sexual abuse and factors associated with sexual abuse. *J Am Acad Child Adolesc Psychiatry* 1996; **35**(10):1355–364.

16. Brown J, Cohen P, Johnson JG, Smailes EM: Childhood abuse and neglect: Specificity of effects on adolescent and young adult depression and suicidality. *J Am Acad Child Adolesc Psychiatry* 1999; **38**(12): 1490–1496.

17. Fergusson DM, Horwood LJ, Lynskey MT: Childhood sexual abuse and psychiatric disorder in young adulthood: II. Psychiatric outcomes of childhood sexual abuse. *J Am Acad Child Adolesc Psychiatry* 1996; **35**(10):1365–1374.

18. Adam BS, Everett BL, O'Neal E: PTSD in physically and sexually abused psychiatrically hospitalized children. *Child Psychiatry Hum Dev* 1992; **23**(1):3–8.

19. Saywitz KJ, Mannarino AP, Berliner L, Cohen JA: Treatment for sexually abused children and adolescents. *Am Psychol* 2000; **55**(9):1040–1049.

20. Wolfe DA, Sas L, Wekerle C: Factors associated with the development of posttraumatic stress disorder among child victims of sexual abuse. *Child Abuse Negl* 1994; **18**(1):37–50.

21. Cohen JA, Deblinger E, Mannarino AP, Steer RA: A multisite, randomized controlled trial for children with sexual abuse-related PTSD symptoms. *J Am Acad Child Adolesc Psychiatry* 2004; **43**(4):393–402.

22. Nelson EC, Heath AC, Madden PA, Cooper ML, Dinwiddie SH, Bucholz KK, et al.: Association between self-reported childhood sexual abuse and adverse psychosocial outcomes: Results from a twin study. *Arch Gen Psychiatry* 2002; **59**(2):139–145.

23. Brent DA, Oquendo M, Birmaher B, Greenhill L, Kolko D, Stanley B, et al.: Familial pathways to early-onset suicide attempt: Risk for suicidal behavior in offspring of mood-disordered suicide attempters. *Arch Gen Psychiatry* 2002; **59**(9):801–807.

24. Jaworowski S: Traffic accident injuries of children: The need for prospective studies of psychiatric sequelae. *Isr J Psychiatry Relat Sci* 1992; **29**(3):174–184.

25. Jones RW, Peterson LW: Post-traumatic stress disorder in a child following an automobile accident. *J Fam Pract* 1993; **36**(2):223–225.

26. Stoddard FJ, Norman DK, Murphy JM, Beardslee WR: Psychiatric outcome of burned children and adolescents. *J Am Acad Child Adolesc Psychiatry* 1989; **28**(4):589–595.

27. Fitzpatrick KM, Boldizar JP: The prevalence and consequences of exposure to violence among African-American youth. *J Am Acad Child Adolesc Psychiatry* 1993; **32**(2):424–430.

28. Youngstrom E, Weist MD, Albus KE: Exploring violence exposure, stress, protective factors and behavioral problems among inner-city youth. *Am J Community Psychol* 2003; **32**(1–2):115–129.

29. Silva RR, Alpert M, Munoz DM, Singh S, Matzner F, Dummit S: Stress and vulnerability to posttraumatic stress disorder in children and adolescents. *Am J Psychiatry* 2000; **157**(8):1229–1235.

30. Wolfe DA, Jaffe P, Wilson SK, Zak L: Children of battered women: The relation of child behavior to family violence and maternal stress. *J Consult Clin Psychol* 1985; **53**(5):657–665.

31. Eth S, Pynoos RS: Children who witness the homicide of a parent. *Psychiatry* 1994; **57**(4):287–306.

32. Burman S, Allen-Meares P: Neglected victims of murder: Children's witness to parental homicide. *Soc Work* 1994; **39**(1):28–34.

33. Freeman LN, Mokros H, Poznanski EO: Violent events reported by normal urban school-aged children: Characteristics and depression correlates. *J Am Acad Child Adolesc Psychiatry* 1993; **32**(2):419–423.

34. Schwab-Stone ME, Ayers TS, Kasprow W, Voyce C, Barone C, Shriver T, et al.: No safe haven: A study of violence exposure in an urban community. *J Am Acad Child Adolesc Psychiatry* 1995; **34**(10):1343–1352.

35. Pynoos RS, Frederick C, Nader K, Arroyo W, Steinberg A, Eth S, et al.: Life threat and posttraumatic stress in school-age children. *Arch Gen Psychiatry* 1987; **44**(12):1057–1063.

36. Lipschitz DS, Rasmusson AM, Anyan W, Cromwell P, Southwick SM: Clinical and functional correlates of posttraumatic stress disorder in urban adolescent girls at a primary care clinic. *J Am Acad Child Adolesc Psychiatry* 2000; **39**(9):1104–1111.

37. Bell CC, Jenkins EJ: Community violence and children on Chicago's southside. *Psychiatry* 1993; **56**(1):46–54.

38. Schubiner H, Scott R, Tzelepis A: Exposure to violence among inner-city youth. *J Adolesc Health* 1993; **14**(3):214–219.

39. Mazza JJ, Reynolds WM: Exposure to violence in young inner-city adolescents: Relationships with suicidal ideation, depression, and PTSD symptomatology. *J Abnorm Child Psychol* 1999; **27**(3):203–213.

40. Fremont WP: Childhood reactions to terrorism-induced trauma: A review of the past 10 years. *J Am Acad Child Adolesc Psychiatry* 2004; **43**(4):381–392.

41. Laor N, Wolmer L, Mayes LC, Golomb A, Silverberg DS, Weizman R, et al.: Israeli preschoolers under Scud missile attacks. A developmental perspective on risk-modifying factors. *Arch Gen Psychiatry* 1996; **53**(5): 416–423.

42. Pfefferbaum B, Nixon SJ, Tucker PM, Tivis RD, Moore VL, Gurwitch RH, et al.: Posttraumatic stress responses in bereaved children after the Oklahoma City bombing. *J Am Acad Child Adolesc Psychiatry* 1999; **38**(11):1372–1379.

43. Koplewicz HS, Vogel JM, Solanto MV, Morrissey RF, Alonso CM, Abikoff H, et al.: Child and parent response to the 1993 World Trade Center bombing. *J Trauma Stress* 2002; **15**(1):77–85.

44. Schuster MA, Stein BD, Jaycox L, Collins RL, Marshall GN, Elliott MN, et al.: A national survey of stress reactions after the September 11, 2001, terrorist attacks. *N Engl J Med* 2001; **345**(20):1507–1512.

45. Sack WH, Clarke G, Him C, Dickason D, Goff B, Lanham K, et al.: A 6-year follow-up study of Cambodian refugee adolescents traumatized as children. *J Am Acad Child Adolesc Psychiatry* 1993; **32**(2):431–437.

46. Sack WH, Clarke GN, Seeley J: Posttraumatic stress disorder across two generations of Cambodian refugees. *J Am Acad Child Adolesc Psychiatry* 1995; **34**(9):1160–1166.

47. Magwaza AS, Killian BJ, Petersen I, Pillay Y: The effects of chronic violence on preschool children living in South African townships. *Child Abuse Negl* 1993; **17**(6):795–803.

48. Nader KO, Pynoos RS, Fairbanks LA, al-Ajeel M, al-Asfour A: A preliminary study of PTSD and grief among the children of Kuwait following the Gulf crisis. *Br J Clin Psychol* 1993; **32**(4):407–416.

49. Dyregrov A, Gupta L, Gjestad R, Mukanoheli E: Trauma exposure and psychological reactions to genocide among Rwandan children. *J Trauma Stress* 2000; **13**(1):3–21.

50. Qouta S, Punamaki RL, El Sarraj E: Prevalence and determinants of PTSD among Palestinian children exposed to military violence. *Eur Child Adolesc Psychiatry* 2003; **12**(6):265–272.

51. Lustig SL, Kia-Keating M, Knight WG, Geltman P, Ellis H, Kinzie JD, *et al.*: Review of child and adolescent refugee mental health. *J Am Acad Child Adolesc Psychiatry* 2004; **43**(1):24–36.

52. Westermeyer J: Psychiatric services for refugee children: an overview. In: Westermeyer J, ed. *Refugee Mental Health in Resettlement Countries: The Series in Clinical and Community Psychology.* Washington, DC: Hemisphere Publishing, 1991:235–245.

53. Rothe EM, Lewis J, Castillo-Matos H, Martinez O, Busquets R, Martinez I: Posttraumatic stress disorder among Cuban children and adolescents after release from a refugee camp. *Psychiatr Serv* 2002; **53**(8):970–976.

54. Punamaki RL: Can ideological commitment protect children's psychological well-being in situations of political violence? *Child Dev* 1996; **67**(1):55–69.

55. Smith P, Perrin S, Yule W, Rabe-Hesketh S: War exposure and maternal reactions in the psychological adjustment of children from Bosnia-Hercegovina. *J Child Psychol Psychiatry* 2001; **42**(3):395–404.

56. Servan-Schreiber D, Le Lin B, Birmaher B: Prevalence of posttraumatic stress disorder and major depressive disorder in Tibetan refugee children. *J Am Acad Child Adolesc Psychiatry* 1998; **37**(8):874–879.

57. Terr LC, Bloch DA, Michel BA, Shi H, Reinhardt JA, Metayer S: Children's symptoms in the wake of Challenger: A field study of distant-traumatic effects and an outline of related conditions. *Am J Psychiatry* 1999; **156**(10):1536–1544.

58. Pfefferbaum B, Nixon SJ, Tivis RD, Doughty DE, Pynoos RS, Gurwitch RH, *et al.*: Television exposure in children after a terrorist incident. *Psychiatry* 2001; **64**(3):202–211.

59. Schlenger WE, Caddell JM, Ebert L, Jordan BK, Rourke KM, Wilson D, *et al.*: Psychological reactions to terrorist attacks: Findings from the National Study of Americans' Reactions to September 11. *JAMA* 2002; **288**(5):581–588.

60. Shannon MP, Lonigan CJ, Finch AJ, Jr., Taylor CM: Children exposed to disaster: I. Epidemiology of posttraumatic symptoms and symptom profiles. *J Am Acad Child Adolesc Psychiatry* 1994; **33**(1):80–93.

61. Lonigan CJ, Shannon MP, Taylor CM, Finch AJ, Jr., Sallee FR: Children exposed to disaster: II. Risk factors

62. Garrison CZ, Bryant ES, Addy CL, Spurrier PG, Freedy JR, Kilpatrick DG: Posttraumatic stress disorder in adolescents after Hurricane Andrew. *J Am Acad Child Adolesc Psychiatry* 1995; **34**(9):1193–1201.

63. Vernberg EM, Silverman WK, La Greca AM, Prinstein MJ: Prediction of posttraumatic stress symptoms in children after hurricane Andrew. *J Abnorm Psychol* 1996; **105**(2):237–248.

64. La Greca AM, Silverman WK, Wasserstein SB: Children's predisaster functioning as a predictor of posttraumatic stress following Hurricane Andrew. *J Consult Clin Psychol* 1998; **66**(6):883–892.

65. Goenjian AK, Pynoos RS, Steinberg AM, Najarian LM, Asarnow JR, Karayan I, *et al.*: Psychiatric comorbidity in children after the 1988 earthquake in Armenia. *J Am Acad Child Adolesc Psychiatry* 1995; **34**(9):1174–1184.

66. Goldstein RD, Wampler NS, Wise PH: War experiences and distress symptoms of Bosnian children. *Pediatrics* 1997; **100**(5):873–878.

67. Najarian LM, Goenjian AK, Pelcovitz D, Mandel F, Najarian B: Relocation after a disaster: Posttraumatic stress disorder in Armenia after the earthquake. *J Am Acad Child Adolesc Psychiatry* 1996; **35**(3):374–383.

68. Laor N, Wolmer L, Cohen DJ: Mothers' functioning and children's symptoms 5 years after a SCUD missile attack. *Am J Psychiatry* 2001; **158**(7):1020–1026.

69. Bryce JW, Walker N, Ghorayeb F, Kanj M: Life experiences, response styles and mental health among mothers and children in Beirut, Lebanon. *Soc Sci Med* 1989; **28**(7):685–695.

70. Breton JJ, Valla JP, Lambert J: Industrial disaster and mental health of children and their parents. *J Am Acad Child Adolesc Psychiatry* 1993; **32**(2):438–445.

71. Garbarino J, Kostelny K: Child maltreatment as a community problem. *Child Abuse Negl* 1992; **16**(4):455–464.

72. Brom D, Kleber RJ, Witztum E: The prevalence of posttraumatic psychopathology in the general and the clinical population. *Isr J Psychiatry Relat Sci* 1992; **28**(4):53–63.

73. Norris FH: Epidemiology of trauma: Frequency and impact of different potentially traumatic events on different demographic groups. *J Consult Clin Psychol* 1992; **60**(3):409–418.

74. Norris FH, Murphy AD, Baker CK, Perilla JL, Rodriguez FG, Rodriguez Jde J: Epidemiology of trauma and posttraumatic stress disorder in Mexico. *J Abnorm Psychol* 2003; **112**(4):646–656.

75. Breslau N, Davis GC, Andreski P, Peterson E: Traumatic events and posttraumatic stress disorder in an urban population of young adults. *Arch Gen Psychiatry* 1991; **48**(3):216–222.

76. Silverman AB, Reinherz HZ, Giaconia RM: The long-term sequelae of child and adolescent abuse: A longitudinal community study. *Child Abuse Negl* 1996; **20**(8):709–723.

77. Cuffe SP, Addy CL, Garrison CZ, Waller JL, Jackson KL, McKeown RE, *et al.*: Prevalence of PTSD in a community sample of older adolescents. *J Am Acad Child Adolesc Psychiatry* 1998; **37**(2):147–154.

78. Steiner H, Garcia IG, Matthews Z: Posttraumatic stress disorder in incarcerated juvenile delinquents. *J Am Acad Child Adolesc Psychiatry* 1997; **36**(3):357–365.

79. Steiner H, Carrion V, Plattner B, Koopman C: Dissociative symptoms in posttraumatic stress disorder: Diagnosis and treatment. *Child Adolesc Psychiatr Clin N Am* 2003; **12**(2):231–249, viii.

80. McLeer SV, Deblinger E, Henry D, Orvaschel H: Sexually abused children at high risk for post-traumatic stress disorder. *J Am Acad Child Adolesc Psychiatry* 1992; **31**(5):875–879.

81. Deblinger E, McLeer SV, Atkins MS, Ralphe D, Foa E: Post-traumatic stress in sexually abused, physically abused, and nonabused children. *Child Abuse Negl* 1989; **13**(3):403–408.

82. McLeer SV, Deblinger E, Atkins MS, Foa EB, Ralphe DL: Post-traumatic stress disorder in sexually abused children. *J Am Acad Child Adolesc Psychiatry* 1988; **27**(5):650–654.

83. Green BL, Korol M, Grace MC, Vary MG, Leonard AC, Gleser GC, *et al.*: Children and disaster: Age, gender, and parental effects on PTSD symptoms. *J Am Acad Child Adolesc Psychiatry* 1991; **30**(6):945–951.

84. Green BL, Lindy JD, Grace MC, Gleser GC, Leonard AC, Korol M, *et al.*: Buffalo Creek survivors in the second decade: Stability of stress symptoms. *Am J Orthopsychiatry* 1990; **60**(1):43–54.

85. Pynoos RS, Goenjian A, Tashjian M, Karakashian M, Manjikian R, Manoukian G, *et al.*: Post-traumatic stress reactions in children after the 1988 Armenian earthquake. *Br J Psychiatry* 1993; **163**:239–247.

86. Yehuda R, McFarlane AC: Conflict between current knowledge about posttraumatic stress disorder and its original conceptual basis. *Am J Psychiatry* 1995; **152**(12):1705–1713.

87. Yehud R, Hallig SL, Grossman R: Childhood trauma and risk for PTSD: Relationship to intergenerational effects of trauma, parental PTSD, and cortisol excretion. *Dev Psychopathol* 2001; **13**(3):733–753.

88. Seligman ME, Csikszentmihalyi M: Positive psychology. An introduction. *Am Psychol* 2000; **55**(1):5–14.

89. Teicher MH, Andersen SL, Polcari A, Anderson CM, Navalta CP, Kim DM: The neurobiological consequences of early stress and childhood maltreatment. *Neurosci Biobehav Rev* 2003; **27**(1–2):33–44.

90. Sapolsky RM, Romero LM, Munck AU: How do glucocorticoids influence stress responses? Integrating permissive, suppressive, stimulatory, and preparative actions. *Endocr Rev* 2000; **21**(1):55–89.

91. Sapolsky RM: Stress and plasticity in the limbic system. *Neurochem Res* 2003; **28**(11):1735–1742.

92. Fletcher K: *Childhood Posttraumatic Stress Disorder.* New York: Guilford Publications, Inc., 1996.

93. Edwards E, Harkins K, Wright G, Henn F: Effects of bilateral adrenalectomy on the induction of learned helplessness behavior. *Neuropsychopharmacology* 1990; **3**(2):109–114.

94. Sapolsky RM, Uno H, Rebert CS, Finch CE: Hippocampal damage associated with prolonged glucocorticoid exposure in primates. *J Neurosci* 1990; **10**(9):2897–2902.

95. Simantov R, Blinder E, Ratovitski T, Tauber M, Gabbay M, Porat S: Dopamine-induced apoptosis in human neuronal cells: Inhibition by nucleic acids antisense to the dopamine transporter. *Neuroscience* 1996; **74**(1):39–50.

96. Dunlop SA, Archer MA, Quinlivan JA, Beazley LD, Newnham JP: Repeated prenatal corticosteroids delay myelination in the ovine central nervous system. *J Matern Fetal Med* 1997; **6**(6):309–313.

97. Sapolsky RM: Stress, glucocorticoids, and damage to the nervous system: The current state of confusion. *Stress* 1996; **1**(1):1–19.

98. Todd RD: Neural development is regulated by classical neurotransmitters: Dopamine D2 receptor stimulation enhances neurite outgrowth. *Biol Psychiatry* 1992; **31**(8):794–807.

99. Gould E, Tanapat P, Cameron HA: Adrenal steroids suppress granule cell death in the developing dentate gyrus through an NMDA receptor-dependent mechanism. *Brain Res Dev Brain Res* 1997; **103**(1):91–93.

100. Gould E, Tanapat P, McEwen BS, Flugge G, Fuchs E: Proliferation of granule cell precursors in the dentate gyrus of adult monkeys is diminished by stress. *Proc Natl Acad Sci USA* 1998; **95**(6):3168–3171.

101. Smith MA, Makino S, Kvetnansky R, Post RM: Effects of stress on neurotrophic factor expression in the rat brain. *Ann N Y Acad Sci* 1995; **771**:234–239.

102. De Bellis MD, Baum AS, Birmaher B, Keshavan MS, Eccard CH, Boring AM, *et al.*: A.E. Bennett Research Award. Developmental traumatology. Part I: Biological stress systems. *Biol Psychiatry* 1999; **45**(10):1259–1270.

103. Queiroz EA, Lombardi AB, Furtado CR, Peixoto CC, Soares TA, Fabre ZL, *et al.*: Biochemical correlate of depression in children. *Arq Neuropsiquiatr* 1991; **49**(4):418–425.

104. De Bellis MD, Chrousos GP, Dorn LD, Burke L, Helmers K, Kling MA, *et al.*: Hypothalamic-pituitary-adrenal axis dysregulation in sexually abused girls. *J Clin Endocrinol Metab* 1994; **78**(2):249–255.

105. Yehuda R, Siever LJ, Teicher MH, Levengood RA, Gerber DK, Schmeidler J, *et al.*: Plasma norepinephrine and 3-methoxy-4-hydroxyphenylglycol concentrations and severity of depression in combat posttraumatic stress disorder and major depressive disorder. *Biol Psychiatry* 1998; **44**(1):56–63.

106. Southwick SM, Krystal JH, Morgan CA, Johnson D, Nagy LM, Nicolaou A, *et al.*: Abnormal noradrenergic function in posttraumatic stress disorder. *Arch Gen Psychiatry* 1993; **50**(4):266–274.

107. Boscarino JA: Posttraumatic stress disorder, exposure to combat, and lower plasma cortisol among Vietnam veterans: Findings and clinical implications. *J Consult Clin Psychol* 1996; **64**(1):191–201.

108. Yehuda R, Kahana B, Binder-Brynes K, Southwick SM, Mason JW, Giller EL: Low urinary cortisol excretion in Holocaust survivors with posttraumatic stress disorder. *Am J Psychiatry* 1995; **152**(7):982–986.

109. Yehuda R, Golier JA, Halligan SL, Meaney M, Bierer LM: The ACTH response to dexamethasone in PTSD. *Am J Psychiatry* 2004; **161**(8):1397–403.

110. Yehuda R, Boisoneau D, Lowy MT, Giller EL, Jr.: Dose-response changes in plasma cortisol and lymphocyte glucocorticoid receptors following dexamethasone administration in combat veterans with and without posttraumatic stress disorder. *Arch Gen Psychiatry* 1995; **52**(7):583–593.

111. Bremner JD, Licinio J, Darnell A, Krystal JH, Owens MJ, Southwick SM, *et al.*: Elevated CSF corticotropin-

releasing factor concentrations in posttraumatic stress disorder. *Am J Psychiatry* 1997; **154**(5):624–629.

112. Smith MA, Davidson J, Ritchie JC, Kudler H, Lipper S, Chappell P, *et al.*: The corticotropin-releasing hormone test in patients with posttraumatic stress disorder. *Biol Psychiatry* 1989; **26**(4):349–355.

113. Yehuda R, Teicher MH, Trestman RL, Levengood RA, Siever LJ: Cortisol regulation in posttraumatic stress disorder and major depression: A chronobiological analysis. *Biol Psychiatry* 1996; **40**(2):79–88.

114. Lemieux AM, Coe CL: Abuse-related posttraumatic stress disorder: Evidence for chronic neuroendocrine activation in women. *Psychosom Med* 1995; **57**(2):105–115.

115. Maes M, Lin A, Bonaccorso S, van Hunsel F, Van Gastel A, Delmeire L, *et al.*: Increased 24-hour urinary cortisol excretion in patients with post-traumatic stress disorder and patients with major depression, but not in patients with fibromyalgia. *Acta Psychiatr Scand* 1998; **98**(4):328–335.

116. Pitman RK, Orr SP. Twenty-four hour urinary cortisol and catecholamine excretion in combat-related post-traumatic stress disorder. *Biol Psychiatry* 1990; **27**(2):245–247.

117. Rasmusson A, Lipschitz DS, Wang S, Hu S, Vojvoda D, Bremner JD, Southwick SM, Charney DS: Increased pituitary and adrenal reactivity in premenopausal women with posttraumatic stress disorder. *Biol Psychiatry* 2001; **50**:965–977.

118. Heim C, Newport DJ, Heit S, Graham YP, Wilcox M, Bonsall R, *et al.*: Pituitary-adrenal and autonomic responses to stress in women after sexual and physical abuse in childhood. *Jama* 2000; **284**(5):592–597.

119. Kanter ED, Wilkinson CW, Radant AD, Petrie EC, Dobie DJ, McFall ME, *et al.*: Glucocorticoid feedback sensitivity and adrenocortical responsiveness in post-traumatic stress disorder. *Biol Psychiatry* 2001; **50**(4):238–245.

120. Carrion VG, Weems CF, Ray RD, Glaser B, Hessl D, Reiss AL: Diurnal salivary cortisol in pediatric post-traumatic stress disorder. *Biological Psychiatry* 2002; **51**:575–582.

121. Gunnar MR, Morison SJ, Chisholm K, Schuder M: Salivary cortisol levels in children adopted from romanian orphanages. *Dev Psychopathol* 2001; **13**(3):611–628.

122. Hart J, Gunnar M, Cichetti D: Altered neuroendocrine activity in maltreated children related to symptoms of depression. *Dev Psychopathol* 1996; **8**:201–214.

123. Goenjian AK, Yehuda R, Pynoos RS, Steinberg AM, Tashjian M, Yang RK, *et al.*: Basal cortisol, dexamethasone suppression of cortisol, and MHPG in adolescents after the 1988 earthquake in Armenia. *Am J Psychiatry* 1996; **153**(7):929–934.

124. King JA, Mandansky D, King S, Fletcher KE, Brewer J: Early sexual abuse and low cortisol. *Psychiatry Clin Neurosci* 2001; **55**(1):71–74.

125. Thomas LA, De Bellis MD: Pituitary volumes in pediatric maltreatment-related posttraumatic stress disorder. *Biol Psychiatry* 2004; **55**(7):752–758.

126. Gertz BJ, Contreras LN, McComb DJ, Kovacs K, Tyrrell JB, Dallman MF: Chronic administration of corticotropin-releasing factor increases pituitary corticotroph number. *Endocrinology* 1987; **120**(1):381–388.

127. Westlund KN, Aguilera G, Childs GV: Quantification of morphological changes in pituitary corticotropes produced by in vivo corticotropin-releasing factor stimulation and adrenalectomy. *Endocrinology* 1985; **116**(1):439–445.

128. Lopez JF, Palkovits M, Arato M, Mansour A, Akil H, Watson SJ: Localization and quantification of pro-opiomelanocortin mRNA and glucocorticoid receptor mRNA in pituitaries of suicide victims. *Neuroendocrinology* 1992; **56**(4):491–501.

129. Sapolsky RM: Glucocorticoids and hippocampal atrophy in neuropsychiatric disorders. *Arch Gen Psychiatry* 2000; **57**(10):925–935.

130. Gurvits TV, Shenton ME, Hokama H, Ohta H, Lasko NB, Gilbertson MW, *et al.*: Magnetic resonance imaging study of hippocampal volume in chronic, combat-related posttraumatic stress disorder. *Biol Psychiatry* 1996; **40**(11):1091–1099.

131. Bremner JD, Randall P, Scott TM, Bronen RA, Seibyl JP, Southwick SM, *et al.*: MRI-based measurement of hippocampal volume in patients with combat-related posttraumatic stress disorder. *Am J Psychiatry* 1995; **152**(7):973–981.

132. Bremner JD, Randall P, Vermetten E, Staib L, Bronen RA, Mazure C, *et al.*: Magnetic resonance imaging-based measurement of hippocampal volume in posttraumatic stress disorder related to childhood physical and sexual abuse–a preliminary report. *Biol Psychiatry* 1997; **41**(1):23–32.

133. Stein MB, Koverola C, Hanna C, Torchia MG, McClarty B: Hippocampal volume in women victimized by childhood sexual abuse. *Psychol Med* 1997; **27**(4):951–959.

134. Starkman MN, Gebarski SS, Berent S, Schteingart DE: Hippocampal formation volume, memory dysfunction, and cortisol levels in patients with Cushing's syndrome. *Biol Psychiatry* 1992; **32**(9):756–765.

135. Starkman MN, Giordani B, Gebarski SS, Berent S, Schork MA, Schteingart DE: Decrease in cortisol reverses human hippocampal atrophy following treatment of Cushing's disease. *Biol Psychiatry* 1999; **46**(12):1595–1602.

136. Bremner JD, Narayan M, Anderson ER, Staib LH, Miller HL, Charney DS: Hippocampal volume reduction in major depression. *Am J Psychiatry* 2000; **157**(1):115–118.

137. Sheline YI, Wang PW, Gado MH, Csernansky JG, Vannier MW: Hippocampal atrophy in recurrent major depression. *Proc Natl Acad Sci USA* 1996; **93**(9):3908–3913.

138. Moghaddam B, Bolinao ML, Stein-Behrens B, Sapolsky R: Glucocorticoids mediate the stress-induced extracellular accumulation of glutamate. *Brain Res* 1994; **655**(1–2):251–254.

139. Carrion VG, Weems CF, Eliez S, Patwardhan A, Brown W, Ray RD, *et al.*: Attenuation of frontal asymmetry in pediatric posttraumatic stress disorder. *Biol Psychiatry* 2001; **50**(12):943–951.

140. De Bellis MD, Keshavan MS, Clark DB, Casey BJ, Giedd JN, Boring AM, *et al.*: A.E. Bennett Research Award. Developmental traumatology. Part II: Brain development. *Biol Psychiatry* 1999; **45**(10):1271–1284.

141. De Bellis MD, Keshavan MS, Shifflett H, Iyengar S, Beers SR, Hall J, *et al.*: Brain structures in pediatric maltreatment-related posttraumatic stress disorder: a sociodemographically matched study. *Biol Psychiatry* 2002; **52**(11):1066–1078.

142. Teicher MH, Ito Y, Glod CA, Andersen SL, Dumont N, Ackerman E: Preliminary evidence for abnormal cortical development in physically and sexually abused children using EEG coherence and MRI. *Ann N Y Acad Sci* 1997; **821**:160–175.

143. De Bellis MD, Clark DB, Beers SR, Soloff PH, Boring AM, Hall J, et al.: Hippocampal volume in adolescent-onset alcohol use disorders. *Am J Psychiatry* 2000; **157**(5):737–744.

144. Purves D, Lichtman JW: Elimination of synapses in the developing nervous system. *Science* 1980; **210**(4466):153–157.

145. Rakic P, Bourgeois JP, Eckenhoff MF, Zecevic N, Goldman-Rakic PS: Concurrent overproduction of synapses in diverse regions of the primate cerebral cortex. *Science* 1986; **232**(4747):232–235.

146. Cowan WM, Fawcett JW, O'Leary DD, Stanfield BB: Regressive events in neurogenesis. *Science* 1984; **225**(4668):1258–1265.

147. Rasmusson AM, Shi L, Duman R: Downregulation of BDNF mRNA in the hippocampal dentate gyrus after re-exposure to cues previously associated with foot-shock. *Neuropsychopharmacology* 2002; **27**(2):133–142.

148. Gilbertson MW, Shenton ME, Ciszewski A, Kasai K, Lasko NB, Orr SP, et al.: Smaller hippocampal volume predicts pathologic vulnerability to psychological trauma. *Nat Neurosci* 2002; **5**(11):1242–1247.

149. Rauch SL, Whalen PJ, Shin LM, McInerney SC, Macklin ML, Lasko NB, et al.: Exaggerated amygdala response to masked facial stimuli in posttraumatic stress disorder: A functional MRI study. *Biol Psychiatry* 2000; **47**(9):769–776.

150. Lieberzon I, Taylor SF, Amdur R. et al.: Brain activation in PTSD in response to trauma-related stimuli. *Biol Psychiatry* 1999; **45**:817–826.

151. Shin LM, McNally RJ, Kosslyn SM, Thompson WL, Rauch SL, Alpert NM, et al.: Regional cerebral blood flow during script-driven imagery in childhood sexual abuse-related PTSD: A PET investigation. *Am J Psychiatry* 1999; **156**(4):575–584.

152. De Bellis MD, Keshavan MS, Spencer S, Hall J: N-Acetylaspartate concentration in the anterior cingulate of maltreated children and adolescents with PTSD. *Am J Psychiatry* 2000; **157**(7):1175–1177.

153. Shaw RJ, Robinson TE, Steiner H: Acute stress disorder following ventilation. *Psychosomatics* 2002; **43**(1):74–76.

154. DePrince AP, Freyd JJ: Forgetting trauma stimuli. *Psychol Sci* 2004; **15**(7):488–492.

155. Freyd JJ: Blind to betrayal: New perspectives on memory for trauma. *Harv Ment Health Lett* 1999; **15**(12):4–6.

156. Williams LM: Recall of childhood trauma: A prospective study of women's memories of child sexual abuse. *J Consult Clin Psychol* 1994; **62**(6):1167–1176.

157. Anderson MC, Ochsner KN, Kuhl B, Cooper J, Robertson E, Gabrieli SW, et al.: Neural systems underlying the suppression of unwanted memories. *Science* 2004; **303**(5655):232–235.

158. Carrion VG, Steiner H: Trauma and dissociation in delinquent adolescents. *J Am Acad Child Adolesc Psychiatry* 2000; **39**(3):353–359.

159. Friedrich WN, Fisher JL, Dittner CA, Acton R, Berliner L, Butler J, et al.: Child Sexual Behavior Inventory: Normative, psychiatric, and sexual abuse comparisons. *Child Maltreat* 2001; **6**(1):37–49.

160. Briere J: *American Professional Society on the Abuse of Children. The APSAC Handbook on Child Maltreatment.* Thousand Oaks: Sage Publications, 1996.

161. Steiner H, Araujo KB, Koopman C: The response evaluation measure [REM-71]: A new instrument for the measurement of defenses in adults and adolescents. *Am J Psychiatry* 2001; **158**(3):467–473.

162. Horowitz M, Wilner N, Alvarez W: Impact of Event Scale: A measure of subjective stress. *Psychosom Med* 1979; **41**(3):209–218.

163. Deblinger E, McLeer SV, Henry D: Cognitive behavioral treatment for sexually abused children suffering post-traumatic stress: Preliminary findings. *J Am Acad Child Adolesc Psychiatry* 1990; **29**(5):747–752.

164. Nurcombe B, Wooding S, Marrington P, Bickman L, Roberts G: Child sexual abuse II: Treatment. *Aust N Z J Psychiatry* 2000; **34**(1):92–97.

165. Ramchandani P, Jones DP: Treating psychological symptoms in sexually abused children: From research findings to service provision. *Br J Psychiatry* 2003; **183**:484–490.

166. Post RM, Weiss SR, Li H, Smith MA, Zhang LX, Xing G, et al.: Neural plasticity and emotional memory. *Biol Psychiatry* 1998; **10**(4):829–855.

167. Post RM, Weiss SRB: Sensitization and kindling phenomena in mood, anxiety, and obsessive-compulsive disorders: The role of serotonergic mechanisms in illness progression. *Biol Psychiatry* 1998; **44**(3):193–206.

168. Seedat S, Lockhat R, Kaminer D, Zungu-Dirwayi N, Stein DJ: An open trial of citalopram in adolescents with post-traumatic stress disorder. *Int Clin Psychopharmacol* 2001; **16**(1):21–25.

169. Steiner H, Petersen ML, Saxena K, Ford S, Matthews Z: Divalproex sodium for the treatment of conduct disorder: A randomized controlled clinical trial. *J Clin Psychiatry* 2003; **64**(10):1183–1191.

170. Silverman M, Carrion V, Chang K, Matthews Z, Peterson M, Steiner H: Divalproex sodium and PTSD treatment: A randomized controlled clinical trial. In: *Annual Meeting of the American Academy of Child and Adolescent Psychiatry 2001*; 2001:132.

171. Famularo R, Kinscherff R, Fenton T: Propranolol treatment for childhood posttraumatic stress disorder, acute type. A pilot study. *Am J Dis Child* 1988; **142**(11):1244–1247.

172. Harmon RJ, Riggs PD: Clonidine for posttraumatic stress disorder in preschool children. *J Am Acad Child Adolesc Psychiatry* 1996; **35**(9):1247–1249.

173. Steiner H: *Handbook of Mental Health Interventions in Children and Adolescents: An Integrated Developmental Approach*, 1st ed. San Francisco, CA: Jossey-Bass Publishers; 2004.

Section III
Developmental Disorders

16

Attachment and Its Disorders

Jerald L. Kay

Introduction

It has been more than a half of century since John Bowlby developed the concept of attachment. Attachment is the affectional connection that a baby develops with its primary caregiver, most often the mothering person, which becomes increasingly discriminating and enduring. It is the availability and responsiveness of the mother or other caretaker that is ultimately the most influential in determining the strength and safety of the attachment system. Bowlby's attachment theory has been integrated into other psychological theories and has experienced an extraordinary growth in its scientific base. His concepts have proved to be persistent and increasingly relevant to a broader and more sophisticated scientific understanding of the centrality of early experience in human development. In addition to the introduction of rigorous methods of assessing attachment, neurobiological studies of humans, primates, and nonprimates have provided strong support for attachment theory concepts. Moreover, psychiatry and psychology have continually demonstrated the impact of attachment and its disruption on childhood, adolescent, and adult stages of life. It is because of its exceptional power to exert influence on the entire life span and subsequent interpersonal relationships in so many dynamically interactive sectors of an individual's life that it especially behooves the child and adolescent mental health professional to become knowledgeable about attachment theory and its helpfulness role in understanding the etiology, prevention, and treatment of psychopathology.

The History of Attachment Theory

Like August Aichhorn and others, John Bowlby's work started with experience involving juvenile delinquency. His retrospective study of 44 such subjects suggested

to him that a distinguishing characteristic of these children appeared to lie in a history of disruptive early experiences with mothering [1]. Although a psychoanalyst, Bowlby's work was greeted initially with strong contempt by the psychoanalytic community [2]. Moreover, his work, even at present, is viewed suspiciously by child and adult psychoanalylists. Criticisms have centered on Bowlby's simplistic and reductionistic model for understanding behavior which was considered by many to have evolved more from the field of ethology than classical psychoanalysis. This included his jettisoning of the dual drive theory, dismissal of the centrality of the Oedipal conflict, underappreciation for the emotional internalized world, exclusive focus on one domain of the parent–infant relationship, and minimization of the specific characteristics the baby contributes to attachment. In essence, his model retained little of analytic metapsychology although Bowlby constantly sought to maintain a relationship with the analytic community in Britain. It is ironic therefore that his contributions instigated the most intense scientific study of any psychoanalytic model and it has produced the strongest research base. As a result, there is now more interest in Bowlby's ideas and newer findings from attachment studies among analysts and child and adolescent psychiatrists that at anytime in the past [2–7].

Core Concepts of Attachment Theory

The infant's attachment behavior is an attempt to bring stability, predictability, and consistency to his or her world through drawing the mother closer. These behaviors include crying, vocalizing, and smiling. Other manifestations are greeting responses, crying when mother leaves, lifting of arms (often expressing the wish to be picked up), following the mother and clinging to her, and later, the rapid return to

Clinical Child Psychiatry, Second Edition. Edited by W.M. Klykylo and J.L. Kay
© 2005 John Wiley & Sons Ltd.

closeness with mother after the child's exploring activities.

Bowlby [8–10] classified attachment in a biologically driven (innate) epigenetic model consisting of four stages, including:

- birth through two months – phase of **limited discrimination** and social responsiveness;
- 2–7 months – phase of **limited preference** toward discriminating familiar figures;
- 7–24 months – phase of **focused attachment** and secure base achievement with initiative in seeking proximity and contact
- 24–36 months – phase of **goal-corrected partnership** with child's attempt to shape mother's ways of relating to accommodate the child's wishes.

Bowlby's tripartite attachment theory consists of: an attachment behavioral system (that attempts to ensure closeness), development of internal models of self and others (internal representation), and the creation of a homeostatic system (to help the child deal with emotional, environmental, and physiological stress). He focused on the impact of levels of deprivation resulting from an infant's broken bond or failure to achieve a secure connection with the mother. The former attachment disorganization was referred to as partial deprivation and the latter was termed complete deprivation, both of which conditions may confer significant and enduring psychological, and in some cases, physical vulnerabilities leading to mental disorders later in life.

Clinicians are most familiar with Bowlby's description of what occurs when the child is separated from the mother for prolonged periods. He spoke of this process as consisting of three phases experienced by the separated or abandoned child: protest, despair, and detachment. These phases are demonstrated powerfully in the Robertsons' movies of children in naturalistic settings who experienced painful separation [11]. Each phase was marked by the child's readily observable behaviors as illustrated in Table 16.1. However, it is important to note that separation is comprised of two distinct processes. The first is the physical act of disruption of the mother–child relationship but undoubtedly more important is the child's appraisal or assessment of the separation experience. In other words, it is the meaning attributed to the phenomenon that is so powerful.

As Solomon and George [12] note, Bowlby's contributions provided a reconceptualization of numerous psychological responses to separation, threat of separation, and loss. For example, some symptoms heretofore attributed to anxiety, phobia, depression, aggression, incomplete mourning, and the failure to establish and maintain healthy interpersonal relationships, could be viewed in an overarching theory more reasonably explaining psychological vulnerability in terms of very early disorganizing and at times traumatizing caretaker–infant experiences.

Table 16.1 Separation behaviors.

Phase	Responses
Protest	Resentment, crying, and attempts to find mother
Despair	Sadness, aggressive behavior towards others, social withdrawal
Detachment	Reaching out to other adults, social reintegration, negative/ambivalent reactions to reunification with mother

The Developmental Significance of Attachment

There is an extensive literature on and theories about what occurs in the mental life of infants and children during the attachment process. At the risk of oversimplifying, the most intriguing and clinically useful of these theories focuses on the process of internalization. Internalization is the mechanism for building psychological structure. More specifically, it is an attempt to describe how the child achieves an increasingly stable and sophisticated view of himself and the world around him. The acquisition of internal representations of the infant and those who care for him are the building blocks of identity formation and individuation. The former includes the capacity for relatedness and cohesiveness of self and the latter refers to the establishment of autonomy or separateness.

Studies have demonstrated how early internal representations are the result of emotional and physical reciprocity between infant and mother [13–15]. That is, primitive representations are products of co-regulation of synchronies and asynchronies in communication patterns (vocalization, gestures, and facial expressions) within the mother–infant dyad. How the mother responds to unintended empathic failures or disengagements is also an important contributor to the representational process. Providing misattunement and separation are not traumatic, they are equally as potent in promoting healthy psychological development.

It is important to note that mirroring the child's affective state does not imply simple reflection [16]. Rather, an attuned mother exaggerates her responses which allow the infant to begin to recognize his own emotional response as being separate from that of his mother's. Fonagy's [2] concept of mentalization is predicated on the mother's ability to promote both relatedness and separateness in the infant through her marked affective responses. Mentalization is the capacity of the infant to ascertain the mental states of the self and of others. It describes a process of the infant's recognition that someone else has a different mind from his own. It is acquired through repeated experiences in judging facial expression, tone of voice, and other nonverbal communications [2,17]. These experiences are encoded in implicit (nondeclarative) memory and in parallel with explicit (declarative) memory which has a temporal dimension. This is a critical accomplishment in that it establishes the basis for secure attachment. Conversely, the failure to mirror the child's affective state results in disorganized attachment through problematic internalization and therefore less than optimal identity formation and individuation.

Recent research has suggested how the attachment process may contribute to the development of empathy. There are a set of motor neurons in the premotor cortex that encodes in procedural memory the actions of others whether they are performed or merely observed passively. Initial research has focused on grasping and reaching movements but [18] have shown that subjects imitate not only hand movements but facial expressions as measured by functional magnetic resonance imaging (fMRI). They found evidence for a common cortical imitation circuit involving, but not limited to, Broca's area, bilateral dorsal and ventral premotor areas, and the superior temporal gyrus. This neuronal circuit facilitates an unconscious recognition of goal detection in another person through shared representations of the observer and the observed and may be a neural substrate for empathy.

Attachment Theory Research

Bowlby's ideas have prompted many different avenues of inquiry. While there has been reinterpretation of some of the findings and explanations of Ainsworth's [19] important studies of attachment types, she nevertheless moved attachment theory forward through the application of rigorous observation. Her most substantial contributions are associated with the development of the Strange Situation test which permitted observation and analysis of clear differentiation between the characteristics of children's attachment patterns or styles. The Strange Situation provides an examination of the response of 1–2-year-old children to being left for two very brief periods. To summarize a large body of data, Ainsworth and colleagues concluded there are distinct ways in which children deal with separation reflecting attachment styles she identified as secure, anxious/avoidant (avoidant), or anxious/resistant (ambivalent). Securely attached infants and toddlers actively seek out their mothers and demonstrate observable relief at reunification. These children are confident that the parent will be available at times of need. A smaller number of children, however, demonstrate some level of indifference to the separation–reunion experience, avoid greeting the parent, and seem not to experience soothing. Ainsworth characterized this group as having anxious/avoidant (avoidant) attachment and associated this style with emotionally restrictive mothering. A third group of children display high levels of distress and anger in an attempt to mobilize the mother and are also unable to be soothed effectively. Ainsworth termed this group anxious/resistant and attributed these characteristics to inconsistent caregiving resulting in the child's failure to integrate emotional responses.

More recent research identified a fourth type of child who attempts to seek proximity through unusual means like hiding or simply denying the presence of the mother. Main and Soloman [20] identified this attachment style as disorganized/disoriented. In addition, these children demonstrate conflicted behaviors upon reunion with their mother including, but not limited to, hitting, freezing, unusual posturing, and nongoal directed activity. A number of clinician–researchers have attributed the disorganized style of the child to experiencing the mother, who is likely to have experienced a major loss or trauma in her life, as either frightened (insecure in her caretaking) or frightening (unreliably comforting and soothing in times of need because of her significant misattunement with the child). This critical body of thought focuses on disorganization of children's behavior after separation and not on resistance or avoidance as patterns of attachment. Although Ainsworth's attachment types were widely accepted for years, some more recent research involving retesting subjects demonstrated poor reliability [21]. Interestingly, it has been the disorganized/disoriented attachment type that has proven more reliable [22] and perhaps a better predictor of future psychopathology [23–25].

Table 16.2 Some measurements of attachment.

Separation Anxiety Test	Pictures of attachment scenes prompt children's responses based on their attachment styles
Attachment interview for childhood and adolescence	Focuses on here and now relationships with parents in preteens and teens
Adult Attachment Interview	Most reliable measure of adult attachment styles as elicited through the narrative construction of significant childhood experiences (parental responses correlate highly with precise attachment style in their child within the Strange Situation)
Inventory of Parent and Peer Attachment Attachment History Questionnaire; Attachment Style Questionnaire	Self-report measures of adult attachment in current relationships

Since the development of the Strange Situation test, numerous new measures of attachment in early and later life have been developed. Table 16.2 summarizes many, but not all of these refinements.

Neurobiological Aspects of Animal Attachment

As noted previously, early in his career Bowlby's work was criticized by many in the psychoanalytic community as being too reliant on ethology. It is ironic, therefore, that some of the most evocative and exciting neurobiological research on attachment and stress in the last decade has involved primates and rodents. This is a very rich and rapidly expanding field that has consistently supported the long-term effects of stressful maternal separation and attachment difficulties in offspring. Because a complete review of this work is beyond the scope of this chapter, discussion will focus on a representative sample of studies.

Studies with monkeys who experience early life separations have revealed life long detrimental neuroendocrine consequences. In one of many of Suomi's studies [26] using rhesus monkeys, he was able to demonstrate that while surrogate mothering and socialization by normally reared peers was helpful in socially integrating monkeys separated from their mothers early after birth, there were nevertheless enduring responses to stress that clearly distinguished the separated monkeys. Most importantly, separated monkeys when exposed to environmental challenges such as separation later in life, responded with more extreme behavioral and physiological reactions, including higher levels of cortisol production, which has been linked repeatedly with such effects as impaired hip-

pocampal neurogenesis [27–29]. Similarly, using the variable foraging model which produces inconsistency and unpredictability in mother feeding [30], anxious mothers disrupt the attachment of their offspring which results in a marked inability to deal with emotions and stress when the offspring reaches adolescence. Kraemer and Clarke [31] noted that peer reared monkeys with inconsistent attachment figures not only demonstrated exaggerated fear response but had high levels of cortisol throughout adulthood.

With respect to rodent research, perinatal separation, even for very short time periods, and abuse, or neglect coupled with genetic variability appears to be associated with enduring changes in many areas of later life functioning including:

- emotional and behavioral regulation;
- cognitive function;
- coping style;
- neuroendocrine response to stress;
- brain morphology [32,33].

As an example, an elegant design was developed by the Emory University group to study the impact of early maternal separation and neglect in rats and its role in depression [34,35]. From day 2 to day 14 after birth, rat pups were separated for three hours each day. The offspring developed anhedonia, and decreased eating, sleeping, and reproductive behavior. They also displayed increased restless activity and withdrawal. Of perhaps even greater significance, the separated rat pups, as opposed to their nonseparated littermates, were treated differently by their mothers. Moreover, at 90 days, the pups were exposed to a stressor consisting of a puff of air into the eye and responded with increased adrenocorticotrophic hormone (ACTH) and double the normal of corticotrophin releasing factor (CRF) in their amygdale.

Early maternal separation in rats has been shown to be associated with both decreased brain derived neurotrophic factor (BDNF) and NMDA receptors [36] as well as increased cell death in the brain [37]. BDNF plays a vital role in neurogenesis but also in the maintenance of neurons and synapses.

Insel [38] has studied another important neurobiological basis for attachment through investigation of the neuropeptides oxytocin and vasopressin in voles and rats. While it would be an oversimplification to attribute the basis for attachment in these animals and humans to these peptides only, this line of inquiry nevertheless has raised some poignant issues, not the least of which is their potential role in understanding the pathophysiology of abnormal social attachment in such conditions as infantile autism.

Insel studied prairie voles and montane voles who display the following characteristics:

Prairie voles
  social
  monogamous/protective of female
  extended mothering
  male parenting of offspring
Montane voles
  asocial
  no partner preference
  females abandon young between days 8 and 14
  minimal parenting of offspring

When the male prairie vole is given a vasopressin antagonist, both the partner preference and aggressivity towards other voles disappeared. After mating, the female prairie vole releases oxytocin vital to establishing the pair bond. However, when the female is given an oxytocin antagonist, she behaves more like the female montane vole. Moreover, upon separation from the mother, the five-day-old prairie vole demonstrates signs of distress through vocalization and corticosterone production. Insel found that prairie and montane voles also have different oxytocin and vasopressin receptor distribution in the brain and that after giving birth, the female montane vole, at least for a short period of time, does possess similar oxytocin receptor configuration of the maternal prairie vole. Last, in Insel's studies of rats, females show little maternal interest when not pregnant. This behavior changes immediately prior to birthing. Insel demonstrated that if oxytocin release is prevented through either lesioning or through the use of antagonist, the onset of maternal care behavior is inhibited. These findings raise provocative questions about a role for oxytocin in human maternal behavior and attachment styles.

There is an additional area of research that has examined the possible reinforcing role of opiod receptors in attachment [39]. Knockout mice, which lack the mu-opiod receptor gene, appear dramatically inhibited in their attachment behavior. For example, when separated briefly from mothers, these offspring showed diminished vocalization but not when exposed to male mice odors or cold. Moreover, these pups also had difficulty in discriminating the smell of their own nests and from those belonging to other mothers. This study raises the possibility of another molecular consequence and basis for attachment disorders.

Recently, animal studies have focused on gene–environment interaction and the impact on subsequent behavioral and emotional changes. This work has examined the role of specific polymorphisms in serotonin transporter genes in conjunction with maternal separation, abuse, and neglect [40,41]. Specifically, the serotonin transporter gene (5-HTT) has variations in the length of its promoter region which is expressed in either short or long allelic forms. Short (ls) allele, unlike the long allele (ll) appears to result in decreased serotonin function, a deficiency which may negatively impact on attachment. The hypothesis is supported by the link between the treatment of anxiety and mood disorders with serotonin reuptake inhibitors and genetic variation in serotonin transporters in humans. Recently, a serotonin knockout mouse with impaired serotonin uptake ability was created [42]. This animal has both exaggerated stress responses as measured by increase hypothalamic–pituitary–adrenal axis (HPA) activity and anxiety-like behaviors. These inquiries support earlier work demonstrating persistent behavioral and social difficulties as a result of separation and other early adverse experiences.

Neurobiological Aspects of Human Attachment

Within the last five years, human studies too have explored the role of gene–environment interaction in the adaptation of children. Caspi et al. [43] have elucidated a representative gene–environment consequence of an abnormally low level of monoamine oxidase A (MAOA) and childhood maltreatment. Low levels of MAOA have been associated with rodents who display increased aggression. Caspi and colleagues studied more than 1000 children in Dunedin who were assessed every two years from the ages of 3 to 15 years and then again at ages 18 and 21 years. This birth cohort was evenly distributed among boys and girls. Moreover, the sample remained intact (96%) even by the age of 26 years. The findings of this study are as follows:

- 64%, 28%, or 8% experienced no, probable, and severe maltreatment respectively;
- males with normal MAOA levels and maltreatment experienced no increase in antisocial behavior;
- 85% of males with low MAOA levels and maltreatment demonstrated significantly more antisocial behavior including;
  - increase in conduct disorders
  - conviction of violent crimes (rape, robbery, assault)

The overarching finding of this study is that neither environmental trauma alone nor low activity of genes by itself is sufficient to cause antisocial behavior. Once again this study emphasizes the role of functional genetic polymorphism and early adverse experience. Recently this finding was replicated in the US as well [44].

Other studies have explored the relationship between attachment problems and developmental issues. Essex *et al.* [45] examined the effect of maternal stress on subsequent childhood pathology. Salivary cortisol levels were measured in 282 4.5-year-old children and more than 150 of their sibs. Measurements of maternal stress were gathered when the children were 1, 4, 12, and 54 months old. Mental health symptoms of the children were assessed when they were in first grade. Children who experienced chronic maternal depression in their infancy were more likely to have elevated cortisol levels and more mental health symptoms in the first grade. Children who were experiencing only concurrent levels of high stress, but not stress during infancy, did not share these symptoms. As is the case with many studies of early stressful experiences, children become sensitized to subsequent stress and demonstrate abnormal glucocorticoid responses. Studies have demonstrated also that exposure to postnatal maternal depression produces abnormally high levels of cortisol that persists into adolescence [46].

Adrenocortical activity among attachment styles has been a fruitful area of study. Since the HPA axis is an integral part of the response to stress and novelty, Spangler and Grossmann [47] studied whether disorganized infants respond differently than securely attached infants. Disorganized infants were examined 30 minutes after the Strange Situation and were found to have significantly elevated cortisol levels. Those with insecure attachment had more moderate increase in cortisol, and securely attached infants showed no increase in HPA activity. Higher levels of cortisol appear to reflect that disorganized children have the least success in developing effective coping response to novelty and stress.

There have been two thrusts in neurobiological research on attachment. Many researchers have examined the behavioral and social responses among attachment styles while others have focused more on brain structure and function as they related to maturation. As noted previously, repeated interaction between mother and infant provides the neural template for the baby's knowledge of himself and his evolving world. These attachment experiences constitute important implicit or procedural memory which shapes brain structure and function. In essence, neurons that fire together, wire together. That is, repeated affect laden interaction between mother and infant provide neuronal organization to the evolving brain through synaptogenesis and pruning. There is a growing body of research addressing the impact of dysfunctional attachment on right–left cortical maturation and functioning [48]. The right brain has been noted to develop earlier than the left and the former plays an important role in the developing capacity to modulate affect, aggression, and stress, all of which are necessary for the acquisition of social skills. It may be that early negative experiences not only disproportionately increase synaptic pruning but leave the infant in a persistent state of vulnerability to stress, as has been demonstrated in animal studies. The studies of child maltreatment and its impact on the corpus callosum also provide support for detrimental effects on brain maturation. The corpus callosum functions as the bridge between the right and left brain. Infants who have been abused or neglected have smaller callossal structures leaving them at a disadvantage regarding the integration of feelings and the developing cognitive capacity of the left brain.

Attachment Disorganization and Psychopathology

For the clinician, perhaps the most clinically relevant research has been that of assessing the impact of attachment problems on the psychological development of children and the likelihood of ensuing psychopathology. This line of inquiry has resulted in some support for the detrimental effects of disorganized attachment on subsequent relationships and adaptive capacity, especially among high risk children. In general, the following family risk factors have been shown to be associated with disorganized attachment:

- alcohol and substance abuse;
- bipolar disorder;
- chronic major depression;

- child maltreatment;
- parental history of abuse or significant loss.

The children of mothers with psychosocial problems have been shown to have higher levels of aggression [49] and more externalizing behavioral problems. Internalizing symptoms appear to be correlated more with avoidant attachment and not disorganized attachment style. The additive component of risk factors is illustrated in a study of disorganized children who also had difficult temperament styles as rated by mothers. These children were noted as exceptionally aggressive by teachers [50]. It seems that disorganized attachment style leads not only to aggression but to controlling behavior in middle childhood with parents frequently feeling helpless and intimidated by the child. The aggressive and controlling child also is less likely to be involved in productive peer relationships. It often appears to the clinician that the disorganized child is more likely to be seen as having poor social skills, less likely to modulate affect and arousal, and have less adaptability and resilience.

Unresolved parental loss appears to be a critical component in the development of attachment disorganization in children [51]. Mothers who have experienced unresolved trauma and or significant loss in their lives relate to their infants in a frightening or hostile manner. Other mothers with unresolved loss and or trauma are often frightened and experience helplessness about caring for their child. Both of these scenarios, despite maternal sensitivity to the child, may result in the mother's inability to control emotions and memories stemming from the loss and or trauma. Frequently, the demands of caring for an infant prompt maternal behaviors that are perceived as threatening to the infant. The infant, in turn, is in an irresolvable situation because of the need to seek comfort from the mother who also becomes a source of danger. Main and Hesse argue that it is this repeated dyadic interaction that engenders the disorganized attachment. Figure 16.1 illustrates the role of unresolved loss and disorganized attachment. This work complements that of Blatt [52] who conceptualizes attachment as a dialectic between two developmental pressures: the need to acquire the capacity to relate to others while at the same time acquiring a sense of identity. If acquiring the ability of relatedness did not go smoothly, later in life the clinician sees patients with dependency and the exaggerated wish for admiration and affirmation.

With respect to explaining disorganized attachment in both clinical studies and treatment, one of the most helpful theories is the relational diathesis model [3]. It

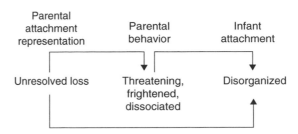

Figure 16.1 The theory of Main and Hesse: linking unresolved loss and infant disorganization. From: Schuengel *et al.*(1999).Unresolved loss and infant disorganization: links to frightening maternal behavior. In: *Attachment Disorganization*. Solomon J, George C, eds. New York: Guilford Press, 1990:73. Reproduced by permission of Guilford Press.

posits that disorganized attachment can be viewed as a product of both the level of safety experienced by the infant as well as the magnitude of his psychological trauma. Moreover, it explains how unresolved loss and trauma often lead to successive traumatic experiences. Figure 16.2 presents this model in schematic form.

There is a growing literature on the effect of disorganized attachment and child and adult pschopathology, but two caveats are in order. First, although studies have supported Bowlby's notions that individual differences in attachment security can be continuous throughout life, they can also change according to experience. Second, the most probable explanation of the contribution of disorganized attachment on psychopathology should include an interaction with other risk factors such as, but not limited to, difficult child temperament, medical illness in the child and family members, family history of mental illness, marital conflict, social and financial adversity, and caretakers with poor parenting skills [53].

Problematic attachment has been correlated with dysfunctional behavior/disorders during infancy and childhood, and the DSM IV-TR diagnostic category of reactive attachment disorder (RAD) recognizes this as is illustrated in Table 16.3.

A number of clinicians and researchers have criticized the DSM criteria for RAD [55]. Criticism has focused on the requirements of persistent disregard of the child's emotional and physical needs, but this is not supported by research. As has been discussed at length, disorganized attachment is not always the result of willful maltreatment. While disorganized children have insecure attachment, the assumption that insecurely attached children are disorganized is incorrect and fails to acknowledge anxious-resistant and

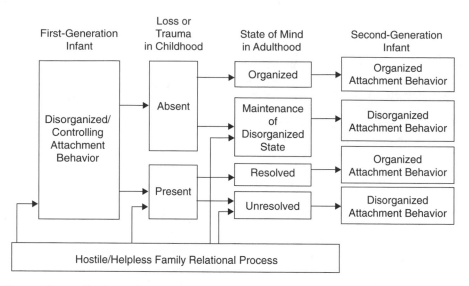

Figure 16.2 Proposed contributions of a relational diathesis. From: Lyons-Ruth *et al.* A relational diathesis model of hostile-helpless states of mind. In: *Attachment Disorganization.* Solomon J, George C, eds. New York: Guilford Press, 1999:44.

Table 16.3 DSM-IV TR criteria for reactive attachment disorder of infancy or early childhood. Reprinted with permission from the Diagnostic and Statistical Manual of Mental Disorders, Copyright 2000. American Psychiatric Association.

Diagnostic criteria for 313.89 Reactive Attachment Disorder of Infancy or Early Childhood

A. Markedly disturbed and developmentally inappropriate social relatedness in most contexts, beginning before age five years, as evidenced by either (1) or (2):
  (1) persistent failure to initiate or respond in a developmentally appropriate fashion to most social interactions, as manifest by excessively inhibited, hypervigilant, or highly ambivalent and contradictory responses (e.g., the child may respond to caregivers with a mixture of approach, avoidance, and resistance to comforting, or may exhibit frozen watchfulness)
  (2) diffuse attachments as manifest by indiscriminate sociability with marked inability to exhibit appropriate selective attachments (e.g., excessive familiarity with relative strangers or lack of selectivity in choice of attachment figures)

B. The disturbance in Criterion A is not accounted for solely by developmental delay (as in mental retardation) and does not meet criteria for a pervasive developmental disorder.

C. Pathogenic care as evidenced by at least one of the following:
  (1) persistent disregard of the child's basic emotional needs for comfort, stimulation, and affection
  (2) persistent disregard of the child's basic physical needs
  (3) repeated changes of primary caregiver that prevent formation of stable attachments (e.g., frequent changes in foster care)

D. There is a presumption that the care in Criterion C is responsible for the disturbed behavior in Criterion A (e.g., the disturbances in Criterion A began following the pathogenic care in Criterion C).

Specify type:
  Inhibited Type: if Criterion A1 predominates in the clinical presentation
  Disinhibited Type: if Criterion A2 predominates in the clinical presentation

---

From: American Psychiatric Association: *Diagnostic and Statistical Manual of Mental Disorders, Fourth Edition, Text Revision.* Washington, DC: American Psychiatric Association, 2000:130.

anxious-avoidant attachment styles. Other clinicians find the Diagnostic Classification of Mental Health and Developmental Disorders of Infancy and Early Childhood (DC:0–3) more comprehensive [56]. In this system, there are primary diagnostic categories for traumatic stress, and mood, anxiety, and regulatory disorders.

Research findings on the association between attachment styles and adaptation later in life is somewhat contradictory. However, there have been a number of studies demonstrating that problematic attachment styles do predict emotional and behavioral disorders in some populations. For example, anxiety symptoms and disorders in adolescence were predicted by an anxious resistant attachment style [57]. In this study, infants were administered the Strange Situation test at one year of age and 172 of these children were assessed by structured clinical interview (The Schedule for Affective Disorders and Schizophrenia for School-Aged Children) at 17.5 years. A birth cohort study of over 1000 subjects in New Zealand tested children at age eight years and then followed them over the course of 21 years [58]. Subjects were assessed in middle childhood for anxious/withdrawn behavior and again at ages 16–18 and 18–21 years for anxiety disorders. Increasing anxious/withdrawn behavior at the age of eight years was associated with higher risk in adolescence and young adulthood for panic disorder with agoraphobia, social and specific phobias, and major depression. Weinfeld *et al.* [59] conducted a 19-year prospective study of 12–18-month old children using the Strange Situation with follow up in 125 subjects in young adulthood using the Adult Attachment Interview. Disorganized attachment in infants was significantly more likely to be insecure or unresolved in late adolescence, and this also predicted unresolved abuse scores for those who experienced childhood abuse.

A prospective study of high risk children found that avoidant and disorganized attachment styles were associated with dissociative symptoms measured at four points in time over 19 years [60]. Carlson [25] too reported that disorganized attachment was associated with dissociation in young adulthood and also with behavioral problems in preschool, primary school, and high school. A study by Lyons-Ruth *et al.* [61] of 62 low-income families assessed attachment in infants at 18 months and at age five through preschool teacher ratings. The most potent predictor of hostile behavior towards classmates was earlier disorganized attachment style, with 71% of aggressive children having been designated as having disorganized attachment earlier in life.

There has been a number of studies of adoptive children with or without deprivation. O'Connor and Rutter [62] conducted a longitudinal examination of 152 Romanian children who experienced significant early hardship and compared them to 52 adoptees from the UK. They found that duration of deprivation correlated highly with severity of attachment disorders. In addition, the attachment disorder behaviors were also associated with conduct and attentional problems. In a study by Roy and Pickles [63] hyperactivity and attentional problems were found to be higher in 19 children from group homes as opposed to a control group of the same number of children from foster care. Another study of these Romanian children [64] demonstrated that secure attachment was highest among the children who spent shorter time in the orphanage. In yet another Romanian study by Smyke *et al.* [65] of 32 toddlers living in a typical unit within a large institution it was found that, compared to 33 toddlers living at home and to 29 children living on a unit designed to provide greater consistency by reducing the number of caretakers, they were more likely to demonstrate emotional withdrawal and indiscriminate social attachment patterns. A Greek study of 86 infants reared in residential care from birth and control group of 41 infants raised with their two biological parents found that 62% of infants from the residential care setting demonstrated disorganized attachment as opposed to 25% of the latter group [66].

Treatment Implications of Disorganized Attachment

Perhaps the most straightforward way to approach this rich topic is by addressing three groups of intervention: prevention, treatment of children, and treatment of parents and other adult patients. In the case of poorly adjusted infants and children, it is assumed that treatment is not limited to the identified patient but frequently may include treatment of families and parents or other caretakers. For example, 30 years ago Selma Frailberg [67] emphasized the importance of recognizing the contribution of unresolved parental childhood conflicts in poor adjustment of their infants. She called these unresolved problems 'ghosts in the nursery,' and described treatment as helping the parents attain insight through examination of the their own childhood experiences and how they affected their ability to care for their infant.

Children with behavior problems and many psychiatric disorders undoubtedly constitute the majority of patients treated by child and adolescent psychiatrists. This book contains chapters that describe the assessment of infants, children and adolescents, as well as treatment approaches to the most common child psychiatric disorders. It also addresses the centrality of those characteristics of the doctor–patient relationship that underlie every treatment situation with children, their parents, and their families. These include, but are not limited to the engagement of patients and their families through establishing a nonjudgmental rapport, an empathic stance, a therapeutic alliance, and attention to a broad range of biological, social, and psychological considerations.

In this concluding section, it seems fitting to return to Bowlby's first interest, criminal and antisocial behavior which frequently is associated with disorganized attachment. A representative example of prevention of these problems is found in the work of Olds and colleagues [69]. They enrolled 400 young (less than 19 years old), unmarried, or of low socioeconomic status high-risk pregnant women with no previous live births. In this randomized controlled trial (RCT) mothers were assigned to standard well-child care in a clinic or to a nurse who made regularly scheduled home visits throughout pregnancy, up to the child's second birthday. The latter group of mothers received on average nine home visits during pregnancy and 23 visits after delivery. In their visits, nurses focused on maternal functioning within three dimensions. These included maternal personal development, health related behaviors, and competent care of their children. A follow up of 15-year-old teenagers of mothers receiving the intervention compared to the former group in the standard well-child care clinic showed:

• less running away;
• fewer arrests;
• fewer convictions;
• fewer sentences to youth corrections;
• less initiation of sexual intercourse;
• fewer sexual partners;
• less illicit substance abuse and;
• fewer school suspensions and teacher reports of disruptive behavior.

This study convincingly demonstrated that prenatal and early childhood intervention can dramatically decrease the likelihood of antisocial behavior among adolescents born into high-risk families. Of equal importance, this study substantiates the benefits of psychotherapy for parents to them and their children. The findings of this RCT complement those of the previously discussed Dunedin study which examined the interaction between low MAOA and adverse childhood experiences [43]. Both studies therefore demonstrate the inextricability of environment and genes in the pathogenesis of antisocial behavior. Other attachment based studies offer promise in the prevention of

the effects of maternal depression and other mental disorders on infants [69–72].

For psychiatrists and other mental health professionals who view psychotherapy, particularly psychodynamic psychotherapy, as a necessary component in the treatment of the many child, adolescent, and adult disorders, attachment theory has provided support for this treatment and highlighted the importance of a patient's attachment to the therapist [73]. It has deepened understanding of the psychological birth of the infant and has reaffirmed important underlying principles about the power of early experience in shaping a person's enduring view of himself, the world around him, the intergenerational transmission of strengths and vulnerabilities, and in some cases, the pathogenesis of mental disorders. Attachment theory has added considerable support to the study of personality development within a social context as expressed through earlier work of British object relationists (Winnicott and Fairbairn), neo-Freudians (Erikson), and self psychologists (Kohut). It has also played an important role in substantiating the effects of psychological trauma on both the mother and her child.

Among other contributions, attachment theory has brought a deeper understanding to the treatment of personality disorders. This is exemplified in some difficult-to-treat patients, very often with significant trauma history, who have an inadequate capacity for mentalization and self-reflection that interferes with the ability to understand mental functioning in themselves as well as the therapist [74]. Not infrequently, there are challenging counter-transference issues in treating such patients who may reenact traumatic situations which define the therapist as unhelpful and persecuting. An understanding of the impact of disorganized attachment and trauma on the ability to reflect provides the child psychiatrist with a nonpunitive and thereby more empathic view of symptoms. From this vantage point, the therapist can conceptualize the patient not in terms of deficits or manipulation, but rather of ultimately unsuccessful adaptation through the attempt to ward off pain from early loss and trauma and insecure attachment [75].

Attachment theory has advanced the understanding of medical treatment and compliance. Using the Bartholomew and Horowitz [76] classification of secure, dismissing, preoccupied, and fearful attachment styles, Ciechanowski and colleagues [77] studied 367 adult patients with type 1 or 2 diabetes within a primary care setting. Patients with dismissing attachment styles tend to undervalue close relationships and present in the doctor–patient relationship as overly self-reliant and minimizing symptoms and the need for other people. Those diabetics with dismissing attachment compared to secure attachment had poorer doctor–patient communication and glucose control, both of which were associated with elevated glycosylated hemoglobin (HbA 1c) levels. (An elevation of HBA 1c of 1% has been shown to be associated over a 10-year-period with an approximate 60% increase in developing diabetic retinopathy.) In addition, those prescribed oral hypoglycemic agents were less likely to take these medications and monitor their blood glucose. This study supports research that has found dismissing attachment style to be associated with greater rejection of health providers, worse use of treatment, less self-disclosure in the treatment context, and fewer visits to health professionals [78,79].

Attachment has also contributed to a richer understanding of cognitive development through its focus on the acquisition of models for internalization and perception. Finally, it has prompted important neurobiological research in animals and humans which has substantiated the wisdom of dispensing with an artificially dichotomous view of nature and nurture and mind and brain.

Conclusion

Despite vehement initial rejection by psychoanalysis, attachment theory has proven to be an increasingly thoughtful contribution to the understanding of human development and psychopathology. Bowlby's theory described the intense innate need of the infant to affectionally connect with the primary caregiver. This connection provides the foundation for biological survival and psychological development and is a powerful motivator in the organization of the infant's mental life and his or her behavior. Moreover, it has a profound effect on all future interpersonal relationships through the establishment of a person's identity and world view. Last, attachment theory has elucidated the contributions to, and the enduring complications of, dysfunctional attachment and deepened the ability of psychiatrists to help their patients resolve these experiences.

References

1. Bowlby J: Forty-four juvenile thieves: Their characters and home life. *Int J Psychoanals* 1944; **25**:19–52.
2. Fonagy P: *Attachment Theory and Psychoanalysis.* New York: Other Press, 2001.
3. Lyons-Ruth K: A relational diathesis model of hostile-helpless states of mind expression in mother–infant interaction. In: Solomon J, George C, eds. *Attachment Disorganization.* New York: Guilford Press, 1999:44.
4. Slade A: Attachment theory and research: Implications for the theory and practice of individual psychotherapy with adults. In: Cassidy J, Shaver PR, eds. *Handbook of Attachment: Theory, Research and Clinical Applications.* New York: Guilford Press, 1999:575–594.
5. Mitchell SA: *Relationality: From Attachment to Intersubjectivity.* Hillsdale, NJ: The Analytic Press, 2000: 79–102.
6. Blatt SJ, Levy KN: Attachment theory, personality development and psychopathology. *Psychoanalytic Inquiry* 2003; **23**:102–150.
7. Diamond D: Attachment disorganization: The reunion of attachment theory and psychoanalysis. *Psychoanalytic Psychol* 2004; **21**(2):276–299.
8. Bowlby J: *Attachment and Loss, Vol. 1: Attachment.* London: Hogarth Press and the Institute of Psycho-Analysis, 1969.
9. Bowlby J: *Attachment and Loss, Vol. 2: Separation: Anxiety and Anger.* London: Hogarth Press and Institute of Psycho-Analysis, 1973.
10. Bowlby J: *Attachment and Loss, Vol. 3: Loss: Sadness and Depression.* London: Hogarth Press and Institute of Psycho-Analysis, 1980.
11. Robertson J, Robertson J: *John, Aged 17 Months [film].* London: Tavistock Institute of Human Relations, 1969.
12. Solomon J, George C: *Attachment Disorganization.* New York: Guilford Press, 1999.
13. Reference deleted.
14. Beebe B, Lachmann F, Jaffe J: Mother-Infant interaction structures and presymbolic self and object representations. *Psychoanalytic Dialog* 1977; **7**:113–182.
15. Stern DN: *The Interpersonal World of the Infant: A View from Psychoanalysis and Developmental Psychology.* New York: Basic Books, 1985.
16. Fonagy P, Target M, Gergely G: Attachment and borderline personality disorder. A theory and some evidence. *Psychiatr Clin North Am* 2000; **23**(1):103–122, vii-viii.
17. Fonagy P: Male perpetrators of violence against women: An attachment theory perspective. *J Appl Psychoanalytic Stud* 1999; **1**:7–27.
18. Leslie KR, Johnson-Frey SH, Grafton ST: Functional imaging of face and hand imitation: Towards a motor theory of empathy. *Neuroimage* 2004; **21**(2):601–607.
19. Ainsworth MDS, Blechar MC, Waters E, Wall S: *Patterns of Attachment: A Psychological Study of the Strange Situation.* Hillside, NJ: Erlbaum, 1978.
20. Main M, Solomon J: Procedures for identifying infants as disorganized/disoriented during the Ainsworth Strange Situation. In: Greenberg M, Ciccetti D, Cummings EM, eds. *Attachment During the Preschool Years: Theory, Research, and Intervention.* Chicago: University of Chicago Press, 1990:121–160.
21. Belsky J, Campbell S, Moore G: Instability of attachment security. *Dev Psychol* 1996; **32**:921–924.
22. Lyons-Ruth K, Repacholi B, McLeod S, Silver E: Disorganized attachment behavior in infancy: Short-term stability, maternal and infant correlates, and risk-related sub-types. *Dev Psychopathol* 1991; **3**:377–396.
23. Shaw DS, Owens EB, Vondra JI, Keenan K, Winslow EB: Early risk factors and pathways in the development of early disruptive behavior problems. *Dev Psychopathol* 1996; **8**:679–699.
24. Lyons-Ruth K: Attachment relationships among children with aggressive behavior problems: The role of dis-

organized early attachment problems. *J Consult Clin Psychol* 1996; **64**:64–73.

25. Carlson EA: A prospective longitudinal study of attachment disorganization/disorientation. *Child Dev* 1998; **69**(4):1107–1128.

26. Suomi SJ: Attachment in rhesus monkeys. In: Cassidy J, Shaver PR, eds. *Handbook of Attachment: Theory, Research and Clinical Applications.* New York: Guilford Press, 1999:181–197.

27. Salpolsky RM, *et al.*: Hippocampal damage associated withprolonged glucocorticoid exposure in primates. *J Neurosci* 1990; **10**(9):2897–2902.

28. Salpolsky RM: Glucocorticoids and hippocampal atrophy in neuropsychiatric disorders. *Arch Gen Psychiatry* 2000; **57**(10):925–935.

29. Heim C, Plotsky PM, Nemeroff C: Importance of studying the contributions of early adverse experience to neurobiological findings in depression. *Neuropsychopharmacology* 2004; **29**(4):641–648.

30. Rosenblum LA, Coplan JD, *et al.*: Adverse early experiences affect noradrenergic and serotonergic functioning in adult primates. *Biol Psychiatry* 1994; **15**(4):221–227.

31. Kraemer GW, Clarke AS: Social attachment, brain function, and aggression. *Ann NY Acad Sci* 1996; **794**:121–135.

32. Sanchez MM, Ladd CO, Plotsky PM: Early adverse experience as a developmental risk factor for later psychopathology: Evidence from rodent and primate models. *Dev Psychopathol* 2001; **13**(3):419–449.

33. Kalinichev M, Easterling KW, Plotsky PM, Holtzman SG: Long-lasting changes in stress-induces corticosterone response and anxiety-like behaviors as a consequence of neonatal maternal separation in Long-Evans rats. *Pharmacol Biochem Behav* 2002; **73**(1):131–140.

34. Nemeroff C: The cortcitropin-releasing factor (CRF) hypothesis of depression: New findings and new directions. *Mol Psychiatry* 1996; **1**:336–342.

35. Nemeroff C: The neurobiology of depression. *Sci Am* 1998; **278**(6):42–49.

36. Roceri M, Hendriks W, Racagni G, Ellenbroek BA, Riva MA: Early maternal deprivation reduces the expression of BDNF and NMDA receptor subunits in rat hippocampus. *Mol Psychiatry* 2002; **7**(6):609–616.

37. Zhang LX, Levine S, Dent G, Zhan Y, Xing G, Okimoto D, Kathleen Gordon M, Post RM, Smith MA: Maternal deprivation increases cell death in the infant rat brain. *Brain Res Dev Brain Res* 2002; **133**(1):1–11.

38. Insel TR: A neurobiological basis of social attachment. *Am J Psychiatry* 1997; **154**(6):726–735.

39. Moles A, Kieffer BL, D'Amato FR: Deficit in attachment behavior in mice lacking the mu-opioid receptor gene. *Science* 2004; **304**(5679):1983–1986.

40. Suomi SJ: Gene-environment interactions and the neurobiology of social conflict. *Ann NY Acad Sci* 2003; **1008**:132–139.

41. Barr CS, Newman TK, Shannon C, *et al.*: Rearing condition and rh5-HTTLPR interact to influence limbic-hypothalmic-pituitary-adrenal axis response to stress in infant macques. *Biol Psychiaty* 2004; **55**:733–738.

42. Holmes A, Murphy DL, Crawley JN: Abnormal behavioral phenotypes of serotonin transporter knockout mice: Parallels with human anxiety and depression. *Biol Psychiatry* 2003; **54**:953–959.

43. Caspi A, *et al.*: Role of genotype in the cycle of violence in maltreated children. *Science* 2002; **297**(5582):851–854.

44. Foley DL, Eaves LJ, Wormley B, Silberg JL, Maes HH, Kuhn J, Riley B: Childhood adversity, monoamine oxidase a genotype, and risk for conduct disorder. *Arch Gen Psychiatry* 2004; **61**(7):738–744.

45. Essex MJ, Klein MH, Cho E, Kalin NH: (2002). Maternal stress beginning in infancy may sensitize children to later stress exposure: Effects on cortisol and behavior. *Biol Psychiatry* 2002; **52**(8):776–784.

46. Halligan SL, Herbert J, Goodyer IM, Murray L: Exposure to postnatal depression predicts elevated cortisol in adolescent offspring. *Biol Psychiatry* 2004; **55**(4):376–381.

47. Spangler G, Grossmann KE: Biobehavioral organization in securely and insecurely attached infants. *Child Development* 1999; **64**:1439–1450.

48. Shore AN: Early organization of the nonlinear right brain and development of a predisposition to psychiatric disorders. *Dev Psychopathol* 1997; **9**:595–631.

49. Lyons-Ruth K: Attachment relationships among children with aggressive behavior problems: The role of disorganized early attachment patterns. *J Consult Clin Psychol* 1996; **64**:32–40.

50. Shaw DS, Owens EB, Vondra JI, Keenan K, Winslow EB: Early risk factors and pathways in the development of early disruptive behavior problems. *Dev Psychopathol* 1997; **8**:679–700.

51. Main M, Hesse E: Parents' unresolved traumatic experiences are related to infant disorganized attachment status: Is frightened and/or frightening parental behavior the linking mechanism? In: Greenberg M, Ciccetti D, Cummings EM, eds. *Attachment in the Preschool Years: Theory Research and Intervention.* Chicago: University of Chicago Press, 1990:161–182.

52. Blatt SJ, Blass R: Relatedness and self definition: A dialectic model of personality development. In: Noam GG, Fischer KW, eds. *Development and Vulnerabilities in Close Relationships.* New York: Erlbaum, 1996, p. 309–338.

53. Rutter ML: Psychosocial adversity and child psychopathology. *Br J Psychiatry* 1999; **174**:480–493.

54. American Psychiatric Association: *Diagnostic and Statistical Manual of Mental Disorders, Fourth Edition, Text Revision.* Washington, DC: American Psychiatric Association, 2000:130.

55. Boris NW, Zeanah CH, Larrieu JA, Sheeringa MS, Heller SS: Attachment disorders in infancy and early childhood: A preliminary investigation of diagnostic criteria. *Am J Psychiatry* 1998; **155**(2):295–297.

56. Greenspan SI, Weider S: *Zero to Three: Diagnostic Classification Task Force.* Arlington, VA: National Center for Clinical Infant Programs, 1994.

57. Warren SL, Huston L, Egeland B, Sroufe LA: Child and adolescent disorders and early attachment. *J Am Acad Child Adolesc Psychiatry* 1997; **36**(5):637–644.

58. Goodwin RD, Fergusson DM, Horwood LJ: Early anxious/withdrawn behaviours predict later internalizing disorders. *J Child Psychiatr* 2004; **45**(4):874–883.

59. Weinfeld NS, Whaley GJ, Egeland B: Continuity, discontinuity, and coherence in attachment from infancy to late adolescence: Sequelae of organization and disorganization. *Attach Hum Dev* 2004; **6**(1):73–97.

60. Ogawa JR, Sroufe LA, Weinfield NS, Carlson EA, Egeland B: Development and the fragmented self: Longitudinal study of dissociative symptomatology in a non-clinical sample: *Dev Psychopathol* 1997; **9**(4):855–879.

61. Lyons-Ruth K, Alpern L, Repacholi B: Disorganized infant attachment classification and maternal psychosocial problems as predictors of hostile-aggressive behavior in the preschool classroom. *Child Dev* 1993; **64**(2): 572–585.

62. O'Conner TG, Rutter M: Attachment disorder behavior following early severe deprivation: Extension and longitudinal follow-up. English and Romanian Adoptees Study Team. *J Am Acad Child Adolesc Psychiatry* 2000; **39**(6):703–712.

63. Roy PR, Pickles A: Institutional care: Risk from family background or pattern of rearing? *J Child Psychol Psychiatry* 2000; **41**(2):139–149.

64. Marvin RS, Britner PA: Normative development: The ontogeny of attachment. In: Cassidy J, Shaver PR, eds. *Handbook of Attachment: Theory, Research and Clinical Application.* New York: Guilford Press, 1999:44–67.

65. Smyke AT, Dumitrescu A, Zeanah CH: Attachment disturbances in young children. I: The continuum of caretaking casualty. *J Am Acad Child Adolesc Psychiatry* 2002; **41**(8):972–982.

66. Vorria P, Papaligoura Z, Dunn J, van IJzendoorn MH, Steele H: Early experiences and attachment relationships of Greek infants raised in residential group care. *J Child Psychol Psychiatry* 2003; **44**(8):1208–1220.

67. Frailberg SH, Adelson E, Shapiro V: Ghosts in the nursery: A psychoanalytic approach to the problem of impaired infant-mother relationships. *J Am Acad Child Psychiatry* 1975; **14**:387–422.

68. Bosquet M, Egeland B: Associations among maternal depressive symptomatology, state of mind and parent and child behaviors: Implications for attachment-based interventions. *Attach Hum Dev* 2001; **3**(2):173–199.

69. Olds D, Henderson CR, Cole R, Echenrode J, Kitzman H, Luckey D, Pettitt, L, Dosora K, Morris P, Powers J: Long-term effects of nurse home visitation on children's criminal and antisocial behavior: 15-year follow-up of a randomized controlled trial. *J Am Med Assoc* 1998; **280**(14):1238–1244.

70. McMahon C, Barnett B, Kowalenko N, Tennant C, Don N: Postnatal depression, anxiety and unsettled infant behaviour. *Aust N Z J Psychiatry* 2001; **35**(5): 581–588.

71. Bifulco A, Figueiredo B, Guedeney N, Gorman LL, Hayes S, Muzik M, Glatigny-Dallay E, Valoriani V, Kammerer MH, Henshaw CA: Maternal attachment style and depression associated with childbirth: Preliminary results from a European and US cross-cultural study. *Br J Psychiatry Suppl* 2004; **46**:s31–s37.

72. Jacobsen, Miller: Compulsive compliance in a young maltreated child. *J Am Acad Child Adolesc Psychiatry* 1998; **37**:462–463.

73. Parish M, Eagle MN: Attachment to the therapist. *Psychoanalytic Psychol* 2003; **20**(2):271–286.

74. Fonagy P. An attachment theory approach to treatment of the difficult patient. *Bull Menniger Clin* 1998; **62**(2): 147–169.

75. Fonagy P, Target M, Steele M, Steele H, Leigh T, Levinson A, Kenedy R: Morality, disruptive behavior, borderline personality disorder, crime and their relationships to security of attachment. In Atkinson L, Zucker KJ, eds. *Attachment and Psychopathology.* New York: Guilford Press, 1997:223–274.

76. Bartholomew K, Horowitz LM: Attachment styles among young adults: A test of a four-category model. *J Pers Soc Psychol* 1991; **61**:226–244.

77. Ciechanowski PS, Katon WJ, Russo JE, Walker EA: The patient-provider relationship: Attachment theory and adherence to treatment in diabetes. *Am J Psychiatry* 2001; **158**:29–35.

78. Feeney J, Ryan S: (1994). Attachment style and affect regulation: Relationships with health behavior and family experiences in illness in a student sample. *Health Psychol* 1994; **13**:334–345.

79. Dozier M: Attachment organization and treatment use for adults with serious psychopathological disorders. *Dev Psychopathol* 1990; **2**:47–60.

17

The Eating Disorders

Randy A. Sansone, Lori A. Sansone

Introduction

We do not know when the first cases of eating disorders initially emerged in human history. However, it is evident that these disorders have asserted their clinical presence in modern times. In this chapter, we review the epidemiology, etiology, diagnosis, treatment, and outcome of these complex disorders. In synthesizing this material, it is important to note that eating disorders seem to truly underscore the relevance of a biopsychosocial perspective in the evaluation and treatment of psychiatric disorders.

Epidemiology

Prevalence Rates

Over the past 50 years, the prevalence of eating disorders has dramatically increased. In a recent review of the literature, Hoek and van Hoeken [1] concluded that the average prevalence rate for anorexia nervosa (AN) and bulimia nervosa (BN) in young women is around 0.3% and 1%, respectively. Other researchers indicate that prevalence rates for AN vary between 0.5% and 1%, with subclinical cases accounting for up to 3.7% [2,3], and for BN between 1.1% and 4.2% [4]. Eating disorders appear to be more prevalent in industrialized and/or affluent countries, so rates vary starkly across the globe.

Age of Onset

Most eating disorder individuals begin to experience symptoms between the ages 12 and 35 years. For AN, the mean age of onset is 17 years, with infrequent inception after the age of 40 years. In our experience, late-onset cases of AN can occur and are often accompanied by parallel psychosocial delays in development (i.e., the developmental position of the individual

essentially conforms with the onset of adolescence, but not with their chronological age). Likewise, BN typically begins in either late adolescence or early adulthood [5].

Gender Distribution

Eating disorders occur more frequently in women, compared with men. Male-to-female ratios vary between 1:6 and 1:10. There appear to be no distinct differences in the diagnostic approach of clinicians to males versus females [6]; however, in our experience, males with eating disorders often suffer from obsessive–compulsive personality features, premorbid weight difficulties, weight pressures related to lean body sports, and/or gender identity issues. We also suspect that the prevalence of BN in males may be underdetected due to both gender patterns related to mental healthcare utilization as well as social stigma.

Racial Distribution

Caucasian women have historically been overrepresented among those with eating disorders and this trend appears to be continuing [7]. However, non-Caucasian women are also affected [8], with some data suggesting that ethnic minorities may experience more difficulties in accessing treatment [9].

Socioeconomic Profiles

The traditional perspective – that eating disorder patients tend to come from middle to upper socioeconomic classes – is controversial. Some studies confirm this impression [10], while others do not [11–13]. It may be that those who present for treatment are individuals with available resources, in effect influencing the conclusions of these types of studies.

Clinical Child Psychiatry, Second Edition. Edited by W.M. Klykylo and J.L. Kay
© 2005 John Wiley & Sons Ltd.

Sports and Professional Influences

In addition to the preceding epidemiological patterns, eating disorders appear to be more frequent among elite performers in specific types of sports and professions (e.g., gymnasts, ballet dancers). This same relationship exists among nonelite performers, as well, particularly in areas that emphasize thinness or muscularity [14]. Eating disorders may also occur at higher rates among occupations that require a specific weight status for initial or continued employment (e.g., historically, flight attendants; the military).

Association with Medical Disorders

Eating disorders may cluster with particular medical disorders such as diabetes mellitus. The prevalence rate for eating disorders among individuals with Type 1 diabetes is twice that of their nondiabetic peers [15]. This comorbidity is associated with an increased risk of diabetic retinopathy [15], which suggests that the medical management of diabetes in individuals with eating disorders may be compromised.

Etiology

The specific etiology of eating disorders remains unknown. However, these disorders appear to be multidetermined, and probably result from the complex intersection of a variety of contributory variables. In our experience, these biopsychosocial variables vary from case to case.

Genetic Factors

Genetic factors appear to influence the development of eating disorders and several studies indicate that eating disorders are more prevalent in the family members of those with eating disorders. For example, the first-degree relatives of individuals with either AN [3,16] or BN [17] have higher rates of eating disorders. In addition, monozygotic twins demonstrate a higher concordance for eating disorders compared with dizygotic twins (approximately 50% versus 14%) [18,19] and the empirically determined heritability of these disorders is as high as 80% [20,21]. However, what exactly is being genetically transmitted through generational lines (i.e., specifically an eating disorder, particular temperaments or personality traits that confer susceptibility, nonspecific factors) remains unclear. It also appears that specific types of psychiatric disorders (i.e., affective disorders, substance abuse [16,22,23]) as well as obsessive–compulsive spectrum disorders [24] and perfectionistic personality traits [25] are more common among the family members of those with eating disorders, suggesting genetic associations.

Neurohormonal Factors

While a variety of neurohormonal abnormalities have been confirmed among those with eating disorders, these generally appear to be secondary to the effects of nutritional deficits or starvation, rather than genuinely causal or etiological in nature. Examples of these secondary abnormalities include changes in luteinizing hormone, follicle-stimulating hormone, cortisol, other hormones, and peptides as well as abnormal opioid and catecholamine metabolism. These biological changes typically normalize with weight restoration.

One genuine causal candidate is brain-derived neurotrophic factor. Alterations in this neural factor may confer susceptibility to restricting AN [26]. Specifically, researchers [26] have determined an association between restricting AN and the *Met* allele of the Val66Met brain-derived neurotrophic factor.

The Self-Perpetuating Starvation State

The starvation state, itself, may initiate or perpetuate some of the symptoms found in eating disordered individuals. As examples, experimental starvation of normal volunteers results in food preoccupation, dysphoria, food hoarding, abnormal taste preferences, binge eating, and compulsive behaviors [27]. These findings suggest that starvation may be the impetus for several notable eating disorder symptoms. On a side note, we have encountered several cases where initial, unintentional weight loss due to medical illness or surgery precipitated eating disorder pathology.

Family Factors

A variety of family factors have been associated with the development of eating disorders. In studies of infants, those with feeding problems tended to have mothers with eating disorders; these mothers demonstrated mealtime disorganization as well as strong controlling behaviors [28]. A parental marital status other than married may confer risk [29]. Parent–child enmeshment (i.e., overinvolvement to the point where it is difficult to distinguish between the needs of the parent versus the wishes of the child) may set the stage for identity struggles, wherein the eating disorder functions as the vehicle for differentiation/individuation. Other family factors may include impaired or poor communication within the family, conflict avoidance, strongly negative emotions within the family, boundary violations manifesting as physical or sexual abuse, and/or the excessive use of food as a soother or mood manager. Family preoccupation with food, body, and weight issues, as well as dieting, exercise, and 'health' preoccupation may also create an environment of risk. Having a parent with an eating disorder may be the culmination of many of these potential risk factors.

Psychological Factors

Both childhood obsessive–compulsive personality traits and perfectionism have been associated with the development of eating disorders [30,31]. In addition, Gowers and Shore [32] underscore the importance of poor impulse control and fears of losing control. Seemingly to coalesce both perspectives, Favaro and Santonastaso [33] describe the coexistence of both impulsivity and compulsivity in relationship to eating disorders.

Psychodynamic Factors

The psychodynamic value of an eating disorder, or the adaptive context, presumes that symptoms result in some benefit to the individual. These psychological benefits vary from individual to individual. For example, severe weight loss may function to disable the individual to the point of successful developmental arrest, thereby containing underlying fears about meeting the demands of an adult role, which may be perceived as overwhelming. Weight loss may be seen as a means of securing popularity or social acceptability (i.e., thinner is better), resolving one's imperfections, engaging a significant other, refocusing parents from marital or other family problems, and/or achieving a sense of empowerment or control in situations or with life stressors that leave one feeling impotent. Sadly, at times, severe weight loss may also function to make one less sexually attractive to a perpetrator.

Among those with comorbid borderline personality disorder, eating disorder symptoms may be viewed as self-injury equivalents and are likely to function in the same manner as other self-destructive behaviors. These functions may include the regulation of overwhelming affects, the consolidation of a self-destructive identity, engagement of others, displacement of anger from others to self, and/or as a means to reorganize oneself from a transient psychotic episode [34]. According to Linehan [35], the primary function of such behaviors is affect regulation or control.

Sociocultural Factors

As the body weights of its citizens increase, thinness becomes increasingly rare and valued within a culture. At least, this appears to be the case in westernized countries. The cultural messages connecting thinness with success resonate with each other and are routinely reflected in the fashion and beauty industry as well as the media. This intense focus on appearance and success seems to have culminated in television shows wherein contestants undergo extensive amounts of plastic surgery and related cosmetic procedures to emerge as 'swans,' or ultimate social successes. The cultural message for success appears to be less on personal development and education, and more on external body appearance. Given the naivety of adolescents, these cultural messages may be very profound and concretely incorporated. Interestingly, one group of investigators determined that while BN is a culture-bound syndrome, AN is not [36]; in keeping with these data, compared with AN, heritability estimates for BN show greater variability across cultures.

Negative Life Events

Whether negative life events actually cause an eating disorder, or act as a psychological trigger, is unknown. However, the McKnight investigators [37] found that an increase in negative life events predicted the onset of eating disorders in a large sample of adolescent girls in grades 6–9. Other investigators have found that childhood adversity, particularly maladaptive paternal behavior, contributes to the development of eating disorders [38].

Summary

To summarize, the risk for (or protection against) the development of eating disorders resides in several domains – biological, psychological, and social [39]. These variables seem to aggregate in specific developmental phases and likely interact with each other to result in symptoms. Eating disorders truly appear to be multidetermined disorders, with antecedent risk factors varying from case to case.

Diagnosis

Anorexia Nervosa

According to the *Diagnostic and Statistical Manual of Mental Disorders, Fourth Edition, Text Revision* (DSM-IV-TR), the criteria for the diagnosis of AN include all of the following:

Diagnostic criteria for Anorexia Nervosa (307.1)

Reprinted with permission from the Diagnostic and Statistical Manual of Mental Disorders, Copyright 2000. American Psychiatric Association.

A. Refusal to maintain body weight at or above a minimally normal weight for age and height (e.g., weight loss leading to maintenance of body weight less than 85% of that expected; or failure to make expected weight gain during a period of growth, leading to body weight less than 85% of that expected).

B. Intense fear of gaining weight or becoming fat, even though underweight.

C. Disturbance in the way in which one's body weight or shape is experienced, undue influence of body weight or shape on self-evaluation, or denial of the seriousness of the current low body weight.

D. In postmenarcheal females, amenorrhea, i.e., the absence of at least three consecutive menstrual cycles. (A woman is considered to have amenorrhea if her periods occur only following hormone, e.g., estrogen, administration.)

Specify type:

  Restricting Type: during the current episode of anorexia nervosa, the person has not regularly engaged in binge-eating or purging behavior (i.e., self-induced vomiting or the misuse of laxatives, diuretics, or enemas)

  Binge-Eating/Purging Type: during the current episode of anorexia nervosa, the person has regularly engaged in binge-eating or purging behavior (i.e., self-induced vomiting or the misuse of laxatives, diuretics, or enemas)

Adjunctive symptoms are noted in Table 17.1. In concluding a diagnosis of AN, significant weight loss, the epidemiological context, and historical evidence of dieting behavior are essential.

Axis I Comorbidity

The starvation state encountered in AN tends to mimic many of the signs and symptoms of depression (e.g., insomnia, irritability, fatigue, dysphoria, psychomotor slowing, social withdrawal). Many of these ameliorate or resolve with weight restoration. Therefore, an accurate assessment for depression is probably most practical when the patient is within 10% of a normal weight for height. In addition, starvation can tend to intensify obsessive thinking and compulsive behavior. Weight restoration tends to improve these symptoms, as well, although genuine obsessive–compulsive disorder may coexist. Milos and colleagues examined the Axis I and II diagnoses in a mixed sample of women with eating disorders and found that about 50% suffered from anxiety disorders and affective disorders. Only 17% had no psychiatric comorbidity [40].

Axis II Comorbidity

In a review of the literature, we determined that the most frequent personality disorder among individuals with AN, restricting type, is obsessive–compulsive personality disorder (about 22%), followed by avoidant personality disorder (about 19%), borderline or dependent personality disorders (around 10%), and Cluster A (i.e., odd cluster) personality disorders (approximately 5%). Overall, Cluster C (i.e., anxious cluster) personality disorders appear predominant among this subgroup [41]. The relationship between

Table 17.1 Adjunctive symptoms and behaviors in anorexia nervosa.

Intense drive for thinness	Relentless body preoccupation
Frequent weighings	Mirror gazing to scrutinize shape
Drive to attain smaller clothing sizes	Anxiety with food ingestion
Fears of becoming fat	Intense scrutiny of 'fat' body areas
Preoccupation with food	Recurrent dreams about food
Cooking for others	Food hoarding
Food-centered conversation	Attempts to conceal weight loss
Denial of weight loss	Slow eating at meals
Rituals with eating	Body size mis-estimation
Irritability	Insomnia
Worry and obsessive thinking	Anxiety
Sexual disinterest	Depression
Light-headedness	Constipation
Amenorrhea	Thin, dry, brittle hair
Low body temperature	Dry skin
Increased body hair (lanugo)	

restrictive AN and obsessive–compulsive personality appears intuitive, given the high levels of restraint and control required to systematically starve oneself.

In those patients suffering from AN, binge-eating/purging type, the most frequent Axis II disorder is borderline personality disorder (25%), followed by avoidant or dependent personality disorders (about 15%), and histrionic personality disorder (10%). Thus, among anorexic individuals with binge-eating/purging symptoms, both Cluster B (i.e., dramatic, impulsive cluster) and Cluster C personality disorders appear predominant, with borderline personality clearly being the most common personality disorder. The relationship between the impulsive behaviors of binge-eating and purging, and borderline personality, also appears logical.

Bulimia Nervosa

According to DSM-IV-TR, the criteria for BN are:

Diagnostic criteria for Bulimia Nervosa (307.51)

Reprinted with permission from the Diagnostic and Statistical Manual of Mental Disorders, Copyright 2000. American Psychiatric Association.

A. Recurrent episodes of binge eating. An episode of binge eating is characterized by both of the following:
   (1) eating, in a discrete period of time (e.g., within any two-hour period), an amount of food that is definitely larger than most people would eat during a similar period of time and under similar circumstances
   (2) a sense of lack of control over eating during the episode (e.g., a feeling that one cannot stop eating or control what or how much one is eating)
B. Recurrent inappropriate compensatory behavior in order to prevent weight gain, such as self-induced vomiting; misuse of laxatives, diuretics, enemas, or other medications; fasting; or excessive exercise.
C. The binge eating and inappropriate compensatory behaviors both occur, on average, at least twice a week for three months.
D. Self-evaluaton is unduly influenced by body shape and weight.
E. The disturbance does not occur exclusively during episodes of anorexia nervosa.

Specify type:
   Purging Type: during the current episode of bulimia nervosa, the person has regularly engaged in self-induced vomiting or the misuse of laxatives, diuretics, or enemas

Nonpurging Type: during the current episode of bulimia nervosa, the person has used other inappropriate compensatory behaviors, such as fasting or excessive exercise, but has not regularly engaged in self-induced vomiting or the misuse of laxatives, diuretics, or enemas

Surprisingly, the exact parameters of a binge are yet to be defined, making the differentiation between overeating and binge eating somewhat challenging. We elicit specific examples and assign binge status based upon the ingestion, in a single sitting, of two and a half times the normal amount of food or 2500 calories.

Adjunctive symptoms and behaviors in BN may relate to either the collection of voluminous amounts of food (e.g., high expenditures for food at the grocery store, excessive use of dormitory food cards, food hoarding), the need for social isolation to undertake a binge (e.g., calculated prompt departures after meals with others), and/or the remnants of purging (e.g., evidence of vomiting in the bathroom). Additional behaviors might include the excessive ingestion of high-calorie foods in a single sitting, the bagging and storage of vomitus, stealing food from others, shoplifting food, and discarding remnants of associated pharmaceuticals in trash cans. According to one study, slightly over one-third of adolescents with eating disorders use herbal products [42]; not surprisingly, about one-third of these herbal users choose products to either decrease their appetites or induce vomiting.

Axis I Comorbidity

Common Axis I disorders in those with BN include mood (e.g., major depression, dysthymia), anxiety, and substance use disorders [43–45]. Likewise, females with substance abuse appear to demonstrate relatively high comorbidity rates with eating disorders (up to 25%) [46]; the majority of these women suffers from BN (nearly two-thirds).

Axis II Comorbidity

In comparison with other eating disorders, including binge eating disorder, BN is the most studied with regard to Axis II comorbidity. According to our review of the literature, borderline personality disorder is the most frequent Axis II disorder (28%), followed by dependent and histrionic personality disorders (20%) [41]. Thus, the Cluster profile for BN subjects in reported studies is predominantly Cluster B followed, to a lesser degree, by Cluster C.

Eating Disorder, Not Otherwise Specified

Individuals who have eating pathology but do not meet the criteria for AN or BN are diagnosed as eating disorder not otherwise specified. Examples might include weight loss of more than 15%, but amenorrhea of less than three months duration; and binge–purge frequencies of less than twice per week in a normal-weight individual. In addition, a number of individuals have partial or subthreshold symptoms that may either progress to full-syndrome disorders, or recede spontaneously or following brief intervention. These syndromes may be classified in this diagnostic category, as well.

Eating Disorder Not Otherwise Specified (307.50)

Reprinted with permission from the Diagnostic and Statistical Manual of Mental Disorders, Copyright 2000. American Psychiatric Association.

The eating eisorder not otherwise Specified category is for disorders of eating that do not meet the criteria for any specific eating disorder. Examples include

1. For females, all of the criteria for anorexia nervosa are met except that the individual has regular menses.
2. All of the criteria for anorexia nervosa are met except that, despite significant weight loss, the individual's current weight is in the normal range.
3. All of the criteria for bulimia nervosa are met except that the binge eating and inappropriate compensatory mechanisms occur at a frequency of less than twice a week or for a duration of less than three months.
4. The regular use of inappropriate compensatory behavior by an individual of normal body weight after eating small amounts of food (e.g., self-induced vomiting after the consumption of two cookies).
5. Repeatedly chewing and spitting out, but not swallowing, large amounts of food.
6. Binge-eating disorder: recurrent episodes of binge eating in the absence of the regular use of inappropriate compensatory behaviors characteristic of bulimia nervosa (see p. 785 for suggested research criteria).

Eating Disorder Assessments

A sampling of the available assessment tools for eating disorders is shown in Table 17.2. These may be utilized as adjunctive tools to the DSM diagnostic criteria. As for laboratory studies, electrolytes, blood urea nitrogen (BUN), creatinine, thyroid assessment, and urinalysis should be considered in all patients [47]. For severely symptomatic or malnourished patients, additional laboratory studies might include calcium, magnesium, and phosphorus levels as well as liver function tests and an electrocardiogram [47]. In surreptitious cases of BN, the ratio of urine sodium to urine chloride is a reasonably good predictor, with ratios greater than 1.16 identifying 52% of cases [48]. Finally, assessment for osteopenia using dual-energy X-ray absorptiometry (DEXA) should be considered in very low-weight patients who have been symptomatic for 6–12 months or longer [47].

Medical Complications

The medical complications encountered in those with eating disorders typically relate to either starvation effects or the methods of purgation. These are summarized in Table 17.3 [49]. In addition, Figure 17.1 illustrates lanugo, a fine downy body hair that emerges with starvation. Figure 17.2 illustrates dental erosion (perimylolysis). In this figure, note that the upper front teeth show marked erosion due to their exposure to gastric acid during vomiting, while the lower teeth remain protected by the tongue. Figure 17.3 illustrates parotid gland enlargement, which occurs in some, but not all patients. The enlargement is typically bilateral, occurs with daily and multiple bouts of vomiting, and recedes with the cessation of vomiting. Although not invariably present in all patients who vomit, when present, vomiting is usually occurring several times per day. Finally, Figure 17.4 illustrates Russell's sign, which is the roughened and calloused skin on the dorsal aspect of the hand due to its repeated impact on the front teeth during gag induction.

Several additional aspects of medical complications are worth noting. First, with the various methods of purgation (e.g., vomiting, laxative abuse, diuretics), serum potassium losses may intensify. Acute potassium losses may cause seizures and cardiac arrhythmias, while longstanding hypokalemia may result in kidney damage or hypokalemic nephropathy.

Second, prolonged amenorrhea, due to malnutrition and starvation, may result in osteoporosis in adulthood. Even with full weight recovery, there appears to be reduced bone mineral density among former anorexic individuals relative to peers [50]. Treatment may entail consultation with a specialist, such as a pediatric endocrinologist or rheumatologist.

Finally, compared with other psychiatric disorders, eating disorders carry a relatively high mortality rate [51]. In AN, mortality is related to the subsequent wasting of the myocardium and cardiac dysfunction; the crude rate is approximately 6% [52]. The mortality rate for BN appears to be considerably less, at 0.3% [53]

Table 17.2 Assessment tools for eating disorders.

Assessment tool	First author	Description
Binge Eating Scale	Gormally	16 Items, self-report, Likert-style response options, binge-eating/purging
The Binge Scale	Hawkins	19 Items, self-report, Likert-style response options, binge-eating/purging
BULIT-R	Thelen	Bulimia Test-Revised, 39 items, self-report, Likert-style response options, binge-eating/purging
EAT-26	Garner	Eating Attitudes Test-26, 26 items, self-report, Likert-style response options, general eating pathology
Eating Disorder Diagnostic Scale	Stice	22 Items, self-report, various response formats, general eating pathology
Eating Disorder Examination	Fairburn	Semistructured interview, graded responses (0–6), eating pathology past 28 days
Eating Disorders Inventory-2	Garner	91 Items, self-report, Likert-style response options, general eating pathology
McKnight Risk Factors Survey	Shisslak	103 Items, self-report, various response formats, eating pathology, depression, perfectionism, risk/protection factors
Revised Restraint Scale	Herman	10 Items, self-report, various response formats, restrained eating/dieting behavior
SCOFF Questionnaire	Morgan	5 Items, self-report, yes/no responses, screening tool for eating disorders
Yale-Brown-Cornell Eating Disorder Scale	Mazure	82 Items, semistructured interview, general eating pathology and rituals
Anorexia Nervosa Stages of Change Questionnaire	Rieger	20 Items, self-report, Likert-style response options, readiness to change

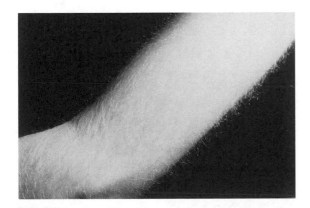

Figure 17.1 Lanugo in a patient with anorexia nervosa.

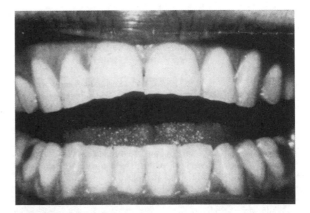

Figure 17.2 Dental erosion (perimylolysis) – a potential complication of self-induced vomiting. Stege P, Visco-Dangler, Rye L: Anorexia nervosa: Review including oral and dental manifestations. *JADA* 1982; **104(5):**648–652. © 1982 American Dental Association. All rights reserved. Reproduced by permission.

Table 17.3 Potential medical complications in eating disorders according to eating-disorder pathology.

Starvation	Self-induced vomiting	Laxative abuse	Diuretic abuse
Emaciation	Dental erosion	Acute-use discomfort	Dehydration
Muscular wasting	↑ parotid/submandibular	Abdominal pain	Light-headedness
Anemia	glands	Nausea	Tachycardia
Leukopenia	Aspiration	Vomiting	Delirium
	Pharyngeal/esophageal	Diarrhea	Seizures
	irritation	Cramping	Cardiac arrhythmias
		Distention	Renal failure
Thrombocytopenia	Esophageal/gastric tears	Bloating	
↓ Erythrocyte sedimentation	Hypokalemia	Laxative dependence	
rate	Hypochloremia	Steatorrhea	
Impaired cell immunity		Protein-losing enteropathy	
Hypercholesterolemia		Cathartic colon	
Hypocalcemia		Fixed drug eruptions	
Hypophosphatemia		(phenolphthalein)	
Hypokalemia		Melanosis coli	
Hypercortisolemia		(senna, cascara)	
Hypoglycemia			
↑ Growth hormone			
↓ Estrogen			
↓ Basal luteinizing hormone			
↓ Basal follicle-stimulating			
hormone			
↑ Liver enzymes			
↑ Amylase			
Bradycardia			
Orthostatic hypotension			
Mitral valve motion			
abnormalities			
↓ Cardiac index			
↓ Left ventricular chamber size			
Systolic dysfunction			

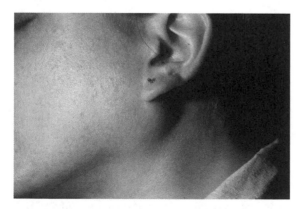

Figure 17.3 Parotid gland enlargement secondary to self-induced vomiting.

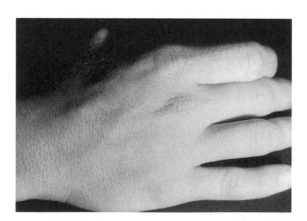

Figure 17.4 Roughened, calloused area on the dorsum of the gag-induction hand (Russell's sign).

and may be related to electrolyte disturbances (e.g., acute hypokalemia).

Treatment

Anorexia Nervosa

Treatment Engagement

At the outset of treatment, it can be very difficult to emotionally engage patients with AN. Such patients seem to have genuine difficulty recognizing or acknowledging their plight because of the intense denial associated with this disorder, the inability to recognize the extent of weight loss (i.e., body-image distortion), and occasional parents who may be reticent to acknowledge that their child has a psychiatric problem. The best approach to building an alliance, in our experience, is to initially validate the patient's physical symptoms. For example, the clinician may empathically acknowledge that the patient may feel dysphoric, cold, isolated, anxious, fearful, exhausted, and overwhelmed. This type of validation helps to establish some level of interpersonal connection and may function as the impetus to establish rapport and build an initial alliance with the patient.

For the patient, the initial treatment encounter is invariably very threatening. From the patient's perspective, the clinician is, in a very pragmatic way, attempting to undermine the arduous efforts at weight loss. So, a high degree of patient resistance can be anticipated. Validating this reality (e.g., 'it must seem like we, the treatment team, are trying to undermine the very goal that you have worked so hard at') can acknowledge this genuine dilemma on a verbal level with the patient.

Determination of the Treatment Environment

During the evaluation, the determination of the initial treatment environment is of the utmost importance. This determination is based upon several factors including the amount of weight lost, the rapidity of the weight loss, how weight loss was achieved, the age of the patient, physical symptoms or laboratory abnormalities, and frankly, local treatment resources. In addition to height and weight measurements, initial laboratory studies should be completed to reveal any existing metabolic imbalances. The primary care physician may have completed laboratory studies and an electrocardiogram, and these should be obtained, if possible, prior to the evaluation. Initial and ongoing weight data are essential and all clinicians should have immediate access to a scale in their office settings.

The determination of the treatment environment is primarily based upon weight status. For those individuals who are 75% or less of expected weight for height, inpatient treatment is indicated and we strongly recommend a milieu-based, eating disorder treatment program. Medical hospitalization is indicated for patients with significant electrolyte disturbances or cardiac arrhythmias (e.g., severe bradycardia, junctional rhythm) and may be undertaken in a general hospital setting. In these settings, the primary care physician or specialist (e.g., cardiologist) manages the patient. For patients with moderate or minimal weight loss, outpatient intervention is recommended.

In designing an overall treatment strategy, comorbid psychiatric conditions will need to be considered (e.g., anxiety disorders, obsessive–compulsive personality disorder), with the realization that comorbidity potentially dampens the overall prognosis. Following a reasonable degree of weight restoration, these comorbid conditions may be more realistically approached with medications as well as various therapies. The initial focus of treatment is weight restoration.

Behavior Modification for Inpatient Weight Restoration

At some point in their careers, many clinicians will face the task of inpatient weight restoration for a patient with AN. While various forms of behavior modification are used, we have had consistent success with the following general approach. After inpatient admission, we collect daily weights (same time of day, usually during the morning just before breakfast; standard garb) for three days and average them to determine a 'starting weight' on a weight graph. From this starting weight, we draw a line on the weight graph that indicates one-quarter pound of weight gain per day. Beginning at 1200 calories per day in six divided feedings, we titrate the patient's daily calorie levels in 300-calorie increments to maintain his or her weight on the anticipated weight-gain schedule according to the weight-gain line. This enables the treatment team to monitor the momentum around weight gain as well as observe for excessive or rapid refeeding. Rapid refeeding may result in refeeding syndrome, which is characterized by severe hypokalemia, hypophosphatemia, and possibly death. During weight restoration, the decisions around food choices, liquid supplements versus solid food, and the number of feedings per day are all negotiated individually. Progress is reinforced with increasing activity levels. At times, patients may be given the choice of a 300-calorie increase or a decrease in activity level. In conjunction with behavioral modification for weight restoration, we have typically used a multiple vitamin as well as calcium supplements that contain vitamin D.

With some minor modifications, this same approach can be used for outpatient weight restoration, as well. Examples of modifications might be weekly weighing at sessions rather than daily weighing in the inpatient setting, less robust expectations around weight gain, and more flexibility around the weighing format. Liquid supplements or puddings may be successfully utilized in the outpatient setting, particularly at the outset of treatment, when control and trust issues are high.

Psychotherapy Treatment

As for the integration of psychotherapy treatment, we emphasize three phases. During the first phase of treatment, when the patient is in an acute starvation state, the ability to abstract well and relate to others is compromised. Because the initial focus of treatment is weight restoration, we recommend cognitive and educational approaches, validation, and rapport building, as well as contracting and negotiation around eating, weight gain, and activity levels.

As weight increases, the next phase of psychotherapy treatment often centers on exploring the various contributory factors that resulted in the eating disorder. During this phase, the psychotherapy focus is somewhat more psychodynamic in nature, with the examination of personal, home, and peer factors. This phase may also entail body-image work, further nutritional education, family work, and continuing cognitive restructuring.

In the final phase of treatment, the psychotherapy focus is more relational – i.e., facilitating reconnection with others. This phase entails developing and practicing skills in social relationships. The patient may require specific interventions in the areas of assertiveness, dealing with the opposite sex, expression of emotional needs with others, boundary issues, compliance versus autonomy in relationships, and various other interpersonal issues.

Because of the multidetermined nature of eating disorders, additional therapies may be elected based upon individual need. For example, all patients should receive educational intervention around nutrition, and almost all young adolescents will benefit from family therapy. When integrated into treatment, family members and significant others benefit from understanding their reactions to the disorder as well as rethinking their responses. In particular cases, specific skills training may be necessary such as assertiveness, conflict management, and stress management. Victims of abuse may benefit from trauma work. Because many patients with AN are young adolescents, developmental (i.e., separation/individuation, dating, peer relationships) as well as academic issues will need to be addressed in the treatment. For married patients, couples therapy may be indicated to address underlying marital conflicts.

Psychotropic Medication

During the acute phase of refeeding, psychotropic medications are not routinely recommended because they appear to have limited efficacy in weight-loss states. Other concerns include the patient's greater susceptibility to side effects because of low body weight, the possible resolution of some mood and anxiety symptoms with weight restoration (e.g., depressive symptoms, obsessive thinking), and patients' fears that the medication is manipulatively intended as a weight-gain ploy by the treatment team. With regard to the latter concern, some studies have shown enhanced weight gain during weight restoration with particular medications for which weight gain is an anticipated side effect, such as olanzapine (Zyprexa). We have intentionally avoided these medications because of the inability to effectively strategize an acceptable weight outcome. In other words, while these medications stimulate weight gain, it is not possible to predict how much weight will eventually be gained.

Given the preceding advisements about medication in low-weight patients with AN, we offer a possible exception. Some patients with severe obsessive–compulsive disorder (OCD) are probably not disadvantaged by early intervention with a selective serotonin reuptake inhibitor (SSRI). The potential side effect risks of this class of antidepressants are low and the potential benefits are high. Severe obsessive–compulsive symptoms that directly relate to food and weight issues (e.g., touching food is perceived as contamination) may so impede a treatment that early intervention with medication is reasonable. There are also other clinical exceptions wherein early medication intervention is indicated (e.g., psychosis).

With regard to medication intervention in low-weight patients, we strongly recommend small, initial doses of medication with slow titration, as well as a credible discussion with the patient about the known weight effects of a prescribed medication. Among psychiatric patients, in general, it is well known that many psychotropic medications cause weight gain, and such suspicions by the patient are not unfounded.

Following weight restoration to within 10% of a normal or previous body weight, we routinely consider medication intervention if adjunctive psychiatric symptoms persist (e.g., anxiety, depression). At the outset, we recommend SSRIs. This class of antidepressants has broad clinical efficacy (i.e., they are effective for various syndromes including depression, anxiety, panic, rumination, worry, obsessive–compulsive symptoms, impulsivity), which is particularly helpful in cases with complex psychiatric comorbidity. SSRIs also have tolerable side effects and reasonable safety in overdose with the possible exception of citalopram (Celexa), which may cause QT prolongation in overdose. In our experience, venlafaxine extended release (Effexor-XR) has also been useful, but has a more limited range of efficacy with regard to polysymptomatic patients. We avoid tricyclic antidepressants (TCAs) due to their cardiovascular effects, the risk of unpredictable weight gain, and high lethality risk in overdose. Bupropion (Wellbutrin) is contraindicated in the treatment of eating disorders because of the heightened risk of seizures. Although there has been emerging concern about the risk of suicidal ideation in adolescents who are exposed to the newer antidepressants including SSRIs, we have not encountered this particular dilemma in our work with patients with eating disorders.

Bulimia Nervosa

Compared with sufferers of AN, those with BN tend to establish an initial and easy rapport with the clinician. This may be related to these patients' later age at clinical presentation (i.e., greater developmental maturity), the type of eating disorder, associated personality features, higher levels of insight, or other related factors. So, typically, at the initial evaluation, there is less resistance by the patient to dialoguing and participating in a treatment plan.

General Treatment Goals

While weight restoration is the initial focus in the treatment of AN, the normalization of eating patterns and interruption of the binge/purge cycle are the initial goals in the treatment of BN. While the definition of normalized eating patterns is speculative, we recommend working towards 1800–2200 calories per day, in four feedings (e.g., breakfast, lunch, dinner, snack). We initially have the patient keep a one-week food record, roughly estimate the daily calorie levels, and then establish an initial menu plan. We gradually advance the daily calorie levels by 300-calorie increments to goal levels and monitor weight status, either formally or informally (patient self-report). We strongly believe that a functional calorie deficit is a major contributory factor to binge eating.

With regard to interrupting binge/purge behavior, we contract for reductions, explore and encourage alternative coping strategies, process behavior chains (i.e., explore thoughts, feelings, and behaviors before, during, and after each event), and examine the interpersonal costs of such behavior. With comorbid substance abuse, we generally recommend initial substance abuse treatment [54]. For patients with comorbid borderline personality disorder, we suggest initially focusing on self-regulation and self-harm behavior, and secondarily focusing on eating disorder issues [55].

Psychotherapy Treatment

Various psychotherapy treatment strategies have been used in BN. In this regard, Richards and colleagues [56] reviewed available treatment studies and concluded that there are substantially more in BN compared with AN. This seemingly adds some confidence to the empirical findings of treatment interventions in BN. However, the authors caution that the treatments in these studies may well be the result of treatment default (i.e., using only techniques confirmed by limited studies) rather than an inherent superiority of such treatments over other types of treatments.

Given the preceding caveat, it is evident that cognitive behavioral therapy is the most studied and empirically supported treatment approach for BN [56]. Interpersonal psychotherapy has also demonstrated efficacy in the treatment of BN. As in the treatment of AN, other types of therapies may be integrated into treatment, depending on individual needs. Psychodynamic psychotherapy may be incorporated into treatment, particularly in an effort to understand how earlier developmental issues are being manifest in adulthood. Acute problem-solving approaches are helpful for emergent issues. Family therapy may be useful in helping members to understand their reactions to the patient's symptoms as well as to intervene in less stressful ways. Family issues may include dealing with blame and guilt, tightening family boundaries, developing healthier responses to the patient's behaviors, and adjusting the expectations of parents and/or significant others. For some older adolescents from highly dysfunctional families, therapeutic emancipation may be in order. Couples or marital therapy may be extremely helpful, if only to develop ways for the couple to neutrally communicate about symptomatic behaviors, actively dialogue home and outside stressors, and work towards healthier ways to deal with negative emotions and feelings. In addition, partners can function as ongoing, full-time home coaches for the patient, when feasible.

These preceding interventions may be undertaken in group or individual settings, including interpersonal psychotherapy [57]. Group treatments offer an efficient and economical means of delivering information and treatment strategies to a number of patients, although many patients benefit from the psychological intimacy of an individual treatment.

In addition, support groups are available in many areas. These are typically open to new participants. Many have group facilitators who are either experienced participants, patients in partial or full recovery, or treatment professionals. These groups vary in philosophy, structure, clinical themes, and their individual screening processes. Rice and Faulkner outline the benefits and risks of such groups [58].

Novel interventions are also emerging for the treatment of eating disorders. These include motivational enhancement therapy, which was developed in the context of addictive disorders; dialectical behavior therapy, which was developed for the treatment of self-harm behavior in borderline personality; and manualized family therapy [59]. Like all new treatments, the efficacy and patient-selection criteria are not explicitly known.

Technology is also augmenting our therapeutic armamentarium. For example, in small practices or practices with few eating disorder patients, the clinician may link patients together into a 'support group' via the internet [60]. In addition, palmtop computers may be effective as 'therapy extension devices' [61]. Finally, Taylor and colleagues discuss the role of Web-based prevention programs as well as online treatment and support groups, and psychoeducation for patients with eating disorders [62].

Medications

Antidepressant medications consistently appear to reduce the frequency of binging and purging, regardless of the presence or not of depression. In our experience, antidepressant therapy initially results in a 50% or better reduction in symptomatology, but complete amelioration of symptoms is rare in the clinical setting. Various types of antidepressants have been used including SSRIs, TCAs, monoamine oxidase inhibitors, and other newer antidepressants (venlafaxine extended release). As in AN, SSRIs are typically an initial starting place because of their mild side effect profiles, general safety, and their unique effects on rumination, worry, and impulsivity. In BN, higher-than-standard doses may be considered. Fluoxetine (Prozac) is the only antidepressant officially indicated by the Food and Drug Administration for the treatment of BN, although all of the SSRIs are effective.

As in AN, we have avoided TCAs in those with BN. These antidepressants have significant side effects including weight gain and cardiovascular effects. The latter potential side effects are particularly problematic in patients with dehydration due to vomiting, laxatives, or diuretics. As noted earlier, TCAs are relatively lethal in overdose. Monoamine oxidase inhibitors are risky interventions because of their potential to interact with various foods and drugs, causing acute hypertension and possibly cerebrovascular bleeds. This risk is particularly heightened in the indiscriminant binge eater or the patient with borderline personality characteristics who engages in self-harm behavior through exposure to contraband food and drugs. For both AN and BN, the only contraindicated antidepressant is bupropion (Wellbutrin) because of the heightened risk of seizures.

Other medications have been helpful in the treatment of BN including the anticonvulsants and psychostimulants. However, these drugs have less empirical support, may be more complicated to use (e.g., laboratory studies with anticonvulsants), and may be potentially hazardous in those patients prone to substance abuse (e.g., the abuse of psychostimulants). In cases of psychiatric comorbidity, the corresponding psychotropic medication would be indicated (e.g., antipsychotics, lithium), although the weight effects of individual drugs may pose more problems for those with eating disorders compared with the general psychiatric patient.

Outcome

Complexities of Outcome Assessment

It is genuinely difficult to draw a general conclusion on the treatment outcome of patients with eating disorders. As expected, outcomes markedly differ because the available empirical studies vary by study populations and methodologies (e.g., different ages of participants, levels of care, treatment settings, levels of psychiatric comorbidity and medical debility, treatment interventions). In addition, there is controversy regarding what constitutes remission versus recovery, and how to measure it.

Four general approaches for assessing treatment outcome have been proposed by Anderson and colleagues [63]: (1) structured interviews; (2) self-report inventories; (3) body mass indices or weights; and (4) the use of test meals to assess comfort with eating. In pragmatic terms, the possibilities for outcome variables seem endless and include the weight and nutritional status of the patient, level of eating difficulties, preoccupation with body weight, persistence of eating disorder symptoms, overall growth and physical development, menstrual functioning, mental state, psychosexual adjustment, psychosocial functioning, and mortality [64].

In an effort to promote a consistent approach to outcome measurement, researchers have developed a brief, self-report inventory, the Multifactorial Assessment of Eating Disorder Symptoms (MAEDS; [65]). The MAEDS assesses six symptom clusters: depression, binge eating, purging behavior, fears of fatness, restrictive eating, and the avoidance of forbidden foods. Only broader use will determine the viability and acceptability among clinicians and patients of this outcome measure.

Outcome of Eating Disorder Symptoms

One statistic that seems to echo throughout the outcome literature is that about one-third of eating-disorder patients experience a poor outcome. In support of this impression, Herzog and colleagues [66], found that at 90 months of follow-up, nearly one-third of patients relapsed. Likewise, Keel [67] found that 10–15 years after presentation for treatment, around 29% of those with BN still retained an eating disorder diagnosis. Herpertz-Dahlmann and colleagues [68] examined the 10-year outcome of adolescents with AN and determined that 31% had not fully recovered; there was a significant association between poor outcome and psychiatric comorbidity. Steinhausen and colleagues [69] reported that after more than six years of follow-up, 30% of patients were unrecovered. In a five-year outcome study, Ben-Tovim and colleagues [70] found that 32% of a mixed sample of patients still had a diagnosable eating disorder. Finally, Nakai and colleagues found that in 4–10-year follow-up, 26%–30% of patients either did not recover or died [71]. Again, the recurring statistic appears to be that about one-third of eating disorder patients experience poor long-term outcomes. Whether poor outcome relates to Axis I or II comorbidity, severity of initial symptoms, history of abuse, age of onset, and/or other variables is unknown. In one study, severity of alcohol use was a predictor of mortality in AN [72]. Conversely, these data indicate that nearly two-thirds of patients achieve partial or full remission, given time.

Fertility and Pregnancy Outcome

Another aspect of outcome is fertility among women with active eating disorders. Crow and colleagues found that although menstrual irregularities were common among women with BN, there was little impact on patients' ability to achieve a pregnancy [73]. Franko and colleagues examined pregnancy complications and neonatal outcomes [74]. While the majority of women had normal pregnancies, 6% of the babies had birth defects. In this prospective study, over one-third of the women experienced postpartum depression and there was also a higher frequency of Caesarean section at delivery. On a side note, Carter and colleagues found that pregnancy did not result in increased eating disorder symptomatology, which is relevant given the dramatic and acute increase in the patient's body size [75]. Protecting the child from the ravages of an eating disorder may be a protective factor for the mother, as well.

Mortality

The crude mortality rates for AN and BN were noted earlier in this chapter. It is important to note that, in addition to succumbing to the physical devastation of eating disorders, a number of individuals surrender to the emotional devastation through suicide. In support of this, AN is empirically associated with a heightened risk of suicide [76]. Again, the variables that contribute to this risk are unknown.

Binge Eating Disorder

Before closing this chapter, we would like to briefly review binge eating disorder (BED), a provisional eating disorder in the *DSM* identified for additional study. Bunnell [77] and Walsh, Wilfrey, and Hudson [78] provide excellent overviews of this disorder, which we now summarize.

BED is characterized by a recurrent pattern of binge eating that occurs at least twice a week for a minimum period of six months. Unlike BN, there is no compensatory behavior (i.e., vomiting, fasting, exercise) to counter these episodes of massive calorie ingestion. Therefore, many BED patients are overweight although weight status, per se, is not a diagnostic criterion. The clinical characteristics of the binge eating behavior are like those encountered in BN; however, women with BED may eat at a normal rate.

The prevalence rate for BED in the community is up to 5%, in weight loss clinics up to 30%, and in those with body mass indices ≥40 up to 50%. These prevalence data indicate that BED is the most common eating disorder. Unlike the preceding eating disorders, a substantial number of males are afflicted, with the female to male ratio being 3:2. The age of onset is typically during the late teens to early 20s, the ethnicity of patients is quite diverse, and the ages of presentation (i.e., 30 to 40 years) for treatment is later than that encountered in AN and BN. Comorbid diabetes occurs in up to 25% of patients with BED.

As in BN, many different types of treatment have been used including cognitive behavioral techniques, interpersonal psychotherapy, weight loss programs, and self-help treatments. Various medications are also being explored including SSRIs, anti-obesity drugs, and topiramate (Topamax). Surprisingly, the elimination of binging does not necessarily result in weight loss.

This diagnostic category remains under investigation. Only additional research and the political atmospheres relating to diagnosis and insurance coverage will determine whether this disorder will attain official ranking with the other DSM eating disorder diagnoses.

Conclusions

Eating disorders are the epitome of the biopsychosocial model of assessment and intervention. They are multidetermined disorders with both psychological and medical sequelae that require creative and diverse therapeutic interventions. These disorders continue to be challenging, with nearly one-third of patients being refractory to treatment. Only additional research, clinician perseverance, and supportive funding will enable the professional community to better understand these complex and intriguing patients.

References

1. Hoek HW, van Hoeken D: Review of the prevalence and incidence of eating disorders. *Int J Eating Disord* 2003; **34**:383–396.
2. Garfinkel PE, Lin E, Goering P, Spegg C, Goldbloom D, Kennedy S, Kaplan AS, *et al.*: Should amenorrhoea be necessary for the diagnosis of anorexia nervosa? Evidence from a Canadian community sample. *Br J Psychiatry* 1996; **168**:500–506.
3. Walters EE, Kendler KS: Anorexia nervosa and anorexic-like syndromes in a population-based female twin sample. *Am J Psychiatry* 1995; **152**:64–71.
4. Garfinkel RE, Lin E, Goering P, Spegg C, Goldbloom DS, Kennedy S, Kaplan AS, *et al.*: Bulimia nervosa in a Canadian community sample: Prevalence and comparison in subgroups. *Am J Psychiatry* 1995; **152**:1052–1058.
5. American Psychiatric Association: *Diagnostic and Statistical Manual of Mental Disorders* (4th ed, Text Revision). Washington, DC: American Psychiatric Association; 2000.
6. Grace GF: Contrasting anorexia nervosa in males cross-nationally in the United States, Canada, and Great Britain. *Diss Abstr Int, Section B* 2003; **64**:2387.
7. Striegel-Moore RH, Dohm FA, Kraemer HC, Taylor DB, Daniels S, Crawford PB, *et al.*: Eating disorders in White and Black women. *Am J Psychiatry* 2003; **160**:1326–1331.
8. Crago M, Shisslak CM, Estes LS: Eating disturbances among American minority groups: A review. *Int J Eating Disord* 1996; **19**:239–248.
9. Becker AE, Franko DL, Speck A, Herzog DB: Ethnicity and differential access to care for eating disorder symptoms. *Int J Eating Disord* 2003; **33**:205–212.
10. Gowers S, McMahon JB: Social class and prognosis in anorexia nervosa. *Int J Eating Disord* 1989; **8**:105–109.
11. Favaro A, Ferrara S, Santonastaso P: The spectrum of eating disorders in young women: A prevalence study in a general population sample. *Psychosom Med* 2003; **65**:701–708.
12. Gard MCE, Freeman CP: Dismantling of a myth: A review of eating disorders and socio-economic status. *Int J Eating Disord* 1996; **20**:1–12.
13. Pope HG, Champoux RF, Hudson JI: Eating disorder and socioeconomic class: Anorexia nervosa and bulimia in nine communities. *J Nerv Ment Dis* 2004; **175**:620–623.
14. Ravaldi C, Vannacci A, Zucchi T, Mannucci E, Cabras PL, Boldrini M, *et al.*: Eating disorders and body image disturbances among ballet dancers, gymnasium users and body builders. *Psychopathology* 2003; **36**:247–254.
15. Rodin G, Olmsted MP, Rydall AC, Maharaj SI, Colton PA, Jones JM, *et al.*: Eating disorders in young women with type 1 diabetes mellitus. *J Psychosom Res* 2002; **53**:943–949.
16. Strober M, Lampert C, Morrell W, Burroughs J, Jacobs C: A controlled family study of anorexia nervosa: Evidence of familial aggregation and lack of shared transmission with affective disorders. *Int J Eat Disord* 1990; **9**:239–253.
17. Stein D, Lilenfeld LR, Plotnicov K, Pollice C, Rao R, Strober M, *et al.*: Familial aggregation of eating disorders: Results from a controlled family study of bulimia nervosa. *Int J Eating Disord* 1999; **26**:211–215.
18. Kendler KS, Maclean C, Neale M, Kessler R, Heath A, Eaves L: The genetic epidemiology of bulimia nervosa. *Am J Psychiatry* 1991; **148**:1627–1637.
19. Crisp AH, Hall A, Holland AJ: Nature and nurture in anorexia nervosa: A study of 34 pairs of twins, one pair of triplets and an adoptive family. *Int J Eating Disord* 1985; **4**:5–29.
20. Lamberg L: Advances in eating disorders offer food for thought. *JAMA* 2003; **290**:1437–1442.
21. Wade TD, Bulik CM, Neale M, Kendler KS: Anorexia nervosa and major depression: Shared genetic and environment risk factors. *Am J Psychiatry* 2000; **157**:469–471.
22. Lilenfeld LR, Kaye WH, Greeno CG, Merikangas KR, Plotnicov K, Pollice C, *et al.*: Psychiatric disorders in women with bulimia nervosa and their first-degree relatives: Effects of comorbid substance dependence. *Int J Eating Disord* 1997; **22**:253–264.
23. Pyle RL, Mitchell JE, Eckert ED: Bulimia: A report of 34 cases. *J Clin Psychiatry* 1981; **42**:60–64.
24. Bellodi L, Cavallini MC, Bertelli S, Chiapparino D, Riboldi C, Smeraldi E: Morbidity risk for obsessive-compulsive spectrum disorders in first-degree relatives of patients with eating disorders. *Am J Psychiatry* 2001; **158**:563–569.
25. Lilenfeld LRR, Stein D, Bulik CM, Strober M, Plotnicov K, Pollice C, *et al.*: Personality traits among current eating disordered, recovered and never ill first-degree female relatives of bulimic and control women. *Psychol Med* 2000; **30**:1399–1410.
26. Ribases M, Gratacos M, Armengol L, de Cid R, Badia A, Jimenez L, *et al.*: Met66 in the brain-derived neu-

rotrophic factor (BDNF) precursor is associated with anorexia nervosa restrictive type. *Mol Psychiatry* 2003; **8**:745–751.

27. Keys A, Brozek J, Henschel A, Mickelsen O, Taylor HL, eds.: *The Biology of Human Starvation*. Minneapolis: University of Minnesota Press; 1950:819–853.

28. Cooper PJ, Whelan E, Woolgar M, Morrell J, Murray L: Association between childhood feeding problems and maternal eating disorder: Role of the family environment. *Br J Psychiatry* 2004; **184**:210–215.

29. Martinez-Gonzalez MA, Gual P, Lahortiga F, Alonso Y, de Irala-Estevez J, Cervera S: Parental factors, mass media influences, and the onset of eating disorders in a prospective population-based cohort. *Pediatrics* 2003; **111**:315–320.

30. Bulik CM, Tozzi F, Anderson C, Mazzeo SE, Aggen S, Sullivan PF: The relation between eating disorders and components of perfectionism. *Am J Psychiatry* 2003; **160**:366–368.

31. Anderluch MB, Tchanturia K, Rabe-Hesketh S, Treasure J: Childhood obsessive-compulsive personality traits in adult women with eating disorders: Defining a broader eating disorder phenotype. *Am J Psychiatry* 2003; **160**:242–247.

32. Gowers SG, Shore A: Development of weight and shape concerns in the aetiology of eating disorders. *Br J Psychiatry* 2001; **179**:236–242.

33. Favaro A, Santonastaso P: The spectrum of self-injurious behavior in eating disorders. *Eating Disord* 2002; **1**:215–225.

34. Gunderson JG: *Borderline Personality Disorder*. Washington, DC: American Psychiatric Press, 1984.

35. Linehan MM: *Cognitive Behavioral Treatment of Borderline Personality*. New York: Guilford, 1993.

36. Keel PK, Klump KL: Are eating disorders culture-bound syndromes: Implications for conceptualizing their etiology. *Psychol Bull* 2003; **129**:747–769.

37. The McKnight Investigators: Risk factors for the onset of eating disorders in adolescent girls: Results of the McKnight Longitudinal Risk Factor Study. *Am J Psychiatry* 2003; **160**:248–254.

38. Johnson JG, Cohen P, Kasen S, Brook JS: Childhood adversities associated with risk for eating disorders or weight problems during adolescence or early adulthood. *Am J Psychiatry* 2002; **159**:394–400.

39. Steiner N, Kwan W, Shaffer TG, Walker S, Miller S, Sagar A, et al.: Risk and protective factors for juvenile eating disorders. *Eur Child Adolesc Psychiatry* 2003; **12**:138–146.

40. Milos GF, Spindler AM, Buddeberg C, Crameri A: Axes I and II comorbidity and treatment experiences in eating disorder subjects. *Psychother Psychosom* 2003; **72**:276–285.

41. Sansone RA, Levitt JL, Sansone LA: The prevalence of personality disorders among those with eating disorders. *Eating Disord* 2005; **13**:7–21.

42. Trigazis L, Tennankore D, Vohra S, Katzman DK: The use of herbal remedies by adolescents with eating disorders. *Int J Eating Disord* 2004; **35**:223–228.

43. Zaider TI, Johnson JG, Cockell SJ: Psychiatric comorbidity associated with eating disorder symptomatology among adolescents in the community. *Int J Eating Disord* 2000; **28**:58–67.

44. Grilo CM, Levy KN, Becker DF, Edell WS, McGlashan TH: Comorbidity of DSM-III-R axis I and II disorders among female inpatients with eating disorders. *Psychiatr Serv* 1996; **47**:426–429.

45. Braun DL, Sunday SR, Halmi KA: Psychiatric comorbidity in patients with eating disorders. *Psychol Med* 1994; **24**:859–867.

46. Matsumoto T, Kosaka K, Yamaguchi A, Kamijo A, Minami K, Endo K, et al.: Eating disorders in female substance use disorders: A preliminary research on the relationship of substances and eating behaviors. *Clin Psychiatry* 2003; **45**:119–127.

47. Work Group on Eating Disorders: Practice guideline for the treatment of patients with eating disorders (revision). *Am J Psychiatry* 2000; **157**:S1–39.

48. Crow SJ, Rosenberg ME, Mitchell JE, Thuras P: Urine electrolytes as markers of bulimia nervosa. *Int J Eating Disord* 2001; **30**:279–287.

49. Sansone RA, Correll TL: Eating disorders. *Hosp Physician* 2001; **5**:1–12.

50. Hartman D, Crisp A, Rooney B, Rackow C, Atkinson R, Patel S: Bone density of women who have recovered from anorexia nervosa. *Int J Eating Disord* 2000; **28**:107–112.

51. Neumaerker K-J: Mortality rates and causes of death. *Eur Eating Disord Rev* 2000; **8**:181–187.

52. Sansone RA, Sansone LA, Wiederman MW: Eating disorders: Diagnosis and management in the primary care setting. *Prim Care Rep* 1998; **4**:43–50.

53. Keel PK, Mitchell JE: Outcome in bulimia nervosa. *Am J Psychiatry* 1997; **154**:313–321.

54. Sansone RA, Dennis AB: The treatment of eating disorder patients with substance abuse and borderline personality disorder. *Eating Disord* 1996; **4**:180–186.

55. Sansone RA, Johnson CL: Treating the eating disorder patient with borderline personality: Theory and technique. In: Barber J, Crits-Christoph P, eds.: *Dynamic Therapies for Psychiatric Disorders (Axis I)*. New York: Basic Books; 1995:230–266.

56. Richards SP, Baldwin BM, Frost HA, Clark-Sly JB, Berrett ME, Hardman RK: What works for treating eating disorders? Conclusions of 28 outcome reviews. *Eating Disord* 2000; **8**:189–206.

57. Wilfley DE, Frank MA, Welch R, Spurrell EB, Rounsaville BJ: Adapting interpersonal psychotherapy to a group format (IPT-G) for binge eating disorder: Toward a model for adapting empirically supported treatments. *Psychother Res* 1998; **8**:379–391.

58. Rice C, Faulkner J: Support and self-help groups. In Harper-Guiffre H, MacKenzie KR, eds.: *Group Psychotherapy for Eating Disorders*. Washington, DC: American Psychiatric Association; 1992:247–260.

59. Kotler LA, Boudreau GS, Devlin MJ: Emerging psychotherapies for eating disorders. *J Psychiatr Pract* 2003; **9**:431–441.

60. Sansone RA: Patient-to-patient e-mail support for clinical practices. *Eating Disord* 2001; **9**:373–375.

61. Norton M, Wonderlich SA, Myers T, Michell JE, Crosby RD: The use of palmtop computers in the treatment of bulimia nervosa. *Eur Eating Disord Rev* 2003; **11**:231–242.

62. Taylor CB, Jobson KO, Winzelberg A, Abascal L: The use of the Internet to provide evidence-based integrated treatment programs for mental health. *Psychiatr Ann* 2002; **32**:671–677.

63. Anderson DA, Williamson DA: Outcome measurement in eating disorders. In IsHak WW, Tal B, Sederer LI, eds.: *Outcome Measurement in Psychiatry: A Critical Review*.

Washington, DC: American Psychiatric Publishing; 2002:289–302.

64. Neiderman M: Prognosis and outcome. In: Lask B, Bryant-Waugh R, eds.: *Anorexia Nervosa and Related Eating Disorders in Childhood and Adolescence,* 2nd ed. Hove, UK: Taylor & Francis; 2000:81–102.

65. Anderson DA, Williamson DA, Duchmann EG, Gleaves DH, Barbin JM: Development and validation of a multifactorial treatment outcome measure for eating disorders. *Assessment* 1999; **6**:7–20.

66. Herzog DB, Dorer DJ, Keel P, Selwyn SE, Ekeblad ER, Flores AT, *et al.*: Recovery and relapse in anorexia and bulimia nervosa: A 7.5-year follow-up study. *J Am Acad Child Adolesc Psychiatry* 1999; **38**:829–837.

67. Keel PK: Long-term outcome of bulimia nervosa. *Diss Abstr Int, Section B* 1998; **58**:6812.

68. Herpertz-Dahlmann B, Muller B, Herpertz S, Heussen N, Hebebrand J, Remschmidt H: Prospective 10-year follow-up in adolescent anorexia nervosa: Course, outcome, psychiatric comorbidity, and psychosocial adaptation. *J Child Psychol Psychiatry* 2001; **42**:603–612.

69. Steinhausen H-C, Boyadjieva S, Griogoroiu-Serbanescu M, Neumaerker K-J: The outcome of adolescent eating disorders: Findings from an international collaborative study. *Eur Child Adolesc Psychiatry* 2003; **12**:191–198.

70. Ben-Tovim B, Walker K, Gilchrist P, Freeman R, Kalucy R, Esterman A: Outcome in patients with eating disorders: A 5-year study. *Lancet* 2001; **357**: 1254–1257.

71. Nakai Y, Hamagaki S, Ishizaka Y, Takagi R, Takagi S, Ishikawa T: Predictors of outcome in eating disorders. *Clin Psychiatry* 2002; **44**:1305–1309.

72. Keel PK, Dorer DJ, Eddy KT, Franko D, Charatan DL, Herzog DB: Predictors of mortality in eating disorders. *Arch Gen Psychiatry* 2003; **60**:179–183.

73. Crow SJ, Thuras P, Keel PK, Mitchell JE: Long-term menstrual and reproductive function in patients with bulimia nervosa. *Am J Psychiatry* 2002; **159**:1048–1050.

74. Franko DL, Blais MA, Becker AE, Delinsky SS, Greenwood DN, Flores AT, *et al.*: Pregnancy complications and neonatal outcomes in women with eating disorders. *Am J Psychiatry* 2001; **158**:1461–1466.

75. Carter FA, McIntosh VVW, Joyce PR, Frampton CM, Bulik CM: Bulimia nervosa, childbirth and psychopathology. *J Psychosom Res* 2003; **55**:357–361.

76. Herzog DB, Greenwood DN, Dorer DJ, Flores AT, Ekeblad ER, Richards A, *et al.*: Mortality in eating disorders: A descriptive study. *Int J Eating Disord* 2000; **28**:20–26.

77. Bunnell D: The "new" eating disorder. *Perspective* 2004; **1**:4–6.

78. Walsh BT, Wilfrey DE, Hudson JI: Binge eating disorder: Progress in understanding and treatment. (Educational monograph). West Wayne, NJ: Health Learning Systems; 2003:1–14.

18

Elimination Disorders:
Enuresis and Encopresis

Daniel J. Feeney

Introduction

It is estimated that less than one-third of US children are completely toilet trained by 24 months of age. The typical progression is for children to attain nighttime bowel control followed by daytime bowel control, daytime bladder control, and ultimately nighttime bladder control. Most children complete these stages by 36 months of age. Problems in achieving and maintaining bowel and bladder continence, however, are generally more common in males than in females, which may in part be explained by the slower physiologic maturation of males. In contrast, the development of daytime bladder continence problems occurs more frequently in females than in males and is also associated with higher comorbidity and psychiatric disturbances [1].

Enuresis

Enuresis is an old disorder: historical reviews have documented bedwetting and its associated social and interpersonal consequences as far back as 1500 B.C. [2]. The actual term 'enuresis' comes from the Greek word 'enourein' which means 'to void urine' [3]. Enuretic symptoms in children (see Box A) can cause significant problems within a family or develop within the context of a family system that is dysfunctional or experiencing significant stress (i.e., parental separation or birth of a child). Parents may see a child's failure to toilet train or the recurrence of continence problems as a reflection of their inadequacy as parents: as a result, the child's symptoms may become a closely guarded secret. Tension may develop between parents and the enuretic child, leading to anger, frustration, and anxiety, which can exacerbate and perpetuate the enuretic symptoms. Issues of control and maladaptive expression of anger may lead to inappropriate voiding as the toilet training setting turns into the battleground on which these issues are acted out. Similarly, the parents may deal with this problem in a harsh and punitive manner that may negatively reinforce and perpetuate the child's enuretic symptoms.

Prevalence

Recent estimates indicate that approximately 5–7 million American children have primary nocturnal enuresis [4]. Enuresis occurs beyond the age of five years in 7%–10% of boys and 3% of girls. This condition is characterized by a 4:1 male-to-female ratio at the age of five years, which declines with age. Approximately 3% of boys and 2% of girls have enuretic symptoms at age 10 years, and the prevalence in the general adult population is 1%. Since 70% of children with enuresis have a first degree relative with the disorder, a genetic component has long been suspected. Some evidence has suggested heterogeneity in chromosomes involved with specific reference to Chromosome 13 [4] and Chomosome 22 in families with a history of multigenerational transmission [3]. The reported modes of transmission have included autosomal dominant, autosomal recessive and sporadic [3].) A connection between socioeconomic status and enuresis has been suggested but not established [5].

Enuresis is often a chronic condition, and it has a spontaneous remission rate of 15%. The chance for spontaneous resolution declines with increasing age, however. Forty percent of two-year-olds with enuresis

Clinical Child Psychiatry, Second Edition. Edited by W.M. Klykylo and J.L. Kay
© 2005 John Wiley & Sons Ltd.

BOX A DSM-IV-TR CRITERIA FOR 307.6 ENURESIS (NOT DUE TO A GENERAL MEDICAL CONDITION)

(A) Repeated voiding of urine into bed or clothes (whether involuntary or intentional).
(B) The behavior is clinically significant as manifested by either a frequency of twice a week for at least three consecutive months or the presence of clinically significant distress or impairment in social, academic (occupational), or other significant areas of functioning.
(C) Chronological age is at least five years (or equivalent developmental level).
(D) The behavior is not due exclusively to the direct physiological effect on a substance (e.g., a diuretic) or a general medical condition (e.g., diabetes, spina bifida, a seizure disorder).

Specify type:
   Nocturnal only: passage of urine only during nighttime sleep.
   Diurnal only: passage of urine during waking hours.
   Nocturnal and diurnal: a combination of the two subtypes.

Reprinted with permission from the Diagnostic and Statistical Manual of Mental Disorders, Copyright 2000. American Psychiatric Association.

Table 18.1 Etiologic considerations for patients with enuretic symptoms.

Urinary tract disease	Endocrine disorders
Infection	Abnormal nighttime release of vasopressin
Urinary outflow obstruction	Diabetes
Anatomic abnormalities	Maturational or developmental disorders
Congenital anomalies of the urinary tract	Emotional or behavioral disorders
Weak bladder or supporting musculature	Familial or genetic considerations
Low bladder pressure threshold causing early emptying	
Neurologic disorders	
Seizure disorder	
Spinal cord disease or trauma	
Sleep disorders	
Mental retardation	
Other cognitive disorders	

achieve continence by three years of age, 20% of three-year-olds by four years of age, 6% of four-year-olds by five years of age, and only 1.5% of five-year-olds by seven years of age. Approximately 1% of male adolescents (and fewer adolescent females) have persisting enuretic symptoms by 18 years of age [5]).

Etiology and Differential Diagnosis

Enuretic symptoms are felt to result from multiple factors (Table 18.1). Nonfunctional enuresis (enuretic symptoms due to an identifiable organic etiology) may be caused by the following conditions:

- urologic conditions (infection or obstruction);
- anatomic abnormalities (spinal cord disease, a weak bladder or supporting bladder musculature, posterior urethral valves in boys and ectopic ureter in girls);

- developmental delay [4];
- physiologic abnormalities (low bladder pressure threshold that causes early emptying);
- metabolic conditions (diabetes);
- urologic mechanisms (seizures).

Some forms of functional enuresis (see enuretic symptoms occurring in the absence of an identifiable organic factor believed to initiate and maintain the disturbance) appear to have a genetic basis. The chance of a child having this condition is 77% if both parents have a history of enuresis and 44% if one parent has such a history. Although a strong genetic factor is suggested in certain cases, the mechanism of transmission is uncertain. For many patients classified as having functional enuresis, hormonal factors and biologic rhythms may actually in part be causing the development of enuretic symptoms. Some patients, for example, may not have a normal nighttime release of vasopressin and consequently may not have the typical nighttime reduction in urine volume. Sleep disorders could also potentially cause enuretic symptoms. Enuretic episodes can occur during any electroencephalogram (EEG) stage. Enuresis occurs in some patients as a result of a maturational disorder (i.e., a deficit existing during a specific developmental period) and is also associated with an over-representation of developmental delays.

Functional enuresis is more prevalent in patients with moderate or severe mental retardation. A psychodynamic cause of functional enuresis is suggested for some patients, owing to its association with other forms of psychopathology such as conduct disorder, mood disorders, and problems with separation. Approximately 50% of children with functional enuresis have comorbid emotional and behavioral symptoms. Functional enuresis may be related to stress (i.e., due to birth of a sibling), trauma, psychosocial crisis (i.e., parental separation or loss) [5]. Psychologic or psychodynamic explanations for children with symptoms of functional enuresis include the following [6]:

- revenge enuresis – a method of retention in response to harsh training practices or a strict parent;
- regressive enuresis – occurring after continence is established in response to a perceived threat to the child's security, for example with the birth of a sibling or with the introduction of a new parental figure;
- enuresis due to fancied injury – occurring after a physically traumatic experience that leaves children with a view of themselves as injured or damaged and no longer in control of their urinary flow;
- enuresis due to lack of training – occurring in families who have decided that because multiple family members have had a history of enuresis, little can be done to improve it.

Clinical Description

Enuretic episodes are most common at night and typically occur 30 minutes to three hours after the onset of sleep; they can, however, occur at any time of day or at night during any EEG or sleep stage. Enuretic episodes may be more frequent in Delta or slow-wave sleep (stages 3 and 4 of nonrapid eye movement sleep, which comprise the deepest sleep stages) or in the post-Delta arousal period of sleep (the transition from Delta sleep to rapid eye movement sleep). Children with daytime enuresis usually have nighttime symptoms as well [5]. A distinction is made not only between enuresis due to a medical condition and functional enuresis but also between primary and secondary enuresis. Primary enuresis refers to patients who have never achieved urinary continence; it is not typically associated with emotional disturbance and is frequently diagnosed in patients with mental retardation. Secondary enuresis refers to patients who have previously achieved at least six months of urinary incontinence and is commonly associated with more severe psychopathology or stress [5].

Assessment, Evaluation, and Work-up

A careful patient history is an essential part of evaluating patients with enuresis (Figure 18.1). The initial evaluation should address issues such as a family history of similar symptoms and, for patients with secondary enuresis, a possible precipitating event. A baseline assessment of symptoms often requires that patients and parents log the symptoms on calendar forms (i.e., wet and dry nights for two or more weeks.) This type of record can provide information on the frequency of symptoms and can help establish chronic from periodic yet sporadic episodes that could be related to seizures. A thorough history should include obtaining answers to such questions as:

- Has your child ever been consistently dry and for how long?
- Is the wetting during the night, day or both night and day and how many times during these periods?
- How often does your child urinate and defecate and does this appear painful for the child?
- Any soiling or the appearance of very hard stools?
- Does your child seem to hold his/her urine until the last minute? [7]

Additional questions to the parents such as:

- Why is this a problem?
- Why is treatment being sought now?
- How has this problem been handled to date?

may reveal additional valuable information and provide direction as to the most appropriate treatment interventions to be used. Details regarding previous treatments and the possible reasons for failure may help prevent similar failures.

The clinician should perform a complete physical examination, including a genital evaluation, assessment for bladder distention and fecal impaction, measurement of maturational indices, and assessment for any congenital malformations that are suggestive of urogenital abnormalities. The physical exam should also include abdominal and flank palpation for masses, inspection of the lower back for cutaneous lesions or an asymmetric gluteal cleft (suggestive of spinal dys-

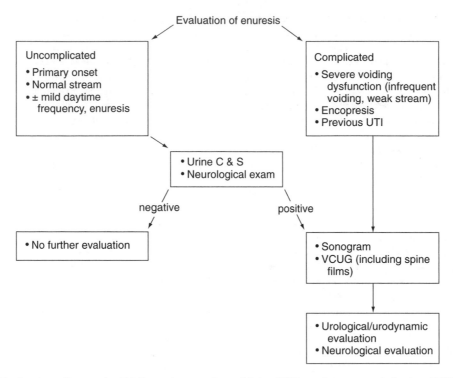

Figure 18.1 Evaluation of enuresis. C&C = culture and sensitivity; UTI = urinary tract infection; VCUG = voiding cystourethrogram. (From Rushton HG: Nocturnal enuresis: Epidemiology, evaluation, and currently available treatment options. *J Pediatr* 1989; **114**[suppl]:691–696.)

paphism and neurologic problem) and evaluation for abnormalities of gait (also suggestive of a neurologic abnormality).

Laboratory evaluation should include a midstream urinalysis at a minimum (assessing for specific gravity, evidence of infection or the presence of blood or glucose) [7]. Depending on clinical suspicions, a chemistry profile, urine culture, and endocrine studies can be obtained. A radiologic evaluation may be indicated in the presence of infected urine, associated symptoms (polyuria, frequency, urgency, dysuria), or a history of recurrent urinary tract infections [1]. Specifically, a work-up for vesicoureteral reflux would be reasonable in such cases and include a voiding cystourethrogram and renal ultrasound [7]. A sleep evaluation in certain instances may be indicated, but an EEG is not a routine part of the evaluation. Referrals to a pediatric urologist or pediatric neurologist may be necessary [5].

Course and Prognosis

As previously stated, enuretic symptoms have a spontaneous remission rate of 15% per year, and the rate is

spontaneous recovery decreases with age to approximately 1% by the age of 18 years. Adolescent-onset enuresis is rare and is typically associated with more psychopathology and a less favorable outcome. Some authors have proposed a relation between this symptom and sexual abuse, particularly in females [9]. Persisting symptoms of enuresis can lead to numerous additional complications, among them severe embarrassment; anger and punishment by parents or other caregivers; teasing or ostracizing by peers; avoidance of overnight activities, group activities (e.g., scouting), age-appropriate heterosexual interactions (e.g., dating); social withdrawal; decreased self-esteem; and emotional and behavioral problems [5].

Treatment

Treatment strategies for this condition can be grouped into three categories: waiting for spontaneous resolution, behavioral therapies (including bladder training exercises and bell and pad moisture sensing devices or alarms), and pharmacologic treatments. Combinations of behavioral interventions and medication management are also frequently employed (Table 18.2).

Behavioral Treatments

Behavioral interventions for nocturnal enuresis often include the restriction of nighttime fluid intake, bladder training exercises and midsleep awakenings for toilet use. Star charting (behavior charting whereby a child receives a special marker or other reward for complying with the desired target behavior) and other systems by which the patient can be rewarded for dry nights are also effective. Night alarms consist of electrodes separated by a device (such as a blanket) that becomes connected when wet, thereby activating a buzzer, bell, or vibrating pad; the device can be set up to awaken even child or the parents. These devices can be readily obtained in most pharmacies, surgical supply stores, or health departments of department stores. Night alarms are reported to be successful in 80%–90% of patients but with high relapse rates (up to 40%) with discontinuation. To be effective, night alarms require significant motivation from patients and parents, and a cure is usually delayed, typically occurring in the second month of treatment. Factors limiting the success of night alarms including failure to understand and follow instructions, frequent false alarms, unintentional awakenings of other family members, and a failure of the child to awaken (or to be awakened by his or her parents). A potential side effect of the treatment is buzzer ulcers that result from laying an ionized urine. Advances in night alarm technology have eliminated this side effect with the use of modern transistorized alarms that do not use continuous, relatively high voltages across the electrodes [1]. Additonal innovations on the alarm strategy have employed the use of ultrasonic monitors mounted on an elastic abdominal belt to replace the pad. The alarm is sounded when the device senses that the bladder capacity has reached a predetermined/preset limit [3]. Measuring success is naturally done in terms of dry nights achieved (for nocturnal symptoms). Improvement is reasonably defined as a 50% reduction in wet nights. Cure of nocturnal enuresis is having only one or two wet nights over a three-month-period and verification that the child has spontaneously awakened in the evening to urinate in the toilet [4]. Websites of interest include: www.nytone.com, www.palcolalabs.com, www.pottypager.com, and www.dri-sleeper.com can be used to order bedwetting alarms [7].

Pharmacologic Treatments

Successful pharmacologic treatments of enuresis include tricyclic antidepressants (imipramine,

Table 18.2 Practical management of nocturnal enuresis.

STAGE 1: ASSESSMENT

Obtain history: frequency, periodicity, and duration of wetting

Why is this a problem? Why now?

Mental status: views and misconceptions (parent and child)

Discover reasons for previous failure or failures

Perform routine physical examination (any minor congenital abnormalities?)

Midstream specimen of urine must be obtained

Radiology and further physical investigation is needed only if symptoms or evidence of urinary tract infection (dysuria and frequency or positive culture results) or polyuria

STAGE 2: ADVICE

Education that enuresis is common and not deliberate

Aim to reduce punitive behavior

Transmit optimism: however, anticipate disappointment at no instant cure

Preview the stepwise recovery and warn of the possibility of relapse

STAGE 3: BASELINE

Use star chart

Focus on positive achievements (be creative)

Examine the effect of simple interventions (e.g., lifting)

STAGE 4

NIGHT ALARM

First-line management unless important to obtain rapid short-term effect

Demonstrate night alarm equipment in the office

Telephone follow-up within a few days of commencing therapy

or

DRUG THERAPY

If rapid suppression of wetting is needed (e.g., before vacation or camp to defuse aggressive or hostile situation between child and parents and siblings)

When family has *proved* incapable of using the equipment

After failure or multiple relapses

Medication of choice: deamino-D-arginine-vasopressin (DDAVP), 20–40 µg at night

---

From Lucas CP, Shaffer D: Elimination disorders. In: Tasman A, Kay J, Lieberman JA, eds. *Psychiatry*. Vol. 1. Philadelphia: WB Saunders; 1997:734.

desipramine, amitriptyline, and nortriptyline), anticholinergic agents (oxybutynin (Ditropan), hyoscyamine (Levsinex), Levsinex Timecaps [8], propantheline, and terodiline), desmopressin (DDAVP; deamino-D-arginine-vasopressin), and psychostimulants (methylphenidate and dextroamphetamine; Dexedrine). There have been limited reports of the effectiveness of indomethacin [10], the oral androgen mesterolone [11] in the treating patients with enuretic symptoms.

Tricyclic Antidepressants
Imipramine (Tofranil) is considered by many to still be the gold-standard medication treatment for enuresis. Imipramine has come to share the spotlight with DDAVP that has increased significantly in its use for the treatment of enuresis over the recent past. Other tricyclic antidepressants (nortriptyline, desipramine, and amitriptyline) are also effective in treating patients with bedwetting symptoms. Although the action mechanism of imipramine's anti-enuretic effect remains unknown, it may exert its therapeutic effect by: anticholinergic-mediated relaxation of the bladder detrusor muscle which inhibits urination and increases bladder filling and capacity; decreasing sleep depth; elevating mood; enhancing voluntary control of the urethral sphincter; or placebo effects. Although 80%–90% of patients show an improvement or elimination of symptoms, there is significant relapse after the discontinuation of treatment, and fewer than 40% of patients experience sustained resolution of symptoms. The use of tricyclic medications requires close monitoring of serum levels and electrocardiogram (ECG) readings, since these agents can produce intracardiac conduction delays. ECG analysis should be obtained prior to initiating a tricyclic medication, after an increase in dosage, as indicated for clinical side effects, and periodically thereafter. Typical doses effective for enuresis usually begin at 25 mg/night and may be gradually increased to 50 mg/night or even 75 mg/night. If necessary, providers are encouraged to seek input from colleagues comfortable in the use of tricyclic agents and who are made aware of the patients medical history before initiating dosing. Tricyclic antidepressants can cause significant problems, owing to their anticholinergic effects (especially constipation and difficults initiating micturition), orthostatic hypotension, sedation and potential cardiac side effects. An important consideration is the possibility for accidental or intentional overdose with these agents in patients or their siblings which can be life threatening.

Anticholinergic Agents
Anticholinergic agents such as oxybutynin, propantheline, terodiline and hyoscyamine are beneficial for those patients with reduced urgency, small bladder capacity, bladder instability, or a neurogenic bladder. Although they are generally ineffective in patients with nocturnal symptoms, anticholinergics may reduce symptoms of daytime enuresis [1]. Significant side effects of these medications include dry mouth, facial flushing, hyperpyrexia, and with excessive doses, blurred vision, and hallucinations [12].

Hormonal Therapy
The synthetic vasopeptide desmopressin (DDAVP), an analog of the antidiuretic hormone vasopressin, has been shown to be successful in treating enuretic symptoms. DDAVP can be administered in oral, rhinal (drops) or intranasal form; the equivalent oral dosage is 10 times the intranasal dosages. The oral form (0.1-mg tablets) is more frequently used in treating patients with the syndrome of inappropriate antidiuretic hormone and diabetes insipidus. The intranasal form is also commonly used; a typical starting dose is two puffs (20 µg) at night and does not exceed four puffs (40 µg) nightly. DDAVP is a relatively more expensive treatment: in the US, a monthly supply (dispensed at the typical starting dosages) costs $87.60 (for oral form) and $95 to just over $100 (for the spray and rhinal/drops). DDAVP may only benefit those children who produce high volumes of urine with low osmolality at night and who lack the normal increase in nighttime secretion of antidiuretic hormone. DDAVP has been known to cause headaches and abdominal pain as well as nasal congestion and epistaxis with the use of the intranasal form. Water intoxication, electrolyte abnormalities, and rare seizures are also potential risks of DDAVP use [13].

Psychostimulant Therapy
When used in combination with education and behavioral therapy, psychostimulants such as Methylphenidate, Adderall and Dextroamphetamine may enhance strategies for learning continence when attention deficit/hyperactivity disorder (ADHD) is a comorbid consideration. Evening doses of stimulants can reduce the depth of sleep in all patients and may facilitate a child's spontaneously awakening in the evening to urinate in the toilet. As a solo treatment strategy, however, psychostimulants have shown no therapeutic efficacy in treating patients with enuresis [1].

Fluoxetine (Prozac)
This author developed an interest in the use of fluoxetine to treat enuretic symptoms based on observations of clinical work (unpublished data). Fluoxetine is now frequently used and has been found to be effective in

treating pediatric patients with depression. The following two case studies illustrate the potential use of the fluoxetine in treating patients with enuresis.

CASE ONE

A 13-year-old boy was initially referred for problems with anxiety and depression and was ultimately diagnosed with ADHD. He had never achieved urinary continence at night and the results from a previous urologic work-up had been negative. He was initially started on a dosage of 20 mg fluoxetine p.o. every morning and experienced a complete resolution of enuretic symptoms within one month of initiating therapy. After a one-year follow-up, the patient continued to be on fluoxetine therapy and continued to be free of enuretic symptoms.

CASE TWO

An 11-year-old girl was referred with a history of oppositional behavior, depression, and an eating disorder not otherwise specified (overeating, binge episodes, and significant obesity). This patient was also diagnosed with ADHD. She had never achieved nocturnal urinary continence and had had a previous urologic work-up with negative results. She was started on 20 mg fluoxetine p.o. every morning and expressed a complete resolution of enuretic symptoms in two weeks. After four weeks of fluoxetine therapy she was started on methylphenidate (Ritalin) for ADHD symptoms and had a recurrence of enuretic symptoms. Two months after initiating fluoxetine therapy, she experienced worsening symptoms of depression that required an increase in her fluoxetine regimen to 40 mg p.o. every morning; this dosage produced another notable improvement in her enuretic symptoms. After nine months of treatment with fluoxetine and methylphenidate, she continued to show improvement in enuretic symptoms over baseline.

The exact mechanism and by which the fluoxetine or other selective serotonin reuptake inhibitors (SSRIs) could benefit patients with enuresis is unknown. Hypothetically, by treating a depressive syndrome, fluoxetine may assist in the resolution of regressive behavior such as enuretic symptoms. Increase peripheral levels of serotonin that result from the use of fluoxetine treatment may directly cause smooth muscle relaxation in the bladder similar to its effects on vascular smooth muscle. There is also the possibility that the indirect role of serotonin on central, spinal, or peripheral mechanisms operates via a functional connection between serotonin and noradrenergic neurons causing an inhibition of noradrenergic input. Alterations in the balance between the adrenergic and cholinergic systems may affect bladder instability capacity. The enhanced serotonin neurotransmission that can occur with the use of SSRIs may increase plasma arginine vasopressin release; this effect has been found in rats [14]. This possible serotonin-mediated increase in plasma vasopressin level may also ameliorate enuretic symptoms. Further research and clinical use will determine if other SSRIs are effective in the treatment of enuresis. At present, a single case study with fluoxetine [15] and a single case study with sertraline [16] indicate potential efficacy in treating patients with enuresis. A growing body of literature suggests that SSRIs may represent relatively safe treatment options for this condition.

Encopresis

Children with encopresis face a terribly embarrassing and stigmatizing condition that may have lifelong negative consequences on their social and personal functioning. The term encopresis was originally coined by Weissenberg in 1926 to refer to a condition of overt psychogenic soiling in children whose involuntary bowel movements occur in abnormal or socially unacceptable situations [17]. Encopresis today is commonly defined according to the *Diagnostic and Statistical Manual of Mental Disorders*, 4th ed. Text Revision (DSM-IV-TR) criteria, which refer to a condition of intentional or involuntary passage of feces into inappropriate places in the absence of any identified physical abnormality in children four years of age and older (Box B) [18]. Encopretic symptoms can be further defined in terms of the presence or absence of constipation and overflow incontinence. Encopresis can be considered as primary, in which patients have never attained bowel continence for a period of six months or more, or secondary, in which patients develop symptoms after achieving bowel continence. There is considerably less literature on recent advancements

---

BOX B DSM IV-TR CRITERIA FOR ENCOPRESIS

(A) Repeated passage of feces into inappropriate places (e.g., clothing or floor) whether involuntary or intentional.

(B) At least one such event a month for at least three months.

(C) Chronological age is at least four years (or equivalent developmental level).

(D) The behavior is not due to the direct physiological effects of a substance (e.g., laxatives) or a general medical condition except through a mechanism involving constipation.

Code as follows:

787.6 – With constipation and overflow incontinence: there is evidence of constipation on physical examination or by history.

307.7 – Without constipation and overflow incontinence: there is no evidence of constipation on physical examination or by history.

Reprinted with permission from the Diagnostic and Statistical Manual of Mental Disorders, Copyright 2000. American Psychiatric Association.

---

and research studies in this area relative to the body of literature that currently exists for enuresis.

Prevalence

Roughly one-third of children are completely toilet trained by 24 months of age, with bowel control preceding bladder control. At age four years, approximately 95% of children have attained bowel continence. The prevalence of encopresis among children varies from 0.3% to 8%, most likely reflecting variations in defining encopresis and in the age ranges sampled [20]. The frequency of this disorder declines with age such that it becomes infrequent after age seven years and quite rare after age 16 years. More specific data indicate that 1.5% of 7–8-year olds and approximately 1% of 10–12-year-olds are encopretic and that boys are four to five times more likely than girls to have this condition. Retentive encopretic patients (having constipation and overflow incontinence) represent 80%–95% of cases with nonretentive encopretic patients making up the remainder [8]. Secondary encopresis is more common than primary encopresis, representing 50%–60% of all cases. Reported data on the prevalence of functional (nonorganically based) encopresis also very among researchers from 0.3% to 8% of children [20].

Etiology and Pathogenesis

A single causative factor or mechanism for encopresis has not been clearly identified. Several possible factors that are felt to contribute to encopresis include anismus, rectal hypersensitivity, oppositional behavior pattern, toilet phobia, limited attention and concentration span, high levels of motor activity [21], developmental delay, toilet skills deficit, and irritable bowel

syndrome [8]. Bowel continence is achieved and maintained through a complex mix of physiologic, psychologic, and behavioral factors, and the presence or absence of constipation also appears to be important. Children show a tendency towards constipation in the first 12 months of life; a reduction of stool frequency with retention between 12 and 24 months of age may indicate a likelihood for developing encopresis [1].

Several theories have attempted to explain the occurrence of encopresis. A once popular psychodynamic model noted that boys particularly value stool as part of themselves when faced with the issues of castration anxiety; the clinical features of the disorder failed to support this model, however [21]. The prevailing theories concerning nonretentive encopresis (encopresis without constipation and overflow incontinence) focus on problematic toilet training. Punitive and coercive training measures can create stress that results in significant anxiety and a resulting pot (toilet) phobia as well as a failure to acquire the appropriate bathroom skills [1]. Encopretic symptoms can occur in response to other life stressors, such as the birth of a sibling or the introduction of a new parental figure, or as a consequence of anger in a child displaying oppositional and negativistic behaviors toward his or her parents [21]. Cultural factors may play a role in the production of symptoms; early toilet training of children, for example, may be emphasized and the quick mastery of toilet skills viewed as a measure of parental competence. Similarly, economic factors may affect the child's production of symptoms; for example, there may be an incentive to toilet train children early to allow parents to pursue other activities such as employment. Finally, some children simply may not receive adequate instruction in toilet skills.

Differential Diagnosis and Organic Considerations

Although the vast majority of children with encopretic symptoms are medically and physically normal, certain organic features can initiate and maintain such a disturbance. Defecation disorders can be grouped as either 'soiling without retention' or 'fecal retention with or without soiling' (Table 18.3). Organic/general medical causes a soiling without retention include the following:

- diarrheal diseases;
- rectal pull through surgery (without stenosis);
- occult spinal dysraphism;
- loss of reservoir capacity after extensive resection of the colorectum;
- spinal cord trauma;

Organic causes of fecal retention with or without soiling include the following [22]:

- motility failure disorders (Hirschsprung disease, pseudo-obstruction syndromes, neuronal dysplasia, multiple endocrine neoplasia type III);
- impaired valsalva maneuver;
- pharmacologic causes (chronic laxative use or abuse, analgesics containing codeine, phenothiazines, chemotherapeutic agents, and lead poisoning);
- endocrine disorders (hypothyroidism, hypokalemia, hypercalcemia, diabetes, uremia, polyuria, pheochromocytoma);
- intestinal smooth muscle disorders (scleroderma and neuropathy or myopathy);
- anal or rectal stenosis (congenital or acquired);
- anterior ectopic anus.

For most of the conditions mentioned above, children are likely to initially present with encopretic symptoms alone. In addition, high rates of comorbid developmental disorders, family dysfunction, and other emotional or behavioral (e.g., oppositional defiant disorder, conduct disorder, mood disorders, and psychosis) often exist in patients with encopresis; when the presence of any of these disorders is suspected, patients should be referred for mental health assessment and treatment.

Assessment, Evaluation, and Work-up

A careful history and physical examination (including a rectal examination) is usually sufficient to rule out any organic causes for encopretic symptoms (Table 18.4; Figure 18.2). If constipation is a symptom, the clinician should inquire about the time of onset, stool frequency, stool consistency and size, fluid and dietary

Table 18.3 Disorders of defecation.

SOILING WITHOUT RETENTION
Organic
    Diarrheal diseases
    Rectal pull-through surgery (without stenosis)
    Occult spinal dysraphism
    Loss of reservoir capacity after extensive resection of colorectum
    Spinal cord trauma
Functional
    Functional nonretentive fecal soiling
    Spock-Bergen syndrome
    Prolonged use of diapers

RETENTION WITH OR WITHOUT SOILING
ORGANIC
Motility failures
    Hirschsprung's disease
    Pseudo-obstruction syndromes
    Neuronal dysplasia
    Multiple endocrine neoplasia type III
Impaired valsalva maneuver
Pharmacologic causes
    Codeine-containing analgesics
    Lead poisoning
    Long-term laxative use (or abuse)
    Phenothiazines
    Chemotherapeutic agents (vincristine)
Endocrine causes of fecal stasis
    Hypothyroidism
    Hypercalcemia
    Hypokalemia
    Diabetes
    Uremia
    Porphyria
    Pheochromocytoma
Diseases of intestinal smooth muscles
    Scleroderma
    Neuropathy/myopathy
Anal or rectal stenosis
Congenital or acquired stenosis or stricture (e.g., secondary to imperforate anus repair, or abscess drainage)
Anterior ectopic anus
FUNCTIONAL
Functional fecal retention syndrome: due to physically and/or emotionally difficult bowel movement

Adapted from Hyman PE, Fleisher DR: A classification of disorders of defecation in infants and children. *Semin Gastrointest Dis* 1994; **5**:20–23 with permission from Elsevier.

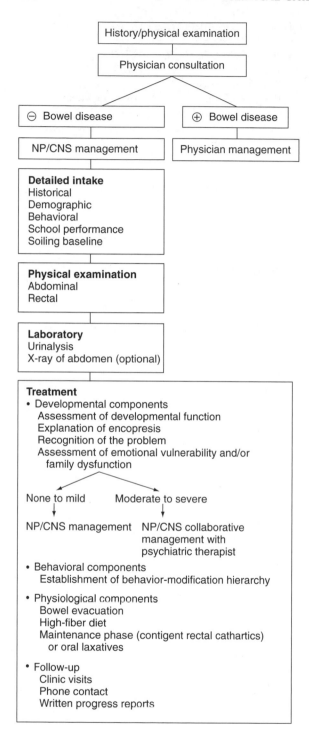

Figure 18.2 Encopretic evaluation and management model. NP/CNS = nurse practitioner/clinical nurse specialist. (From Sprague-McRae JM: Encopresis: Developmental, behavioral and physiological considerations for treatment. *Nurse Pract* 1990; **15**[6]:8–24.)

Table 18.4 History and physical examination of the encopretic patient [8].

(I)   History
(A)   Stool pattern
      Size
      Consistency
      Interval between bowel movements
(B)   Hisory of constipation
      Age of onset
(C)   History of soiling
      Age of onset
      Type and amount of fecal material
(D)   Dietary history
      Type and amount of food
      Changes in diet
(E)   Decrease in appetite
(F)   Abdominal pain
(G)   Medications
(H)   Urinary symptoms
      Day or night enuresis
      Urinary tract infection
(I)   Family history of constipation
(J)   Family or personal stressors

(II) Physical examination
(A)   Height
(B)   Weight
(C)   Abdominal examination
      Distention
      Mass, especially suprapubic
(D)   Rectal examination
      Sacral dimple
      Position of anus
      Anal fissures
      Anal wink
      Sphincter tone
      Rectal vault size
      Presence or absence of stool in rectum
      Pelvic mass

(III) Neurologic examination

habits, the patient's perception of the urge to deficate, withholding behavior, and toilet training procedures with therapeutic measures previously employed. The use of medications and a family history of constipation should be assessed. Associated symptoms such as abdominal pain and distention, nausea or emesis, and failure to thrive need to be elicited, since such symptoms may have an underlying organic cause [22].

Physical examination findings that suggest an organic cause of encopretic symptoms include a patulous anus (neurologic disease), flat buttocks (sacral agenesis), and a pilonidal dimple (spina bifida occulta and associated tethered cord). An anteriorly displaced anus is considered a normal variant in most patients but can cause problems with defecation in some children. Constipation can be confirmed by a plain abdominal X-ray evaluation. If initial treatment efforts fail, further work-up can include a stool analysis (fecal fat, ova, parasites, and white blood cells) to evaluate for malabsorption and infectious diseases. Tests such as a rectal biopsy, anal manometry, and a barium enema can be helpful if Hirschsprung disease is suspected. Defecography (evacuation proctography) can be useful when rectal intussusceptions, rectoceles, or outlet-obstruction constipation is suspected. Pelvic floor electromyography can reveal abnormal pelvic floor function during defecation, which is considered a functional cause of encopresis likely to respond to biofeedback. Rectal compliance can be assessed using a pressure probe placed between the rectal wall and an inflated latex balloon in the rectum. Colonic manometry can distinguish between myopathic and neuropathic etiologies in patients with abnormal transit times [23].

Course and Prognosis

Substantial follow-up studies are currently unavailable. As previously noted, encopresis diminishes with age and is very rare in adolescence and adults. For those patients with associated medical conditions, developmental delays, mental retardation or mental health disorders, the prognosis depends on how successfully such comorbid conditions are identified and treated. The presence of significant parental disinterest or family dysfunction is likely to lead to a more chronic and persisting course, since the encopretic symptoms may serve a stabilizing or homeostatic function for these pathologic family environments [5]. Comorbid mental health disorders/coexisting behavioral problems predict a poorer outcome to toilet-training behavioral protocols [8].

Treatment

In the literature regarding treatment of encopresis – which is far less developed than that regarding enuresis – all treatment rests on the fundamental assumption that an empty bowel cannot soil. Specific treatment methods can include one or a combination of the following methods: behavioral strategies, medications, cathartics, dietary and fluid intake alterations, biofeedback, relaxation techniques, psy-

chotherapy, hypnotherapy, and hospitalization (Table 18.5) [17].

Behavioral Treatments

Behavioral therapy is commonly considered the mainstay of treating patients with encopresis. Parents and other care providers need to be educated regarding the need to display to the child significant and consistent motivation and interests, to focus and praise appropriate efforts by the child, and to make the bathroom a pleasant and nonthreatening place. The toilet should be made easy to use. Children should be educated in toilet-use skills such as being shown where to obtain necessities such as toilet paper. For those children whose feet cannot reach the floor when they are on the toilet, they should be provided with a step that allows for bracing when straining. Initially, a warm bath prior to use of the toilet may allow for easier defecation in an anxious child. The child should be made to use the toilet for up to 15 minutes in the morning after breakfast (the time of the day during which the colon is most ready to function for defecation) and after each meal.

Emphasis should be placed on recognizing and rewarding only accomplishments and other positive behavior as well as identifying and eliminating sources of secondary gain that may perpetuate encopretic symptoms. Some clinicians advocate mildly adverse intervention such as requiring the patient to clean soiled clothing or other soiling messes; care should be taken, however, to prevent such interventions from becoming too harsh. Graded exposure schemes for toilet phobia symptoms for particularly anxious children have been shown to be effective [19]. The use of star charts that target aspects of appropriate toilet use in need of improvement have produced positive results. Parents should use a tangible reward with this technique (e.g., a sticker) to highlight days in which the desired behavior has been achieved. It is best to also emphasize accomplishments with positive verbal comments and to refrain from lecturing or providing any kind of reward on those days when the desired behavior has not been achieved. Parents should place the chart where many people can see it, mark the chart when the child is present, and consider a suitable additional reward for maintaining the given behavior for an agreed on number of days, which can be lengthened as achievements are made [1].

Pharmacologic Treatments

In patients with retention and significant constipation, valuable treatments include an increased fluid intake,

Table 18.5 Practical management of encopresis.

STAGE 1: ASSESSMENT

Whether primary or secondary

Presence or physical cause

Presence or absence of constipation

Presence or absence of acute stress

Presence or absence of psychiatric disorder including phobic symptoms or smearing

ABC (antecedents, behavior, consequences) of encopresis, including secondary gain

Discover reasons for previous failure or failures

STAGE 2: ADVICE

Education regarding diet, constipation, and toileting

Aim to reduce punitive or coercive behavior

Transmit optimism; however, anticipate disappointment at no instant cure

Preview the stepwise recovery and warn of the possibility of relapse

STAGE 3

TOILETING

Baseline observation using star chart

Focus on positive achievements (e.g., toileting, rather than soiling)

High-fiber diet (try bran in soup, milk shakes)

Toilet after meals, 15 minutes maximum

Check that adequately rising intra-abdominal pressure is present

Graded exposure scheme if 'not phobic'

with

LAXATIVES

Indicated if physical examination or abdominal radiograph shows fecal loading

Medication of choice: Senokot syrup (senna) up to 10 mL twice daily, lacrulose syrup up to 30 mL (20 mg) twice daily

Dosage will be reduced over time; titrate with bowel frequency

ENEMAS

Microenema (e.g., bisacodyl 30 mL) if the bowel is excessively loaded with rocklike feces

STAGE 4: BIOFEEDBACK

Consider after relapse or failure to respond to toileting or laxatives

---

From Lucas CP, Shaffer D: Elimination disorders. In: Tasman A, Kay J, Lieberman JA, eds. *Psychiatry.* Vol. 1. Philadelphia: WB Saunders; 1997:739.

dietary changes, and the use of laxatives, suppositories, and enemas to ensure well-formed and soft stools. Encopretic patients should be placed on a high-fiber diet consisting of increased amounts of vegetables, fruits and fruit juices, grains, cereals, legumes, nuts, and seeds (Table 18.6). Raw bran or wheat germ can be added or sprinkled on to other foods or cooked into foods. A reduction (not the complete elimination) of dairy products may also be a beneficial change. Enemas and laxatives should be used briefly to initially evacuate the bowel. Mineral oil can be initiated concurrently with a multivitamin supplement given 2–3 hours after meals (to reduce the impact mineral oil has on the absorption of fat-soluble vitamins). The use of mineral oil should be continued until regular bowel movements have been attained (typically after several weeks) and then gradually tapered and discontinued [17]. Mineral oil is contraindicated in patients at risk for aspiration. Other regimens include propylene glycol, lactulose, Milk of Magnesia (1–3 ml/kg/day) or sorbitol (1–3 mg/kg/day) [8]. Prolonged use of the above laxative agents should be considered safe as there does not exist credible evidence to suggest otherwise [23]. Reports exist regarding the beneficial use of imipramine, amitriptyline and propulsid for encopretic symptoms. While tricyclic antidepressants have played a major role in the treatment of enuresis, the impact of such pharmacologic agents in the treatment of encopresis has been much more modest. Certainly, due consideration should be given to the anticholinergic/constipating potential of tricyclic antidepressants before using in patients with encopresis [3].

Psychotherapy

Psychotherapeutic intervention such as traditional individual therapies, play therapy, and family therapy have been used to treat patients with encopresis; individual and play therapies, however, have not been demonstrated as effective in treating these patients [14]. Most investigators agree that family interventions are essential and that extensive formal family therapy may be required in instances of severely dysfunctional family dynamics.

Hypnosis

A few case studies and small group studies have documented encouraging results with the use of hypnosis to treat children with encopresis, although large sample studies have not been conducted. Suggestions used during hypnosis stress the child's ability to control his or her bowel functioning. In addition, self-control and

Table 18.6 Dietary sources of high-fiber foods (100 g = 3.5 oz).

VEGETABLES

1–1.9 g fiber/100 g edible portion

Beans, snap, raw/canned
Beets, canned
Cabbage, Chinese, raw/cooked
Carrots, canned
Celery, raw
Corn, canned
Cucumbers, raw
Lettuce
Mushrooms, raw
Onions, raw
Peppers, sweet, raw
Pickles
Potatoes, raw, flesh/skin
Potatoes, baked, flesh
Potatoes, boiled, flesh
Squash, summer, raw/cooked
Squash, winter, raw
Sweet potatoes, canned
Tomatoes, raw
Turnips, raw

≥2 g fiber/100 g edible portion

Broccoli
Cabbage, red/white, raw/cooked
Cauliflower, raw/cooked
Mushrooms, boiled
Onions, spring, raw
Peas, podded, raw/cooked
Potatoes, hashbrowned
Spinach, raw/cooked
Squash, winter, cooked
Tomato puree
Turnip, greens, raw
Turnips boiled
Water chestnuts, canned
Watercress

≥3 g fiber/100 g edible portion

Artichokes, raw
Brussels sprouts, boiled
Carrots, raw
Chives
Corn, raw/cooked
French fries, frozen
Parsley, raw

Peas, canned
Potatoes, baked with skin
Sweet potatoes, raw/cooked
Turnip greens, cooked
Mixed vegetables, frozen/cooked

FRUITS

1–1.9 g fiber/100 g edible portion

Apples without skin
Applesauce
Bananas
Fruit cocktail, canned
Nectarines, raw
Peaches, raw/canned
Pineapple, raw/canned
Prune juice

2–4.9 g fiber/100 g edible portion

Apples, raw with skin
Blueberries, raw
Kiwifruit, raw
Olives
Oranges, raw
Pears, raw
Strawberries

≥5 g fiber/100 g edible portion

Apricots, dried
Figs, dried
Peaches, dried
Prunes, stewed/dried
Raisins

GRAINS/CEREALS/ LEGUMES/NUTS/SEEDS

≥2–3.9 g fiber/100 g edible portion

Bagel, plain
Bread, French
Bread, Italian
Bread, oatmeal
Bread, Vienna
Bread, wheat
Bread, white toasted
Bread stuffing
Brownies with nuts
Cereal, cornflakes plain/frosted
Cereal, farina, dry
Cereal, oatflakes

Cookies, butter
Cookies, chocolate chip
Cookies, chocolate sandwich
Cookies, oatmeal
Cornbread
Crackers, graham
Crackers, Matzo
Crackers, saltine
Doughnuts, leavened
Flour, arrowroot
Flour, rice, white
Flour, wheat, white
French toast, frozen
Fruitcake
Hominy, canned
Muffins, blueberry
Noodles, chow mein
Noodles, egg
Pie, pecan
Pie, pumpkin
Pretzels
Rice, brown, long-grained, raw
Rice, white, glutinous
Rolls, dinner (egg)
Semolina
Spaghetti, dry
Tortillas, whole wheat
Waffles, frozen

≥4 g fiber/100 g edible portion

Baked beans, canned
Bread, Boston brown
Bread, bran
Bread, cracked wheat
Bread, Hollywood-type, light
Bread, mixed grain
Bread, pita, whole wheat
Bread, pumpernickel
Bread, rye
Bread, white, high-fiber
Bread, whole wheat
Bread crumbs
Cashews
Cereal, wheat flakes
Cereal, wheat/malted barley
Chickpeas, canned
Chips, corn

Chips, potato
Chips, tortilla
Coconut
Corn, toasted
Cornmeal, degermed
Cowpeas, cooked
Crackers, Matzo egg/onion
Crackers, wheat
Fig bars
Flour, oat
Flour, rice, brown
Granola bars
Hazelnuts
Ice cream cones
Lima beans, cooked
Macaroni
Melba toast
Millet, hulled/raw
Mixed nuts
Muffins, English, whole wheat
Muffins, oat bran
Noodles, Japanese, udon/somen, dry
Noodles, spinach
Peanut butter
Peanuts
Pecans
Rice, wild, raw
Sunflower seeds
Taco shells
Tortillas, corn
Walnuts

≥10 g fiber/100 g edible portion

Almonds
Amaranth/amaranth flour
Barley
Beans, Great Northern, raw
Bulgur
Bread, crisp, rye
Bread, high-fiber whole wheat
Cereal, bran, high-fiber
Cereal, bran flakes
Cereal, fruit with fiber
Cereal, granola
Cereal, oatmeal
Corn bran, crude

Table 18.6 *Continued*

Cornmeal, whole germ	Flour, corn	Popcorn	Triticale/triticale flour
Cowpeas, raw	Flour, rye	Rice bran, crude	Wheat bran, crude
Crackers, rye	Flour, whole wheat	Spaghetti, spinach, dry	Wheat germ, crude
Crackers, Matzo whole wheat	Lima beans, raw	Spaghetti, whole wheat, dry	Wheat germ, toasted
Crackers, whole wheat	Oat bran		
	Pistachios		

Adapted from US Department of Agriculture: Provisional Table on the Dietary Fiber Content of Selected Foods; September 1988.

the use of imagery to assist the child in attaining bowel control appear to be the most effective aspects of such treatment [17].

Biofeedback

Biofeedback is a type of behavior modification in which the patient is provided with the measure of a particular bodily function during a given activity to allow for the initiation and maintenance of the desired change [20]. It has been reported to be successful in teaching encopretic patients to learn sphincter control, particularly in individuals who develop encopresis secondary to an underlying organic cause [17]. However, in Loenig-Baucke's study of 129 children with encopresis, constipation, or abnormal defecation dynamics, those receiving biofeedback in addition to a conventional treatment regimen (nearly one-half of the subjects) exhibited no difference or improvement in long-term recovery rates over control subjects [24,25]. Clearly, more research needs to be conducted in this area.

Other Alternative/Unconventional Treaments

There is some documentation in the literature of the effectiveness of acupuncture in the treatment of encopretic children. Additional studies need to be perfomed in this area as well before such a treatment can be recommended [25].

References

1. Lucas CP, Shaffer D: Elimination disorders. In: Tasman A, Kay J, Lieberman JA, eds.: *Psychiatry*. Vol.1. Philadelphia: WB Saunders; 1997:731–742.
2. Monda JM, Husmann DA: Primary nocturnal enuresis: A comparison among observation, imipramine, desmopressin acetate and bed-wetting alarm systems. *J Urol* 1995; **154**:745–748.
3. Mikkelsen EJ: Enuresis and encopresis: Ten years of progress. *J Am Acad Child Adolesc Psychiatry* 2001; **40**(10):1146–1158.
4. Cendron M: Primary nocturnal enuresis: Current. *Am Fam Physician* 1999; **59**(5):1205–1214.
5. Lucas, CP, Shaffer,D: Enuresis. In: Tasman A, Kay J, Lieberman DA, eds.: *Psychiatry*, 2nd ed. John Wiley and Sons; 2003:842–849.
6. English OS, Finch SM: *Introduction to Psychiatry*. WW Norton and Company, 1964.
7. Thiedke CC: Nocturnal enuresis. *Am Fam Physician* 2003, **67**(7):1499–1506.
8. Kuhn BR, Marcus BA, Pitner SL: Treatment guidelines for primary nonretentive encopresis and stool toileting refusal. *Am Fam Physician* 1999; **59**(8):2171–2178.
9. Kendall-Tackett KA, Williams LM, Finkelhor D: Impact of sexual abuse on children: A review and synthesis of recent empirical studies. *Psycholog Bull* 1993; **113**(1):164–180.
10. Al-Wali NS: Indomethacin suppository to treat primary nocturnal enuresis: Double-blind study. *J Urol* 1989; **142**:1290–1292.
11. el-Sadir A, Sabry AA, Abdel-Rahman M, *et al.*: Treatment of primary nocturnal enuresis by the oral androgen mesterolone: A clinical and cystometric study. *Urology* 1990; **36**(4):331–335.
12. Rushton HG: Older pharmacologic therapy for nocturnal enuresis. *Clin Pediatr* 1993:10–13.
13. Moffatt ME, Harlos S, Kirshen AJ, Burd L: Desmopressin acetate and nocturnal enuresis: How much do we know? *Pediatrics* 1993; **92**(3):420–425.
14. Altemas M, Pigott T, Kalogeras KT, *et al.*: Abnormalities in the regulation of vasopressin and corticotropin-releasing factor secretion in obsessive-compulsive disorder. *Arch Gen Psychiatry* 1992; **49**:9–20.
15. Mesaros JD: Fluoxetine for primary enuresis. *J Am Acad Child Adolesc Psychiatry* 1993; **32**:877–878.
16. Sprenger D: Sertraline for nocturnal enuresis. *J Am Acad Child Adolesc Psychiatry* 1997; **36**(3):304–305.
17. Becker JH: An approach to the treatment of encopresis. *Surg Annu* 1994; **26**:49–66.
18. American Psychiatric Association: *Diagnostic and Statistical Manual of Mental Disorders*, 4th ed, Text Revision. Washington, DC: American Psychiatric Association; 2000:116–121.
19. Stallard P: Cognitive behaviour therapy with children: A selective review of key issues. *Behav Cog Psychother* 2002; **30**:297–309.

20. Howe AC, Walker CE: Behavioral management of toilet training, enuresis, and encopresis. *Pediatr Clin North Am* 1992; **39**(3):413–432.
21. Nolan T, Oberklaid F: New concepts in the management of encopresis. *Pediatr Rev* 1993; **14**(11):447–451.
22. Seth R, Heyman MB: Management of constipation and encopresis in infants and children. *Pediatr Gastroenterol* 1994; **23**(4):621–636.
23. Youssef NN, DiLorenzo C: Childhood constipation. *J Clin Gastroenterol* 2001; **33**(3):199–205.
24. Loening-Baucke V: Biofeedback treatment for chronic constipation and encopresis in childhood: Long-term outcome. *Pediatrics* 1995; **96**(1):105–110.
25. Loening-Baucke V: Encopresis. *Curr Opin Pediatrics* 2002, **14**:570–575.

Suggested Readings

Ambrosini PJ: Mechanism for effect of benztropine on bedwetting [letter]. *Am J Psychiatry* 1991; **148**:280.
Benninga MA, Butler HA, Heymans HS, *et al.*: Is encopresis always the result of constipation? *Arch Dis Child* 1994; **71**:186–193.
Bloom DA: The American experience with desmopressin. *Clin Pediatr* special edition 1993:28–31.
Boon FF, Singh NN: A model for the treatment of encopresis. *Behav Modif* 1991; **15**:355–371.
Castiglia PT: Encopresis. *J Pediatr Health Care* 1987; **1**(6):335–337.
Davis RC, Morris DS, Briggs JE: Nocturnal enuresis. *Lancet* 1992; **340**:1550.
Fraser AM: Childhood encopresis extended into adult life. *Br J Psychiatry* 1986; **149**:370–371.

Hyman PE, Fleisher DR: A classification of disorders of defecation in infants and children. *Semin Gastrointest Dis* 1994; **5**:20–23.
Montanari G, Baraldo M, Zara G, *et al.*: Side effects of imipramine therapy in enuretic children. *Pharmacol Res* 1990; **22**:103–104.
O'Brien S, Ross LV, Christopherson ER: Primary encopresis: Evaluation and treatment. *J Appl Behav Anal* 1986; **19**:137–145.
Rapoport L: The treatment of nocturnal enuresis – where are we now? *Pediatrics* 1993; **92**:465–466.
Rushton HG: Nocturnal enuresis: Epidemiology, evaluation, and currently available treatment options. *J Pediatr* 1989; **114**(Suppl):691–696.
Sureshkumar P, Bower W, Craig JC, Knight JF: Treatment of daytime urinary incontinence in children: Systematic review of randomized controlled trials. *J Urol* 2003; **170**:196–200.
Sprague-McRae JM: Encopresis: Developmental, behavioral and physiological considerations for treatment. *Nurse Pract* 1990; **15**(6):8–24.
Sprague-McRae JM, Lamb W, Homer D: Encopresis: A study of treatment alternatives and historical and behavioral characteristics. *Nurse Pract* 1993; **18**(10):52–53, 56–63.
Stenberg A, Lackgren G: Desmopressin tablets in the treatment of severe nocturnal enuresis in adolescents. *Pediatrics* 1994; **94**:841–846.
Thapar A, Davies G, Jones T, Rivett M: Treatment of childhood encopresis – a review. *Child Care Health Dev* 1992; **18**:343–353.
Warzak MH, Brennan LC, Baker RD, Baker SS: Functional encopresis: Symptom reduction and behavioral improvement. *J Dev Behav Pediatr* 1995; **16**:226–232.

19

Sexual Development and the Treatment of Sexual Disorders in Children and Adolescents

James Lock, Jennifer Couturier

Introduction

In this chapter, we review sexual development and discuss sexual disorders whose origins are in childhood. Although the central role of sexuality in theoretical models of psychologic health and development originated with the psychoanalytic work of Sigmund Freud, sexuality has always played key roles in the biologic and social activities of humans. These roles have varied significantly over time and across cultures. What seems natural and correct to the Balinese would likely astonish the Saudis, and what would be commonplace in ancient Greece would be stigmatized in modern Greece. Biology seems to have established a mandate for sexual behavior within humans, both for procreation and for pleasure, but the structure of this behavior is extremely varied and has an ongoing and lively interaction with historical and cultural beliefs and values.

It is important for the clinician to keep these historical [1] and cultural [2] factors in mind when working on issues of sexual behavior. Today, especially in regions where many cultures interface, variations between and among cultures can increase children's confusion about sexuality and sexual behavior. Parental attitudes, which are based in various cultural belief systems, can be at odds with the prevailing peer group attitudes of their children, thus adding to the confusion. Clinicians working with child and adolescent sexual problems need to be aware of these cultural belief systems to better facilitate solutions to conflicts that arise among family members in these areas. Although this chapter's perspective and approach

largely draw from Western contemporary culture, it is hoped that most readers work primarily in this context themselves so will benefit from this perspective.

Sex and Gender Development

An understanding of the relationship between sexual development and gender development – which encapsulates the relationship between the biologic and cultural aspects of sexuality – is central to the evaluation of sexual behavior. A review of the behavioral, cognitive, and biologic dimensions of this topic provides a basis for understanding both normal and unusual sexual behavior within a developmental scheme.

Infancy and Early Childhood

During early infancy, both sexes enjoy the sensations associated with nursing, diapering, and the cleansing of the genitals. It is not unusual for infants to begin to play with their genitals in the first year of life. Boys are likely to discover the genitals earlier than girls. Masturbation develops from genital play gradually to the second year of life. Self-stimulation in girls is less frequent and less focused than that of boys. Self-stimulation and pleasure contributes to feelings of autonomy, control, and mastery.

By the age of two years, self-stimulation is more focused, intense, and frequent. There is increased genital pride, which may be accompanied by exhibitionism. The child may begin to develop a primitive form of fantasy life associated with self-stimulation. In

Clinical Child Psychiatry, Second Edition. Edited by W.M. Klykylo and J.L. Kay
© 2005 John Wiley & Sons Ltd.

girls, masturbation usually involves indirect methods and may begin by using legs, thighs, or toys, for example. In the US, sexual socialization of the two-year-old mixes issues of autonomy, sexuality, and toileting and may create confusion in the child's mind by superimposing issues of control and autonomy over sexual pleasure and activity.

Erotic interests become more diverse as children develop. Games such as 'mommy and daddy' or 'playing doctor' are common, and by age four years, one half of US preschoolers are involved in sex games or masturbation. Parental concerns with gender, and investment in gender behavior, are an important part of a child's perception of how to behave along these lines. Both direct and subtle messages about self-worth are contained in these parental and familial messages. Achievement, competition, and the control of emotional expression are the norm for parents when raising boys, as is an intolerance of behaviors that deviate from the traditional male stereotype. Parents predict atypical outcomes (such as homosexuality) in boys with feminine behaviors more often than in girls with masculine behaviors.

Kohlberg postulated a sequence of development of gender processes that progress through a series of sequential stages [3]. The first stage starts when children become aware that there are two sexes. Somewhat later, they become aware of differences between the sexes and can self-identify, but the difference has no meaningful content. In the next stage, children learn specific content regarding differences between the sexes. Children who master this stage can be said to have achieved gender identification. The next task for the child is to understand that gender is a stable and consistent aspect of their identity. Finally – usually in the early school-age years – they achieve the stage of gender constancy.

School-Age Years

When children enter school, significant behavioral changes occur to their family's interactions. Children tend to bathe alone as they grow older. It is uncommon for mothers to bathe with sons who are over eight years old, or for fathers to bathe with daughters more than nine years old. Although there is some reduction in sexual activity and apparent erotic interest in children at about age five years, children continue to be concerned with sexuality. In Kinsey's 1953 study, 57% of males and 48% of females who were interviewed as adults remembered sexual play occurring between the ages of 8 and 13 years [4]. Among males interviewed

when they were prepubescent, 70% claimed that they engaged in some sex play. After age seven years, relationships tend to be with same-sex peers. On the playground, sexual topics are common, especially among boys. By this time, children are well aware of adult prohibitions around sex and try not to be caught. Nonetheless, games of Truth or Dare or strip poker remain common.

During the school-age years, group behavior is divided clearly along gender lines. Those who do not engage in such behavior risk being ostracized and ridiculed. Boys are particularly intolerant of deviation from gender norms. Some studies, however, indicate that boys' peer groups (ages 9–11 years) use their group activities to achieve varying levels of sexual arousal and use all-male groups to practice using sexually oriented language, viewing erotic materials, and disparaging other males with sexually laden terms, usually with negative homosexual content [4].

Adolescence

Although Offer [5] and others have argued persuasively against the 'storm and stress' or 'turmoil-ridden' notions of adolescence and have claimed that approximately 80% of teenagers report a generally smooth and uneventful passage through adolescence, many nonetheless experience difficulty and anxiety around sexual behavior and development. It is therefore important for the clinician working with sexual issues to conduct a brief review of pertinent biologic and sexual behavioral norms in adolescents. Physical changes associated with puberty are the external marker of profound emotional changes that lead to the development of social and behavioral changes. When compared with other biologic changes that occur over a lifetime, the changes associated with puberty are rapid and dramatic and second only to those in the first year of life. The most observable changes emerge over a four-year-period and begin and end approximately two years earlier for girls than for boys. Hormonal systems are established prenatally but are reactivated at puberty. It has been observed in both sexes that children reach a critical fat-to-lean ratio roughly represented by weight, that appears to be correlated with the onset of puberty.

Boys

The average age of the first penis and testes growth begins between ages 10 and 11 years. This is followed by the development of pubic hair about age 12–13 years. Rapid growth of the penis and testes occurs in the 13th and 14th year, followed by the development of axillary hair, down on the lip, and voice changes in the 14th to 15th years. By ages 15–16 years, boys have mature spermatozoa, and by age 16–17 years, facial hair and body hair are present. Improved health and nutrition are causing puberty to begin earlier. Studies of the psychologic effects of the timing of puberty in boys indicate that those who mature early have an advantage, at least in the teen years, over those who mature late. In adolescence, the former are more athletic, socially valued, and are perceived to be leaders. Their maturity is generally perceived positively by adults, and they tend to experience less guilt, anxiety, or other emotional problems. In adulthood, they continue to hold leadership positions, but they also seem to take conventional approaches to problems, which sometimes limits their leadership and social relations. Boys who mature late, in contrast, are less confident, hold more negative self-concepts, and are viewed less positively by peers and adults. In adulthood, however, these men display greater intellectual curiosity, more social initiative, and are more creative problem solvers. A recent study supports some of these views, finding that in early adulthood, young men who matured late had increased rates of disruptive behavior and substance use disorders during the transition to adulthood, but that early maturation was not linked to any lifetime or current disorders among young men [6].

Masturbation is the most common source of orgasm in boys. By age 14 years, 80% have masturbated, and by age 18 years, 90%–98% have masturbated. At the same time, more than 50% of boys experience guilt in relation to this activity. Studies of first coitus in males show that by age 19 years, 79% have had intercourse. First intercourse at age 13 years is experienced by 5% of males. Approximately one-half of these experiences occur in the context of a romantic partnership, but one third occur with friends or new acquaintances. About two-thirds of boys find this first experience to some degree satisfying; the remaining one-third are disappointed.

Girls

Puberty typically begins in girls between the ages of 9 and 14 years. It is initiated by the release of gonadotropin-releasing hormone, which is produced by the hypothalamus. Between the ages of 8 and 13 years, breast buds appear, and pubic hair begins to develop on the labia as breast buds enlarge. Later, when the breast areolae and nipples begin to form, menstruation first occurs. Menarche starts at an average age of 12.5 years. These first menstrual cycles are usually painless, because they are not accompanied by ovulation. During this time, asymmetry of breast development is common and vaginal secretions increase, both of which cause concern in some girls. Growth rate slows after the onset of menstruation, and most girls gain about 11.4 kg. The timing of maturation in girls also has an effect on social and sexual behaviors. In contrast to the trend in boys, girls who mature early are more likely than those who mature late to be viewed negatively by peers and adults, to initiate sexual interactions earlier, and to become pregnant in the teen years. In young adulthood, women who mature early report elevated lifetime rates of major depressive disorder, anxiety, and disruptive behavior disorder compared with those who mature on time [6]. They also report poorer quality of relationships as young adults. Girls who mature late do not appear to be at a disadvantage, and do not have elevated rates of disorder. In fact, women who are late maturers were more likely to complete college in a recent study [6].

According to the few reports available, masturbation occurs less frequently in girls than in boys. Sexual intercourse is generally unplanned and unprotected. Adolescent sexual activity has steadily increased over the past five decades. Studies indicate that about 60% of girls have intercourse by age 18 years, and 47%–53% of US teenage females engage in sexual intercourse; 58% of these girls have had two or more partners. Approximately 89% of US adult women have had sexual intercourse. However, the adolescent sexual climate appears to be changing with the advent of the internet. Adolescents have more privacy with this medium than ever before which may aid the phenomenon of 'hooking up' (sexual experimentation without dating), along with a shift to oral sex rather than intercourse [7].

A significant issue during adolescence is pregnancy. Every year, about one million adolescent girls become pregnant. Of these, one-half give birth, accounting for 18% of firstborns in the US. The remainder obtain abortions (40%) or miscarry (10%). Birth rates among teens are rising. Medical complications of teenage pregnancy include inadequate or excessive weight gain, hypertension, anemia, sexually transmitted diseases, and cephalopelvic disproportion. Most of these complications are a result of poor nutrition and poor prenatal care. In comparison to other adolescent girls, those who become teenage mothers are more likely to receive less education, have lower adult incomes, and have higher rates of depression. They are also less likely to be with the father after two years. Developmental issues of adolescence may be so foreshortened that identity issues remain unresolved; this may result from a continued dependency on families of origin or from the loss of opportunities for peer relations.

Sexuality and the Developmental Tasks of Adolescence

Adolescence can be viewed as comprising three phases, each of which has a specific relationship to sexual development and behaviors. The first of these is the early phase (ages 12–14 years), which primarily involves the dramatic physical changes associated with puberty. The middle phase of adolescence (ages 14–16 years) is dominated by adolescents' increasing use of peers and abstracting abilities to distinguish themselves from parents. The late phase of adolescence (ages 16–19 years) is associated with setting patterns and plans for work and establishing patterns of more intimate interpersonal relationships.

In the early phase, the most significant issues involve the changes associated with puberty itself. These are specifically related to attractiveness, size, and maturation rate and the relationship of these issues to self-esteem and body image. As noted earlier, these issues are processed somewhat differently for boys than for girls, at least in our culture. Girls generally are more concerned with maturing too early, being overweight or too tall, and not being perceived as attractive. Boys, conversely, are more concerned with maturing late, being too small or too short, and not being strong enough.

In the middle phase, sexual issues intensify and more strongly affect peer relationships. General themes of these sexual issues include dating competence, sexual orientation, and exploratory sexual experiences. Other issues that can complicate sexual development in this period involve separation from one's family and can include guilt, fears of abandonment, and angry and rebellious feelings. Repression, avoidance, and the isolation of sexual impulses may be one approach to this difficulty, whereas acting out, promiscuity, and other reckless sexual behavior may be another. This phase is further complicated by increasing comparisons of oneself to the peer group. When these comparisons cause lowered self-esteem and self-worth, this can lead to problems with sexual development.

In the late phase of adolescence, sexual issues principally involve practicing for true sexual intimacy. This phase is characterized by increasing wishes and ability for emotional and sexual intimacy and fewer needs for a familial base. Sexual problems that might arise during this phase are derived from residual problems in these areas, such as continued excessive emotional or physical dependency on parents or family, continued anxiety about sexual abilities or body image and anxiety about the meaning of personal intimacy in terms of procreation.

Medical Illness and Sexual Development

Physical illnesses affect sexual development and behavior in a variety of ways that include physical, social, and emotional components. For physically ill children, the type of problems with sexual issues experienced during the early phase of adolescence is governed largely by the impact their illness or its treatment has on their pubertal development. These effects might include influences on the timing of puberty and associated secondary sex characteristics, body size, or the development of dysmorphic physical features. There are several examples of medical illnesses that affect the timing of puberty, such as endocrinopathies and intersex genetic anomalies. In addition, medical treatments of a variety of illnesses can include agents such as steroids and can thus affect the timing of puberty. A secondary effect of changing the timing of puberty is the impact this may have on height and weight, which can also be affected by specific illnesses and medical treatments. For boys, especially at this phase, body size is a significant source of sexual and gender role anxiety. Illnesses that make them shorter or thinner have a powerfully negative impact on their developing image of themselves as sexual and male. For girls, illnesses or treatments that cause weight gain or facial changes are particularly troubling during this phase.

During the middle phase, sexual problems arise as a result of impediments to developing peer groups. Medically ill adolescents can experience difficulties in sexual development for many reasons that include dependency on family members and institutions for care, increased periods of isolation from peers due to physical illness, decreased capacities for sexual action due to acute or chronic health limitations (e.g., infections, injury, energy, and medication side effects), and increased shame surrounding illness and its impact on psychosocial functioning. If a genetic cause is suspected, increased familial guilt and patient anger can become particularly evident. These emotions can lead to a kind of angry enmeshed familial dynamic that effectively stifles the sexual emancipation and exploration that are key to working through this phase of adolescence.

Seizure disorders, chronic illnesses, and oncologic disorders are examples of illnesses that can have a particularly negative effect on sexual development during the middle phase. Adolescents with seizure disorders are often ashamed of an illness that can cause them to lose bowel and bladder control at unpredictable times. In addition, the medications required can interfere with social activities, and their side effects can inhibit both physical and sexual functioning. These adolescents are sometimes not allowed to drive, which can interfere with social activities, especially dating, leading to avoidance or counterphobic sexual behavior. Teenagers with oncologic illness demonstrate another aspect of difficulties during this developmental stage: these teens often have increased dependency on family members, become socially isolated from their peers because of hospitalization and shame, and experience side effects of treatment that alter appearance and can lead to body image distortions. As a result, these teens can exhibit avoidance, family enmeshment and infantilization of sexual drives, shame about their body, lower sexual self-esteem, higher sexual anxiety, and a reluctance to explore sexual intimacy.

In the late phase of adolescence, sexual issues are associated with an increasing need and desire for intimate personal relationships and decreasing emotional ties with the family. Key sexual issues for the medically ill adolescent include concern about decreased life span, fertility, transferring dependency needs from families to intimate partners, and the potential for the genetic transmission of illness. Because of chronic dependency on their family and then disability and pain, these teenagers experience extreme difficulty in finding and developing young adult roles for sexual intimacy. Families are often overprotective and infantilize them, which adds to the burden. In addition, some patients worry about the genetic transmission of their illness to their offspring, which may inhibit desire. The case below illustrates how hemophilia is an illness affecting the issues of this phase. For a comprehensive review of psychosexual development in adolescents with chronic medical illnesses see Lock [8].

CASE ONE

Tony was an 18-year-old male with hemophilia who had experienced repeated hospitalizations for pain and bleeding throughout his adolescence. He had missed most of high school because of this, although he had completed an equivalent educational process at home. His father had abandoned the family when Tony was a boy and he and his mother

had developed a close, if sometimes turbulent, relationship that veered from overprotection to threats of abandonment. At age 18 years, Tony had no sexual experiences and had few friends. He was aware of his own anger at his parents for 'giving me this illness,' and he felt a deep ambivalence about procreation. He felt that he was unattractive and unlikely to ever find a mate. He was increasingly despondent and refused to interact with anyone who he had not known for many years. The therapist working with Tony avoided talking to him about his sexual needs and development because of feeling unprepared about how to help him. With supervision and education, however, the therapist ultimately helped Tony discuss sexual issues and developed some strategies to help him with his questions and need for love and sexual interactions.

Intersex Conditions and Sex Chromosome Disorders

A variety of medical conditions directly or indirectly affect sexual development via biologic processes that control sexual maturity, sexual organs, and sexual capacities. Many of these disorders are inherited, but few systematic studies have examined the sexual behaviors and concerns of these patients. In the area of sex chromosome disorders, we do know that girls with Turner's syndrome (karyotype 45, X) have greater problems with socialization and peer relationships leading to increased difficulties with sexual immaturity. Among boys with endocrinopathies, those with Klinefelter syndrome have been reported as having significant psychosexual implications, including transsexualism, body image problems, and low sexual self-esteem.

In regard to intersex conditions, females born with masculinized genitalia or pseudohermaphroditism caused by virilizing congenital adrenal hyperplasia have greater bodily concerns, higher androgyny scores, difficulties with gender identity, and delays in dating and sexual relations as adolescents and adults. Boys who are genetically males but who are born with agenesis of the penis or only partial genesis of the penis experience special problems. Many are surgically castrated and raised as females and are therefore socialized into female gender roles. Unfortunately, many do not accept this categorization and end up seeking sex reassignment during adolescence or young adulthood. For example, Reiner and Gearhart [9] studied 16 genetic males born with cloacal exstrophy, a defect in pelvic embryogenesis that results in severe genital inadequacy along with urological and gastrointestinal malformations. Of these 16 genetically male children, 14 were reassigned to female sex (two subjects were reared as males because the parents refused to have them reassigned). At the time of the study, subjects were 5–16 years old, and six of the 14 subjects reassigned female at birth had declared themselves male and were living as males. The sexual behavior and attitudes of all 16 subjects reflected strong male-typical characteristics. This research calls for a reconsideration of reassignment of genetically male infants to female sex, and suggests reassignment may only complicate already complex neonatal conditions [9].

Sex reassignment surgery creates great upheaval in families who may feel guilt about their original decision as well as anxiety about the life their child will lead after reassignment. For those boys who are brought up as males, other problems develop, mostly related to self-esteem, sexual anxiety, and inhibition. Surgical enhancement of the penis is possible, but this is only a cosmetic change and may lead to other frustrations. These young men are ashamed of their genitalia and avoid any occasions in which others, even those they are attracted to, would see them. Naturally, this inhibits any sexual experimentation and seriously curtails even the social aspects of dating relationships. Therapeutic involvement is helpful and should focus on differentiating the concept of masculinity from the concrete presence or absence of a penis. With older adolescents, it may help to associate this condition with other males who because of injury, illness, or paralysis are no longer sexually functional.

Fortunately, intersex conditions are rare. However, there remains much controversy over the urgency of sex assignment in these conditions, and attitudes in the medical profession are changing after many intersex individuals have condemned infant genital surgery [10]. In the 1960s, newborn penile size charts were used and if the stretched penis was less than 2.5 cm, gender was likely to be assigned as female, and surgery performed within the first few months of life. It was thought that infants were gender neutral at birth and that gender development occurred by interaction with the environment, relying on appearance of the genitalia. Thus, early surgery was preferred in order to reduce parental anxiety and align genital appearance to sex of rearing [10]. However, no studies have confirmed that psychological functioning of parents or children is improved by early surgery.

A recent set of guidelines published by a multidisplinary team working with children born with atypical genitalia concluded that none of the appearance altering surgeries need to be done urgently, and that surgery to normalize appearance done without the consent of the patient lacks ethical justification [11]. This is in contrast to a recent document produced by the American Academy of Pediatrics suggesting that the birth of a child with ambiguous genitalia constitutes a social emergency and that a diagnosis and treatment plan be established as quickly as possible to minimize medical, psychological and social complications [12]. However, waiting for surgery brings forth another ethical dilemma of whether the child should be raised as male, female, or an intersex person. There are many differing views on this subject as well. In any case, Frader et al. [11] suggest that the available data do not provide reasons for using surgery in most cases before the child has the capacity to participate in decision making. They also suggest that the field undertake a comprehensive assessment of practice, that rigorous follow-up studies are essential, that health professionals need considerably more education in this area, that children have the right to know about their bodies in an age-appropriate fashion, and that families with children with an intersex condition require a comprehensive package of services immediately following diagnosis including access to mental health professionals and support groups [11].

CASE TWO

Matt was a 17-year-old football star and straight A student referred to a psychiatrist by his urologist because of depression. Matt was tall, good-looking, and muscular. He had trouble making eye contact with the psychiatrist but described his problem as a 'masculinity problem.' Matt disclosed that his erect penis was only about one and a half inches long and that he was ashamed of it. He described how even though he was an athlete, he had managed to avoid being seen by male peers all through high school. In addition, he had recently broken up with a girl that he loved because one evening she had attempted to touch him between the legs. He said he left her then and never spoke to her again. Matt was very depressed and felt hopeless about his situation. He understood his achievements were in many way attempts to compensate for his feeling of inadequacy, but he could see no way to feel better about himself.

Homosexuality

One of the most common issues of adolescence is a concern with sexual orientation. Data do not support the formulation of the world into homosexuals and heterosexuals. Kinsey's scale that rated sexual orientation from 1 to 6 – exclusive heterosexual to exclusive homosexual – found that a significant percentage fall in the 3–4 range [4]. In addition, the few existing studies suggest that many people, especially males, participate in homosexual behavior at some point. Solitary or group masturbation and same-sex sexual experiences are well-known components of male adolescent sexual histories. These activities seem to serve as a means of expressing manhood and masculinity, by demonstrating a capacity for, frequency of, and rapidity of ejaculation. Girls do not appear to use these strategies as boys do. Nonetheless, homosexual behavior and varying levels of heterosexual and homosexual desire may complicate a person's sense of their sexual orientation and gender role performance. Some adolescents, rather than experience this same-sex behavior as expressive of their masculinity or femininity, may experience increased anxiety about these issues and as a result develop homophobic avoidance and defensiveness. In other words, although homosexual activity is apparently naturally occurring and common, it may be difficult for some people to integrate it into their need to conform to gender and gender role expectations.

Adolescents who are gay or lesbian can develop significant problems secondary to internalized homophobia (the self-hatred that develops as a result of being a socially stigmatized person) or externalized homophobia (the irrational hatred of a person because he or she is believed to be homosexual). Estimates of the overall homosexual population range from 2% to 4% to more than 10%. Few studies have examined the impact of homophobia on gay and lesbian youth. One recent study of gay and lesbian youth aged 15–21 years found that, as a result of their sexual orientation, 80% had experienced verbal insults, 44% had been threatened with violence, 33% had had objects thrown at them, 31% had been chased or followed, and 17% had been physically assaulted [13]. Numerous studies have identified an increased rate of suicide attempts among gay and lesbian youth. Risk factors for suicide attempts before age 20 years in gay and lesbian youth include:

- discovering same-sex preference early in adolescence;
- experiencing violence due to gay or lesbian identity;
- using alcohol or drugs to cope; and
- being rejected by family members as a result of being homosexual [14].

Other studies have reported increased high school drop-out rates, substance abuse, and family discord among gay and lesbian youth and adolescents. In studies attempting to predict patterns of sexual acts among homosexual and bisexual youth, researchers have found that improved patterns of sexual risk-taking behaviors are associated with decreased levels of internalized homophobia, as demonstrated by high self-esteem and low levels of anxiety, depression, and substance abuse [15]. Another study found self-acceptance, a corollary of decreased internalized homophobia, to be the single largest predictor of mental health – more important, for example, than either family support or victimization alone [16].

Adolescents and young adults often need assistance with problems that develop as a result of internalized homophobia. Therapeutic work with sexual minority youth has employed both individual and group approaches. Key elements of psychodynamic treatments include neutralizing internalized homophobia through education, interpreting anxieties about passivity, dependency, masculinity, and femininity, and using techniques that are supportive and affirm homosexual identity [17]. Group approaches for teens and young adults aim to diminish isolation, create supportive communities, and serve as psychoeducational forums [18]. Although intervention with families seems advisable, because of the lack of support provided by society as a whole, only limited clinical research has addressed the family factors that play a role in the difficulties faced by gay and lesbian youth. Overall, there is a lack of research specific to the needs of gay and lesbian youth. Reports do indicate, however, that they have been coming out at younger ages: 10 years ago the average age was 21 years in women and 19 in men, whereas the average ages are now 19 years in women and 16 years in men. Other studies have focused on the societal origins of homophobia and have attempted to provide prevention and intervention for gay and lesbian youth in high schools or community centers [19–21]. These approaches to the prevention of internalized and externalized homophobia have been difficult to develop and maintain, in large measure because of parental and societal fears about homosexuality.

Sex and Gender Disorders

Taking a Sexual History

One of the most neglected aspects of training, perhaps especially in child psychiatry, is the process of taking a sexual history. It is presumed that clinicians have learned to take an appropriate and detailed history, but more often than not clinicians are uncomfortable with taking a sexual history or have not determined how best to conduct such a history. An understanding of a patient's sexual history is especially important for those clinicians who work with children and adolescents who have sexual problems. Interviewing may be done face to face with patients and families and through the use of questionnaires. The clinician must be able to sensitively interview children and adolescents to determine if the child has been sexually abused or is at risk for such abuse. Unfortunately, the legal mandate to report such findings may contribute to some clinicians' hesitancy to take thorough sexual histories. In addition, since sexual behavior poses increasing risks to general health concerns, because of sexually transmitted diseases and human immunodeficiency virus, clinicians need to be aware of their adolescent patients' sexual behaviors to educate and help them manage these behaviors more safely.

To successfully interview children and adolescents, the clinician should approach the patient with an awareness of his or her developmental capacities. Questions should be straightforward, direct, and posed without embarrassment. The correct terminology for all body parts should be used. For younger children, anatomically correct dolls may be employed as an aid. Adolescents sometimes prefer a self-administered format that allows them to respond with less embarrassment. However, there are no self-report questionnaires on adolescent sexual behavior that are commonly used for clinical purposes. The Youth Risk Behavior Survey has been used in epidemiological studies [22]. Confidentiality of adolescent responses should be assured. Patience and support are also necessary, since children and adolescents may require extra time and encouragement to answer these types of inquiries.

Gender Identity Disorder (GID)

Definition
Diagnostic and Statistical Manual of Mental Disorders, 4th ed., Text Revision (DSM-IV-TR) [23] criteria require the presence of a strong and persistent cross-gender identification that is manifested by four of the following:

- repeatedly stated desire to be of the other sex;
- in boys, preference for cross-dressing or simulating female attire; in girls, insistence on wearing only stereotypical masculine clothing;
- strong preference for cross-sex play and fantasies;
- strong preference for playmates of the other sex;
- intense desire to participate in games of other sex.

This must be accompanied by persistent discomfort with one's own sex or gender role.

Epidemiology, Etiology, and Pathology
Sexual identity is the biologic sex, gender identity is the identification of oneself as belonging to a gender, and gender roles are the behaviors associated with a particular sex within a culture or group. GID is concerned with each of these to a degree, but the principal problems psychologically are the dysphoria a child experiences with his or her biologic sex and the behavioral manifestations of this dissatisfaction, most typically as gender role nonconformity.

Diagnostic criteria for GID have evolved. In early formulations, there was considerable variation between the criteria for boys and girls, which generally allowed girls more gender role variation than boys. The more recent criteria are gender neutral [23]. The referral rates for GID, however, continue to range from 6 to 30 boys for every girl. The sex ratio for referred adolescents appears less skewed, with a male to female ratio of 1.4:1 [24]. What may simply be increased concern by parents and social institutions about femininity in boys, make some critical of this diagnostic category's scientific basis. Critics of the diagnostic criteria for GID contend that the behaviors such children exhibit are not in themselves psychopathologic but are labeled as such from parental and social intolerance of them, and that distress results from such intolerance [25]. They suggest that cross-gender behavior may be a normal developmental pathway to later homosexuality and point out that there is very little research on the validity of this diagnosis [25]. A study of cross-gendered behaviors among children, in which mothers reported their perception of their son's wishes to be of the opposite sex, found that at age 4–5 years, about 15% of clinically referred boys wished to be of the opposite sex, compared to about 1% of nonreferred boys [26]. This study suggests that a substantial number of males without GID nonetheless experience opposite-gendered behavior during early childhood. The rates in this study were also higher for referred than for nonreferred girls but were stable at much lower rates of 4%–8% [26].

There are no formal estimates of the prevalence of GID. If it is assumed that GID leads to adult transsexualism, it would constitute a rare disorder – one in 24 000–37 000 men and one in 103 000–150 000 women become transsexual [27]. Others assume that GID ultimately ends in homosexuality. Estimates of the homosexual population are also contested, however. In addition, although some homosexuals recall engaging in cross-gendered behavior, it is doubtful that most ever met the criteria for GID. One is left to conclude that cross-gendered behavior is common but that GID is relatively rare.

Etiologic theories for GID fall into two major classes: biologic and psychoanalytic. The biologic theories cite genetic and hormonal studies or medical conditions that support a biologic basis for GID. The support for a genetic etiology draws from studies that indicate a hereditary basis for homosexuality. The most compelling data on this issue are from Pillard and Bailey's study of 56 monozygotic twins, 54 dizygotic twins, and 57 genetically unrelated adopted brothers. The researchers found that 11% of the adoptive brothers, 22% of the dizygotic twins, and 52% of the monozygotic twins were concordant for homosexuality [28]. Other studies have indicated that up to 70% of the variation may be accounted for genetically [29]. Similar, though somewhat less dramatic, findings have also been found in lesbians. Nonetheless, the presumption that GID is genetically determined is a leap from these data because, as noted earlier, GID is not a precondition of homosexuality and does not itself necessarily lead to homosexuality.

Another etiologic hypothesis is derived from studies of psychoendocrine research. This research examined sexual orientation in the context of psychosexual development as it is influenced by hormones. No association between systemic sex hormone levels during adolescence and adulthood and GID or homosexuality was found, however. More recent research is based only on a theory that prenatal exposure to androgens promotes the development of attraction to females whereas nonresponsiveness to androgens is associated with erotic attraction to males. Some support for this theory comes from studies on girls and women with congenital adrenal hyperplasia in which female fetuses are exposed to increased levels of androgens *in utero*. These girls display some gender role behaviors that are more similar to those of boys. In addition, compared to control women, adult women with this condition have less heterosexual involvement and more homosexual fantasy (see review by Bradley and Zucker [24]). In boys, it has been hypothesized that some pregnant mothers expose the male fetus to risk of incomplete androgenization of the brain, resulting in homosexual attraction. Possible mechanisms for this include antibodies to testosterone from previous pregnancy with a male fetus and androgen insufficiency caused by stress. Support for this hypothesis comes from studies that demonstrate later birth order for male homosexuals and an increased number of male older siblings [30,31]. Problems arise with this hypothesis because of the genetic studies already cited and the lack of compara-

ble data for female homosexuality. The tenuous link between homosexuality and GID also continues to be a limitation.

Brain anatomy studies attempting to find similarities between homosexual men and heterosexual women to support the prenatal exposure theory have been inconclusive and unreplicated. In addition, cognitive performance in untreated patients with GID has been investigated in order to support this theory. Results have been inconsistent. Haraldsen *et al.* [32] found that performance appears to be consistent with biologic sex and not gender identity, while Cohen-Kettenis *et al.* [33] found that male patients with GID had an advantage in verbalization more similar to female controls. More recent studies are investigating the possibility that the brain begins to develop differently in males and females even before sex hormones come into play, and that perhaps in the future genes may be identified that predict the likely gender identity of an individual [34].

Psychoanalytic theories examine familial, especially parental, factors as the root cause of GID. Family studies have shown that fathers are absent in 34%–85% of the families of boys with GID; in those families with a father present, he spent notably less time than is typical interacting with the son in early childhood [35]. Mothers in these families were found to be hostile toward males and viewed their husbands as potentially violent and out of control. These mothers discouraged 'rough and tumble' play and were often harsh and authoritarian disciplinarians [35]. Many of these mothers had themselves experienced traumatic experiences during the early years of their child's life (e.g., rape, or death of another child or parent). Theoretically, then, mothers' anxiety about masculine violence, their poor management of stress, and their ambivalent and hostile relationship with the fathers could lead the parents to promote cross-gender behaviors in their sons. Conversely, the sons are anxious about maternal withdrawal and abandonment (over 60% meet criteria for separation anxiety disorder) and identify with the mother to assuage the anxieties associated with separation and loss [35]. In accordance with a more behavioral theory, one of the strongest findings in children with GID is the lack of parental discouragement of cross-sex behavior [24].

Differential Diagnosis

The most important distinction to make in an assessment of GID is between predictable cross-gender exploration and play and cross-gendered behaviors that are rooted in persistent and intense distress about one's biologic sex. An example of predictable cross-gendered play might involve a boy putting on a wig or a dress temporarily, whereas an elaboration of this play, along with enthusiasm and persistence might be of more concern. The quality of persistence is best assessed by several factors, including the age of the child, the length of time the behavior or belief has existed, and the determination with which the behavior is maintained. In general, an increased age of the child, duration of the cross-gendered behaviors, and resistance to changing the behaviors all indicate a more likely diagnosis of true GID. Factors such as familial stress, the death of a parent, the birth of a sibling, and other traumas may be associated with brief periods of cross-gendered behaviors. These adjustment factors should be considered in any assessment.

Course and Natural History

Studies of the outcome of boys with gender nonconformity in childhood are conflicting. In a study of existing longitudinal data, Kohlberg found little or no correlation between childhood masculinity or femininity and heterosexuality in adulthood [36]. Studies have shown that a large proportion of boys referred for gender nonconformity grow up to become homosexuals; these studies, however, may represent a particular subset of homosexuals. Studies examining the childhood memories of adult homosexuals indicate that some degree of gender nonconformity may predict later homosexuality. A meta-analysis of retrospective literature found a very strong relationship between the extent of childhood cross-gender behavior and later homosexual orientation for both men and women [37].

The child with GID is likely to develop significant problems with peer relations. School-age children are anxious about gender role behavior and are often intolerant of variations from stereotypes. Thus children, especially boys, with GID are likely to be teased and harassed by their peers. This can result in school avoidance, truancy, and other behavior problems. They are also likely to develop lower self-esteem, which is to some degree dependent on social approval. Separation anxiety is a common confounding condition for those individuals with GID and can add to the burden of both familial and peer interactions. Zucker and Bradley [38] found that children with GID had less social competence on the Child Behavior Checklist (CBCL), and that boys had a predominance of internalizing, as opposed to the typical externalizing behavioral difficulties seen in clinical samples of boys. Girls with GID had both internalizing and externalizing elevations on the CBCL. A more recent international study found that boys with GID had even more problems with peer relations than girls with GID, and that poor peer relations were the strongest predictor of

behavior problems [39]. When present, any comorbid conditions, such as depression and separation anxiety should be treated in conjunction with the GID.

By the time gender identity-disordered children reach puberty and high school, approximately two-thirds of them are likely to have developed a homosexual orientation. A new set of social problems emerges as sexual and aggressive impulses of peers are now near adult levels. Exposure to this now physically threatening level of harassment leads to significant risk of depression, truancy, and substance abuse. In those families that are intolerant of homosexuality, runaway behavior and homelessness are common. For those adolescents who do not become homosexual as adults, harassment for continued cross-gendered behavior is likely to result, even though they are heterosexual, and may be similar to problems that homosexuals experience. Others with GID may become transsexuals and decide to live their lives as members of the opposite biologic sex. Some of these individuals seek hormonal and surgical treatments to physically augment their psychologic and behavioral cross-gender condition. A prospective follow-up study of 20 adolescents with GID who underwent hormone treatment and sex reassignment surgery over a 4–5-year period found that at one year postsurgery they were no longer gender dysphoric and were functioning well [40]. No one expressed regret about the surgery. The authors suggest that with careful diagnosis and strict criteria, earlier treatment may have some benefits over later treatment including improved social and psychological functioning.

Treatment

Treatment for GID is a conflict-ridden area of child and adolescent psychiatric practice. As discussed earlier, some practitioners argue that children with gender nonconformity are treated inappropriately because the problem is not their behavior so much as others' responses to it. These practitioners argue that educating the parents and communities about the acceptability of these behaviors is preferable to teaching children to hide or change what comes naturally to them. More conventional approaches try to help the child find safe opportunities to play however he or she chooses, help parents understand their need to protect, support and love their child, and help the child understand the reactions of peers and others. Other practitioners use a variety of psychoanalytic approaches, such as working with concepts of enmeshment and overidentification with the mother figure and trying to change core gender identity. No systematic data are available on the effectiveness of any of these treatments, whatever their explicit aims.

Goals and Phases of Treatment

The principal goal of psychotherapeutic treatment for GID is to reduce the patient's anxiety and dysphoria. Often these problems are not associated with the cross-gendered behaviors themselves but with parental and social reactions to them. Thus, the first task is to address the family's reactions to the behavior of the gender-disordered child. This often involves a thorough assessment of the familial variables, including parental hostility, paternal avoidance, maternal dependence on the patient, and the identification of traumatic injuries in parents that remain unresolved and contribute to the child's difficulties. In addition, education about the prognosis and likely outcome of their child is an important part of the treatment. When the patient is male, involving the father in more interactions with him may be another important intervention. The goal is not to change the child's behaviors but rather to change the dynamics of familial issues. The reinforcement of cross-gendered behaviors should be limited, but punishment, ridicule, and other methods of criticizing the child should cease. Often it is helpful to provide the child with a safe alternative place to play and thereby to ultimately encourage the exploration of other less cross-gendered activities. This technique increases the likelihood that the child will find ways to better relate to peers and may thus assist the child in maintaining a positive self-image.

Some practitioners have used behavioral approaches to discourage cross-gendered behaviors. Although these approaches have not been studied systematically, some improvements have been noted on specific behaviors. A technical problem with this approach is that specific behavioral treatments do not generalize to other cross-gender behaviors (e.g., the cessation of cross-dressing does not lead to decreased play with dolls). Ethical problems with this treatment emerge if one considers that biologic bases for these disorders exist in many cases. Efforts to partially modify these behaviors – without being able to ultimately change the overall disorder – can therefore add to the child's burden by reinforcing negative and judgmental appraisals of his or her interests and behaviors. This approach is generally not recommended. Many suggest that the focus of clinical work should be the dysphoria accompanying the gender identity rather than treating gender role behavior itself [25].

Common Problems in Management

Clinicians face a variety of common problems when treating patients with GID. Resistance to change on the part of the family and the child are predictable. Embarrassment and shame, especially among fathers, is another common difficulty. Work with group child-care settings and schools, when appropriate, should also be undertaken to protect and support the child. Occasionally countertransference problems can contribute to an inability to empathize and assist children and families with this disorder. Religious and moral beliefs about sex roles and homosexuality, whether in families or therapists, may confound the treatment of these patients.

CASE THREE

Tommy's mother brought him in for an evaluation at her husband's insistence. Tommy was four years old and according to his mother was a wonderful child with an active interest in dolls, dressing up in her clothing, and playing with girls and an active disinterest in playing with other boys, whom he considered too rough and mean. During the interview, Tommy appeared developmentally appropriate on all measures. His appearance was noteworthy for wearing pink plastic sandals and carrying a tin lunch box with Cinderella on the cover. Tommy was polite and deferential to the male evaluator. As the evaluation proceeded, it became clear that Tommy's mother and father were having marital problems. He was an only child and languished in their discord. The father was an overworked physician who had little time or interest in his son and was clearly displeased with his feminine appearance and behaviors. Work with Tommy was supportive and consisted of play therapy intended to explore the meaning of his play interests. He was clearly anxious about both his parents. He wanted his father's attention, but his mother was the only parent consistently available to him. He both enjoyed her attention and felt anxious about her approval. The mother reported that she enjoyed her son's cross-gender play and in some ways encouraged it. The therapist began to work with her on being more neutral in her reaction to Tommy's behavior and also encouraged the family to develop opportunities for the father and son to interact more frequently. Although Tommy remained interested in many feminine things, over time he also clearly enjoyed a broader range of play. When he started kindergarten the following year, he was not teased or routinely harassed.

Paraphilias

Definition

The DSM-IV-TR lists the following paraphilias: exhibitionism, fetishism, transvestic fetishism, frotteurism, pedophilia, masochism, sadism, and voyeurism.

Epidemiology, Etiology, and Pathology

These disorders all share the diagnostic criteria that patients experience recurrent, intense, and sexually arousing fantasies, sexual urges, or behaviors for at least six months that lead to clinically significant distress or impairment in social, occupational, or other important areas of functioning. Although there are specific characteristics for each major subtype of paraphilia, general characteristics of paraphilias include the use of nonhuman objects, suffering, the humiliation of self or a sexual partner, or children or nonconsensual sexual interactions.

Our scientific understanding of paraphilia is extremely limited. Paraphilias are rarely diagnosed clinically, but the large commercial market in paraphilia-related materials suggests that it is more prevalent than clinical samples indicate. Paraphilias, with the exception of sexual masochism, are only rarely diagnosed in females. The most common presenting paraphilias in clinical populations are pedophilia, voyeurism, and exhibitionism – but this may be simply a result of these patients coming to the attention of clinicians because of legal involvements resulting from these sexual behaviors. About 50% of the patients with paraphilia are married. Most paraphilias are chronic, lifelong disorders. They usually begin in childhood and adolescence and diminish in intensity with advancing age. Multiple paraphilias are the rule, not the exception. Most paraphilias are exacerbated with other psychiatric illness, stress, or additional free time. Personality disorders and depression are common among patients with a paraphilia.

The etiology of paraphilias is unclear. Paraphilias have been a part of the psychiatric literature since the time of Freud, but reports of paraphilic behaviors stretch back centuries. Psychoanalytic, behavioral, traumatic, and biologic theories have all been suggested to explain the origin of paraphilias. The most developed theories are psychoanalytic. Freud thought that paraphilia was based on a childhood belief that women had penises and that individuals with paraphilias were preoccupied with the fantasy that they would be castrated [41]. Stoller thought that hatred and hostility, which resulted from past humiliation, were eroticized in paraphilic behaviors [42]. He pre-ferred the term perversion rather than paraphilia, explaining that this term better represents the desire to harm, hurt, be cruel to, or humiliate someone. Cooper's related theory suggested that paraphiliacs attempt to manage a deeply traumatizing relationship with primary maternal figures through efforts to absolutely control sexual interactions [43]. Others have viewed paraphilia as the result of gender instability and a form of intimacy dysfunction [44]. Behavioral theorists contend that paraphilias are learned behaviors that are strongly reinforced by intermittent sexual rewards. Because there is considerable evidence that men with paraphilia have a high incidence of sexual abuse histories, often intrafamilial, some theories suggest that a specific trauma may lead to paraphiliac behavior.

The biologic bases for paraphilia were examined during the 1980s and 1990s. The original hypothesis was based on a theory of excessive testosterone in pedophiles, since castration, either chemical or physical, was found to be effective in curtailing pedophilic behaviors. Other studies have focused on the comorbid psychiatric conditions found among paraphiliacs, including depression, obsessive–compulsive disorders, anxiety disorders, and substance abuse, as the basis for biologic origin. Recent evidence that paraphiliacs respond to serotonin reuptake inhibitors (SSRIs) suggests a neurotransmitter dysregulation of the serotonin system as the root cause of paraphilia [45,46].

Diagnosis, Course, and Natural History of Specific Paraphilia

Exhibitionism

Exhibitionism is characterized by intense sexually arousing activities or fantasies that involve exposure of one's genitalia to strangers. Usually no other sexual activity is sought with these strangers. These urges to expose seem to occur in waves, perhaps associated with an increase in either free time or stress. Exhibitionism is rare in females. The typical exhibitionist has hundreds of exposures before seeking treatment. About 20% of adult females have been targets for exhibitionists or voyeurs.

Fetish and Transvestic Fetish

The fetishist uses a nonhuman object for sexual gratification but does not cross-dress whereas the transvestic fetishist finds the cross-dressing process itself sexually arousing. Most fetishes begin in adolescence and involve males. The fetishist may develop erectile difficulties without the fetish present. Most problems develop for the fetishist because they exclude their sexual partners in their erotic activities. Transvestic fetishists are usually heterosexual, but a few of them have had occasional homosexual experiences. Transvestic fetishes usually begin in childhood and progress in adolescence. Cross-dressing appears to not only be sexually arousing but also mitigates symptoms of anxiety and depression. Both of these disorders result in feelings of shame and guilt, which complicate their presentations and treatment.

Frotteurism

Frotteurism is rubbing or touching an unsuspecting person for sexual arousal. Most frotteurers operate in crowded situations, attempting to touch the body of a female through clothing with an erect penis. Most frotteurers are passive, nonassertive men. The behavior starts in adolescence and is most frequent when the patient is between the ages of 15 and 24 years. As with any of the paraphilias, frotteurism may not be considered pathological in some cultures, and the cultural context must be taken into account [23].

Pedophilia

Pedophilia is the most socially disapproved of the paraphilias because the victims are children. Pedophilia generally involves older males engaging females in sexual acts – usually genital fondling or oral sex. Ninety-five percent of pedophiles are heterosexual, although they may engage in pedophiliac sexual interactions with either sex. Female victims are usually between the ages of 8 and 10 years, and male victims are usually slightly older. The primary motive behind these actions appears to be achieving sexual arousal and activity without the threat of an adult partner. Most pedophiles have low self-esteem and begin the behavior in adolescence. Recidivism is extremely high among pedophiles and can be predicted by a preference for male victims and an exclusive attraction to children. Ten to 20% of all children have been sexually molested by the age of 18 years.

Masochism

Sexual masochism is the only perversion for which females are also commonly diagnosed. Still, the male-to-female ratio is 20:1. Masochists are sexually stimulated by fantasies and activities that can include humiliation, the infliction of pain, and suffering. Examples of such activities include bondage, blindfolding, paddling, whipping, cutting, being urinated or defecated on, and being verbally abused. Two additional variations are *infantism*, in which the masochist is diapered and bottle fed, and *hypoxyphilia*, which involves near strangulation or oxygen deprivation.

Approximately one-third of masochists have played the sadist role as well. Most sexual masochism begins in early adulthood.

Sadism

Most sexually sadistic behavior starts before the age of 18 years. Fantasies of sadistic activities, however, begin in childhood well before such behaviors. Sadists are sexually aroused by fantasies and behaviors that cause real suffering. Most sadists work with one or only a few partners, who may be consenting or nonconsenting. Sadists do not necessarily need to increase the level of suffering over time to achieve arousal and sexual satisfaction. About 8% of rapists have a sadistic sexual interest.

Voyeurism

Voyeurs find it sexually exciting to observe an unsuspecting person undressing or having sex. This is the earliest type of paraphilia to develop and usually begins before the age of 15 years. Usually the voyeur masturbates while others are undressing or engaged in sexual activity. Because there are few consequences of this behavior and victims are not likely to know they are being watched, it can go undetected for an extended period. This can reinforce the behavior and make it more difficult to treat. As with other paraphilias, voyeurism can also increase in waves associated with mood, stress, and available time.

Treatment

Most information about treating patients with paraphilias is derived from work with adults, because most patients are not identified until adulthood. There are three major approaches to working with patients with paraphilia. The oldest and most common approach uses psychotherapy, usually with a psychoanalytic base, the next is a behavioral approach, and the most recent is the use of medications. Combinations of treatments are also common, because the effectiveness of any of these approaches is limited.

Psychotherapy

The first assumption of the psychotherapies used to treat paraphilia is that the paraphilia serves a function in the patient's life. The goal is to find other ways to meet the need that the paraphilic behavior is masking. Paraphilia is, in this sense, a way to avoid insight. Paraphilias are perceived as a means of preventing the recall of past trauma, poor parenting relationships, or past victimization. Paraphilia may also temporarily help sexually insecure males with a fragile sense of masculinity. Other evidence suggests that paraphilias help these individuals manage emotional states other than cognitive and developmental distortions – particularly anger, depression, anxiety, sadness, guilt, and loneliness. Thus, paraphilias can be seen as a means of avoiding the realities of life and the demands of intimacy and human relations. Therapeutic approaches to these issues include identifying underlying motivations behind the behaviors; clarifying the relationship of these behaviors to the patient's emotional states; interpreting any resistance to changing behaviors; and helping the patient progress into the often frightening areas of more intimate human relationships without depending on or relapsing into paraphilic behaviors and fantasies.

Specific approaches to working with adolescents with paraphilia require an awareness of the overall challenges of adolescent psychotherapeutic work. Adolescents have varying developmental capacities and motivations for psychotherapy. In addition, they are often more invested in erotic interest than older adults. Conversely, patterns of personal relationships and defensive management of emotional needs are not as fixed as in adults and may therefore be more malleable to treatment. The family may also play a part in the treatment of this age group. Because many of these patients only come to the attention of a psychiatrist if a victim has come forward – sometimes with the force of law – family members feel shame, anger, and guilt, and their wishes to punish and avoid the child often need to be addressed. In addition, since issues of relationships with parental figures are almost always a part of the history of these patients, the therapist will likely encounter significant efforts to deny or distort family dynamics. The younger the patient, the more important it is to keep the family involved.

One of the most important problems that therapists face when working with these adolescents is countertransference. It is often difficult for therapists to manage their own feelings of disgust, anger, and fear of the fantasies and behaviors of patients with paraphilias. Identification with the victims and their families is common and can limit the development of an empathic relationship with the patient. The younger the victim and the more physically aggressive the sexual assault, the more likely the therapist will experience these difficulties. Therapists may need to work to overcome these reactions. Those that do can find meaningful and rewarding work in developing a therapeutic relationship that not only assists the particular patient but also prevents further victimization.

Behavioral Treatment

Behavior therapy is used to interrupt a learned paraphilic behavioral pattern. Approaches include cognitive behavior therapy, social skills learning, and relapse-prevention strategies. A cognitive behavioral approach aims to identify and elucidate the sequence of events that lead to paraphilic behavior. Usually, both an initial event and a sequence of subsequent events are required to support the ultimate expression of the paraphiliac behavior. By learning to identify these events and developing an increased awareness of the pattern, patients can identify opportunities to disrupt the ultimate behavioral outcome. Cognitive awareness is sometimes coupled with noxious stimuli, such as electric shocks and bad odors, to recondition the behavior and prevent its reinforcement. It is often helpful if these treatments can be self-administered, because it allows the patient to assess and interrupt the chain of events leading to paraphilic behavior when therapists are unavailable. Group cognitive work can support the individual cognitive behavioral approach by adding a supportive element as well as providing the patient with perspectives from others with similar difficulties. Most of the research on these behavioral treatments is directed toward the treatment of pedophilia. No substantive empirical studies have been published on the behavioral treatment of adolescents with paraphilia.

Medication

Biological approaches to treating paraphilia have been developed for many years. The basic goal of the initial approaches was to decrease testosterone levels and thereby reduce the sexual drive and arousal that motivated paraphilic behaviors. Although castration is an effective method of limiting these behaviors, surgical castration is intrusive and irreversible. Chemical castration may be a reasonable alternative for treatment-resistant patients with severe paraphilia that results in the chronic victimization of others. In the early 1980s, medroxyprogesterone acetate (MPA)(Depo-Provera) and cyproterone acetate (CPA) began to be used to treat paraphilia of a severe and persistent nature (e.g., constant masturbation, committing sex offenses, and high-risk sexual behaviors). MPA inhibits gonadotropin secretions whereas CPA antagonizes the effects of testosterone through competitive inhibition at androgen receptors. Weekly injection of MPA was highly successful in reducing these behaviors, but a significant number of patients experienced side effects of weight gain, hypertension, muscle cramps, and gynecomastia. In the late 1980s, oral MPA, in doses of

30–80 mg/day, was also found effective, and with fewer side effects. Currently, the intramuscular route of administration is only recommended for the most severe of cases often accompanied by treatment non-compliance [47].

More recently, studies using long-lasting luteinizing hormone-releasing hormone (LHRH) agonists have shown similar results, with decreases in paraphiliac behaviors paralleling the decrease of plasma testosterone levels. These agents (leuprolide, nafarelin, goserelin, treptorelin) work by exerting a continuous, rather than the physiologic pulsatile effect, on the pituitary–gonadal axis thereby downregulating the gonadotroph cells. Although effective, these medications are not without serious side effects including bone demineralization with osteoporosis, gynecomastia, erectile dysfunction, nausea, and depression [47]. Due to the side effects of MPA, CPA, and LHRH agonists, they are generally considered in adults for a moderate to severe disorder, or after other treatments have been tried (for review and treatment algorithm see Briken *et al.* [47]). In adolescents, these drugs are rarely used due to these side effects [48]. In fact, psychotherapeutic interventions are commonly first line treatments in adolescent patients.

The most recent breakthrough in psychopharmacologic management is the use of SSRIs to treat paraphilia. In case reports in the 1980s and early 1990s as well as clinical trials currently being conducted, these agents are showing promising effects. Clomipramine, fluoxetine, fluvoxamine, paroxetine and sertraline all are medications under investigation [45,46]. In their algorithm of medication treatment for paraphilias in adults, Briken *et al.* [47] suggest that SSRIs be first-line treatments for adults with mild symptoms, or for those with comorbid depressive, anxious, or obsessive–compulsive symptoms, and that for moderate to severe symptoms with or without comorbid mood or anxiety symptoms, a combination of SSRIs and CPA, MPA or LHRH could be used. They suggest that all pharmacological interventions should be accompanied by supportive or intensive psychotherapy. The relationship between paraphilia, obsessive–compulsive disorder, and depression, is also under exploration, since the latter two are also responsive to SSRIs. Although these medications are promising, and perhaps safer in adolescents due to a better side effect profile, rigorous studies of their effectiveness are not yet available.

CASE FOUR

An 18-year-old male high school senior was brought in by his professional father for an evaluation for a transvestic fetish. The boy described himself as hypermasculine, with interests in every sport and a wish to join the air force to become a pilot. Over the past two years, however, he had begun to cross-dress and masturbate. He felt ashamed of this behavior and wanted to end it so he could join the military. The onset of this behavior was after the divorce of his parents and his subsequent decision to live with his father, which he had made about three years prior to the evaluation. His father was a heterosexual man who was powerful, good-looking, charming, and seductive. From early childhood the boy had wished to be close to this man who was at once powerful and unavailable. Although the young man was heterosexual, his wish to have a closer relationship with his father, now that his mother was out of the picture, apparently increased and led to the transvestic fetish. Although there was clearly a sexual component, the real purpose of the transvestism was to allure and involve the father, who was both fascinated and overinvolved with his son during his treatment. This relationship during therapy allowed the son to control the father and reverse the dynamic that had been humiliating to the son. When the son's therapist gave him permission to openly participate in his transvestic fetish, it apparently lost some of its appeal; he gave it up and joined the military. It is likely, however, that this paraphilia will return or another will take its place.

The Effect of Sexual Abuse on Sexual Development and Behavior

The subject of sexual abuse and its treatment are covered elsewhere in this book. Some specific discussion of the impact of sexual abuse on sexual development and behavior is warranted here, however. As with any abuse, sexual abuse is likely to have the most severe effects on persons who are otherwise vulnerable or young, when the abuser is a close relative, or when the abuse is violent and ongoing.

Victim Psychologic Responses

Although sexual abuse can assume many possible manifestations in later sexual development two of the most hazardous are becoming an offender oneself and repeating the experience of being a sexual victim. Although there is no definitive rule, abused boys often take the former course and abused girls take the latter. Boys may be socially and otherwise conditioned to find the role of victim particularly ego dystonic. In other words, no matter how abused they may have been, it may seem that the best way to manage these painful experiences is to identify with the sexual aggressor. They thus become seemingly free from the past trauma. Girls may find the role of being a sexual aggressor less socially acceptable and may instead find a familiarity with the role of victim, which frees them from past traumas because these repetitions override past memories.

Either of these ways of managing sexual abuse can lead to abnormal sexual behaviors. Sexually abused children may initiate sexual activities earlier than others, seek out much older or much younger partners, and find sexual experiences to be dissociated from feelings of intimacy. As a result, they may struggle to achieve real emotional connection with their sexual partners. Some may find it impossible to have sexual relationships with people they love. Some sexually abused children grow up to be sexually avoidant and unusually anxious about sexual development; they, too, may be unable to achieve real emotional intimacy with those they love. Children who are sexually abused by someone of the same sex may feel that this predetermines their sexual orientation. Although this is not the case, this feeling can be reinforced by peers and by misinformation in the culture which supports this view.

Treatment of Sexually Abused Children

Assisting a child or adolescent with issues surrounding sexual abuse requires unusual sensitivity and patience on the part of therapists. Although medications might alleviate some aspects of post-traumatic experiences, medication has little to offer in the specific area of sexual development. A variety of approaches have been attempted and include individual therapy aimed at revisiting the past trauma and group therapy aimed at reducing the child's or adolescent's feeling of isolation and shame. Clearly, the first goal is to ensure that the abuse has stopped and that the child is safe. It is also necessary to ensure that the possibility of contact with the abuser has ended. This sets a framework in which the therapist can establish safe parameters to conduct exploratory work. It is essential for the therapist to recognize that sexual abuse is clearly about aggression and minimally about sex; sex is the vehicle for aggression. In the child's eye, sex and aggression are merged. This leads to both emotional and cognitive confusion that underlies many of the behavioral and emotional difficulties that may develop. The goals of therapy are to assist the child or adolescent with sexual difficulties that have resulted from abuse to help them understand why this confusion exists, and to help them to change these feelings as much as possible.

Shame is another result of sexual abuse that can complicate later sexual functioning. Shame may result in feelings of being unlovable, damaged and worthless, and different from peers because of this sexual experience. Helping a child or adolescent resolve this sexual shame requires addressing fundamental ideas of the self and how it has been damaged by abuse. Psychotherapeutic exploration of these issues is currently best formulated with techniques of empathy, mirroring, and other reflecting tools. Issues of provocative sexual behavior, dress, and language by sexually abused children should be anticipated as part of sexually abused children's therapy. Therapists need to be available and empathic, while also maintaining an extraordinary awareness of their boundaries to keep the patient safe from any hint of violation. Even the most experienced clinicians find it beneficial to get supervision with such cases.

Group treatments have been used in therapy for sexual abuse but have received mixed reviews. Some abused children find them helpful; others find that they are intrusive and increase their feelings of shame. When timed appropriately, these group treatments can be a helpful adjunct to individual work, because they allow for a level of peer support around sexual activity and exploration that is normative for peers. Although such groups are even used for younger children, this seems inadvisable because of the developmental limitation of younger peer groups to provide reliable support and guidance.

Sex Offenders

Sex offenders have sometimes been victims themselves. They have become perpetrators, perhaps in an effort to manage some of the anxieties that their own abuse continues to provoke. Becker summarized the data on male adolescent sexual assault: each year, between 200 000 and 450 000 sexual assaults using force occur [49]. About 20% of these are rapes, and 30%–50% involve child abuse. About three-quarters of adolescent sex offenders have assaulted someone before their twelfth birthday. Overall, about 2% of adolescent males engage in aggressive sexual assaults and as many as 15% are estimated to engage in some type of forced sexual contact. Approximately one-third of females and one-tenth of males report sexual abuse before the age of 18 years.

Sex offenders have been described as loners, underachievers, impulsive, having low frustration tolerance, and tending to rely on external regulators of behaviors. In comparison to other nonsexual violent offenders, sex offenders live more often with their birth parents, have lower self-reported delinquency, and use fewer drugs and alcohol; they do, however, have more familial violence and abuse, especially sexual abuse, and are more socially and sexually isolated. A history of childhood sexual abuse seems to be particularly high among those sex offenders whose victims are boys. Some studies have shown that there is also an increased rate of depressive symptomatology in this group [49]. Among incarcerated male teens who had been perpetrators of sexual assault, there were four predictors of sexual assault: living with violence at home, being a victim of sexual assault, parents encouraging violence, and knowing a role model for sexual assault [50]. There is evidence that the management of sexual aggression, considered a learned restraint, is mediated by family interaction patterns.

Treatment of Sex Offenders

Treatment of child and adolescent sex offenders includes individual, family, and group work and is aimed at preventing recurrence of the behavior. A recent review of treatment approaches for this group found a paucity of empirically based research [51]. To date there have only been two controlled outcome studies in this area, one on multisystemic therapy, and the other of a court-based sexual offender outpatient treatment program. Although the results from multisystemic therapy were encouraging, the sample size was small, and the study has not yet been replicated (see review by Becker and Hicks [51]). There have been many other uncontrolled studies using various therapies including cognitive behavioral interventions, relapse prevention models, group therapy, and family therapy. However, there is no clear evidence for the efficacy of any treatment approaches for adolescent sex offenders. Another critique of existing treatment studies concludes that the treatment outcome literature is still developing, although preliminary reports indicate that juvenile sex offenders appear responsive to treatment [52].

References

1. Yates A: Childhood sexuality. In: Lewis M, ed. *Child and Adolescent Psychiatry; A Comprehensive Textbook*. Baltimore: Williams & Wilkins, 1991:195–214.
2. Currier RL: Juvenile sexuality in global perspective. In: Constantine LL, Marinson FM, eds. *Children and Sex: New Findings, New Perspectives*. Boston: Liule, Brown & Co., 1981.
3. Kohlberg L: A cognitive developmental analysis of children's sex roles and attitudes. In Maccoby EE, ed. *The Development of Sex Differences,* Stanford: Stanford University Press, 1966.
4. Kinsey AC, Wardell BP, Martin CE: *Sexual Behavior in the Human Male*. Philadelphia: WB Saunders Co., 1948.
5. Offer D: In defense of adolescents. *JAMA* 1987; **257**:3407.
6. Graber JA, Seeley JR, Brooks-Gunn J, Lewinsohn PM: Is pubertal timing associated with psychopathology in young adulthood? *J Am Acad Child Adolesc Psychiatry* 2004; **43**:718–726.
7. Denizet-Lewis B: Friends, friends with benefits and the benefits of the local mall. *NY Times Magazine* 2004.
8. Lock J: Psychosexual development in adolescents with chronic medical illnesses. *Psychosomatics* 1998; **39**: 340–349.
9. Reiner WG, Gearhart JP: Discordant sexual identity in some genetic males with cloacal exstrophy assigned to female sex at birth. *New Engl J Med* 2004; **350**:333–341.
10. Creighton SM, Liao LM: Changing attitudes to sex assignment in intersex. *BJU Int* 2004; **93**:659–664.
11. Frader J, Alderson P, Asch A, Aspinall C, Davis D, Dreger A, Edwards J, Feder E, Frank A, Abelow Hedley L, Kittay E, Marsh J, Miller P, Mouradianh W, Nelson H, Parens E: Health care professionals and intersex conditions. *Arch Pediatr Adolesc Med* 2004; **158**: 426–428.
12. American Academy of Pediatrics: Evaluation of the newborn with developmental anomalies of the external genitalia. *Pediatrics* 2000; **106**:138–142.
13. Pilkington NW, D'Augelli AR: Victimization of lesbian, gay, and bisexual youth in community sellings. *Community Psychol* 1995; **23**:34–56.
14. Hammelman TL: Gay and lesbian youth: Contributing factors to serious attempts or considerations of suicide. *J Gay Lesbian Psychother* 1993; **2**:77–89.
15. Rotheram-Borus MJ, Rosario M, Reid H, Koopman C: Predicting patterns of sexual acts among homosexual and bisexual youths. *Am J Psychiatry* 1995; **152**:588–595.
16. Hershberger SL, D'Augelli AR: The impact of victimization on the mental health and suicidality of lesbian, gay, and bisexual youth. *Dev Psychol* 1995; **31**:65–74.
17. Troiden RR: *Gay and Lesbian Identity*. Dix Hills NY: General Hall, 1988.
18. Hetrick ES, Martin AD: Developmental issues and their resolution for gay and lesbian adolescents. *J Homosex* 1987; **14**:25–44.
19. Uribe V: Project 10: A School-based outreach to gay and lesbian youth. *High School J* 1993; **77**(special issue): 108–112.
20. Stanley JL: An applied collaborative training program for graduate students in community psychology: A case study of a community project working with lesbian, gay, bisexual, transgender, and questioning youth. *Am J Commun Psychol* 2003; **31**:253–265.

21. Lasser J, D. Tharinger D: Visibility management in school and beyond: A qualitative study of gay, lesbian, bisexual youth. *J Adolesc* 2003; **26**:233–244.

22. Brenner ND, Collins JL, Kann L, *et al.*: Reliability of the Youth Risk Behavior Survey questionnaire. *Am J Epidemiol* 1995; **141**:575–580.

23. American Psychiatric Association: *Diagnostic and Statistical Manual of Mental Disorders*, 4th ed., Text Revision. Washington DC: American Psychiatric Association, 2000.

24. Bradley SJ, Zucker KJ: Gender Identity Disorder: A review of the past 10 years. *J Am Acad Child Adolesc Psychiatry* 1997; **36**:872–880.

25. Wilson I, Griffin C, Wren B: The validity of the diagnosis of gender identity disorder (child and adolescent criteria). *Clin Child Psychol Psychiatry* 2002; **7**(3):335–351.

26. Zucker KJ: Cross-gender-identified children. In: Steiner BW, ed. *Gender Dysphoria: Development, Research, and Management*. New York: Plenum Publishing Corp., 1985:75–174.

27. Zucker KJ, Green R: Psychosexual disorders in children and adolescents. *J Child Psychol Psychiatry* 1992; **33**:107–151.

28. Pillard RC: Kinsey Scale: Is it familial? In: McWhirter DP, Sanders SA, Reinisch JM, eds.: *Homosexuality/ Heterosexuality: Concepts of Sexual Orientation*. New York: Oxford University Press, 1990:88–100.

29. Meyer-Bahlburg HFL: Sex hormone changes during puberty and sexual behavior. In: Samson J, ed.: *Childhood and Sexuality*. Montreal: Editions Etudes Vivantes, 1980: 113–122.

30. Blanchard R, Zucker K, Bradley S, Hume C: Birth order and sibling sex ratio in homosexual male adolescents and probably prehomosexual feminine boys. *Dev Psychol* 1995; **31**:22–30.

31. Blanchard R: Fraternal birth order and the maternal immune hypothesis of male homosexuality. *Hormones and Behavior* 2001; **40**:105–114.

32. Haraldsen IR, Opjordsmoen S, Egeland T, Finset A: Sex-sensitive cognitive performance in untreated patients with early onset gender identity disorder. *Psychoneuroendocrinology* 2003; **28**:906–915.

33. Cohen-Kettenis PT, van Goozen SH, Doorn CD, Gooren LJ: Cognitive ability and cerebral lateralisation in transsexuals. *Psychoneuroendocrinology* 1998; **23**: 631–641.

34. Dennis C: The most important sexual organ. *Nature* 2004; **427**:390–392.

35. Coates S, Person ES: Extreme boyhood femininity: Isolated behavior or pervasive disorder? *J Am Acad Child Psychiatry* 1985; **24**:702–709.

36. Kohlberg L, Ricks D, Snarey J: Childhood development as a predictor of adaptation in adulthood. *Genet Psychol Monogr* 1984; **110**:91–172.

37. Bailey JM, Zucker KJ: Childhood sex-typed behavior and sexual orientation: A conceptual analysis and quantitative review. *Dev Psychol* 1995; **31**:43–55.

38. Zucker KJ, Bradley SJ: *Gender Identity Disorder and Psychosexual Problems in Children and Adolescents*. New York: Guilford Press, 1995.

39. Cohen-Kettenis PT, Owen A, Kaijser VG, Bradley SJ, Zucker KJ: Demographic characteristics, social competence, and behavior problems in children with gender identity disorder: A cross-national, cross-clinic comparative analysis. *J Abnormal Child Psychol* 2003; **31**: 41–53.

40. Smith YL, Goozen SH, Cohen-Kettenis PT: Adolescents with gender identity disorder who were accepted or rejected for sex reassignment surgery: A prospective follow-up study. *J Am Acad Child Adolesc Psychiatry* 2001; **40**:472–481.

41. Freud S: *Three Essays on the Theory of Sexuality*. Standard Edition 7. London: Hogarth, 1905:130–243.

42. Stoller RJ: *Observing the Erotic Imagination*. New Haven CT: Yale University Press, 1985.

43. Cooper AM, Sack MH: Sadism and masochism in character disorder and resistance. In: Fogel GI, Myers WA, eds.: *Perversions and Near Perversions in Clinical Practice: New Psychoanalytic Perspectives*. New Haven, CT: Yale University Press, 1991:17–25.

44. Kaplan LJ: *Female Perversions: The Temptations of Emma Bovary*. New York: Doubleday & Co., 1991.

45. Kafka MP: Sertraline pharmacotherapy for paraphilias and paraphilia-related disorders: An open trial. *Ann Clin Psychiatry* 1994; **6**:189–195.

46. Abouesh A, Clayton A: Compulsive voyeurism and exhibitionism: A clinical response to paroxetine. *Arch Sex Behav* 1999; **28**:23–30.

47. Briken P, Hill A, Berner W: Pharmacotherapy of paraphilias with long-acting agonists of luteinizing hormone-releasing hormone: A systematic review. *J Clin Psychiatry* 2003; **64**:890–897.

48. Gerardin P, Thibaut F: Epidemiology and treatment of juvenile sexual offending. *Paediatric Drugs* 2004; **6**: 79–91.

49. Becker JV: Offenders: Characteristics and treatment. *Future Child* 1994; **4**(2):176–197.

50. Morris RE, Anderson MM, Knox GW: Incarcerated adolescents' experiences as perpetrators of sexual assault. *Arch Pediatr Adolesc Med* 2002; **156**:831–835.

51. Becker JV, Hicks SJ: Juvenile sexual offenders: Characteristics, interventions, and policy issues. *Ann N Y Acad Sci* 2003; **989**:397–410.

52. Brown EJ, Kolko DG: Treatment efficacy and program evaluation with juvenile sexual abusers: A critique with directions for service delivery and research. *Child Maltreatment* 1998; **3**(4):362–373.

20

Learning and Communications Disorders

Pamela A. Gulley

Introduction

The American Psychiatric Association's 1987 decision to move from a single diagnostic criterion to multiaxial diagnostic criteria for these disorders afforded clinicians an opportunity to use a more holistic approach to determine pathology [1]. This was a particularly important change with respect to our current understanding of the nature of childhood psychiatric disorders. Pathology in children does not consist of a discrete series of behaviors that fit easily into designated areas. Rather, the child's difficulties are manifested as behaviors that could be mislabeled and misdiagnosed depending on the system that is used to first identify the atypical behaviors. The child who is slow to develop language skills, for example, may be classified as mentally retarded, but with further investigation, it may be discovered that a trauma occurred that resulted in elective mutism. This chapter discusses the educational aspects of clinical diagnosis as well as the impact of communication disorders on a 'child's ability to function effectively in his or her environment.'

Educational disorders coded on Axis I relate to reading, writing, and mathematical abilities as measured on individually administered achievement tests. A child is identified as having a disorder in an academic area if his or her academic achievement is not commensurate with the standards for the child's chronologic age, measured cognitive ability, and age-appropriate education. The term learning disability has been used in the educational field since the early 1970s. Learning disorders appeared as a part of the clinical criteria of the *Diagnostic and Statistical Manual of Mental Disorders* (DSM) system in 1987. Much controversy has surrounded the definition and the diagnosis of children's learning problems. In the educational arena, the concept of learning disability has gone through several phases of definition, which are delimited as follows [2,3]:

- Foundation phase – involved basic research in the area of brain function and dysfunction that led to a definition of learning disabilities that was based on a neurologic handicap.
- Transition phase – focused on the information processing aspect of the disorder. Learning disabilities were considered to be related to perceptual disorders; this led to many theories of the relationships among the various sensory systems auditory, visual, tactile, and kinetic. If the sensory systems did not communicate effectively with each other, then a learning disability was identified.
- Integration phase – recognized that children with learning disorders would require specialized educational services to achieve better success in school. It also became evident that children with learning disorders were not fitting into categories for special educational services because they were not mentally retarded or behaviorally handicapped. Legislation enacted to rectify this problem (the 1969 Children with Specific Learning Disabilities Act) began the establishment of appropriate educational programs for children with learning disabilities [4].

With program options in place, other controversies ensued related to the definition, identification, and proper diagnosis of a learning disability. The term 'learning disability' became a catch-all 'diagnosis' for any child who had academic difficulties. Controversy also centered around methods for determining whether a child's learning problems are related to a disorder, a dysfunction, or behavioral, emotional, or environmental influences. Related issues included the reliability and validity of assessment measures as well as the pro-

Clinical Child Psychiatry, Second Edition. Edited by W.M. Klykylo and J.L. Kay
© 2005 John Wiley & Sons Ltd.

fessional training required to determine whether a person has a disability.

The Education for All Handicapped Act of 1975 was enacted to provide federal guidelines clarifying the inconsistency and controversy created by the original law [5]. This law defined the various disabilities, established the general provisions from which programs were developed, and determined the funding of such programs. In 1990, the Individuals with Disabilities Education Act (IDEA) amended the 1972 laws [6]. The entire language of the original law was amended to reflect 'person-first' language and to establish the use of the term 'disability.' The term 'handicapped' was dropped from the law. This was an important step for people with disabilities: they were recognized as individuals with many needs rather than as people who were placed into established categories in the name of available educational programming.

In 2004, the 'Improving Education Results for Children with Disabilities Act' which reforms the 1997 IDEA, raised the bar on accountability not only for those identified as having a disability, by including them in state assessment accountability systems, but for those teaching in special needs settings, using highly qualified teacher standards [7]. In the US, the federal definition of learning disabilities (Table 20.1) parallels the clinical diagnostic categories of the DSM-IV (Box A). Each state using the federal definition must develop specific definitions that are consistent and appropriate for determining educational services and interventions in the public school system. The funding of such programs is linked to an accurate interpretation and implementation of the IDEA. When determining an accurate diagnosis for a child, therefore, it is important that clinicians be aware of the specific laws of the state in which they work. It can create confusion if a parent or guardian is told that the child has a disability only to be informed by educational personnel that the child does not meet the appropriate criteria to receive services within the school setting. (See Table 20.1 for the IDEA's definition of specific learning disabilities.)

Diagnostic Categories

From a clinical viewpoint, the definition of specific learning disabilities translates into the following DSM-IV diagnostic categories [8]:

- Mathematics Disorder 315.1
- Reading Disorder 315.00
- Disorder of Written Expression 315.2

Table 20.1 Specific learning disability. A disorder in one or more of the basic psychological processes involved in understanding or in using language, spoken or written, that may manifest itself in an imperfect ability to listen, think, speak, read, write, spell, or to do mathematical calculations. This includes such conditions as perceptual disabilities, brain injury, minimal brain dysfunction, dyslexia, and developmental aphasia. This does not apply to children who have learning problems that are primarily the result of visual, hearing, or motor disabilities, mental retardation, emotional disturbance, or environmental, cultural, or economic disadvantages.

Documentation must provide evidence of the following:

(1) a severe discrepancy between ability and achievement that is not correctable without special education and/or related services
(2) the determination that the discrepancy is not primarily the result of a visual, hearing, or motor impairment; mental retardation; emotional disturbance; or environmental, cultural, or economic disadvantage
(3) the relationship of observed behavior to the child's academic functioning

---

From Individuals with Disabilities Education Act of 1990. Public Law 91-230, Title 20, U.S. Code Section 1401(a)15; 1997.

- Learning Disorder Not Otherwise Specified 315.9 (see Box A).

When coding any of these disorders, it is important to note on Axis III any sensory deficits or related medical conditions, such as a neurologic disorder.

To determine the existence of an academically based disorder, the results of an individually administered achievement test are compared with the individual's expected academic aptitude. Achievement tests measure reading accuracy and comprehension, mathematics and calculation ability, and writing skills. A child's performance on such measures determines if he or she is performing 'substantially below' what is expected given the individual's intelligence, which is measured on an individual standardized test, chronologic age, and age-appropriate education. Such a discrepancy between a child's expected academic level and actual academic performance might result in impaired academic achievement or daily living skills [9].

The qualifier substantially below is typically defined as two standard deviations below the expected level of

---

BOX A DSM-IV DIAGNOSTIC CRITERIA FOR 315.1 MATHEMATICS DISORDER; 315.00 READING DISORDER; AND 315.2 DISORDER OF WRITTEN EXPRESSION

(A) Mathematical ability, reading achievement, and writing skills, as measured by individually administered standardized tests, is substantially below that expected given chronological age, measured intelligence, and age-appropriate education.

(B) The disturbance in Criterion A significantly interferes with academic achievement or activities of daily living requiring mathematical ability, reading skills, or the composition of written texts (e.g., writing grammatically correct sentences and organizing paragraphs).

(C) If a sensory deficit is present, the difficulties in mathematical ability, reading ability, or writing skills are in excess of those usually associated with it. Coding note: If a general medical (e.g., neurological) condition or sensory deficit is present, code the condition on Axis III.

Reprinted with permission from the *Diagnostic and Statistical Manual of Mental Disorders*, Fourth Edition. Copyright 1994 American Psychiatric Association.

---

performance. Typically, 15 points represents one standard deviation in a quotient score. With an intelligence quotient (IQ) of 115, for example, a child would be eligible for special education services if he or she obtained a standard score of 85 or below on a measure of academic achievement. In most states this qualifier is determined by the local education agency; it is important for clinicians to understand a particular state's criteria prior to diagnosing a learning disorder.

A child with a learning disability may present behaviors such as sadness, irritability, anger, and nonmotivation, especially regarding activities related to school tasks. This disorder does not mean that the child cannot perform academically, however; it means that the child is not performing up to an expected academic level. This lack of achievement is first evident in an educational setting; therefore, unless associated developmental problems exist, a learning disability may not be identified until the child reaches school age and enters the educational arena.

This disorder is typically first manifest in a child as a reluctance to complete school work or homework, a disinterest in going to school, and possibly even school refusal. Acting out or oppositional behavior may also be evident. The child with a specific learning disability is aware that school is difficult and can feel much stigma because he or she cannot compete in the classroom. Children with learning disabilities are easily singled out as the subjects of a teacher's efforts to assist them with individual instruction, retention, or specialized programs. Although these interventions may be truly academically appropriate for the child, they can also lead to emotional and behavioral difficulties related to the frustration of the disorder and the social consequence of not being as competent as one's peers.

Learning disorders may also coexist with other disorders, such as attention deficit hyperactivity disorder (ADHD), oppositional defiant disorder (ODD), conduct disorder, and depression. This complicates not only the diagnostic process but also treatment planning. Children with ADHD frequently have an associated learning disorder, even though learning disorders and attention deficit disorders can exist by themselves. Except on the most difficult tasks, the academic performance of children with both a learning disability and ADHD may not differ from that of children with only a learning disability [10]. Children who have a diagnosis related to disruptive behaviors such as a conduct disorder or an ODD may also be found to have associated learning problems. In many of these instances, it is difficult to discern the primary diagnosis, since it is often unclear whether the behavior or the poor school performance was first present. However the behavior initially presented itself, it must be identified and appropriate treatment strategies implemented for the child to begin to change behavior and integrate more effectively into his or her environment [11,12].

Depression in childhood is often presents in children with learning disabilities. It is frequently manifested as a lack of motivation, a pervasive sense of unhappiness, and a general apathy toward school.

Specific Learning Disabilities

Reading

To determine what a reading disorder is, the clinician must have a general understanding of the process of reading. Reading is a complex set of behaviors composed of many specific skills and an audiovisual task that involves obtaining meaning from symbols (letters and words) [9]. It involves two basic processes. The first process is understanding the relationship between a phoneme (a basic unit of sound) and a grapheme (a writing symbol) and then translating the printed symbols – words – into oral language. This basic process enables the individual to decode and then pronounce words correctly. The second process, comprehension, involves understanding the meaning of words both in the context of other words and in isolation. Reading is the integration of the two processes into a fluid application of these skills. Reading skills are critical to success in an educational environment. Difficulties in reading are the principal cause of school failure and strongly influence a child's self-concept and feelings of competency.

The best way to screen a child for the presence of reading difficulties is to ask him or her to read. First, observe the child's reaction to the task. If the child eagerly approaches a stack of children's books and begins to choose a favorite, chances are that reading is not a chore. If the child becomes oppositional or reluctant, this should be noted for further consideration. Second, listen to how the child reads. If the child struggles to pronounce every word or hesitates and needs assistance, an assessment of specific skills may be warranted. Mispronunciation, substitution of words, and insertion of words not on the printed page are also indicators of reading problems.

Older children often easily disclose academic difficulties in the process of the clinical interview. To determine if reading should be further assessed, it may help to ask children if they like to read, what they like to read, or to remember a favorite book. The education system is typically ahead of clinicians in detecting reading problems; therefore, the parents should request school records to provide to the clinician. Parents typically keep report cards and school group achievement results that can also be shared. If the child is presenting with a history of school difficulties, the results of a previous psychoeducational assessment by the school psychologist are often available.

Mathematics

This is a process that is based on logical structure. It involves skill development that occurs in a hierarchical manner from the ability to sort objects by size, to match objects, to compute, and to understand fractions, decimals, and percentages. A disability in mathematics usually involves an inability first to construct simple relationships and then to move on to more complex tasks. Particularly in mathematics, lower-level skills are essential for learning higher order math skills [9]. The most effective way of recognizing a mathematics disability in a clinical setting is to review educational records or to conduct an interview or an assessment in mathematics.

Written Language

Written expression requires the use of a variety of cognitive activities. One must first conceive ideas, integrate the ideas into logical thought, and finally express the thoughts in written form. One's ability to use these cognitive activities to engage readers in a written format requires much more than the mechanical aspects of spelling, punctuation, capitalization, grammar, word use, penmanship, outlining, and organizational skills. Written expression also requires basic psychologic processes such that if a disorder is present, the individual can be identified as having a learning disability in this specific area. To determine if a disability exists in written expression, the assessment should focus on the mechanics taught in an educational setting, such as spelling and sentence structure. Standardized instruments can be used; however, a careful review of a person's actual writing is the most effective screening measure. Writing a journal is frequently used as an effective technique in therapy. A review of both writing mechanics and content of the writing can indicate whether further assessment for a disorder in this area is warranted.

Learning Disorder Not Otherwise Specified

The DSM-IV provides a category to identify learning disorders that do not meet the criteria of any specific categories. This diagnosis is appropriate if a disability exists in all three areas and significantly interferes with the academic functioning of the individual. This diagnosis can be used even if performance on standardized tests is not substantially below the level expected for a given chronologic age, intellectual level, and age-appropriate education. Making a diagnosis of learning disabilities not otherwise specified can also help the clinician indicate that the client as a learner has specific needs that must be considered in the treatment planning process.

Communication Disorders

The assessment and diagnosis of communication disorders are unfamiliar to many clinicians. These disorders are typically identified by family physicians, pediatricians, or school personnel if a child exhibits slow development in either the expression or reception of language. How a child develops oral language is crucial to his or her overall emotional health and can affect both the existence and treatment of a psychiatric disturbance. Communication disorders are frequently linked with additional educational disorders. When a child with a communication disorder exhibits a psychiatric disorder, the psychiatric disorder can be overlooked by mental health clinicians because of the child's inability to tell someone how he or she is thinking and feeling. Any behavior that exists because of a communication problem may be considered 'treatable' in the realm of speech and language services without consideration of possible psychiatric needs; this follows the logic that if a child can understand and communicate language more effectively, the problematic behavior will diminish.

Communication disorders are categorized into difficulties with expressive language and those with receptive language. Expressive language difficulties are manifest as a limited vocabulary, grammar errors (e.g., incorrect tense usage), and syntax errors (e.g., word recall and language structure). Receptive language disorders are manifest as an inability to understand the meaning of individual words, whole statements, or the relationships of specific words in a phrase (e.g., the relationship of the two words Mommy's keys means that these keys belong to Mommy) [10].

The diagnosis of a communication disorder typically follows a battery of standardized tests that measure whether a child is functioning substantially below the performance expected for a given chronologic age and level of cognitive functioning. The federal definition of speech or language impairment is shown in Table 20.2 and the DSM-IV categories include expressive language disorder, mixed receptive-expressive disorder, phonologic disorder, stuttering, and communication disorder not otherwise specified (Box B and Box C).

A phonologic disorder exists when a child does not produce the developmentally appropriate speech sounds for his or her age and dialect. It is evident in a clinical setting when the child is difficult to understand and is reluctant to repeat a word or phrase when asked. A disorder in this area is typically evaluated and diagnosed early in a child's development, owing to a general awareness that the child is not speaking normally. Programs that typically screen for delays in articulation include Head Start programs and pre-school and kindergarten programs. Speech intervention programs are also readily available to identified children through the IDEA [5].

Table 20.2 Speech or language impairment.

A communication disorder such as stuttering, impaired articulation, a language impairment, or a voice impairment that adversely affects a child's educational performance.

From Individuals with Disabilities Act; 1990. Public Law 91-230, Title 20, U.S. Code Section 1401(a)15; 1997.

BOX B DSM-1V DIAGNOSTIC CRITERIA FOR 315.31 EXPRESSIVE LANGUAGE DISORDER; 315.31 MIXED RECEPTIVE-EXPRESSIVE LANGUAGE DISORDER

(A) The scores obtained from standardized individually administered measures of expressive language development are substantially below those obtained from standardized measures of nonverbal intellectual capacity. The expressive language disturbance may be manifest clinically by symptoms that include having markedly limited vocabulary, making errors in tense, or having difficulty recalling words or producing sentences with developmentally appropriate length or complexity.

(B) Symptoms for mixed receptive-expressive language disorder include those for expressive language disorder as well as difficulty understanding words, sentences, or specific types of words, such as spatial terms.

(C) The difficulties with expressive language interfere with academic or occupational achievement or with social communication.

(D) Criteria are not met for a pervasive developmental disorder.

(E) If mental retardation, a speech-motor or sensory deficit, or environmental deprivation is present, the language difficulties are in excess of those usually associated with these problems.

Reprinted with permission from the *Diagnostic and Statistical Manual of Mental Disorders*, 4th ed. Copyright 1994 American Psychiatric Association.

BOX C DSM-IV DIAGNOSTIC CRITERIA FOR 315.39 PHONOLOGICAL DISORDER

(A) Failure to use developmentally expected speech sounds that are appropriate for age and dialect (errors in sound production, use, representation, or organization not limited to substitutions of one sound for another [use of /b for target /k/ sound] or omissions of sounds such as final consonants).

(B) Difficulties in speech sound production interfere with academic or occupational achievement or with social communication.

(C) If mental retardation, a speech-motor or sensory deficit, or environmental deprivation is present, the speech difficulties are in excess of those usually associated with these problems. (Coding note: If a speech-motor or sensory deficit or a neurological condition is present, code the condition on Axis III.)

Reprinted with permission from the *Diagnostic and Statistical Manual of Mental Disorders*, 4th ed. Copyright 1994 American Psychiatric Association.

Stuttering is a developmentally inappropriate interruption of the normal fluency and pacing of an individual's speech. It is categorized as the frequent occurrence of one or more of the following: sound and syllable repetition, sound prolongation, interjections, pauses within words, filled or unfilled pauses in speech (known as silent blocking), words produced with an excess of physical tension, and monosyllabic whole-word repetitions (e.g., 'my-my-my book').

Communication disorder not otherwise specified includes a voice disorder or other disorder that does not meet the criteria of the other communication disorder categories (Table 20.3).

When considered in relationship to a psychiatric disorder, the critical aspect of a language disorder is that oral language is a behavior that enables individuals to generate ideas and to transmit those ideas to other people in their community. When a disruption occurs in this process and a person is not understood, an emotional component takes hold. If a person experiences a significant life stressor or trauma and because of a language disorder cannot tell others accurately or process the experience symbolically, there will be some effect on his or her psychic structure. Language disorders make it difficult to interview individuals not only because of their inability to communicate but also because of their own awareness of not being understood. It may help to use alternative methods of collecting information regarding mental health needs. This could take the form of interviewing significant caretakers or using inventories and checklists such as the Children's Depression Inventory [13], the Incomplete Sentences test [14], and the Child Behavior Checklist [15].

Diagnostic Comorbidity

Comorbidity, defined as the coexistence of two or more distinct psychiatric diagnoses in the same indi-

Table 20.3 Features common to all communication disorders.

---

(1) Inadequate development of some aspect of communication

(2) Absence (in developmental types) of any demonstrable etiology of physical disorder, neurologic disorder, global mental retardation, or severe environmental deprivation

(3) Onset in childhood

(4) Long duration

(5) Clinical features resembling the functional levels of younger normal children

(6) Impairments in adaptive functioning, especially in school

(7) Tendency to run in families

(8) Predisposition toward males

(9) Multiple presumed etiologic factors

(10) Increased prevalence in younger ages

(11) Diagnosis requiring a range of standardized techniques

(12) Tendency toward certain specific associated problems, such as attention deficit hyperactivity disorder

(13) Wide range of subtype and severity

Adapted from: Baker L: Specific communication disorders. In: Garfinkel BD, Carlson GA, Weller EB, eds. *Psychiatric Disorders in Children and Adolescents*. Philadelphia: WB Saunders Co., 1990:258.

vidual, is of significant concern to clinicians when it is evident in individuals with learning or language disorders [16]. An understanding of the comorbidity between distinct diagnostic categories will assist clinicians in choosing an appropriate treatment approach, since individuals with comorbid disorders respond differently to specific therapeutic approaches.

Cantwell and Baker [17] demonstrated that approximately half of children identified with learning or language disorders also exhibited other behavioral characteristics that could lead to a psychiatric diagnosis, and in 1988, Camarata and colleagues reported a direct correlation between difficulties in oral language and behavior disorders [18]. ADHD, for example, has consistently been reported in the literature as having a high level of comorbidity with learning and language disorders. The degree of overlap has been measured as high as 92% and as low as 10%, with variation dependent on selection criteria, sampling, and measurement instruments as well as inconsistencies in the criteria used to define both ADHD and learning disorders [19,20]. Studies have shown that children with ADHD who also perform poorly in academic areas are more likely to require placement in special education programs and additional assistance to complete homework and meet the requirements of the grade-appropriate curriculum. Not all children with learning and language difficulties have ADHD, however.

There is also a correlation in children between learning or language disorders and disruptive behavior disorders. If a child is ineffective in the school environment, he or she may learn quickly to draw attention away from the learning difficulty and to his or her behavior. Comorbidities that exist between ODD, conduct disorder, and learning disorders complicate the clinician's efforts to discern the most effective course of treatment. Even if the child's behavioral symptoms are minimized through psychiatric intervention, educational issues may persist, and the child's behavior at school may not be affected by only one type of treatment. To address the multiple needs of the child, it may be necessary to involve many aspects of the child's environment, such as school, family, and community.

Comorbidity with mood disorders is more complicated. Depression is reported as a high-risk factor for children with psychiatric diagnoses of ADHD, ODD, and conduct disorder as well as learning or language disorders, thus making diagnostic conundrum inevitable.

The following are basic principles that will help clinicians gather the information needed to make accurate diagnoses that will guide the treatment of children with learning and language disorders.

(1) Past historical information and traditional developmental data are especially important in the diagnostic assessment of children. The history needs to focus on behavioral observation and the child's history of approach to printed material, interest in books, interest in listening to stories, and making up stories. Information surrounding the child's first exposure to the educational environment should include whether the child was ever excited about going to school or played school either in pretend play or with peers or family members. The caregiver should also provide information about the child's initial reaction to the school experience. In general, children present a history of looking forward to school and being interested and enthusiastic about learning. When this is not apparent, a learning difficulty may be underlying the presenting symptoms.

(2) Current history regarding the child's reaction to the educational environment is helpful to determine if a child's behavioral symptoms are related to learning issues. If school performance has been typical and there is a sudden change in the child's reaction to school, learning disorders are less likely to be an underlying factor.

(3) Collateral information from educational personnel as well as school records will augment a caregiver's description of the child's behavioral symptoms. It is helpful for the clinician to have access to any papers that the child has completed and to ask the child to complete age-appropriate tasks. Materials such as workbooks [21] that provide tasks appropriate for various age groups are available in most bookstores. Observing the child's reaction to being given an educationally based task can be not only an informational strategy but also an effective means of establishing rapport.

(4) Observation is one of the clinician's most effective diagnostic tools for evaluating a child. An understanding of the behaviors and reactions to learning of typical children can provide the benchmark for determining if learning is an issue. Beihler and Snowman have provided an excellent resource for characteristics that are related to age and grade-level expectations [22] (Table 20.4).

Objective assessments are the most common means of determining if a learning problem exists. Table 20.5 provides currently used assessment measures that can assist in diagnosing learning problems. School personnel can also help the clinician by obtaining specific assessment data through curriculum-based measurement techniques and learning style inventories.

To formulate an accurate diagnosis for children with learning disorders, the clinician must be conscious of many factors. The following basic rules for formulating a diagnosis can help clinicians decide what to treat

Table 20.4 Learning characteristics of school-age children.

Kindergarten (ages 5–6 years)
- Skillful with language and like to use it
- Talk a lot and like to talk in front of a group
- Stick to their own language rules (e.g., 'Mommy holded the doggie and I patted him')
- Competence encouraged by interaction, interest, opportunities, urging, adoration, and signs of affection

Primary School (1st through 3rd Grade)
- Eager to learn
- Like to talk; more ability in speech than in writing
- Have a literal interpretation of rules (may tend to be tattletales)

Elementary School (4th through 6th Grade)
- Gender differences become evident in specific cognitive abilities
- Differences in cognitive (learning) styles become apparent

Junior High (7th through 9th Grade)
- Transition from operational to formal thought
- Transition from the moralities of constraint to cooperation
- Political thinking more abstract, liberal (flexible?), and knowledgeable

High School (10th through 12th Grade)
- Increasingly capable of engaging in formal thought, although may not use process without prompting
- May engage in unrestrained theorizing
- Become overwhelmed with the awareness of life's possibilities
- May exhibit adolescent egocentrism

Beihler RF, Snowman J: *Psychology Applied to Teaching*, 6th ed. Boston: Houghton Mifflin, 1990:98.

Table 20.5 Commonly used achievement tests (arranged by type).

Group Administered
California Achievement Test, Iowa Test of Basic Skills, Metropolitan Achievement Test, Stanford Achievement Test, Science Research Associates (SRA) Achievement Series
Individually Administered
Comprehensive
Basic Achievement Skills Individual-Screener (BASIS)
Kaufman Test of Educational Achievement
Weschler Individual Achievement Test-Second Edition (WIAT-II)
Woodcock-Johnson Psychoeducational Battery
Specific
Durrell Analysis of Reading Difficulty Third Edition (DARD)
Stanford Diagnostic Reading Test, Fourth Edition (SDRT-4)
Boehm Test of Basic Concepts, Third Edition (BOEHM-3)
Stanford Diagnostic Mathematics Test, Fourth Edition (SDRT-4)

- start with the diagnosis that is the most treatable and has the best prognosis.

Taking all of these factors into consideration provides the foundation upon which the clinical decision making process can be built. As children grow and their disorder become more complicated this basic strategy will continue to guide the clinical process.

first, plan further diagnostic efforts, and determine the likely prognosis [23]:

- disorders due to general medical conditions or cognitive disorders preempt all other diagnoses that could produce the same symptoms;
- use the fewest possible diagnoses to explain the presenting symptoms;
- consider first those disorders that have been present the longest;
- family history is a primary guide;

References

1. American Psychiatric Association: *Diagnostic and Statistical Manual of Mental Disorders*, 4th ed revised. Washington, DC: American Psychiatric Association, 2000.
2. Singh NN, Beale IL, eds.: *Learning Disabilities: Nature, Theory, and Treatment*. New York: Springer-Verlag, 1992.
3. Swanson HL, Harris KR, Graham S, eds.: *Handbook of Learning Disabilities*. New York: Guilford Press, 2003.
4. *Children with Specific Learning Disabilities Act of 1969*. Public Law 91–230. 91st U.S. Congress; 1969.
5. *Education for All Handicapped Children Act of 1975*. Public Law 94–142. 94th U.S. Congress; 1975.
6. *Individuals with Disabilities Education Act of 1990*. Public Law 91–230, Title 20, U.S. Code Section 1401(a)15; 1997.
7. *Individuals with Disabilities Education Act of 2004*. Public Law, Title, U.S.

8. American Psychiatric Association: *Diagnostic and Statistical Manual of Mental Disorders.* 4th ed. Washington, DC: American Psychiatric Association, 1997.

9. Lerner JW: *Learning Disabilities: Theories, Diagnosis, and Teaching Strategies,* 5th ed. Chicago: Houghton Mifflin Company, 1989.

10. Felton RH, Wood FB, Brown IS, *et al.*: Separate verbal memory and naming deficits in attention deficit disorders and reading disability. *Brain Lang* 1987; **31**(1): 171–184.

11. Mercer CD, Mercer AR: *Teaching Students with Learning Problems.* Columbus, OH: Charles E. Merrill, 1985.

12. Lovinger SL, Brandell ME, Seestedt-Stanford L: *Language Learning Disabilities: A New and Practical Approach for Those Who Work with Children and Their Families.* New York: Continuum Press; 1991.

13. Kovaks M: *Children's Depression Inventory.* University of Pittsburgh, PA: Western Psychiatric Institute and Clinic, 1985.

14. Lanyon BP, Lanyon R: *Incomplete Sentences Task: Manual.* Chicago: Stoelling, 1980.

15. Achenbach TM: *Child Behavior Checklist for Ages 4–16.* San Antonio, TX: The Psychological Corporation, 1981.

16. Bird HR, Gould MS, Staghezza BM: Patterns of diagnostic comorbidity in a community sample of children aged 9 through 16 years. *J Am Acad Child Adolesc Psychiatry* 1993; **32**:2.

17. Cantwell DP, Baker L: *Psychiatric and Developmental Disorders in Children with Communication Disorders.* Washington, DC: American Psychiatric Association, 1991.

18. Camarata SM, Hughes CA, Ruhl KL: Mild/moderate behaviorally disordered students: A population at risk for language disorders. *Lang Speech Hear Serv Schools* 1988; **19**:191–200.

19. Biederman J, Newcom J, Spich S: Comorbidity of attention-deficit disorder with conduct, depressive, anxiety and other disorders. *Am J Psychiatry* 1991; **148**(5): 564–577.

20. Maser JD, Cloninger CR: Comorbidity of anxiety and mood disorders: Introduction and overview. In: Maser JD, Cloninger CR, eds. *Comorbidity of Mood and Anxiety Disorders.* Washington, DC: American Psychiatric Press, 1990.

21. The Original Workbook Series. Grand Rapids, MI: School Zone Publishing Co; 1990.

22. Beihler RF, Snowman J: *Psychology Applied to Teaching.* Sixth Edition. Boston: Houghton Mifflin, 1990..

23. Morrison J: *DSM-IV Made Easy: The Clinician's Guide to Diagnosis.* New York: Guilford Press, 1995.

21

The Autistic Spectrum Disorders

Tom Owley, Bennett L. Leventhal, Edwin H. Cook, Jr.

Introduction

The autism spectrum disorders (ASDs) are a group of clinical syndromes that have varying degrees of two fundamental elements: developmental delays and developmental deviations. Two-thirds of cases have evidence of atypical development before 12 months, and one-third of cases have a regression in speech and language before 18 months. Onset should occur before 30 months for all but childhood disintegrative disorder. The core syndrome includes deficits in social interactions and communication, along with presence of stereotyped behaviors, activities and interests. The prototypic ASD is autistic disorder. The other ASDs, including Rett disorder, childhood disintegrative disorder, Asperger disorder, and pervasive developmental disorder not otherwise specified (PDD NOS), share many of the core features of autistic disorder.

Epidemiology

ASDs are relatively common, with prevalence rates in the range of two per 1000 children [1]. Review of studies across cultures reveals similar rates of autistic disorder and consistent phenomenology, and ASDs are seen throughout all socioeconomic levels [2,3].

Autistic disorder is four times more prevalent in males than females [2,4]. The other ASDs seem to be similar to autistic disorder with a greater ratio of affected males, except in the case of Rett disorder, which is diagnosed almost exclusively in females.

About half of children with autistic disorder are mentally retarded. Overall, intelligence levels range from profoundly retarded to above average in autistic disorder and the other ASDs [2,5]. A notable exception is in childhood disintegrative disorder, in which all affected children are mentally retarded [6]. In addition, follow-up studies of autistic disorder have demonstrated that mental retardation, when present, persists from the time of diagnosis onward [7]. Intelligence quotients (IQ) tend to be stable over time and are felt to be one of the most important predictors of outcome in autism [8]. Relative strengths lie in visuospatial skills and rote memory skills [9]. A small number of autistic individuals have phenomenal abilities in particular areas such as in memory, calendar calculation or artistic endeavors. These so-called 'savant' talents are also seen in individuals with other developmental disorders [10].

Etiology and Pathophysiology

At this time, the precise etiology and pathogenesis of ASDs is unknown. However, the continued search for etiologies has led to an enormous shift in perspectives over the past two decades. There is now overwhelming evidence for a strong, yet complex, genetic contribution to this neurodevelopmental disease process.

Early biological hypotheses focused on neurotransmitter abnormalities as a cause of autistic disorder, starting with Freedman's early observation of hyperserotonemia in many individuals with autism [11]. This has been replicated numerous times [12], proving to be one of the most enduring biological findings in psychiatry. Hyperserotonemia is most likely due to genetic variations leading to abnormalities in the functioning of proteins involved in serotonergic regulation, such as the serotonin transporter and serotonin 5-HT$_{2A}$ receptor, which are expressed in both the developing brain and platelet [13,14].

Since the ASDs are often (~50%) associated with mental retardation, the search for etiology has included common factors. For example, individuals with fragile X syndrome are considered to have a

Clinical Child Psychiatry, Second Edition. Edited by W.M. Klykylo and J.L. Kay

higher prevalence rate of autism [15]. While fragile X syndrome may account for only a small number of cases of PDD, most children with fragile X syndrome have an ASD [16]. Other genetic disorders have been associated with ASDs, including duplications of the proximal portion of the long arm of chromosome 15 [17,18,], phenylketonuria [19], and tuberous sclerosis [20]. Perhaps the most progress has occurred in relation to finding a genetic basis for Rett disorder: mutations in the gene, MECP2, encoding X-linked methyl-CpG-binding protein 2 (MeCP2) have been identified as the cause of more than 80% of classic cases of Rett syndrome [21].

Twin and family studies have yielded some useful information about genetic aspects of autism. Concordance in monozygotic twin pairs has ranged from 60% to over 90% while dizygotic twin pairs in these studies have generally found a concordance rate similar to that found in siblings of unaffected children [22,23]. When considered as a spectrum disorder, twin studies suggest that at least 92% of monozygotic twin pairs are concordant for at least milder but similar deficits in the social and communication realms, compared to a 10% rate in these studies for dizygotic twin pairs [24]. A range of 30% to 75% of autistic individuals have nonspecific neurologic abnormalities including: poor coordination, hypo- or hypertonicity, choreiform movements, abnormal posture and gait, tremor, and myoclonic jerking [25]. About 25% of autistic individuals develop seizures or EEG abnormalities by the end of adolescence [26]. This phenomenon has been highly correlated with mental retardation and may be more correlated with mental impairment than the presence of PDD or autism [26,27]. Seizures with onset in adolescence often generalize, but are typically infrequent [28].

Using direct neuroradiologic or neuropathologic evidence or well-documented lesions from other cases with specific neuroanatomical or neurophysiological abnormalities, there has been a search for a lesion that underlies autism. Arguments for very specific, highly localized deficits (e.g., in facial recognition or processing of gaze) have been made as well as those that propose broader deficits in information processing and cognition that have less clear implications for neurobiology. Whatever the primary deficit or deficits in autism, these deficits must affect the way in which a child acquires information and skills from very early in development. In addition, the hypothesized deficits must allow for relative sparing of some domains (e.g., early gross motor development, sequence of development of syntax and lexical semantics, object permanence).

There is evidence for neuropathologic changes in ASDs. Postmortem studies have shown abnormalities in the cerebellum [29,30], hippocampus, and amygdala [30]. More recently, small studies have found a reduction in the size of cortical minicolumns, as well as an increased number of these minicolumns in both subjects with autism [31] and Asperger disorder [32].

In terms of structural studies of the brain in subjects with autism, a consistent finding is that young subjects with autism have larger brains than matched controls; more precisely, there appears to be an acceleration in brain growth that subsequently slows by late childhood [33]. Magnetic resonance imaging (MRI) studies have shown cerebellar hypoplasia in some but not all studies [34,35]. Other studies have found decreased cross-sectional area of the area dentata [36], increased amygdala volumes [33] as well as differences in cortical asymmetries [37]. MRI studies have revealed increased brain and lateral ventricular volume in autistic disorder [38].

Functional imaging studies have also been undertaken in autism. Positron-emission tomography (PET) revealed generalized hypermetabolism in one [39], but not another study [40]. Using PET scans on patients with infantile spasms, 10 of 14 children that had bitemporal hypometabolism met criteria for an ASD at follow up [41]. The same group [42] found asymmetries in serotonin synthesis in the brains of children with autism, as well as a global increase in cerebral serotonin synthesis capacity in children with ASDs (versus controls that show a steady decrease with age towards adult levels) [43]. Subjects with ASD show decreased activation in the amygdala while undergoing a facial processing task [44]. Magnetic resonance spectroscopy (MRS) revealed decreased levels of phosphocreatine and αATP in dorsolateral frontal cortex [45].

Diagnosis

Phenomenology

The central feature of these disorders is disturbance of social development, including difficulty in developing meaningful attachments and social reciprocity [46,47]. There is clearly some variation in the clinical presentation (Table 21.1). Typically, a child with autistic disorder has abnormal patterns of eye contact and facial expression. The child with autism is less apt to engage in these behaviors, seeming to be less capable of coordinating social cues. They seem to lack empathy or the ability to perceive other's moods or anticipate others' responses. This may lead the child to act in a socially inappropriate manner or lack the social responsiveness

Table 21.1 DSM IV diagnosis of autistic disorder and other pervasive developmental disorders. Reprinted with permission from the Diagnostic and Statistical Manual of Mental Disorders, Copyright 2000. American Psychiatric Association.

	Autistic disorder	Rett disorder	Childhood disintegrative disorder	Asperger disorder	PDD NOS
Age of onset	Delays or abnormal functioning in social interaction, language, or play by age three years; 6 of 12 of criteria below must be met at time of diagnosis	Apparently normal prenatal development; apparently normal motor development for first five months; normal head circumference at birth; deceleration of head growth between 5 months and 48 months	Apparently normal development for at least the first two years of birth; clinically significant loss of previously acquired skills before age 10	No clinically significant delay in language, cognitive development or development of age-appropriate self-help skills, adaptive behavior, and environment in childhood	This diagnosis is to be used in cases of pervasive impairment in social interaction and communication, with presence of stereotyped behaviors or interests when criteria for a specific PDD are not met
Social interaction	Qualitative impairment in social interaction, as manifested by at least two of the following: (a) marked impairment in the use of multiple nonverbal behaviors, i.e., eye-to-eye gaze, facial expression (b) failure to develop peer relationships appropriate to developmental level (c) lack of spontaneous seeking to share enjoyment, interests or achievements with other people (d) lack of social or emotional reciprocity	Loss of social engagement early in the course (although often social interaction develops later)	Qualitative impairment along with loss of social skills or adaptive behavior	Same as autistic disorder	
Communication	Qualitative impairments of communication as manifested by at least one of the following: (a) delay in, or total lack of, the	Severely impaired expressive and receptive language development with	Qualitative impairment in communication along with	No clinically significant delay in language (single words	

Table 21.1 *Continued*

	Autistic disorder	Rett disorder	Childhood disintegrative disorder	Asperger disorder	PDD NOS
	development of spoken language (without attempt to compensate with gesture) (b) marked impairment in initiating or sustaining a conversation with others in individuals with adequate speech (c) stereotyped and repetitive use of language or idiosyncratic language (d) lack of varied, spontaneous make-believe or imitative play appropriate to developmental level	severe psychomotor retardation	loss of expressive or receptive language	by age two years and communicative phrases by three years)	
Restricted and Repetitive Interests	Restricted, repetitive and stereotyped patterns of behavior, as manifested by one of the following: (a) preoccupation with one or more stereotyped or restricted patterns of interest that is abnormal in either intensity or focus (b) apparently inflexible adherence to nonfunctional routines or rituals (c) stereotyped and repetitive motor mannerisms (d) persistent preoccupation with parts of objects	Loss of previously acquired purposeful hand movements with the subsequent development of stereotyped hand movements; appearance of poorly coordinated gait or trunk movements	Restricted, repetitive and stereotyped patterns of behavior with loss of bowel or bladder control, play motor skills previously acquired	Same as autistic disorder	
Exclusions	Disturbance not better accounted for by Rett disorder or childhood disintegrative disorder		Disturbance not better accounted for by another PDD or schizophrenia	Criteria are not met for another PDD or schizophrenia	

needed to succeed in social settings. Because of these difficulties, there may be a subsequent difficulty in developing close, meaningful relationships. However, some autistic youth eventually develop warm, friendly relationships with family while their relationships with peers lag behind considerably.

Another area of difficulty is in the acquisition and proper use of language for communication. It is estimated that only about half of children with autism develop functional speech. If a child with autism does begin to speak, their babble is decreased in quantity and lacking in vocal experimentation. On the other hand, some children with autism are even loquacious; however, their speech tends to be repetitious and focused on preoccupations rather than aimed at maintaining a dialogue. People with autistic disorder commonly use stereotyped speech including immediate and delayed echolalia, pronoun reversal, and neologisms. Speech usage is idiosyncratic, may consist of concrete and poorly constructed grammar may lack social meaning, and often lacks in inference and imagination. The delivery of speech is frequently abnormal with atypical tone, pitch, and prosody (accent and cadence).

Individuals with autistic disorder frequently engage in unusual patterns of behavior. Most people with autistic disorder also resist, or have significant difficulty with, new experiences or transitions. At younger mental ages, they often perform stereotyped motor acts again and again, such as hand clapping or flapping, or peculiar finger movements. These movements often occur at the periphery of their vision near the face. Some children with autism engage in self-injurious behaviors including biting or striking themselves, or banging their heads. Self-injury is most likely to occur in children with autism with moderate, severe, or profound mental retardation, but is also found in children with autism without mental retardation [48]. Their play only occasionally involves traditional toys and typically includes unusual preoccupations. Individuals with autistic disorder seem to have unusual sensitivity to some sensory experiences, particularly sounds.

Other problems in autistic disorder and other ASDs include deficits in shifting of attention and joint attention [49,50]. Joint attention is normally present by 12 months. At that developmental level, it is characterized by children shifting their gaze to follow verbal and nonverbal cues of the parent to look at the same object together. Many children also have symptoms of hyperactivity and difficulty sustaining attention, but these should be distinguished from the joint attentional dysfunction found in all patients with autistic disorder.

Examples of joint attention include social exchanges that include pointing, referential gaze, and gestures showing interest.

Asperger disorder and autistic disorder share many common features. Asperger remarked that the children he studied began to speak at about the same time as other children and eventually gained a full complement of language and syntax. However, he noted exhaustive focus on particular topics. Asperger also described that the children he studied had difficulty in social reciprocity, and focused on certain interests excessively [51]. DSM-IV diagnosis of Asperger disorder is made if criteria for social deficits and repetitive stereotyped interests and behaviors of autistic disorder are met, but language is normal at three years of age by history, and full criteria for autistic disorder are not met.

Rett disorder is a developmental disorder that occurs almost exclusively in females and typically differs substantially from autistic disorder after the toddler stage. Typically, the child with Rett disorder has an uneventful pre- and perinatal course that continues through at least the first six months. With onset of the disease, there is typically deceleration of head growth, usually between five months and four years of age. In toddlerhood, the manifestations can be similar to autistic disorder in that there is frequently impairment in language and social development along with presence of stereotyped motor movements. In particular, there is loss of acquired language, restricted interest in social contact or interactions, and the start of hand wringing, clapping or tapping in the midline of the body. Purposeful hand movement is typically lost. Another common symptom is hyperventilation. The child with Rett disorder actually may improve in social capabilities as time passes while progressively deteriorating in cognitive and motor function. The disorder is relatively easily differentiated from other ASDs after the child has reached the age of four or five years [52]. Mutations in the gene MECP2 have been identified as the cause of more than 80% of classic cases of Rett syndrome [21]. Different mutations are likely responsible for much of the phenotypic variation seen in the disorder [53], including cases with preserved speech and normal head circumference [54].

Childhood disintegrative disorder and autistic disorder have some similarities in that they both involve deficits in social interaction and communication, as well as repetitive behaviors. However, the symptoms of childhood disintegrative disorder appear abruptly or over a few months' time after two years or more of normal development. There is generally no prior serious illness or insult although a few cases have been linked to certain organic brain ailments such as measles encephalitis, leukodystrophies, or other diseases. With onset of childhood disintegrative disorder, the child loses previously mastered cognitive, language, and motor skills and regresses to such a degree that there is loss of bowel and bladder control [6,55]. Children with childhood disintegrative disorder tend to lose abilities that would normally allow them to take care of themselves, and their motor activity contains fewer complex, repetitive behaviors than in autism. Some children with this disorder experience regression that occurs over a period of time and then becomes stable. Another group of children afflicted with childhood disintegrative disorder have a poorer outcome with onset of focal neurological findings, and seizures, in the face of a worsening course and greater motor impairment [56]. The vast majority of children with this disorder deteriorate to a severe level of mental retardation with a few retaining selected abilities in specific areas. Differential diagnosis of childhood disintegrative disorder requires obtaining a particularly thorough developmental history, history of course of illness, and neurological evaluation to rule out disorders including acquired epileptic aphasia. (See Differential Diagnosis.)

Pervasive developmental disorder not otherwise specified (PDD NOS) or atypical autism should be reserved for cases in which there are qualitative impairments in reciprocal social development, communication, and imaginative and flexible interests, but criteria for a specific pervasive developmental disorder described above are not met. It is important in the education of parents, teachers, and colleagues to be clear that PDD NOS is closely related to autistic disorder, since many families that have been given diagnoses of autistic disorder and PDD NOS have the mistaken impression that this represents strong diagnostic disagreement between clinicians.

Differential Diagnosis

Diagnosis of autistic disorder and other pervasive developmental disorders requires distinguishing amongst several disorders that consist of deviations in socialization, language, and play. One systematic approach would be to examine the course of the patient from birth, and in so doing, determine if there had ever been a period of normal development. Disorders to be considered in the differential diagnosis include developmental language disorder, mental retardation, acquired epileptic aphasia (Landau–Kleffner syndrome), schizophrenia, selective mutism, psychosocial deprivation, as well as other conditions listed in Table 21.2.

Table 21.2 Differential diagnosis of autistic disorder and other PDDs.

Developmental language disorder
Mental retardation
Acquired epileptic aphasia (Landau–Kleffner syndrome)
Fragile X syndrome
Chromosome 15 q11-13 duplication
Schizophrenia
Selective mutism
Psychosocial deprivation
Hearing impairment
Visual impairment
Traumatic brain injury
Dementia
Metabolic disorders (inborn errors of metabolism, e.g., phenylketonuria)

Children with developmental language delay can appear to have symptoms related to autistic disorder at early ages. Because of their language deficits, these children may seem to have communication problems, and may be socially immature. However, children with language delay use relatively normal patterns of language, engage in imaginative play, and demonstrate appropriate attachment behaviors and social interactions with family and friends [57]. These children do not tend to have obsessive interests, or restricted and repetitive behaviors like those seen in children with autism. They also do not respond unusually to sensory experiences as children with autism frequently do [58].

Approximately one-half of severely and profoundly mentally retarded children have symptoms consistent with a pervasive developmental disorder, and it is unclear whether this is due to a high rate of pervasive developmental disorders in this group or a consequence of severe and profound mental retardation having some phenomenological overlap with ASD in terms of the presence of developmental delays. It is useful for planning interventions to add the additional diagnosis of a pervasive developmental disorder, if present. Individuals with profound retardation without a pervasive developmental disorder have social skills expected for their mental age. Many of the social and communication skills not seen in profoundly retarded individuals with autistic disorder, such as eye-to-eye gaze, are typically seen as early as 6–8 weeks of life in normally developing infants. Acquired epileptic aphasia (Landau–Kleffner syndrome) is very rare compared to autistic disorder and other ASDs. A high index of suspicion for this disorder is raised by the loss of phrase speech after the age of 24 months with EEG confirmation. Since the typical regression in pervasive developmental disorder occurs before 18 months, children who regress in language skills between 18 months and 30 months should also be evaluated by EEG, preferably with unmedicated sleep to rule out an atypical acquired epileptic aphasia syndrome. Diagnosis of acquired epileptic aphasia is important because language may return after anticonvulsant or corticosteroid treatment [59].

Schizophrenia is differentiated from autism on the basis of symptom presentation. While some children with autism may have disorganized speech or behavior, they will not exhibit the hallucinations or delusions that characterize childhood schizophrenia. In terms of thought processes, higher functioning autistic people tend to be ruminative, and may be so preoccupied as to appear illogical or thought disordered. Again, however, delusions and hallucinations will not be present, except in rare cases where older adolescents or young adults with autism develop schizophrenia.

In selective mutism, the child is unable to speak in certain situations. As in autistic disorder, the child may seem socially isolative and nonresponsive to his environment outside of the home. The child with selective mutism child usually can converse with family members and engage in imaginative play. Some selectively mute children do have articulation problems, and/or language delay, but do not have deviations of speech such as those found in children with autism [60].

Children with severe psychosocial deprivation can present with broad language deficiencies, stunted social development, and odd motor movements and habits [61]. However, this triad is qualitatively distinct from that seen in autistic disorder. Fortunately, many children subjected to extreme neglect, even over periods of years, can resume the developmental process at a rapid rate when exposed to nurturing and stimulating surroundings [62]. A child with a significant abuse and/or neglect history, as well as other children, should not be presumed to have autistic disorder unless a diligent assessment as described below has been completed.

Evaluation

The diagnosis of autism is carried out by gathering information about the child's historical background, behavior, and cognitive abilities. Appropriate sources for this information include parents, teachers, and anyone who has had meaningful contact with the child. Other means of obtaining needed information include direct observation of the child and standardized assessment. A crucial step in evaluating developmental disorders lies in procuring a solid account of the developmental history. Special heed should be taken with regard to developmental phases of language, social interactions, and play [46]. Also, an investigation of any chronic illnesses or illnesses with a neurological bearing in the child should be performed, as well the medical history of the family. Clinicians should inquire about family history of neurological disease, psychiatric disorder, history of developmental delay, social, language, and learning problems (Table 21.3).

There are structured interviews available for use in evaluating children specifically for autism that help clinicians collect and organize historical information in a reliable manner. One such instrument is the Autism Diagnostic Interview-Revised (ADI-R), which is a standardized, semistructured interview that can be administered to parents to help determine if the child has an ASD [47].

An essential piece of the overall evaluation is gained through direct observation of the child. Ideally, this should be done in a variety of settings to obtain an overall view of the child's behaviors and functioning under differing environmental conditions. The Autism Diagnostic Observation Schedule (ADOS) is recommended to structure observation of children, adolescents, and adults with suspected autism [63]. There is also a variety of other instruments available for evaluative purposes, including the Childhood Autism Rating Scale [64], and the Autism Behavior Checklist [65]. Another useful instrument is the Aberrant Behavior Checklist – Community Version (ABC-CV), which is useful for following response of irritability and hyperactivity to interventions [66].

A complete physical examination, including a thorough neurological exam, is an essential component of any evaluation. Medical and dental problems that could be contributing to, or exacerbating, a child's psychiatric symptoms are important to identify and treat. Overall physical health should be assessed and particular attention should be paid to those findings that could be related to pervasive developmental disorders. For instance, cardiac and other congenital physical anomalies should be noted, and a skin (visual and Wood's lamp exam) and dysmorphology exam should be done to search for lesions consistent with genetic, metabolic, or structural disorders. All children with speech delay or articulation problems should have audiological testing, as even subtle hearing loss can

Table 21.3 Suggested components of an evaluation of suspected autism.

History
Sources: parents, teachers, other caregivers, anyone
    with regular meaningful contact
Developmental history
    Semistructured interview with primary caregiver(s)
        strongly suggested: Autism Diagnostic
        Interview-Revised (ADI-R)
    Past medical history
    Family history
Examination
    Direct observation of child's social,
        communication, and imaginative skills
    Autism Diagnostic Observation Schedule (ADOS)
        suggested
    Psychological testing (nonverbal and verbal
        intellectual testing)
    Speech and language evaluation
    Tests of adaptive functioning, e.g., Vineland
        Adaptive Behavior Scales
    Vocational assessment
    Physical examination including particular attention
        to the neurological examination, dysmorphology
        examination, and examination of the skin
        (preferably with a Wood's lamp to rule out
        hypopigmented macules of tuberous sclerosis)
    Audiological testing
Laboratory testing
    Lead level
    Quantitative urinary amino acids
    Other tests depending on clinical situation
    EEG if suspicion of history of possible seizures or
        speech regression after 24 months
    Chromosomal analysis and fragile X DNA testing
        if dysmorphology, family history of
        chromosomal disorders, or as part of genetic
        counseling
    MRI if findings in history or examination to
        suggest potential therapeutic yield
    Other laboratory testing based on findings from
        history and physical examination (e.g., organic
        acids, thyroid function tests, etc.)

affect development. Vision testing should be performed if there is any suggestion of visual deficit. There are no specific, diagnostic laboratory tests for autism. A high index of suspicion should be maintained for seizure disorder. Specialized laboratory tests are warranted only with specific indications but these might include chromosomal analysis, amino

acid studies, and/or EEG. Although one-quarter of children have nonspecific findings on structural neuroimaging scans, MRI should only be performed if there are findings from history and physical examination that suggest a potentially treatable structural lesion.

Chromosomal studies are indicated for children with history and physical examination suggestive of fragile X syndrome or other specific chromosomal abnormalities. Although genetic counseling, including chromosomal analysis to exclude fragile X syndrome, interstitial 15q 11q 13 duplications and other chromosomal anomalies is most obviously indicated for families considering a subsequent pregnancy, 25% of the boys born to maternal aunts of children with fragile X syndrome will have fragile X syndrome. Currently, there is no specific treatment for fragile X syndrome or duplications of the Prader–Willi/Angelman syndrome region of chromosome 15, but chromosomal testing will have implications beyond genetic counseling if treatments are developed for these disorders in the future.

Psychological Testing

Various psychological instruments can be administered to develop a detailed picture of a child's intellectual performance. Tests should never stand alone as conclusive evidence of a child's skills. The most useful measures are those that yield data about adaptive functioning, language skills, and intelligence. The Vineland Adaptive Behavior Scales [67,68] provide valuable information about adaptive functioning while language and communication abilities can be assessed using a number of specific measures. Intelligence tests used in this population should allow for separating out verbal from nonverbal scores, as there is usually a disparity between these values in people with autism (e.g., Merrill–Palmer Scale [69], Leiter International Performance Scale [70], Bayley Scales of Infant Development [71], and Differential Abilities Scales [72]).

Course and Natural History

As a child with autism grows older, some aspects of the disorder also change. Those with a lower mental age may be completely socially removed, with virtually no speech or only echolalic speech, motor stereotypies, and little ability to adapt to change. As a child enters the school years, the echolalic speech patterns sometimes lessen and the child may begin speaking a bit more spontaneously. During the school years, the child may begin to tolerate play near other children, and there can be formation of rudimentary social relations in less impaired individuals. Many bothersome preschool behaviors often later subside. Further, the child with autism learns to adjust to regular demands or expectations placed on him. Peculiar interests and ritualistic behaviors, however, can and often do persist into adolescence and adulthood. With the advent of adolescence, a small number of children with autism demonstrate significant improvement in symptoms, and this is indicative of a good outcome in the adult years. In some adolescents, however, there is an increase in aggression with the onset of puberty; if this occurs, it is worthwhile to have an EEG done, as there is an increased possibility of seizures in children with autism in this age group, and significant regression may accompany this epileptogenic activity. However, clinical, seizures with this late onset are typically few in number and the behavioral symptoms respond to psychotropic medication. Aspects of puberty such as sexual drive and menstruation are handled without much difficulty by many autistic adolescents with appropriate education. Some autistic individuals, however, do not understand the social implications of public masturbation or exhibitionism and engage in these behaviors. Higher-functioning, autistic adolescents may become aware of the fact that they differ significantly from their peers. They may even develop some interest in others and a desire to make friendships, but they lack the 'know-how' to accomplish this. This may lead to demoralization and even depression. In terms of language, receptive and expressive abilities can gradually improve over the adolescent years [28,48,73–76].

Follow-up studies of children with autism into adulthood show that approximately two-thirds remain seriously impaired and are incapable of caring for their own needs. In fact, the vast majority of these individuals live in long-term institutional settings during their adult years, although there is a positive trend toward placement in group homes in the community. Between 5% and 17% of autistic adults are able to work with minimal support. In spite of social improvement in about half of children with autism over periods of years, most autistic individuals have abnormal social relationships. Except for higher functioning individuals, it is unusual for an autistic adult to marry or sustain a long-term sexual relationship. Outcome in autism is largely determined by IQ and language abilities, with IQ being the most powerful predictor. Good or fair outcomes are almost always associated with full-scale IQs of greater than 60. Acquisition of useful speech by five years of age is another important predictor of positive outcome. Even when an individual has an IQ and language abilities within a relatively normal range, there is nearly always residual social impairment that is persistent into adulthood.

Goals of Treatment

Initially, attempts were made to treat autism via psychoanalytic interventions. There was little evidence that these treatments were of benefit. Behavioral treatments brought a great deal of hope for the prognosis of autism based on the premise that behavior is learned. The use of behavioral methods has not had a curative effect on autism, though it has beneficial effects [77]. Unfortunately, behaviors learned by children with autism in one particular setting are not necessarily carried over to other contexts or retained well [78].

The use of a variety of treatments and educational interventions are thought to be most useful in treatment of individuals with autistic disorder. Additionally, autistic disorder is recognized as a chronic disorder with a changing course requiring long-term intervention with implementation of various treatments at any given point in time. Given that there is no current cure for autistic disorder or the other pervasive developmental disorders, goals of treatment should encompass short-term and long-term needs of the individual and his/her family. Rutter has defined goals for treatment in terms of four quintessential aims. These include the following:

(1) the advancement of development, particularly regarding cognition, language, and socialization;
(2) the promotion of learning and problem-solving;
(3) the reduction of behaviors that impede the learning process;
(4) the assistance of families coping with autism.

Since these goals are broad, it is useful to separate these goals into immediate and long-term needs. Each goal likely will require a distinct scheme of its own. It is best to maintain an autistic child as an outpatient because institutionalization may hinder a child's ability to learn means of functioning in normal society. This can usually be accomplished, except in times of extreme stress or need, during which a child could benefit from respite care or brief hospitalization. Effective treatment often entails setting appropriate expectations for the child and adjusting the child's environment to foster success [46] (Table 21.4).

Approach to Treatment

Since the individual with ASD often requires diverse treatment and services simultaneously during his or

Table 21.4 Goals for treatment.

Advancement of normal development, particularly
  regarding cognition, language, and socialization
Promotion of learning and problem-solving
Reduction of behaviors that impede learning
Assistance of families coping with autistic disorder
Treatment of comorbid psychiatric disorders

---

her lifetime [79], an imperative role of the primary clinician is that of coordinator of services. Frequent visits with the child and his caretakers initially allows the clinician to assess the individual needs of the child while establishing a therapeutic alliance. An effective approach often calls for the services of a number of professionals working in a multidisciplinary fashion. This group may include psychiatrists, pediatricians, psychologists, pediatric neurologists, special educators, speech and language therapists, social workers, and other specialized therapists.

Psychosocial Interventions

Some of the most beneficial interventions for children with autism have been achieved through the educational process. With the passage of the Education for All Handicapped Children Act of 1975 (Public Law 94-142), all handicapped children, including those with autistic disorder, were guaranteed the right to a free, appropriate public education. This right was guaranteed notwithstanding the severity or nature of the child's disability. Further, this law mandated that the education of a handicapped child must take place in the least restrictive environment while still meeting the needs of the child. Improvement in the educational experience afforded children with autistic disorder in recent years has resulted in fewer children requiring long stays in institutional settings [80]. With regard to lower-functioning or severely mentally retarded children with autism, no single educational approach has been identified as superlative in improving a specific area of weakness.

A debate has been ongoing during the last several years regarding the issue of mainstreaming of handicapped children within the schools. Although there has been a move toward implementation of mainstreaming, many children with autism remain in homogeneous classrooms with children of similar needs. Currently, there is little data on the performance of children with autism within various stages of integration. It is generally felt that few children with autism will be able to function academically or behaviorally at

their best if placed totally within a regular classroom setting with no other supports. However, there can be distinct advantages in the placement of mild-to-moderately functioning children with autistic disorder in a regular classroom for at least part of the day. These include social exposure to children who are not on the autistic spectrum, and greater intellectual stimulation than is sometimes available in highly structured, special education classrooms.

Curricula that encourage and teach appropriate communication can be beneficial to the majority of children with autism. This can be done individually with even very young children, and also can involve teaching parents and others how to encourage communication in an autistic child. Behavioral techniques derived from operant conditioning theory are used routinely by teachers and clinicians working with children with autism. Reinforcing positive behaviors, failing to reinforce unwanted behaviors, and using simple techniques to replace an undesirable behavior with a more adaptive one are standard behavioral procedures. Organizing a milieu that is predictable and promotes understanding and learning for the child with autism often alleviates the need for intensive behavior programs.

Success has been achieved in placing adults with autism in jobs and workshops in the community. How successful one is in securing a job for an autistic adult depends on the resources in the community, and the ability of the adult's parents or others to advocate for them. Work placement and training as well as encouragement and consistent support on the job have contributed to success in the workplace for the individual with autism.

Depending on the specific needs of the individual autistic child, a child can benefit from many different therapies or interventions. Among these are speech and language therapy, occupational therapy, and physical therapy. Some programs offer art and or music therapy as a means of encouraging communication and self-expression. Brief individual psychotherapies may be helpful to those who are verbal and have a focused problem or are experiencing symptoms of anxiety or depression. Social skills groups or training may be especially beneficial for higher-functioning children, adolescents, and adults. These interventions can serve to give the individual social experience in a positive, supportive setting.

Doctor–Patient Relationship

As with any clinical relationship, respect for the patient is the cornerstone of assessment and treatment. Many of the difficulties faced by persons with autistic disorder are not a consequence of their lack of empathy but rather a function of the lack of empathy concerning their unique deficits by those around them. In many ways, this stems from countertransference issues towards people with culturally defined 'defects' [81]. It is essential that the clinician keep in mind that every person, regardless of presence or absence of any diagnosis, is sensitive to their treatment by others. One must be cognizant that drives for mastery and development of autonomy are not reduced by the presence of an ASD.

Literally all families can benefit from supportive measures from their child's clinician, and some families need structured family therapy involving either their primary clinician or another health professional skilled in this area. Helping families deal with frustration, disappointment, fear and ambivalence with regard to their handicapped family member is essential. Other crucial steps include aiding families in arranging for special services or respite care in addition to providing behavior management techniques and emotional support. Many individuals with autistic disorder and families draw support and services through local and national organizations, as well. Such agencies include the Association for Retarded Citizens, Autism Society of America, and other community support groups. Books are also available to assist families [82] and peers [83] in learning about pervasive developmental disorders and to assist families in adapting to having a child with autistic disorder [84].

Pharmacotherapy

There is a paucity of an adequate number of controlled trials in all areas of pediatric psychopharmacology. There are no pharmacologic agents with Food and Drugs Administration (FDA)-approved labeling specific for the treatment of autistic disorder or other pervasive developmental disorders in either children or adults. This is problematic, because many of the symptoms commonly seen in autistic disorder and other ASDs (rituals, aggressive behavior, and hyperactivity) are also common in mentally retarded children and adolescents, without a pervasive developmental disorder. Some of the pharmacologic strategies for the treatment of autistic disorder have been extrapolated from studies of other neuropsychiatric conditions, including attention deficit hyperactivity disorder (ADHD) and OCD.

It is important to remember that the current state-of-the-art is empirical treatment of target symptoms. One should not use psychopharmacological agents with the expectation that they will cure children with autistic disorder. Some parents and teachers of chil-

dren with autistic disorder may have the misconception that medication can eliminate core social and cognitive dysfunction. There is no pharmacological substitute for appropriate educational, behavioral, psychotherapeutic, vocational, and recreational programming. It is essential to remember and remind parents, teachers, and others that medication should always be seen as an adjunct to the core interventions that address the primary developmental challenges associated with these disorders.

The use of medications to treat autistic disorder and other pervasive developmental disorders appears to have significant potential as an adjunct to educational, environmental and social interventions. Regrettably, there is no diagnosis-specific treatment at the present time. Nonetheless, individuals with autistic disorder still have significant impairments as well as the all-too-often forgotten potential to gain skills and levels of functioning compatible with living in the community. It is a reasonable goal for clinicians to adopt the judicious use of psychopharmacologic agents to assist in this adaptation. Out of necessity, this focus on facilitating adaptation, requires attention to six important principles:

(1) Environmental manipulations, including behavioral treatment, may be as effective, if not more effective, than medication for symptom treatment.
(2) It is essential that the living arrangement for the individual is capable of safely and consistently administering and monitoring the medication to be used.
(3) Individuals with autistic disorder and other pervasive developmental disorders are at as much, if not greater, risk for DSM-IV Axis I disorders. If a comorbid DSM-IV Axis I disorder is present, standard treatment for that disorder should be initiated.
(4) There must be an established way of specifically monitoring the response to treatment over time.
(5) A careful assessment of the risk–benefit ratio must be made before initiating treatment and, to the extent possible, the patient's caretakers and the patient must understand the risks and benefits of the treatment.
(6) The risk–benefit ratio must be regularly assessed over the course of treatment.

Potent Serotonin Transporter Inhibitors

This class of agents includes selective and potent serotonin reuptake inhibitors (fluoxetine, sertraline, paroxetine, fluvoxamine, citalopram and escitalopram) as well as the less selective but potent clomipramine, a tricyclic antidepressant (Table 21.5). This group of

Table 21.5 Summary of treatment principles.

Psychosocial interventions
    Educational
        curricula that target communication
        behavioral techniques
        structured milieu
        vocational training and placement
        other specialized interventions such as speech
           and therapy, physical, and occupational
           therapy
    Social skills training
    Individual psychotherapy for high-functioning
        individuals
Medical interventions
    cohesive doctor–patient relationship
    supportive measures with families coping with
        autistic disorder
    behavioral treatment
    pharmacotherapy to address problematic signs and
        symptoms

medications is most effective when insistence on routines or rituals are present to the point of manifest anxiety or aggression in response to interruption of the routines or rituals [85–89], or after the onset of another disorder such as major depressive disorder or obsesive-compulsive disorder (OCD) [90]. The common side effects associated with selective serotonin reuptake inhibitors (SSRIs) are motor restlessness, insomnia, elation, irritability, and decreased appetite, each of which may occur alone or, more often, together. These side effects are dose-related; however, for unclear reasons (perhaps having to do with the well-replicated findings serotonergic dysmodulation in ASDs), there is very wide variation in the dose that this population can tolerate before these side effects emerge [91]. In particular, weight does not appear to predict for the dose at which side effects will emerge [94]. Because many of these symptoms may be present in the often cyclical natural course of autistic disorder before the medication is initiated, the emergence of new symptoms, a different quality of the symptom, and occurrence of these symptoms in a new cluster are clues that the symptoms are side effects of medication rather than part of the natural course of the disorder [86]. Until genetic variation or some other marker is discovered that allows us to predict for the final dose, it is best to begin at a very low dose in this population, and push the dose in a forced titration fashion. When the dose-related side

effects are encountered, the dose should be decreased to the highest previously tolerated dose [91]. Interestingly, a recent study suggests that insomnia may not be nearly as likely a side effect with the SSRI escitalopram [94].

Stimulants

Small, but significant, reductions in hyperactivity ratings may be seen in children with autistic disorder in response to stimulants such as methylphenidate [92], dextroamphetamine, and pemoline. In a placebo-controlled crossover study, 8 of 13 subjects showed a reduction of at least 50% on methylphendate [93]. Stereotypies may worsen, so drug trials for the individual patient must always be assessed to determine that therapeutic effects outweigh side effects. A key distinction in assessing attentional problems of children with autistic disorder is the distinction between poor sustained attention (characteristic of children with ADHD) and poor joint attention (characteristic of children with autistic disorder). Problems in joint attention require educational and behavioral interventions or treatment of compulsions or rituals with a potent serotonin transporter inhibitor. Problems in maintenance of attention of the type seen in ADIID are more likely to respond to stimulants. Interestingly, significant experience in our clinic suggests that Adderall products (mixed dextroamphetamine salts) tend to be more effective in this population than the methylphenidate products (unpublished observation; [85]), although direct comparative trials are needed to document this observation.

Sympatholytics

The alpha$_2$-adrenergic receptor agonist clonidine reduced irritability as well as hyperactivity and impulsivity in two double-blind, placebo-controlled trials [95,96]. However, tolerance developed several months after initiation of the treatment in each child who was treated long-term [96]. Tolerance was not prevented by transdermal skin patch administration of the drug. If tolerance does develop, the dose should not be increased because tolerance to sedation does not occur, and sedation may lead to increased aggression due to decreased cognitive control of impulses. Adrenergic receptor antagonists, such as propranolol and naldolol, have not been tested in double-blind trials in autistic disorder. However, open trials have reported the use of these medications in the treatment of aggression and impulsivity in developmental disorders [97] including autistic disorder [98].

Neuroleptics

Typical Neuroleptics

Because they were among the first developed psychopharmacological classes, typical neuroleptics have been among the most extensively studied drugs in autistic disorder. Trifluoperazine, haloperidol, and pimozide have been studied in double-blind, controlled trials lasting from two to six months. Reduction of fidgetiness, interpersonal withdrawal, speech deviance, and stereotypies has been documented in response to these treatments [99–106]. However, patients with autistic disorder are as vulnerable to potentially irreversible tardive dyskinesia as any other group of young patients [107,108]. Owing to the often earlier age at initiation of pharmacotherapy, patients with autistic disorder treated with typical neuroleptics may be at higher risk because of the potential increased lifetime exposure.

Atypical Neuroleptics

Because of the positive response of many children with autistic disorder to typical neuroleptics, similar medications with reduced risk of extrapyramidal symptoms must be considered. In addition, atypical neuroleptics are often effective in treating the negative symptoms of schizophrenia, which seem similar to several of the social deficits in autistic disorder. Both risperidone and olanzapine have shown promise in open label trials in reducing hyperactivity, impulsivity, aggressiveness, and obsessive preoccupations [109–114]. A large double-blind, placebo-controlled study found risperidone to be more effective than placebo in the treatment of repetitive behavior, aggression, and irritability [115,116], and these gains appear to hold up over time [117]. Weight gain has been a significant problem in longer term studies [117,118]. Open-label outcomes with olanzapine for similar target symptoms have been mixed, with positive results being found by some [110,113], but not others [119]; weight gain was also a severe problem in these studies. The perceived effectiveness of these medications coupled with the problems with weight gain have led some to look at ziprasidone (which is not thought to cause weight gain) in this population. In one study [120], a retrospective chart review was undertaken of adult subjects that had been on an atypical agent and were then switched to the atypical ziprasidone. Seven of 10 subjects did better or as well on ziprasidone, and there was a net weight loss. Another study with youths also found positive outcomes in 6 of 12 subjects with autism and also reported no weight gain. However, ongoing concern about QTc prolongation exists for ziprasidone without more safety data for children and adolescents in general and ASD more specifically.

Anticonvulsants

Because 25% to 33% of patients with autistic disorder have seizures, the psychopharmacological management of patients with autistic disorder or other ASD must take into consideration the past or current history of epilepsy and the potential role of anticonvulsants [26]. Unfortunately, very few studies have been undertaken in this area. In an open trial of divalproex, 10 of 14 patients responded favorably, including improvements in affective stability, impulsivity, and aggression [121]. The anticonvulsant class to be avoided, when possible, is the barbiturate class (e.g., phenobarbital). Because barbiturates have been associated with hyperactivity, depression, and cognitive impairment, they should be changed to an alternative drug, depending on the seizure type [122,123]. In addition, phenytoin (Dilantin) is sedating and causes hypertrophy of the gums and hirsutism, which may contribute to the social challenges for people with autistic disorder.

Carbamazepine and valproate may have positive psychotropic effects, particularly when cyclical irritability, insomnia, and hyperactivity are present. Several children with autistic disorder were treated with valproic acid after EEG abnormalities were found. These children had an improvement in behavioral symptoms associated with autistic disorder after valproate treatment [124]. Oxcarbazepine may have some of the positive psychotropic effects of carbamazepine, with less risk of agranulocytosis, but concern about uncommon hyponatremia remains.

Naltrexone

The opiate antagonist, naltrexone, was suggested as a specific treatment for autistic disorder. However, double-blind trials have suggested that naltrexone has little efficacy in treating the core social and cognitive symptoms of autistic disorder [125]. Whereas the use of naltrexone as a treatment of core symptoms of autistic disorder no longer seems to be likely, it may have a role in the treatment of self-injurious behavior, although the controlled data are equivocal [125,126]. Controlled trials have shown a modest reduction in symptoms of hyperactivity and restlessness sometimes associated with autistic disorder [125,127–130]. Potential side effects include nausea and vomiting. Controlled trials in autistic disorder have not shown liver dysfunction or other physical side effects. Naltrexone may have an adverse effect on the outcome of Rett disorder on the basis of a relatively large, randomized, double-blind, placebo-controlled trial [131].

Lithium

Adolescents and adults with autistic disorder often exhibit symptoms in a cyclic manner and so there is much interest in how these patients might respond to agents typically used in bipolar disorder. A single open trial of lithium revealed no significant improvement in symptoms in patients with autistic disorder without bipolar disorder [132].

Anxiolytics

Benzodiazepines have not been studied systematically in children and adolescents with autistic disorder. However, their use to reduce anxiety in short-term treatment, such as before dental procedures, is similar to their use in management of anxiety in people without a PDD. One open-label study has found a decrease in anxiety and irritability in patients receiving the anxiolytic buspirone [133].

Glutamatergic Antagonists

Interest in these agents has been sparked by the hypothesis that ASDs may be a disorder of hypoglutaminergic activity [134]. In a double-blind, placebo-controlled study of the glutamatergic antagonist amantadine hydrochloride, there were substantial improvements in clinician-rated hyperactivity and irritability, although parental reports did not reach statistical significance (which may have been partially due to a strong placebo response) [135]. Further study of this medication and consideration of this hypothesis is warranted.

Pyridoxine and Dietary Supplements

Pyridoxine, the water-soluble essential vitamin B6, has been used extensively as a pharmacological treatment in autistic disorder. In the doses used for autistic disorder, it is not being used as a cofactor for normally regulated enzyme function or as a vitamin; rather, it is used as a pharmacological agent to modulate the function of neurotransmitter enzymes, such as tryptophan hydroxylase and tyrosine hydroxylase. While Martineau [136] showed modest improvements in about 30% of children, recent reviews have concluded that there are little data to support the claim that vitamin B6 improves developmental course [137,138].

Fenfluramine

Although fenfluramine originally showed promise in the treatment of autistic disorder and associated cognitive dysfunction [139], double-blind controlled trials did not confirm an improvement in cognitive function or a reduction in core autistic symptoms [140,141].

However, much like naltrexone, fenfluramine may reduce hyperactivity and impulsivity commonly present in autistic disorder and other developmental disorders [142]. The potential changes in neurochemical regulation after long-term administration [141], which *may* represent neurotoxic effects [143] and potential for acquired cardiac valvular disease when coadministered with phenteramine suggests that fenfluramine no longer be used in autistic disorder.

Secretin

A case series of three autistic patients that showed improvement in core symptoms after receiving the gastrointestinal hormone secretin [144], led to a series of studies on this substance as a possible treatment for ASD. The results have been disappointing, with all studies done so far [145–153] showing the substance to be no more useful than placebo. These studies, along with the negative studies that followed the initial excitement after open-label studies of naltrexone and fenfluramine, point to the necessity of performing double-blind, placebo-controlled studies of any putative treatments to ensure safety and establish effectiveness.

Summary

Autistic disorder and other pervasive developmental disorders are complex, early-onset disorders that usually lead to moderate-to-severe disability in domains of social, communicative, and flexible behavior. A more thorough understanding of these conditions and their treatment has developed over the past two decades. A coordinated, multidisciplinary approach to treatment, that focuses on development of adaptive, social, and communicative functioning, yields the best results.

References

1. Chakrabarti S, Fombonne E: Pervasive developmental disorders in preschool children. *JAMA* 2001; **285**:3093–3099.
2. Fombonne E: The epidemiology of autism: A review. *Psychol Med* 1999; **29**:769–786.
3. Zahner G, Pauls D: Epidemiological surveys of infantile autism. In: Cohen D, Donnellan A, eds. *Handbook of Autism and Pervasive Developmental Disorders*. New York: John Wiley and Sons, 1987:199–210.
4. Ritvo ER, Jorde LB, Mason-Brothers A, Freeman BJ, Pingree C, Jones MB, McMahon WM, Peterson PB, Jenson WR, Mo A: The UCLA-University of Utah epidemiologic survey of autism: Recurrent risk estimates and genetic counseling. *Am J Psych* 1989; **146**:1032–1036.

5. Volkmar F, Klin A, Siegel B, Szatmari P, Lord C, Campbell M, Freeman B, Cicchetti D, Rutter M, Kline W, Buitelaar J, Hattab Y, Fombonne E, Fuentes J, Werry J, Stone W, Kerbeshian J, Hoshino Y, Bregman J, Loveland K, et al.: Field trial for autistic disorder in DSM-IV. Am J Psychiatry 1994; 151:1361–1367.

6. Kurita H, Kita M, Miyake Y: A comparative study of development and symptoms among disintegrative psychosis and infantile autism with and without speech loss. J Autism Dev Disord 1992; 22:175–188.

7. Freeman BJ, Ritvo ER, Needleman R, Yokota A: The stability of cognitive and linguistic parameters in autism: A five-year prospective study. J Am Acad Child Psychiatry 1985; 24:459–464.

8. Venter A, Lord C, Schopler E: A follow-up study of high-functioning autistic children. J Child Psychol Psychiat 1992; 33:489–507.

9. Rutter M: Cognitive deficits in the pathogenesis of autism. J Child Psychol Psychiat 1993; 24:513–532.

10. Frith U: Autism: Explaining the Enigma. New York: Blackwell, 1989.

11. Schain RJ, Freedman DX: Studies on 5-hydroxyindole metabolism in autistic and other mentally retarded children. J Pediatrics 1961; 58:315–320.

12. Anderson GM, Freedman DX, Cohen DJ, Volkmar FR, Hoder EL, McPhedran P, Minderaa RB, Hansen CR, Young JG: Whole blood serotonin in autistic and normal subjects. J Child Psychol Psychiatry 1987; 28:885–900.

13. Cook E, Arora R, Anderson G, Berry-Kravis E, Yan S-Y, Yeoh H, Sklena P, Charak D, Leventhal B: Platelet serotonin studies in hyperserotonemic relatives of children with autistic disorder. Life Sci 1993; 52:2005–2015.

14. Cook EH, Fletcher KE, Wainwright M, Marks N, Yan S-Y, Leventhal BL: Primary structure of the human platelet serotonin 5-HT$_{2A}$ receptor: Identity with frontal cortex serotonin 5-HT$_{2A}$ receptor. J Neurochem 1994; 63:465–469.

15. Bailey A, Bolton P, Butler L, Le Couteur A, Murphy M, Scott S, Webb T, Rutter M: Prevalence of the fragile X anomaly amongst autistic twins and singletons. J Child Psychol Psychiatry 1993; 34(5):673–688.

16. Reiss AL, Freund L: Fragile X syndrome, DSM-III-R, and autism. J Am Acad Child Adolesc Psychiatry 1990; 29:885–891.

17. Gillberg C, Steffenburg S, Wahlström J, Gillberg I, Sjöstedt A, Martinsson T, Liedgren S, Eeg-Olofsson O: Autism associated with marker chromosome. J Am Acad Child Adolesc Psychiatry 1991; 30:489–494.

18. Cook E, Lindgren V, Leventhal B, Courchesne R, Lincoln A, Shulman C, Lord C, Courchesne E: Autism or atypical autism in maternally but not paternally derived proximal 15q duplication. Am J Hum Genet 1997; 60:928–934.

19. Knoblock H, Pasamanick B: Some etiologic and prognostic factors in early infantile autism and psychosis. Pediatrics 1975; 55:182–191.

20. Smalley SL, Tanguay PE, Smith M, Gutierrez G: Autism and tuberous sclerosis. J Autism Dev Disord 1992; 22:339–355.

21. Buyse IM, Fang P, Hoon KT, Amir RE, Zoghbi HY, Roa BB: Diagnostic testing for Rett syndrome by DHPLC and direct sequencing analysis of the MECP2 gene: Identification of several novel mutations and polymorphisms. Am J Hum Genet 2000; 67:1428–1436.

22. Bailey A, Le Couteur A, Gottesman I, Bolton P, Simonoff E, Yuzda E, Rutter M: Autism as a strong genetic disorder: Evidence from a British twin study. Psychol Med 1995; 25:63–77.

23. Steffenburg S, Gillberg C, Hellgren L, Andersson L, Gillberg IC, Jakobsson G, Bohman M: A twin study of autism in Denmark, Finland, Iceland, Norway and Sweden. J Child Psychol Psychiat 1989; 30:405–416.

24. Bailey A, Le Couteur A, Gottesman I, Bolton P, Simonoff E, Yuzda E, Rutter M: Autism as a strongly genetic disorder: Evidence from a British twin study. Psychol Med 1995; 25(1):63–77.

25. Damasio AR, Maurer RG: A neurological model of childhood autism. Arch Neurol 1978; 35:777–786.

26. Volkmar FR, Nelson DS: Seizure disorders in autism. J Am Acad Child Adolesc Psychiatry 1990; 29:127–129.

27. Deykin EY, Macmahon B: The incidence of seizures among children with autistic symptoms. Am J Psychiatry 1979; 136:1310–1312.

28. Rutter M, Greenfield D, Lockyer L: A five to fifteen year follow-up study of infantile psychosis. II. Social and behavioural outcome. Br J Psychiatry 1967; 113:1183–1199.

29. Ritvo ER, Freeman BJ, Scheibel AB, Duong T, Robinson H, Guthrie D, Ritvo A: Lower Purkinje cell counts in the cerebella of four autistic subjects: Initial findings of the UCLA-NSAC autopsy research report. Am J Psychiatry 1986; 143:862–866.

30. Bauman M, Kemper T: Neuroanatomic observations of the brain in autism. In: Bauman M, Kemper T, eds. The Neurobiology of Autism. Baltimore: Johns Hopkins University Press, 1994:119–145.

31. Casanova MF, Buxhoeveden DP, Switala AE, Roy E: Neuronal density and architecture (Grey Level Index) in the brains of autistic patients. J Child Neurol 2002; 17:515–521.

32. Casanova MF, Buxhoeveden DP, Switala AE, Roy E: Asperger's syndrome and cortical neuropathology. J Child Neurol 2002; 17:142–145.

33. Sparks BF, Friedman SD, Shaw DW, Aylward EH, Echelard D, Artru AA, Maravilla B, Giedd JN, Munson J, Dawson G, Dager SR: Brain structural abnormalities in young children with autism spectrum disorder. Neurology 2002; 59:184–192.

34. Courchesne E, Yeung CR, Press GA, Hesselink JR, Jernigan TL: Hypoplasia of cerebellar vermal lobules VI and VII in autism. N Engl J Med 1988; 318:1349–1354.

35. Holttum J, Minshew N, Sanders R, Philips N: Magnetic resonance imaging of the posterior fossa in autism. Biol Psychiatry 1992; 32:1091–1101.

36. Saitoh O, Karns CM, Courchesne E: Development of the hippocampal formation from 2 to 42 years: MRI evidence of smaller area dentata in autism. Brain 2001; 124:1317–1324.

37. Herbert MR, Harris GJ, Adrien KT, Ziegler DA, Makris N, Kennedy DN, Lange NT, Chabris CF, Bakardjiev A, Hodgson J, Takeoka M, Tager-Flusberg H, Caviness VS Jr.: Abnormal asymmetry in language association cortex in autism. Ann Neurol 2002; 52:588–596.

38. Piven J, Arndt S, Bailey J, Havercamp S, Andreasen NC, Palmer P: An MRI study of brain size in autism. *Am J Psychiatry* 1995; **152**:1145–1149.

39. Rumsey JM, Duara R, Grady C, Rapoport JL, Margolin RA, Rapoport SI, Cutler NR: Brain metabolism in autism: Resting cerebral glucose utilization rates as measured with positron emission tomography. *Arch Gen Psychiatry* 1985; **42**:448–455.

40. Herold S, Frackowiak RSJ, Le Couteur A, Rutter M, Howlin P: Cerebral blood flow and metabolism of oxygen and glucose in young autistic adults. *Psychol Med* 1988; **18**:823–831.

41. Chugani HT, Da Silva E, Chugani DC: Infantile spasms: III. Prognostic implications of bitemporal hypometabolism on positron emission tomography. *Ann Neurol* 1996; **39**:943–649.

42. Chugani DC, Muzik O, Rothermel R, Behen M, Chakraborty P, Mangner T, Da Silva E, Chugani HT: Altered serotonin synthesis in the dentatothalamocortical pathway in autism boys. *Ann Neuro* 1997; **42**:666–669.

43. Chugani DC, Muzik O, Behen M, Rothermel R, Janisse JJ, Lee J, Chugani HT: Developmental changes in brain serotonin synthesis capacity in autistic and nonautistic children. *Ann Neurol* 1999; **45**:287–295.

44. Pierce K, Muller RA, Ambrose J, Allen G, Courchesne E: Face processing occurs outside the fusiform 'face area' in autism: Evidence from functional MRI. *Brain* 2001; **124**:2059–2073.

45. Minshew N: In vivo brain chemistry in autism: ^{31}P magnetic resonance spectroscopy studies. In: Bauman M, Kemper T, eds. *The Neurobiology of Autism.* Baltimore: Johns Hopkins University Press, 1994:86–101.

46. Rutter M: Infantile autism. In: Shaffer D, Ehrhardt AA, Greenhill LL, eds. *The Clinical Guide to Child Psychiatry.* New York: The Free Press, 1985:48–78.

47. Lord C, Rutter M, Le Couteur A: Autism Diagnostic Interview – Revised: A revised version of a diagnostic interview for caregivers of individuals with possible pervasive developmental disorders. *J Autism Dev Disord* 1994; **24**:659–685.

48. Rumsey JM, Rapoport JL, Sceery WR: Autistic children as adults: Psychiatric, social, and behavioral outcomes. *J Am Acad Child Psychiatry* 1985; **24**:465–473.

49. Mundy P, Sigman M: The theoretical implications of joint-attention deficits in autism. *Dev Psychopathol* 1989; **1**:173–183.

50. Kasari C, Sigman M, Mundy P, Yirmiya N: Affective sharing in the context of joint attention interactions of normal, autistic, and mentally retarded children. *J Autism Dev Disord* 1990; **20**:87–94.

51. Asperger H: Die 'Autistischen Psychopathen' kindesalter. *Arch Psychiatr Nervenkr* 1944; **117**:76–136.

52. Olsson B, Rett A: A review of the Rett syndrome with a theory of autism. *Brain Dev* 1990; **12**:11–15.

53. Naidu S, Bibat G, Kratz L, Kelley RI, Pevsner J, Hoffman E, Cuffari C, Rohde C, Blue C, Johnson MV: Clinical variability in Rett's syndrome. *J Child Neurol* 2003; **18**:662–668.

54. Kim SJ, Cook EH Jr: Novel de novo nonsense mutation of MECP2 in a patient with Rett Syndrome. *Hum Mutat* 2000; **15**:382–383.

55. Volkmar F, Cohen D: Disintegrative disorder or 'late onset' autism. *J Child Psychol Psychiat* 1989; **30**:717–724.

56. Corbett J, Harris R: Progressive disintegrative psychosis of childhood. *J Child Psychol Psychiat* 1977; **18**:211–219.

57. Bartak L, Rutter M, Cox A: A comparative study of infantile autism and specific developmental receptive language disorder. I: The children. *Br J Psychiatry* 1975; **126**:127–145.

58. Ornitz E, Ritvo E: The syndrome of autism: A critical review. *Am J Psychiatry* 1976; **133**:609–621.

59. Lerman P, Lerman-Sagie T, Kivity S: Effect of early corticosteroid therapy for Landau–Kleffner syndrome. *Dev Med Child Neurol* 1991; **33**:257–260.

60. Kolvin I, Fundudis T: Elective mute children: Psychological development and background factors. *J Child Psychol Psychiat* 1981; **22**:219–232.

61. Hoffman-Plotkin D, Twentyman C: A multimodal assessment of behavioral and cognitive deficits in abused and neglected preschoolers. *Child Dev* 1984; **55**:794–802.

62. Rutter M, Andersen-Wood L, Beckett C, Bredenkamp D, Castle J, Groothues C, Keaveney L, Lord C, O'Connor TG: Quasi-autistic patterns following severe early global privation. English and Romanian Adoptees (ERA) Study Team. *J Child Psychol Psychiatry* 1999; **40**:537–549.

63. Lord C, Risi S, Lambrecht L, Cook EH Jr, Leventhal BL, DiLavore, Pickles A, Rutter M: The Autism Diagnostic Observation Schedule-Generic: A standard measure of social and communication deficits associated with the spectrum of autism. *J Autism Dev Disor* 2000; **30**:205–223.

64. Schopler E, Reichler RJ, Renner BR: *The Childhood Autism Rating Scale (CARS).* Los Angeles, CA: Western Psychological Services, 1988.

65. Krug D, Arick J, Almond P: Behavior checklist for identifying severely handicapped individuals with high levels of autistic behavior. *J Child Psychol Psychiat* 1980; **21**:221–229.

66. Aman M: *Aberrant Behavior Checklist – Community Version.* East Aurora, NY: Slosson Educational Publications, 1994.

67. de Bildt A, Kraijer D, Sytema S, Minderaa R: The psychometric properties of the Vineland Adaptive Behavior Scales in children and adolescents with mental retardation. *J Autism Dev Disord* 2005; **35**(1):53–62.

68. Sparrow S, Balla D, Cicchetti D: *Vineland Scales of Adaptive Behavior, Survey Form Manual.* Circle Pines, MN: American Guidance Service, 1984.

69. Stutsman R: *Merrill-Palmer Scale of Mental Tests.* New York: Harcourt, Brace, and World, 1948.

70. Shah A, Holmes N: The use of the Leiter International Performance Scale with autistic children. *J Autism Dev Disord* 1985; **15**:195–204.

71. Bayley N: *Manual for the Bayley Scales of Infant Development.* New York: Psychological Corporation, 1969.

72. Elliott C: *Differential Abilities Scales.* Pensacola, FL: Psychological Corporation, 1990.

73. Brown J: Adolescent development of children with infantile psychosis. *Sem Psychiatry* 1969; **1**:79–89.

74. Kanner L, Rodriguez A, Ashenden B: How far can autistic children go in matters of social adaptation. *J Aut Child Schizo* 1972; **2**:9–33.

75. Lotter V: Social adjustment and placement of autistic children in Middlesex: A follow-up study. *J Aut Child Schizo* 1974; **4**:11–32.

76. Gillberg C: Autistic children growing up: Problems during puberty and adolescence. *Dev Med Child Neurol* 1984; **26**:125–129.

77. Carr E: The motivation of self-injurious behavior: A review of some hypotheses. *Psychological Bulletin* 1977; **84**:800–816.

78. Lord C: The development of peer relations in children with autism. In: Morrison F, Lord C, Keating D, eds. *Applied Developmental Psychology*. New York: Academic Press, 1984:165–229.

79. Campbell M, Schopler E, Cueva J, Hallin A: Treatment of autistic disorder. *J Am Acad Child Adolesc Psychiatry* 1996; **35**:134–143.

80. Schopler E, Olley G: Comprehensive educational services for autistic children: The TEACCH model. In: Reynolds C, Gutkin T, eds. *The Handbook of School Psychology*. New York: John Wiley & Sons, 1982: 629–643.

81. Solnit A, Stark M: Mourning and the birth of a defective child. *Psychoanalytic Study Child* 1961; **16**: 523–537.

82. Powers M: *Children with Autism: A Parent's Guide.* Bethesda, MD: Woodbine House, 1989.

83. Amenta C: *Russell is Extra Special: A Book about Autism for Children.* New York: Brunner/Mazel, 1992.

84. Siegel B, Silverstein S: *What About Me? Growing Up with a Developmentally Disabled Sibling.* New York: Plenum, 1994.

85. Cook E, Rowlett R, Jaselskis C, Leventhal B: Fluoxetine treatment of patients with autism and mental retardation. *J Am Acad Child Adolesc Psychiatry* 1992; **31**:739–745.

86. Gordon C, State R, Nelson J, Hamburger S, Rapoport J: A double-blind comparison of clomipramine, desipramine, and placebo in the treatment of autistic disorder. *Arch Gen Psychiatry* 1993; **50**:441–447.

87. McDougle C, Naylor S, Cohen D, Volkmar F, Heninger G, Price L: A double-blind, placebo-controlled study of fluvoxamine in adults with autistic disorder. *Arch Gen Psychiatry* 1996; **53**:1001–1008.

88. Posey DJ, Litwiller M, Koburn A, McDougle CJ: Paroxetine in autism. *J Am Acad Child Adolesc Psychiatry* 1999; **38**:111–112.

89. Namerow LB, Thomas P, Bostic JQ, Prince J, Monuteaux MC: Use of citalopram in pervasive developmental disorders. *J Dev Behav Pediatr* 2003; **24**:104–108.

90. Ghaziuddin M, Tsai L, Ghaziuddin N: Fluoxetine in autism with depression. *J Am Acad Child Adolesc Psychiatry* 1991; **30**:508–509.

91. Owley T: The Pharmacological Treatment of Autistic Spectrum Disorders. *CNS Spectrums* 2002; **7**:663–669

92. Quintana H, Birmaher B, Stedge D, Lennon S, Freed J, Bridge J, Greenhill L: Use of methylphenidate in the treatment of children with autistic disorder. *J Autism Dev Disord* 1995; **25**:283–294.

93. Handen BL, Johnson CR, Lubetsky M: Efficacy of methylphenidate among children with autism and symptoms of attention-deficit hyperactivity disorder. *J Autism Dev Disord* 2000; **30**:245–255.

94. Owley T, Walton L, Salt J, Guter S, Winnega M, Leventhal BL, Cook EH Jr: An open label trial of escitalopram in autistic spectrum disorders. *J Am Acad Child Adolesc Psychiatry* 2005; **44**(4):343–348.

95. Fankhauser MP, Karumanchi VC, German ML, Yates A, Karumanchi SD: A double-blind, placebo-controlled study of the efficacy of transdermal clonidine in autism. *J Clin Psychiatry* 1992; **53**:77–82.

96. Jaselskis CA, Cook EH, Fletcher KE, Leventhal BL: Clonidine treatment of hyperactive and impulsive children with autistic disorder. *J Clin Psychopharm* 1992; **12**:322–327.

97. Williams DT, Mehl R, Yudofsky S, Adams D, Roseman B: The effect of propranolol on uncontrolled rage outbursts in children and adolescents with organic brain dysfunction. *J Am Acad Child Psychiatry* 1982 **21**(2): 129–135.

98. Ratey JJ, Mikkelsen E, Sorgi, P, Zuckerman HS, Polakoff S, Bemporad J, Bick P, Kadish W: Autism: The treatment of aggressive behaviors. *J Clin Psychopharmacol* 1987; **7**(1):35–41.

99. Anderson LT, Campbell M, Adams P, Small AM, Perry R, Shell J: The effects of haloperidol on discrimination learning and behavioral symptoms in autistic children. *J Aut Develop Disord* 1989; **9**:227–239.

100. Anderson LT, Campbell M, Grega DM, Perry R, Small AM, Green WH: Haloperidol in the treatment of infantile autism: Effects on learning and behavioral symptoms. *Am J Psychiatry* 1984; **141**:1195–1202.

101. Campbell M, Anderson LT, Meier M, Cohen IL, Small AM, Samit C, Sachar EJ: A comparison of haloperidol and behavior therapy and their interaction in autistic children. *J Am Acad Child Psychiatry* 1976; **17**:640–655.

102. Cohen IL, Campbell M, Posner D, Small AM, Triebel D, Anderson LT: Behavioral effects of haloperidol in young autistic children. An objective analysis using a within subject reversal design. *J Am Acad Child Psychiatry* 1980; **19**:665–677.

103. Ernst M, Magee HJ, Gonzalez NM, Locascio JJ, Rosenberg CR, Campbell M: Pimozide in autistic children. *Psychopharmacol Bull* 1992; **28**:187–191.

104. Fish B, Shapiro T, Campbell M: Long-term prognosis and the response of schizophrenic children to drug therapy: A controlled study of trifluoperazine. *Am J Psychiatry* 1966; **123**:32–39.

105. Naruse H, Nagahata M, Nakane Y, Shirahashi K, Takesada M, Yamazaki K: A multi-center double-blind trial of pimozide (Orap), haloperidol and placebo in children with behavioral disorders, using crossover design. *Acta Paedopsychiat* 1982; **48**:173–184.

106. Perry R, Campbell M, Adams P, Lynch N, Spencer EK, Curren EL, Overall JE: Long-term efficacy of haloperidol in autistic children: Continuous versus discontinuous drug administration. *J Am Acad Child Adolesc Psychiatry* 1989; **28**(1):87–92.

107. Campbell M, Adams P, Perry R, Spencer EK, Overall JE: Tardive and withdrawal dyskinesia in autistic children: A prospective study. *Psychopharm Bull* 1988; **24**:251–255

108. Campbell M, Armenteros JL, Malone RP, Adams PB, Eisenberg ZW, Overall JE: Neuroleptic-related dyskinesias in autistic children: A prospective, longitudinal study. *J Am Acad Child Adolesc Psychiatry* 1997;**36**(6): 835–843.

109. O'Brien J, Barber R: Marked improvement in tardive dyskinesia following treatment with olanzapine in an elderly subject. *Br J Psychiatry* 1998; **172**:186.

110. Malone RP, Cater J, Sheikh RM, Choudhury MS, Delaney MA: Olanzapine versus haloperidol in children with autistic disorder: An open pilot study. *J Am Acad Child Adolesc Psychiatry* 2001; **40**:887–894.

111. Masi G, Cosenza A, Mucci M, Brovedani P: Open trial of risperidone in 24 young children with pervasive developmental disorders. *J Am Acad Child Adolesc Psychiatry* 2001; **40**:1206–1214.

112. McDougle CJ, Holmes JP, Bronson MR, Anderson GM, Volkmar FR, Price LH, Cohen DJ: Risperidone treatment of children and adolescents with pervasive developmental disorders: A prospective open-label study. *J Am Acad Child Adolesc Psychiatry* 1997; **36**:685–693.

113. Potenza MN, Holmes JP, Kanes SJ, McDougle CJ: Olanzapine treatment of children, adolescents, and adults with pervasive developmental disorders: An open-label pilot study. *J Clin Psychopharmacol* 1999; **19**:37–44.

114. Nicolson R, Awad G, Sloman L: An open trial of risperidone in young autistic children. *J Am Acad Child Adolesc Psychiatry* 1998; **37**(4):372–376.

115. McDougle CJ, Holmes JP, Carlson DC, Pelton GH, Cohen DJ, Price LH: A double-blind, placebo-controlled study of risperidone in adults with autistic disorder and other pervasive developmental disorders. *Arch Gen Psychiatry* 1998; **55**:633–641.

116. McCracken JT, McGough J, Shah B, Cronin P, Hong D, Aman MG, Arnold LE, Lindsay R, Nash P, Hollway J, McDougle CJ, Posey D, Swiezy N, Kohn A, Scahill L, Martin A, Koenig K, Volkmar F, Carroll D, Lancor A, Tierney E, Ghuman J, Gonzalez NM, Grados M, Vitiello B, Ritz L, Davies M, Robinson J, McMahon D: Risperidone in children with autism and serious behavioral problems. *N Engl J Med* 2002; **347**:314–321.

117. Masi G, Cosenza A, Mucci M, Brovedani P: A 3-year naturalistic study of 53 preschool children with pervasive developmental disorders treated with risperidone. *J Clin Psychiatry* 2003; **64**(9):1039–1047.

118. Gagliano A, Germano E, Pustorino G, Impallomeni C, D'Arrigo C, Calamoneri F, Spina E: Risperidone treatment of children with autistic disorder: Effectiveness, tolerability, and pharmacokinetic implications. *J Child Adolesc Psychopharmacol* 2004; **14**(1):39–47.

119. Kemner C, Willemsen-Swinkels SH, de Jonge M, Tuynman-Qua H, van Engeland H: Open-label study olanzapine in children with pervasive developmental disorder. *J Clin Psychopharmacol* 2002; **22**:455–460.

120. Cohen SA, Fitzgerald BJ, Khan SR, Khan A: The effect of a switch to ziprasidone in an adult population with autistic disorder: Chart review of naturalistic, open-label treatment. *J Clin Psychiatry* 2004; **65**:110–113.

121. Hollander E, Dolgoff-Kaspar R, Cartwright C, Rawitt R, Novotny S: An open trial of divalproex sodium in autism spectrum disorders. *J Clin Psychiatry* 2001; **62**:530–534.

122. Brent DA, Crumrine PK, Varma RR, Allan M, Allman C: Phenobarbital treatment and major depressive disorder in children with epilepsy. *Pediatrics* 1987; **80**:909–917.

123. Vining EPG, Mellits D, Dorsen MM, Cataldo MF, Quaskey SA, Spielberg SP, Freeman JM: Psychologic and behavioral effects of antiepileptic drugs in children: A double-blind comparison between phenobarbital and valproic acid. *Pediatrics* 1987; **80**:165–174.

124. Plioplys AV: Autism: electroencephalogram abnormalities and clinical improvement with valproic acid. *Arch Pediatrics Adolesc Med* 1994; **24**(1):23–37.

125. Campbell M, Anderson L, Small A, Adams P, Gonzalez N, Ernst M: Naltrexone in autistic children: Behavioral symptoms and attentional learning. *J Am Acad Child Adolesc Psychiatry* 1993; **32**:1283–1291.

126. Willemsen-Swinkels SHN, Buitelaar JK, Weijnen FG, Van Engeland H: Placebo-controlled acute dosage naltrexone study in young autistic children. *Psychiatry Res* 1995; **58**:203–215.

127. Feldman HM, Kolmen BK, Gonzaga AM: Naltrexone and communication skills in young children with autism. *J Am Acad Child Adolesc Psychiatry* 1999; **38**(5):587–593.

128. Herman BH, Hammock MK, Egan J, Arthur-Smith A, Chatoor I, Werner A: Peptides in self-injurious behavior: Dissociation from autonomic nervous system functioning. *Dev Pharmacol Therapeut* 1989; **12**:81–89.

129. Willemsen-Swinkels SH, Buitelaar JK, van Berckelaer-Onnes IA, van Engeland H: Brief report: Six months continuation treatment in naltrexone-responsive children with autism: An open-label case-control design. *J Autism Dev Disord* 1999; **29**:167–169.

130. Willemsen-Swinkels SHN, Buitelaar JK, Van Engeland H: The effects of chronic naltrexone treatment in young autistic children: A double-blind placebo-controlled crossover study. *Biol Psychiatry* 1996; **39**: 1023–1031.

131. Percy AK, Glaze DG, Schultz RJ, Zoghbi HY, Williamson D, Frost J Jr., Jankovic JJ, del Junco D, Skender M, Waring S, *et al.*: Rett syndrome: Controlled study of an oral opiate antagonist, naltrexone. *Ann Neurol* 1994; **35**:464–470.

132. Campbell M, Fish B, Korein J, Shapiro T, Collins P, Koh C: Lithium and chlorpromazine: A controlled crossover study of hyperactive severely disturbed young children. *J Autism Child Schizophr* 1972; **2**:234–263.

133. Buitelaar JK, van der Gaag RJ, van der Hoeven J: Buspirone in the management of anxiety and irritability in children with pervasive developmental disorders: Results of an open label study. *J Clin Psychiatry* 1998; **56**:56–59.

134. Carlsson ML: Hypothesis: is infantile autism a hypoglutamatergic disorder? Relevance of glutamate – serotonin interactions for pharmacotherapy. *J Neural Transm* 1998; **105**:525–35.

135. King B, Wright D, Handen B, Sikich L, Zimmerman A, McMahon W, Cantwell E, *et al.*: A double-blind, placebo-controlled study of amantidine hydrochloride in the treatment of children with autistic disorder. *J Am Acad Child Adolesc Psychiatry* 2001; **40**:658–665.

136. Martineau J, Barthelemy C, Cheliakine C, Lelord G: Brief report: An open middle-term study of combined vitamin B6-magnesium in a subgroup of autistic children selected on their sensitivity to this treatment. *J Autism Dev Disord* 1988; **18**(3):435–447.

137. Kleijnen J, Knipschild P: Niacin and vitamin B6 in mental functioning: A review of controlled trials in humans. *Biol Psychiatry* 1991; **29**:931–941.

138. Pfeiffer SI, Norton J, Nelson L, Shott S: Efficacy of vitamin B6 and magnesium in the treatment of autism: A methodology review and summary of outcomes. *J Autism Dev Disord* 1995; **25**:481–493.

139. Geller E, Ritvo ER, Freeman BJ, Yuwiler A: Preliminary observations on the effect of fenfluramine on blood serotonin and symptoms in three autistic boys. *N Engl J Med* 1982; **307**(3):165–169.

140. Aman MG, Kern RA: Review of fenfluramine in the treatment of the developmental disabilities. *J Am Acad Child and Adolesc Psychiatry* 1989; **28**: 549–565.

141. Leventhal B, Cook E, Morford M, Ravitz A, Heller W, Freedman D: Fenfluramine: Clinical and neurochemical effects in children with autism. *J Neuropsychiatry Clin Neurosci* 1993; **5**:307–315.

142. Aman MG, Kern RA, Arnold LE, McGhee DE: Fenfluramine and mental retardation. *J Am Acad Child Adolesc Psychiatry* 1991; **30**:507–508.

143. Schuster CR, Lewis M, Seiden LS: Fenfluramine: Neurotoxicity. *Psychopharm Bull* 1986; **22**:148–151.

144. Horvath K, Stefanatos G, Sokolski KN, Wachtel R, Nabors L, Tildon JT: Improved social and language skills after secretin administration in patients with autistic spectrum disorders. *J Assoc Acad Minor Phys* 1998; **9**:9–15.

145. Chez MG, Buchanan CP, Bagan BT, Hammer MS, McCarthy KS, Ovrutskaya I, Nowinski CV, *et al.*: Secretin and autism: A two-part clinical investigation. *J Autism Dev Disord* 2000; **30**:87–94.

146. Coniglio SJ, Lewis JD, Lang C, Burns TG, Subhani-Siddique R, Weintraub A, Schub H, *et al.*: A randomized, double-blind, placebo-controlled trial of single-dose intravenous secretin as treatment for children with autism. *J Pediatr* 2001; **138**:649–655.

147. Dunn-Geier J, Ho HH, Auersperg E, Doyle D, Eaves L, Matsuba C, Orrbine E, *et al.*: Effect of secretin on children with autism: A randomized controlled trial. *Dev Med Child Neurol* 2000; **42**:796–802.

148. Levy SE, Souders MC, Wray J, Jawad AF, Gallagher PR, Coplan J, Belchic JK, Gerdes M, Mitchell R, Mulberg AE: Children with autistic spectrum disorders. I: Comparison of placebo and single dose of human synthetic secretin. *Arch Dis Child* 2003; **88**(8):731–736.

149. Molloy CA, Manning-Courtney P, Swayne S, Bean J, Brown JM, Murray DS, Kinsman AM, Brasington M, Ulrich CD 2nd: Lack of benefit of intravenous synthetic human secretin in the treatment of autism. *J Autism Dev Disord* 2002; **32**(6):545–551.

150. Owley T, McMahon W, Cook EH, Laulhere TM, South M, Mays LZ, Shernoff ES, *et al.*: Multi-site, double-blind, placebo-controlled trial of porcine secretin in autism. *J Am Acad Child Adolesc Psychiatry* 2001; **40**:1293–1299.

151. Roberts W, Weaver L, Brian J, Bryson S, Emelianova S, Griffiths AM, MacKinnon B, *et al.*: Repeated doses of porcine secretin in the treatment of autism: A randomized, placebo-controlled trial. *Pediatrics* 2001; **107**:E71.

152. Sandler AD, Sutton KA, DeWeese J, Girardi MA, Sheppard V, Bodfish JW: Lack of benefit of a single dose of synthetic human secretin in the treatment of autism and pervasive developmental disorder. *N Engl J Med* 1999; **341**:1801–1806.

153. Unis AS, Munson JA, Rogers SJ, Goldson E, Osterling J, Gabriels R, Abbott RD, Dawson G: A randomized, double-blind, placebo-controlled trial of porcine versus synthetic secretin for reducing symptoms of autism. *J Am Acad Child Adolesc Psychiatry* 2002; **41**(11): 1315–1321.

22

Mental Retardation

Bryan H. King, Matthew W. State, Arthur Maerlender

Introduction

Some 50 years ago, Tredgold wrote that the literature had come to be so extensive, and to relate to so many different disciplines, that a single textbook could scarcely contain it all [1]. Knowledge relating to mental retardation (MR), from definition to assessment, and from etiology to treatment, now fills many books. The aim of this chapter will be to provide an overview for the child psychiatrist.

At the outset it is worth highlighting the fact that the population with MR is heterogeneous. There are no personality traits that are unique to persons with intellectual disability, and insofar as generalizations are possible, it is perhaps worthwhile to remember that a person's intelligence quotient (IQ) is as useful as his age in terms of inferring his personality. Just as a group of senior citizens might include both the bedridden and skydivers, so, also, a group of persons with intelligence quotients of 60 will include persons representing an enormous range of talents and temperaments.

Definition of Mental Retardation (Intellectual Disability)

The landscape regarding both the diagnosis and the use of the 'label' of MR continues to be, and perhaps always has been, in a state of flux. Current terminology appears to be in the process of change from 'mental retardation' to 'intellectual disability.' As of 1992, the American Association on Mental Retardation (AAMR) definition of MR required a multidimensional approach, with emphasis on functioning and environmental considerations, rather than previously used medical or statistical frameworks [2]. How MR severity is described has also changed. Rather than using IQ cutoff scores, both AAMR and *International Classification of Disease, Tenth Edition,* (ICD-

10) use intensity of supports needed by an individual to define severity, which is believed to be more functional, relevant, and service-oriented [3]. Given that the *Diagnostic and Statistical Manual of Mental Disorders,* 4th ed. [4] of the American Psychiatric Association continues to use IQ cutoff points to define severity, there still remains no universally agreed upon definition or classification system for MR [5] (Box A).

Arguably, MR or intellectual disability is arbitrarily defined along the continuum of intellectual abilities, and its definition has challenged both medicine and society. Esquirol [6] is credited as being the first medical writer to have defined 'idiocy' as a disorder in which the mental faculties fail to develop. He provided an important distinction between intellectual disability and mental disorders on the one hand, and dementia on the other. Modern definitions retain this differentiation by requiring that the age at onset is less than 18 years (Figure 22.1).

Functional impairment has historically been an additional defining criterion for intellectual disability, with sixteenth-century legal standards being the ability to count to 20 pence, tell one's age, to name one's parents [7], or the ability to name the days of the week and to measure a yard of cloth [8]. Today, adaptive functioning is assessed with the use of standardized tests. The most widely used instruments are the Vineland Adaptive Behavior Scales [9] and the AAMR Adaptive Behavior Scale – School, or Residential and Community, 2nd ed. [10]. The Vineland provides indices of function in the domains of communication, daily living skills, motor skills, and socialization. A composite score can also be generated which expresses global adaptive function referenced to that expected for an individual of a given chronological age.

The third criterion which must be met to satisfy the definition of MR is that of below average intellectual functioning. Formal tests of intelligence are typically

Clinical Child Psychiatry, Second Edition. Edited by W.M. Klykylo and J.L. Kay
© 2005 John Wiley & Sons Ltd.

BOX A DSM-IV-TR DIAGNOSTIC CRITERIA FOR MENTAL RETARDATION

Notes: This is coded on Axis II
Mental retardation

(A) Significantly subaverage intellectual functioning: an IQ of approximately 70 or below on an individually administered IQ test (for infants, a clinical judgment of significantly subaverage intellectual functioning)

(B) Concurrent deficits or impairments in present adaptive functioning (i.e., the person's effectiveness in meeting the standards expected for his or her age by his to her cultural group) in at least two of the following areas: communication, self-care, home living, social/interpersonal skills, use of community resources, self-direction, functional academic skills, work, leisure, health, and safety

(C) The onset is before age 18 years

Code based on degree of severity reflecting level of intellectual impairment:

317	Mild mental retardation IQ level 50–55 to approximately 70
318.0	Moderate mental retardation IQ level 35–40 to 50–55
318.1	Severe mental retardation IQ level 20–25 to 35–40
318.2	Profound mental retardation IQ level below 20 or 25
319	Mental retardation, severity unspecified, when there is a strong presumption of mental retardation but the person's intelligence is untestable by standard tests (e.g., for individuals too impaired or uncooperative, or with infants)

Reprinted with permission from American Psychiatric Association: *Diagnostic and Statistical Manual of Mental Disorders*, 4th ed. Text Revision. Washington, DC: American Psychiatric Association, 2000.

Mental retardation refers to substantial limitations in present functioning. It is characterized by significantly subaverage intellectual functioning, existing concurrently with related limitations in two or more of the following applicable adaptive skill areas: communication, self-care, home living, social skills, community use, self-direction, health and safety, functional academics, leisure, and work. Mental retardation manifests before the age of 18 years.

From American Association on Mental Retardation: *Mental Retardation: Definition, Classification, and Systems of Support.* 9th ed. Washington, DC: American Association on Mental Retardation, 1992

Figure 22.1 The American Association on Mental Retardation's definition of mental retardation.

expressed as a ratio of measured performance (expressed in terms of developmental age) to chronological age, which defines the intelligence 'quotient' or IQ. The most widely used instruments for measuring IQ are the Weschler Intelligence Scales for Children – Revised and the Stanford–Binet. A modification of the Stanford–Binet, the Kuhlman–Binet, may be useful for individuals with profound intellectual disability.

For the population as a whole, IQ follows a normal distribution or 'bell-shaped curve.' For most IQ tests, each standard deviation is approximately 15 points, so an IQ of 70 is approximately two standard deviations from the mean. Fifty-five would be three standard deviations below the mean; 40 is four standard deviations, and so on. This successive marching of standard deviations out from the mean corresponds to the traditional categories of, 'mild, moderate, severe, and profound,' which form a measure of the severity of intellectual disability [4]. Alternatively, these categories might also represent the level of intervention needed to support the habilitation of an affected individual [2].

Not surprisingly, there are more ways to go wrong than right, and pathways to disability outnumber pathways to giftedness. As a result, the distribution of the population in terms of IQ is not perfectly bell shaped. It is believed that as intellectual disability increases in severity, the probability of an identifiable organic etiology also increases. Furthermore, because of the unique demands placed upon a child's attention and concentration by school, it is not infrequent that MR first becomes a consideration as part of the evaluation of poor school performance. On the other hand, persons given the diagnosis of MR during school-age years may disappear into society and function well enough so as no longer to meet criteria later in life.

There is also evidence that cognitive differences exist between individuals with the same IQ [11,12]. Reitan and Wolfson [13] thus argue that use of IQ scores alone to diagnose MR is insufficient. A more detailed neuropsychological battery may provide important insights about brain dysfunction as well as account for inter- and intra-individual differences. A neuropsychological battery can reveal differences in severity of particular impairments and may facilitate differential diagnosis.

Indeed, specific forms of MR have different cognitive profiles. Many patients with Turner syndrome show parietal lobe dysfunction and do poorly on visual-perceptual and visual-constructional tasks.

In Down syndrome, although cognitive development and learning can continue beyond adolescence and into adulthood, particularly with appropriate learning experiences [14], there is evidence that cognitive development declines with age [15]. Children with mosaicism tend to score higher on IQ tests, and better on tests of visual-perceptual skills than do children with complete trisomy [16].

Pulsifer [17] reviewed the literature concerning MR from a neuropsychological perspective, with particular attention to idiopathic MR and five major identifiable prenatal causes of MR: fetal alcohol syndrome, Down syndrome, fragile X syndrome, Prader–Willi syndrome, and Angelman syndrome. Cognitive deficits common to all disorders were demonstrated for attention, short-term memory, and sequential information processing, whereas language and visuospatial abilities were varied. Neuroanatomical abnormalities common to all disorders are identifiable in the hippocampus and cerebellum; individual disorders typically showed a unique pattern of other neurological abnormalities.

That a person could have MR in one setting and not another fuels the controversy as to what constitutes real 'intelligence' and whether it can be reduced to a single number. As neuropsychological testing demonstrates, individuals may have certain 'splinter' skills that are not adequately captured in a global IQ measure. Others may have substantially different verbal and nonverbal abilities and perform poorly on some standardized tests, but relatively better on others. And at the end of the day, the utility or significance of an IQ test must be placed into a real world context. In certain neighborhoods, for example, the survival value of knowing how to interpret gang slogans and what

colors not to wear is clearly greater than being able to recognize or define 'a limpet.' Taken together, clinicians must take into account the range of strengths and deficits with which a patient presents in considering the diagnosis of mental retardation.

Incidence and Prevalence of Mental Retardation

The considerable variations in the estimates of prevalence of intellectual disability across countries and regions, from 2 to 85 per 1000, may be attributable to the variations in major classification systems and to diversity in operational definitions and methodologies [18]. Nevertheless, many reviews of international epidemiological studies suggest that the prevalence of severe MR (SMR) is approximately 3–4 per 1000 in children [18,19]. This rate has been fairly stable over time. What has changed is the prevalence of what is defined as mild MR (MMR) which has almost doubled from 5.4 to 10.6 per 1000 by the inclusion of education department data using record linkage [20].

Regardless of the definition, males are between 1.6 to 1.7 times more likely to experience MMR, SMR, isolated MR or MR accompanied by other neurological disorders [21]. Croen and colleagues [22] found that the relative risk for males for MMR (1.9) was greater than for SMR (1.4) for MR of unknown etiology. Both genetic (X-linked) and neonatal mortality factors (that is, the likelihood of prenatal or neonatal mortality increases as the significance of the brain pathology increases) could explain some of this difference [20].

The current consensus is that mental retardation affects approximately 1%–2% of the population in developed countries. Again, because of the importance of significant impairments in both cognitive and adaptive abilities in meeting diagnostic criteria, the prevalence of mental retardation appears to be less than that which would be predicted on the basis of IQ distribution alone (2.28%).

Etiological Considerations

As noted by Esquirol, intellectual disability is not a disease in and of itself, but the developmental outcome of a pathogenic process. With advances in medicine generally and in molecular genetics in particular, new causes of mental retardation, or the genetic etiologies of formerly unspecified syndromes are identified at an extraordinary pace. In the previous version of this chapter, it was noted that over 350 causes of mental retardation had been identified [23]. Currently, a keyword search of 'mental retardation' in the Online

Mendelian Inheritance in Man database [24] yields some 1231 entries, and there are over 300 X-linked mental retardation syndromes alone.

As clinicians approach the etiology of mental retardation for a particular patient, it is helpful to work from a broad framework initially. A straightforward initial distinction might be drawn in terms of congenital versus acquired etiologies. For the latter, the timing of the insult which led to disability may be further broken down into perinatal or postnatal causes. Congenital causes might be divided into genetic disorders or developmental disorders of brain formation, or still more specifically into inborn errors of metabolism and so on.

Etiological factors associated with mild MR are typically more difficult to ascertain. Mild intellectual disability is significantly higher, for example, in individuals from lower socioeconomic situations. Often, other family members may have similar intellectual profiles. Adverse conditions such as environmental toxins, and traumatic living situations are more common in this group.

Behavioral Phenotypes

Interest in the association between behavior and underlying chromosomal abnormalities has grown over the past 30 years, when, for example, a review of behavioral aspects of chromosomal disorders included just five syndromes [25]. Nowadays, such lists are much longer, and eventually, the number of disorders for which a 'behavioral phenotype' is suggested will likely approach the number of disorders for which a specific genetic etiology is known. Dykens [26], proposed that a 'behavioral phenotype' exists for a genetic disorder when the probability of the expression of certain behaviors, or constellations of behaviors, is greater than that which would otherwise be expected. Stereotyped hand movements, for example, have been described in many contexts, but a particular form of stereotyped hand wringing is almost invariably seen in Rett syndrome. Obesity is certainly nonspecific, but the probability of an individual with Prader–Willi Syndrome becoming obese is nearly 100%. Penrose [27] anticipated modern neuropsychological characterization when he observed that persons with Down syndrome were typified by '... cheerful and friendly personalities. Their capacities for imitation and their memories for people, for music and for complex situations may be found to range far beyond their other abilities. They are incapable of abstract reasoning. They cannot do arithmetic although they may sometimes be able to read and write.'([27] p. 206).

Table 22.1 lists a representative sample of syndromes for which behavioral phenotypes have been described. These disorders are still being studied with respect to their behavioral and neuropsychological profiles. In some cases, particular aspects of a behavioral phenotype are already widely accepted and have been carefully validated using standardized measures. In other instances, the proposed phenotypes are suggested by only a relatively small number of descriptive case series.

The ongoing process of identifying and clarifying behavioral phenotypes brings with it considerable potential benefit. From a clinical standpoint, recognition of certain behavioral patterns may suggest a diagnosis, and thus provide valuable information regarding the course, prognosis, treatment, and expected areas of relative strength and difficulty associated with a syndrome. From a research perspective, the elaboration of behavioral phenotypes is equally important. As basic and clinical sciences continue rapidly to advance, individuals with known genetic lesions and well-defined behavioral manifestations may provide scientists with critical insights into the complex interaction of nature and nurture.

Mental Retardation and Mental Disorders

In his text on *The Biology of Mental Defect*, Penrose [27] observed that mental illness needed to be distinguished from intellectual defect. Further, that 'a person of any level of intellectual capacity can suffer from any degree of mental illness' ([27] p. 248). He also observed that 'the susceptibility to [mental] illness may indeed be correlated with intelligence level, in that certain kinds of defect may predispose to epilepsy or psychosis' ([27] p. 248). The situation of epiloia (tuberous sclerosis complex), interestingly, was specifically singled out as one in which mental illness seemed inextricably linked to the syndrome itself.

The literature since Penrose has repeatedly confirmed that children with MR are at a higher risk for psychiatric problems than the general population. In the case of Down syndrome, the risk for externalizing problems [attention deficit hyperactivity disorder (ADHD), oppositional defiant disorder (ODD), conduct disorder (CD)] and aggressive behaviors) is higher than for internalizing problems. Children with Down syndrome are at a lower risk for developing psychiatric disorders than are other children with MR, but their risk is still higher than the general population [28].

The presence of intellectual disability is a significant risk factor for mental disorders. However, the problem

Table 22.1 Mental retardation and representative behavioral phenotypes.

Disorder	Pathogenic features	Clinical features/behavioral phenotype
Down syndrome	Trisomy 21, most often associated with nondisjunction (95%); the remainder are generally translocations involving chromosome 21. Frequency of occurrence is 1:1000 live births, but increases dramatically with maternal age to 1:2500 in women <30 years old, 1:80 <40 years old	Some level of impaired cognitive development. Children with mosaicism tend to have higher IQ scores than those with trisomy 21. Visual short-term memory better than auditory Cognitive development declines with age Children with mosaicism tend to score higher on IQ tests than those with trisomy 21 Some indication of average visual-perceptual skills in mosaicism children as well Evidence that cognitive development and learning can continue beyond adolescence and into adulthood, particularly with appropriate learning experiences
Fragile X syndrome	Inactivation of *FMR-1* gene at X q27.3 is generally due to >200 CCG base repeats and associated methylation Inheritance is recessive Frequency of occurrence is 1:1000 male births and 1:3000 female FraX accounts for 10%–12% of MR in males and remains the most common heritable cause of MR	Strengths in verbal memory Executive dysfunction including attention deficits, short-attention span, hyperactivity, perseverative behaviors Females with normal IQ often have learning disabilities, attention and organizational problems and math difficulties
Prader–Willi syndrome	Deletion in 15q11–15q13 region of paternal origin (75%) Some cases of maternal uniparental disomy (22%) and imprinting errors and translocations (3%) A number of genes within the critical region may contribute to specific features of the phenotype Incidence of PWS ranges from 1:10 000 to 1:25 000 live births	Hypotonia, often failure to thrive in infancy, later obesity, small hands, and feet, microorchidism, cryptorchidism, short stature, almond shaped eyes, fair hair and light skin, flat face, scoliosis, orthopaedic problems, prominent forehead and bitemporal narrowing OCD is common Relative strengths in spatial-perceptual organization and visual processing (puzzles) Relative weaknesses in short-term processing Considerable variability in profiles Findings support the reports of cognitive differences between deletion and disomy genetic subgroups with higher verbal abilities in those with chromosome 15 disomy, while those

Table 22.1 *Continued*

Disorder	Pathogenic features	Clinical features/behavioral phenotype
		with deletions are similar to the general LD group A new finding is that the disomy groups have particular difficulty with graphomotor control
Angelman syndrome	Deletion in 15q11–15q13 (same region as for PWS above) but of maternal origin (70%) Some cases of paternal uniparental disomy (3%), and intragenic mutations Approximately 20% of cases have an unknown genetic etiology As with PWS, many candidate genes could contribute to aspects of the phenotype Involvement of a gamma-aminobutyric acid receptor subunit gene may be important in the pathogenesis of epilepsy in AS Estimated incidence is 1 : 20 000 live births Prevalence in populations of individuals with severe MR is 1.4%	Fair hair and blue eyes (66%), dysmorphic facies including wide mouth, thin upper lip, pointed chin, epilepsy (90%) with characteristic EEG, ataxia, small head circumphrence, 25% microcephalic Happy disposition, paroxysmal laughter, hand flapping, clapping, sleep disturbance with nighttime waking Developmental delay, which becomes apparent by 6–12 months of age, severely impaired expressive language, ataxic gait, tremulousness of limbs, and a typical behavioral profile, including a happy demeanor, hypermotoric behavior, and low attention span Receptive language somewhat better than expressive, in part due to oral-motor dyspraxia
Cornelia de Lange syndrome	Deletion in NIPBL gene (human homolog of *Drosophila* 'Nipped-B' gene) at 5p13.1 Similar phenotype has been associated with other chromosomal deletions including one at 3q26.3 Prevalence is estimated to be as high as 1 : 10 000	Continuous eyebrows, thin down-turning upper lip, microcephaly, short stature, small hands and feet, small upturned nose, anteverted nostrils, malformed upper lips, failure to thrive Language delays, avoidance of being held, stereotypic movements, twirling behaviors Degree of MR from borderline (10%), through mild (8%), moderate (18%), and severe (20%) to profound (43%) A wide variety of symptoms occur frequently, notably hyperactivity (40%), self-injury (44%), daily aggression (49%), and sleep disturbance (55%) These behaviors correlate closely with the presence of an autistic like syndrome and with the degree of MR

Table 22.1 *Continued*

Disorder	Pathogenic features	Clinical features/behavioral phenotype
		The frequency and severity of disturbance, continuing beyond childhood, is important when planning the amount and duration of support required by parents
Williams syndrome	Hemizygous (autosomal dominant) deletion in chromosome 7q11.23, often including the gene for elastin (*ELN*) Prevalence may be as high as 1 : 7500, or 6% of individuals with identifiable genetic causes for MR	Short stature, unusual facial features including broad forehead, depressed nasal bridge, stellate pattern of the iris, widely spaced teeth, full lips; renal and cardiovascular abnormalities, hypercalcemia ADHD, poor peer relationships, loquaciousness, excessive anxiety and sleep disturbance, increased mimicry, socially outgoing and disinhibited Verbal abilities typically better than nonverbal Visual-spatial construction very weak, with improvement over time, but more protracted development rarely reaching average levels Auditory rote memory better than might be expected given overall cognitive ability Oral language skills are relative strengths Overall IQ scores variable, but typically below average
Cri du Chat syndrome	Autosomal dominant deletion in chromosome 5p15.2, probably involving the adherens junction protein, delta-catenin (*CTNND2*) This protein is expressed early in neuronal development and plays a role in cell motility Estimated prevalence is between 1 : 15 000 and 1 : 45 000 live births	Round face; moderate to severe MR Significantly better receptive language than expressive (but still delayed)
Tuberous Sclerosis Complex, 1 and 2	Autosomal dominant disorder caused by a mutation in either the *TSC1* gene (hamartin) on chromosome 9q34 or the *TSC2* gene (tuberin) on chromosome 16p13. These proteins form a TSC1–TSC2 tumor suppressor	Epilepsy Autism is common (as many as 40% of individuals) Hyperactivity, impulsivity, aggression The spectrum of MR ranges from none (30%) to profound

Table 22.1 *Continued*

Disorder	Pathogenic features	Clinical features/behavioral phenotype
	complex, providing an explanation for the similar phenotype in individuals with mutations in either of these genes. Prevalence is approximately 1:6000 individuals, *TSC1* (50%) and *TSC2* (50%), but *TSC1* may be associated with a milder phenotype	Self-injurious behaviors, sleep disturbances including nightmare waking and early morning waking have all been described
Neurofibromatosis Type 1	One of the most common autosomal dominant disorders in humans, located at 17q11.2, and affecting 1:3000 individuals *NF1* is a large gene that codes for neurofibromin Loss of *NF1* gene expression results in enhanced cell proliferation and tumor formation *NF2* is much rarer, estimated to occur in 1:33 000, and the majority of these cases are asymptomatic The gene for *NF2* appears to be at chromosome 22q12.2	Full scale IQs ranged from 70 to 130 among children with NF1 and from 99 to 139 among unaffected sibs Scores of parents with NF1 range from 85 to 114 compared to 80 to 134 in unaffected parents Children with NF1 may show significant deficits in language and reading abilities compared to sibs, but not in mathematics They also can have impaired visuospatial and neuromotor skills A statistically significant correlation has been found between lowering of IQ and visuospatial deficits and the number of foci seen on MRI Speech difficulties, verbal IQ > performance IQ, distractible, impulsive, hyperactive, anxious Possible association with increased incidence of mood and anxiety disorders Variable physical manifestations may include café au lait spots, cutaneous neurofibromas, Lisch nodules, short stature and macrocephaly
Lesch–Nyhan syndrome	Single gene defect in hypoxanthine guanine phosphoribosyltransferase (Xq26–q27.2) with possible secondary dopamine supersensitivity in the striatum LNS is recessive, and rare, with incidence estimated to be 1:38 000	Variability in cognitive compromise with the majority below 70 IQ Difficulty with multistep reasoning and working memory demands; also cognitive flexibility sequential skills and environmental monitoring Focused attention seems strong Motor skills are impaired, with visual-motor integration less so Some indication that visual-spatial skills are a strength

Table 22.1 *Continued*

Disorder	Pathogenic features	Clinical features/behavioral phenotype
		Severe (compulsive) self-biting behavior is common Aggression and anxiety are also frequent Ataxia, chorea, kidney failure, gout
Galactosemia	Autosomal recessive defect in galactose-1-phosphate uridylyltransferase gene located at 9p13. The disorder is quite rare, occurring in as few as 1 : 62 000 births (slightly more common in Caucasians)	MR is a diagnostic feature In children with galactosemia, cognitive outcome appears to relate to genotype rather than metabolic control There is evidence that variability in neurocognitive outcome is at least in part dependent on allelic heterogeneity Vomiting in early infancy, jaundice, hepatosplenomegaly, later cataracts, weight loss, food refusal, increased intracranial pressure and increased risk for sepsis, ovarian failure, failure to thrive, renal tubular damage Visuospatial deficits, language disorders, reports of increased behavioral problems, anxiety, social withdrawal, and shyness
Phenylketonuria	Autosomal recessive defect in phenylalanine hydroxylase (PAH) located at 12q.24.1, or cofactor (biopterin synthetase, 11q22.3–q23.3) with toxic accumulation of phenylalanine Prevalence is approximately 1 : 12 000	While early treated PKU children exhibit IQ levels within the normal range, it appears that they do not reach levels predicted by parent and sibling levels Declines possible, particularly with poor dietary control Symptoms absent neonatally, later development of seizures (25% grand mal), fair skin, blue eyes, blond hair, rash Untreated: mild to profound MR, language delay, destructiveness, self-injury, rage attacks, hyperactivity Treated: possible increase in hyperactivity and anxiety
Hurler syndrome	Rare autosomal recessive deficiency in alpha-L-iduronidase, located at 4p16.3 Estimated prevalence is 1 : 144 000 births	Decline in cognition after first year Sensory impairments with language delays secondary to hearing loss Loss of skills by age three years CNS deterioration accompanied by hydrocephalus

Table 22.1 *Continued*

Disorder	Pathogenic features	Clinical features/behavioral phenotype
		Early onset, short stature, hepatosplenomegaly, hirsutism, corneal clouding, death before 10 years of age; dwarfism, coarse facial features, recurrent respiratory infections Moderate to severe MR, anxious, fearful, rarely aggressive
Hunter syndrome	Rare deficiency in iduronate sulfatase, located at Xq28 Estimated prevalence is 1:111000 births	Normal infancy; symptom onset 2–4 years old Typical coarse facies with flat nasal bridge, flaring nostrils, hearing loss, ataxia, hernia common, enlarged liver and spleen, joint stiffness, recurrent infections, growth retardation, cardiovascular abnormalities Death in first or second decade Hyperactivity MR evident by two years old Speech delay, loss of speech at 8–10 years old Restless, aggressive, inattentive, abnormal sleep Apathetic, sedentary with disease progression
Sanfilipo syndrome Type A, B, C, and D	Autosomal recessive (1:24000 live births) Heparin-N-sulfatase deficiency (type A) Chromosome 12q is implicated in type D	Normal early development, recurrent ear, nose, throat and bowel problems CNS deterioration by six years, hearing loss, mild skeletal abnormalities, death in second or third decade MR mild to profound Biting, hyperactivity, unprovoked aggression, sleep disturbance, second decade increasingly immobile and quiet, dementia, mood liability
Fetal alcohol syndrome	Maternal alcohol consumption (third trimester > second > first trimester), 1:3000 live births in Western countries (most common preventable cause of MR) As many as 1:300 children may have fetal alcohol effects (FAE)	MR is possible Often learning disabilities, attention deficits, hyperactivity, memory loss and conduct problems due to poor awareness of consequences of behavior Irritability, decreased abstracting ability, impulsivity, speech and

Table 22.1 *Continued*

Disorder	Pathogenic features	Clinical features/behavioral phenotype
		language delays; fetal alcohol effects = incomplete syndrome Microcephaly, short stature, midface hypoplasia, short palpebral fissure, thin upper lip, retrognathia in infancy, micrognathia in adolescence, hypoplastic long and smooth philtrum
Smith–Magenis syndrome	Most cases of SMS have a large deletion within chromosome 17p11.2 Several candidate genes have been suggested Disturbed melatonin secretion may be implicated in the sleep disturbance associated with this syndrome Estimated prevalence is approximately 1 : 25 000 live births	Broad face, flat midface, short broad hands, small toes and hoarse, deep voice Severe self-injury including hand biting, head banging, and pulling out finger and toe nails Autistic features Initial and middle insomnia Measured IQ ranges between 20 and 78, most patients falling in the moderate range of MR (between 40 and 54), although scores in the mild or borderline range are not uncommon Simultaneous processing is generally stronger than sequential processing A strength in visual-Gestalt closure and reading/decoding has been identified Expressive vocabulary is stronger than receptive vocabulary Relative weaknesses in arithmetic and in understanding riddles have also been identified Longer term memory processes appear to be relatively stronger than short-term processes, which also impact attentional functioning Hyperactivity in 75%
Rubinstein–Taybi syndrome	Autosomal dominant deletion involving the cyclic adenosine monophosphate (cAMP) response element binding (CREB) protein gene (*CBP*) located at 16.13.3 Estimated prevalence is 1 : 10 000 live births and RTS may account for approximately 0.2% of individuals with MR in institutional settings	Short stature and microcephaly, broad thumb and big toes Prominent nose, broad nasal bridge, hypertelorism, ptosis, frequent fractures, feeding difficulties in infancy, congenital heart disease, EEG abnormalities in 75%, seizures in 25% Poor concentration, distractible, expressive language difficulties, PIQ > VIQ

Table 22.1 *Continued*

Disorder	Pathogenic features	Clinical features/behavioral phenotype
		Anecdotally happy, loving sociable, responsive to music, self-stimulating behavior Older individuals with mood lability and temper tantrums
Velocardiofacial syndrome (VCFS), DiGeorge syndrome, CATCH 22	Several candidate genes have been identified at the 22q11.2 locus for VCFS including the T-box gene, *TBX1* T-box genes are transcription factors involved in the regulation of developmental processes The catechol-O-methyltransferase gene, *COMT*, is also located at the 22q11.2 region, and its importance in the catabolism of catecholamines, including the neurotransmitters dopamine, epinephrine, and norepinephrine, may be important in the high incidence of psychosis associated with VCFS Prevalence is 1 : 4000 VCFS is the second most common cause of congenital cardiac anomalies after Down syndrome	VCFS is the most common MR syndrome that has palatal anomalies as a major feature Cleft palate, cardiac anomalies, typical facies Less frequent features include microcephaly, MR, short stature, slender hands and digits, minor auricular anomalies, and inguinal hernia. Prominent tubular nose, narrow palpebral fissures, and slightly retruded mandible Ophthalmologic abnormalities including tortuous retinal vessels, small optic discs, or bilateral cataracts (70%). Neonatal hypocalcemia requiring treatment may occur (13%) Cardiac pathology, most commonly tetralogy of Fallot, ventricular septal defect, interrupted aortic arch, apulmonary atresia/ventricular septal defect, and truncus arteriosus Higher verbal than nonverbal IQ scores, assets in verbal memory, and deficits in the areas of attention, story memory, visuospatial memory, arithmetic performance relative to other areas of achievement, and psychosocial functioning Learning disabilities characterized by difficulty with abstraction, reading comprehension, and mathematics Children with VCFS may have characteristic personality features of blunt or inappropriate affect, with a greater than expected number of children developing severe psychiatric illnesses as they approached adolescence

of what to consider a mental disorder, and how to diagnose it, is one that has long challenged psychiatrists working with persons with MR. How does one diagnose psychosis in a patient who cannot endorse hallucinations or delusions? How does depression or anxiety manifest itself when these feelings cannot be communicated verbally? When is a behavior problem evidence of a mental disorder and not just an example of 'mental retardation'?

The approach to these challenges is similar to the approach child psychiatrists utilize in evaluating young patients who similarly may be unable to understand or articulate feelings, and whose behavior may even be attributed to their young age by parents or careproviders. When it comes to children and adults with intellectual disability, clinicians must determine how a particular symptom or pattern of behavior relates to what could be expected from a person of a given developmental age, and to appreciate how certain subjective feeling states might be communicated in the context of a limited repertoire for such expression.

With this strategy in hand, it is possible to make psychiatric diagnoses in persons with intellectual disability using the Diagnostic and Statistical Manual with some practical allowances. The National Association for the Dually Diagnosed ('dual diagnosis' refers to mental retardation and mental illness) is currently collaborating with the American Psychiatric Association to develop modified diagnostic criteria to assist in this process. The Royal College of Psychiatrists has similarly developed criteria for the diagnosis of mental disorders for adults with intellectual disability [29].

Adaptation of Diagnostic Criteria

Disruptive Behavior Disorders

Attention Deficit Hyperactivity Disorder

For persons with MR, the diagnosis of ADHD currently requires that symptoms are excessive for an individual's mental age. In the context of profound MR, attention span, distractibility, or 'on-task' behavior are predictably quite variable and could be influenced not only by cognitive limitations but also by motivational factors. Individuals given the diagnosis of ADHD in this context should, in comparison to their peers with similar levels of disability, exhibit unusually short attention span (even for activities of interest), excessive psychomotor activity level, remarkable impulsivity, and so on.

In some cases, the clinician will encounter a situation in which an individual does not evidence remarkable psychomotor activity, nor attention difficulties, but may be unusually impulsive. In these situations, most commonly exemplified by an individual who might inexplicably strike out at a peer in the absence of any identifiable environmental stressor, the diagnosis of an impulse control disorder [not otherwise specified (NOS)] should be entertained. The problem with such a diagnosis is that the criteria upon which it is based are arguably in the eye of the beholder. On the other hand, the value in rendering such a diagnosis is that it indicates that other disorders (for which criteria are arguably better established) like depression, anxiety, and so on, have been considered and ruled out. The diagnosis of a 'specific' disorder of impulse control also identifies a target for intervention beyond 'mental retardation'.

Oppositional Defiant Disorder/Conduct Disorder

The DSM-IV diagnosis of ODD or CD also requires comparisons be made to others of similar mental age. In addition, both diagnoses assume some degree of willfulness on the part of the individual in question (for example, disobedience motivated by spite or resentment) which can be very difficult to discern in nonverbal subjects with profound cognitive deficits. This point also has been made by Reid [30]. As with many psychiatric illnesses in this context, the certainty with which the disorder is diagnosed will tend to evaporate with greater severity of intellectual disability.

Anxiety Disorders

Anxiety disorders are probably more often overlooked than many other mental illnesses in this population, but there is clear evidence that the full range of anxiety disorders can occur in the context of intellectual disability [31]. Specific anxiety disorders like separation anxiety, overanxious disorder, obsessive–compulsive disorder (OCD), panic disorder, generalized anxiety disorder, and so on, rely heavily on an individual's ability to describe subjective symptoms of anxiety. According to DSM-IV, concurrent pervasive developmental disorder specifically trumps the diagnosis of most of these disorders as well. Nevertheless, many children with autism spectrum disorders in particular, and intellectual disability in general, are referred with constellations of signs and symptoms that best are captured in the anxiety disorder spectrum.

Children and adolescents who are clearly avoidant, who exhibit autonomic arousal in the face of stimuli that most of their peers would not find aversive, who present with other features of anxiety might be given a diagnosis of anxiety disorder NOS when they cannot articulate their subjective states. In some cases individuals engage in behavior that appears compulsive or driven, and even ego-alien. The diagnosis of OCD NOS might be considered under such circumstances.

Recently, an empirically derived, behaviorally based instrument has been described which may become particularly useful in identifying mood and anxiety disorders in persons with intellectual disability. The Anxiety, Depression, And Mood Scale (ADAMS), is a 28-item survey that demonstrates both reliability and validity in preliminary study [32], and could become an important adjunct in differential diagnosis in this population.

Repetitive behaviors are not uncommon in persons with mental retardation. These behaviors should not be equated with compulsions necessarily. For example, a child may quite enjoy flipping light switches on and off; or swinging in a swing. These behaviors may be innately reinforcing for sensory or other reasons, and would not satisfy an anxiolytic or 'ego-alien' criterion thought to be at the core of OCD. Such behaviors are perhaps better viewed on a continuum with stereotyped movements, but in some cases may be more goal directed. The discrimination between repetitive behaviors in terms of their etiology and their treatment (if appropriate) should be a focus of additional research in this population.

Another form of repetitive behavior includes self-injury. For some of these individuals, there may also be evidence of self-restraint. They may, for example, securing their extremities in their clothing or hold on to objects such that their hands are functionally unavailable. Alternatively, they might cling to their parents or care-providers – seemingly to prevent self-injurious behaviors [33]. In these cases, the self-injury appears to be compulsive or 'driven' and a diagnosis of OCD might be considered.

Eating Disorders

The diagnoses of anorexia nervosa and bulimia are effectively precluded for individuals with severe or profound mental retardation because of the near total reliance of diagnostic criteria upon the subjective experience of the patient with the eating disorder. For example, it would be a challenge at best to identify classic distortions in body image, or guilt feelings associated with bingeing in nonverbal subjects. Food refusal or self-induced vomiting would have to be viewed as atypical eating disorders if such symptoms were to occur in the absence of other diagnosable disorders (for example depression, rumination, etc.). Pica is likely to be among the most common of the eating disorders diagnosed among persons with intellectual disability, however psychogenic overeating, vomiting, rumination, and simple food refusal may be relatively common [34].

Disorders Associated with a General Medical Condition

Strictly speaking, one might submit that everyone with MR retardation has some 'organic' cerebral dysfunction, by definition, and thus any psychiatric illness should be regarded as organic or due to a general medical condition. In his study of psychiatric illness in a sample of institutionalized patients with Down syndrome, Menolascino [35] argued that psychiatric nosology did not have to be reinvented to accommodate individuals with a 'tissue diagnosis.' Moreover, patients with so-called 'dual diagnoses' of mental illness and Down syndrome need to be distinguished from others with Down syndrome alone. Thus, the application of the diagnoses of organic mental syndromes and disorders is probably best approached as if patients do not have MR. The same principle should apply to Axis II personality disorders. The diagnosis of 'organic' personality disorder is best reserved for individuals whose preexisting personality was altered in a pathological way by some additional cerebral insult. In essence, this category (due to a medical condition) is best reserved for patients whose MR is acquired and results in a change in personality, usually secondary to central nervous system (CNS) trauma experienced in childhood or early adolescence.

Psychosis

The diagnosis of schizophrenia essentially requires that a patient relate the experience of delusions or hallucinations. As has been suggested by others [36–38] persons with profound MR and limited communicative ability pose particular problems with it comes to diagnosing classic schizophrenia. Nonetheless, the display of presumptive evidence of response to hallucinations (e.g., striking or shouting at empty space, throwing imaginary peers from furniture) or the adoption of catatonic postures can appear to be psychotic in origin. In these cases the diagnosis of psychosis NOS should be considered if these signs exist in the absence of sufficient evidence to warrant the diagnosis of a supervening mood disorder.

Mood Disorders

The diagnosis of mood disorders is fairly straightforward even in profound MR. Generally, a change in mood from baseline is obvious (recent onset lability, tearfulness, mood elevation, irritability). If coupled with changes in interests, in activity level, sleep, appetite, or sexual behavior, of sufficient duration and causing sufficient impairment in function, the diagnoses of mania or of depression can be made in nonverbal patients [39,40].

Other Disorders

The diagnosis of Tourette syndrome is made difficult in persons with severe MR because of the common coexistence of stereotyped or other repetitive movements [41,42]. Additionally, it can be quite difficult to discriminate between intentional and unintentional movements, or vocal tics from spontaneous, stereotyped, or echolalic vocalizations. The diagnosis of stereotyped movement disorder might be considered in such circumstances. Since elimination disorders require a mental age of four years in order to be considered, the diagnoses of functional encopresis or functional enuresis are seldom made in the context of severe intellectual disability. Where there is evidence for the loss of previously acquired skills, for example, urinary continence, but such losses typically do not occur in isolation, alternate diagnoses (e.g., delirium, depression, etc.) should be considered under such circumstances. Somatoform disorders, depersonalization disorders, and sexual disorders are less frequently diagnosed in the context of mental retardation though certainly not precluded.

Sleep disorders ultimately require the subjective input of the patient regarding the adequacy of rest, occurrence of nightmares, and so on, and given the frequent history of abuse reported for people with MR as a group, one should not overlook the possibility of post-traumatic stress disorder when sleep disturbance is a presenting problem. Sleep disturbances are a common reason for referral for treatment or evaluation, and have received relatively little study in this population.

Provisional Diagnoses

Comorbidity is common. Additionally, some individuals may have psychiatric symptoms that significantly interfere with function, but which do not allow for a clear distinction between diagnoses. An impulse control disorder NOS, perhaps characterized by an individual who engages in impulsive aggressive acts, versus an anxiety disorder NOS, perhaps suggested by an individual who strikes out in the context of a stressor which would go unnoticed by most people, may be very difficult to discriminate from one another. The clinician should always make a best effort at a working diagnosis, and be prepared to make modifications as indicated by data gathered through collateral sources and from increasing familiarity with a particular patient. It should be acknowledged that the diagnostic process is a 'work in progress,' and the certainty with which a clinician comes to a diagnosis will in most cases be inversely proportionate to the patient's degree of disability [43].

Approach to Maladaptive Behavior

As with child psychiatry in general, there is little specificity that can be attached to a given symptom. Persons with MR will typically be referred for evaluation because of self-injurious, aggressive, impulsive, or hyperactive behavior. Because of the lack of diagnostic specificity for each of these symptoms, a diagnostic decision tree with any utility cannot be constructed. Instead, it is perhaps more useful to ask a series of questions about the expression of a particular behavior. If the behavior is of recent onset, one is more likely to consider an acute medical or psychiatric etiology. If the behavior is highly situational, occurring primarily in the context of the stress of task demands, the likelihood of a psychosis or mood disorder is probably reduced. If attempts are made to avoid the behavior by self-restraint, the inference of some compulsive features may be tenable. Assessing the sum of these and collateral data will lead the clinician to a presumptive diagnosis that will form the basis for a treatment plan.

For self-injurious and other maladaptive behavior, if the behavior becomes the focus of a treatment intervention, a diagnosable psychiatric disorder is present by definition. On the other hand, a given behavior, in and of itself, does not constitute grounds for a diagnosis. Just as 'shopping' may be normal in most contexts, unrestrained buying may come to be recognized as harmful to an individual. In the absence of any other clear psychopathology, excessive shopping will likely be diagnosed as a disorder of impulse control. The same principle applies for many behaviors in the context of MR. The Royal College's Diagnostic Criteria for Adults with Learning Disabilities (Mental Retardation) actually offers 'problem behavior' as an available diagnosis in its own right, but imposes criteria to ensure that such behavior is of sufficient importance that clinical involvement is necessary, that the problem is not due to other psychiatric or medical conditions, that the behavior exerts a significant negative impact on quality of life or puts the individual or others at risk, and that it is present across a range of situations [44].

Treatment

An array of therapeutic techniques have been employed in the treatment of mental disorders among persons with MR. Of these, the most widely utilized and investigated have been: behavioral treatments, psychopharmacological interventions, so-called 'ecological' or environmentally mediated interventions, and psychotherapy, including individual, group, and family-oriented approaches.

As for child psychiatry generally, it is clear is that no single therapeutic modality is indicated exclusively for any given problem. One should assume that most patients experience the same complex interaction of biological, psychological and environmental forces that characterizes psychic disturbance in patients without developmental delays. Perhaps even more so than in patients without intellectual disability, optimal care must include a comprehensive, multidimensional, and multidisciplinary approach [45].

Behavioral Techniques

Didden and colleagues [46] reviewed the effectiveness of treatment for problem behaviors for individuals with MR. Sorting treatment effectiveness into four categories including 'quite effective,' 'fairly effective,' 'questionably effective,' and 'unreliable' or ineffective, the investigators observed that nearly three-fourths of behaviors could be treated fairly or quite effectively. Only 3% of behaviors fell into the unreliably treated group. The investigators also observed that behaviors defined as externally destructive tend to be less successfully treated than are behaviors defined as internally maladaptive or as socially disruptive. Additionally, response contingent procedures tend to be more effective than are other categories of treatment. An element of caution should be taken when interpreting these results as the review did not examine the effects of study design, allocation of patients, disease severity, or heterogeneity on the validity and generalizability of the results.

Investigations over the past two decades have thus supported the effectiveness of behavioral therapies in managing many difficulties in patients with MR. The theoretical basis and clinical practice of behavioral treatments are reviewed extensively elsewhere. Briefly, efforts at altering behaviors for patients with MR are generally divided into two main categories, those aimed at increasing or enhancing desired behaviors and those aimed at reducing or eliminating behavioral excesses [43].

In the clinical setting, the most commonly studied approaches have been those based upon principles of operant conditioning. With respect to enhancing behavior, common operant techniques include differential reinforcement of other behaviors (DRO), differential reinforcement of incompatible behaviors (DRI), and differential reinforcement of low rates of behavior (DRL). These approaches reward patients either for not engaging in behaviors that have been identified as problematic (DRO and DRI) or for reducing the frequency of unwanted behaviors (DRL). In DRO, a patient is observed over a predetermined time period and rewarded for engaging in any behavior other than that which has been targeted for elimination. In DRI, a patient is rewarded for engaging in a particular behavior that is physically incompatible with the targeted behavior, for instance, making a fist instead of biting one's nails. In DRL the patient is rewarded for reducing the frequency of unwanted behaviors, for example, only getting out of his or her seat once in a given time-frame.

A sizeable collection of operant strategies exists for reducing unwanted behaviors. The most widely cited group of strategies are based on punishment; applying or responding with aversive consequences to an undesired behavior. Time out (removal from the preferred environment or activity and prevention of access to reinforcement) is probably the most common of these interventions. Overcorrection is another strategy, wherein the individual is required to restore an environment to its original state after a disruption (such as cleaning up a spill). Response cost is yet another strategy – losing a privilege for an unwanted behavior (being 'grounded'). Other behavior reduction strategies, for example, the use of aversive stimuli like a brief application of an electrical shock, should arguably be reserved only for reduction of the most dangerous types of behavioral problems, if ever.

Punishment-oriented strategies are the subject of intense public debate. Some argue that treatment based upon punishment is unethical, cruel and dehumanizing, especially when applied to those with intellectual disability. These critics also highlight the existence of alternative techniques to manage behavioral problems, and observe that punishment may simply lead to the substitution of one unwanted behavior for another. Concerns about possible inappropriate application of these techniques and thus the risks for abuse, either by professional or nonprofessional staff, are entirely appropriate.

Advocates of punishment techniques have maintained that these interventions have been shown to be rapid and effective tools in managing behavioral problems and are an important option, especially for cases of aggressive and self-injurious patients. Moreover, they point out that most of the strategies used are minimally aversive – even a harshly spoken 'no!' is aversive – and behavior reduction techniques may be particularly effective adjuncts to behavior reinforcing strategies. Finally, proponents point out that, as with other medical interventions that pose some risk of harm to a patient, these types of interventions may in certain circumstances be worth the inherent risks, and must be considered in the context of the patient's overall clinical situation.

In 1989, a Consensus Development Conference at the NIH addressed the issue of aversive treatments for the management of destructive behaviors and reached the following conclusions: 'Behavior reduction strategies should be selected for their rapid effectiveness *only* if the exigencies of the clinical situation require short term use of the restrictive interventions and *only* after appropriate review and informed consent are obtained . . . Behavior reduction procedures make little or no direct contribution to providing constructive alternatives to the destructive behaviors targeted for elimination. Thus the interventions should be used only if they are incorporated in the context of a comprehensive and individualized behavior enhancement treatment package' [47].

In addition to the approaches noted above, other types of behavior-oriented interventions have been used, some based on theories of social learning and others based on theories of respondent conditioning. Included among the many that have been reported are desensitization, modeling, patient rehearsal, self-reinforcement, and various cognitive behavioral techniques, such as problem-solving and social-skills training.

Many of these interventions are aimed at providing patients with MR with alternatives to unwanted behaviors. The rationale is that as individuals acquire more appropriate means of obtaining desired ends, the frequency of aberrant behaviors might be reduced. A number of investigators have found these strategies to be quite successful in patients with mild and moderate impairment. Especially in light of the criticisms of behavior reduction techniques, these approaches have been the subject of increasing attention of late.

Positive behavior support (PBS), for example, is a collaborative, assessment-based process to develop effective, individualized interventions for individuals with challenging behavior. Support plans focus on proactive and educative approaches. It involves the assessment and reengineering of environments so people with problem behaviors experience reductions in their problem behaviors and increase social, personal, and professional quality in their lives. Positive behavior support is the application of behavior analysis and systems change perspectives within the context of person-centered values to the intensely social problems created by behaviors such as self-injury, aggression, property destruction, pica, defiance, and disruption.

The overriding goal of PBS is to enhance quality of life for individuals and their support providers in home, school, and community settings [48]. Positive behavior support has three primary features: (1) functional (behavioral) assessment; (2) comprehensive intervention; and (3) lifestyle enhancement.

Carr and colleagues [48] completed a comprehensive literature review on PBS in response to a request from the US Department of Education, Office of Special Education Programs. The principal findings included that PBS is widely applicable to people with developmental disabilities and severe problem behavior, and within typical settings by direct support providers. Positive behavior support appeared to be effective in one-half to two-thirds of the cases, although long term quality of life outcomes were typically not reported.

Pharmacotherapy

Several recent reviews have noted that in the order of 60% of institutionalized persons with MR and more than 40% of patients seen in community based clinics are treated with psychotropic medication [49–51]. Antipsychotic drugs may be prescribed to as many as 40% of individuals with MR in some surveys [51]. Still the empirical evidence base for the efficacy of psychotropic agents in this population remains relatively limited.

As is the case for children generally, though significant advances have been made over the past decade, there remain relatively few rigorous, well-controlled studies of medication management of psychiatric problems in those with developmental delays.

Just as in the case of treatment of behavior problems, pharmacologic treatments of common psychiatric syndromes in patients with MR have received too little study. Despite this, conventional wisdom holds that patients generally respond in a fashion similar to that expected for the general population when treated for common psychopathology. There is a considerable number of case studies to support this contention. However, rigorous validation of this consensus is lacking. The reliable literature on the treatment of depression, anxiety, OCD and psychosis is minimal and ultimately limited by a lack of consensus with respect to the criteria used to characterize these disorders.

One area that might be regarded as an exception to this rule is the treatment of ADHD. Several groups of investigators have demonstrated that stimulants are efficacious in the treatment of hyperactivity to a degree that seems to match that in populations without intellectual disability [52,53]. There has been some suggestion that these effects may be most robust for patients with mild to moderate mental retardation, with patients with greatest cognitive disability showing either little effect or adverse response to the medication [54].

Across diagnostic categories, the most common clinical justification for the use of psychotropic medication is destructive behavior. Three of the most commonly identified types, self-injurious behaviors, stereotyped behaviors, and aggression, have been the subject of considerable attention. While these symptoms are often grouped together as outcomes variables in studies, their pathogenesis is likely to be quite different, and their responsiveness to particular pharmacologic agents varies considerably. Increasingly, a dimensional approach to the use of pharmacotherapy in these situations is being articulated [55].

Neuroleptics have been the most commonly prescribed and most widely used agents in the treatment of destructive behaviors. With respect to both self-injury and aggression, the vast majority of studies, admittedly of widely varying quality, have concluded that such behaviors may be effectively suppressed by these agents. Overall, the number of controlled, blinded investigations is very limited with the recent exception of risperidone. Presently there are over 50 studies involving various numbers of subjects with developmental disabilities, including two relatively large controlled studies, that support the consideration of risperidone for the treatment of a variety of disruptive behaviors [56,57]. One of the criticisms of studies published over the past two decades is that such effects may be nonspecific in that improvement has been reported for many different target behaviors simultaneously. Such a concern is important, but the available evidence does not support the notion that the therapeutic effect of these drugs is merely indiscriminate behavioral suppression, for example, via sedation.

Studies of stereotyped behaviors have arguably produced more consistent and reliable results. Neuroleptics have been shown to be clearly and specifically effective in decreasing these behaviors [58]. The finding of specificity is difficult to interpret in light of the evidence from studies noted above. One possible explanation is that effective doses used in the treatment of stereotypies have been lower on average than those used in studies of self-injurious behavior.

Despite some demonstrated utility, substantial concerns have been raised regarding the side effects of neuroleptics, including tardive dyskinesia, sedation, dystonia, and weight gain. Moreover it is possible that adaptive, as well as maladaptive, behaviors are suppressed by higher-dose neuroleptic treatments. Conse-

quently, there has been widespread interest in finding alternatives to these agents for the control of destructive behaviors.

The opiate receptor antagonist, naltrexone, has received more attention specifically for a possible effect on self-injurious behavior than any other drug to date. Early indications were favorable with respect to self-injury [59,60]. However, subsequent results have not been uniformly encouraging. Some authors have observed that self-injurious behavior may initially be worsened by opiate blockers [61], and a relatively large double-blind study found no positive clinical effects in more than 30 adult subjects with self-injurious or autistic behaviors. In fact, the patients in a lower dose (50 mg/day) arm of the study fared significantly worse based on the Clinical Global Impression Scale in comparison to those on placebo. Moreover, naltrexone appeared to exacerbate stereotypic behaviors in some of the individuals studied [62].

Interest in the role of serotonergic agents in moderating aggression, stereotypy, self-injurious behavior and compulsive behaviors has been increasing. Several studies have demonstrated the efficacy of clomipramine in the treatment of repetitive behaviors in children with autism [63], and persons with MR [64]. These findings have spurred interest in the use of the newer serotonin reuptake inhibitors for patients with developmental delays. Well-controlled, double-blinded studies are still pending, however, preliminary reports have been promising [65,66]. Perhaps more so than for patients without intellectual disability, a tendency to become disinhibited, and more impulsive and aggressive, has been observed in some patients with MR treated with serotonin reuptake inhibitors [67,68].

Additional medications with promise in the treatment of aggression include lithium and β-blockers. Several investigations, some methodologically sound, have shown high rates of response to lithium [69]. In the case of adrenergics, reported successes in patients without MR generated interest [70] but have perhaps curiously disappeared from the radar screen of clinical literature over the past decade.

Buspirone has similarly disappeared from view in the literature, but studies for the treatment of aggression yielded mixed effects [71,72]. Additional medications that have been implicated as possible treatments include anticonvulsants and benzodiazepines, about which there is little evidence [73]. The experience with tricyclic antidepressants is best characterized as disappointing [74].

One area of potential pharmacotherapy that is particularly of interest in cognitive disability concerns the class of medications known as nootropics, or cognitive enhancing agents. In a placebo-controlled crossover trial, Lobaugh and colleagues found that piracetam therapy does not enhance cognitive functioning in children with Down syndrome [75].

All told, psychopharmacology for patients with MR, while widely practiced, remains in its infancy. A growing body of literature suggests that judicious use of medication does have a place in the overall treatment of persons with intellectual disability. With regard to destructive behaviors, the existing evidence would suggest that attempting to identify underlying psychiatric syndromes is an essential first step in the rational use of medications. In those cases where underlying psychopathology is not clear, there is still some evidence to suggest that a number of agents, including lithium, opiate-receptor blockers, beta blockers, serotonin reuptake inhibitors, and in certain cases neuroleptics, may be useful for some patients. Clearly the consideration of any medication, and especially those with significant side effects, must be taken carefully and in the context of a comprehensive treatment approach.

Ecological Approaches

It seems self-evident that the environmental conditions in which patients find themselves would have important impact. Yet, until fairly recently, issues of quality of life for those with developmental delays were largely ignored. Starting in the 1960s and 1970s, the individuals with MR began to have increasing opportunities to integrate into society and were encouraged to lead as normal a life as possible. Structured interventions and living arrangements which support this type of integration have become the rule. Whereas in 1987, nearly half of the individuals with autism in the state of California resided out of home, that percentage was upwards of 85% in 2002 [76].

Despite the seemingly self-evident impact of environment, its effect on aberrant behaviors and psychopathology has not been widely studied. Still, it seems likely that positive changes in a patient's surround might reduce behavioral excesses and minimize stresses associated with the development of affective and anxiety syndromes. Recently, there has been an increasing recognition of the importance of comprehensive functional analysis of behavior for patients with MR. Associated with this has been an interest in studying the systematic manipulation of potential environmental precipitants in efforts to minimize psychosocial problems.

School Interventions

Strategy training has been identified as providing improvement in learning for individuals with MR [77]. Verbal elaboration (use of complex verbal devices to amplify stimuli to enhance discrimination or recall), mediation (use of simple verbal devices to link together stimuli to enhance subsequent discrimination or recall) and imagery (use of visual devices to link together one or more stimuli to enhance subsequent discrimination or recall) have been shown to provide significant results for increasing on-task behavior as well as targeted academic skills. Verbal rehearsal (repetition of serially presented stimuli after presentation – vocal or subvocal), input organization (systematic ordering of presentation of stimuli by salient dimensions), verbal labeling (naming stimuli to be discriminated or recalled by salient dimensions during presentation), and combinations of these also can be effective.

Studies of reading development in children with mental retardation are beginning to demonstrate that progress in word recognition and comprehension can be significant [78,79]. Teachers are using phonetic approaches along with functional reading approaches [80,81] and are creating literacy-rich environments in classrooms [82]. However, there is still very little research on the cognitive processes underlying reading ability in children with intellectual disability. It is still not known which early skills predict literacy acquisition in children with intellectual disability, or if the dominant theories of reading development and reading difficulties apply to children with intellectual disability.

Psychotherapy

Interest in psychotherapeutic approaches to mental retardation has been varied. In the 1930s, there was some consideration of the role that psychoanalysis might play in the treatment of developmentally delayed patients. However, efforts at systematically studying this issue waned in the ensuing decades, with the majority of attention focused on the putative reasons for not including patients with mental retardation in analysis. These exclusionary criteria included problems with transference, lack of potential for insight, poor impulse control, and a reduced capacity for change [83].

While rote learning and more crystallized cognitive functions can benefit from structured and behavioral intervention strategies, more flexible, abstract thought processes are often resistant to interventions. This is consistent with neuropsychological findings as well as analysis of intellectual test profiles. Thus, behavioral treatments have predominated, although interest in psychotherapeutic techniques continues.

But as the psychotherapeutic landscape has changed over the last decade, there has been a resurgence of interest in the application of these techniques in patients with MR. Of course, the notion of what constitutes appropriate treatment has broadened over the years. Contemporary discussions of psychotherapeutic options for patients with low IQ include dynamic-oriented approaches, cognitive behavioral treatments, group psychotherapy, and family therapy.

Dagnan and Chadwick [84] considered cognitive behavioral therapies to fall into two broad categories when used for people with MR: self-management approaches and cognitive therapy. Self-management interventions include self-monitoring, self-instruction, problem solving and decision making. They are used in conjunction with relaxation techniques, education, skill acquisition and social-skills training. Cognitive behavior therapy is aimed at controlling distorted cognitions. The studies reported are with adults, and most are uncontrolled trials and case reports, and primarily with incarcerated. It is unclear how well these interventions would translate to children. Similarly, the evidence for psychodynamic therapies is limited to adult populations and involves primarily case reports and uncontrolled trials.

There are numerous case studies suggesting the benefits of each of these types of strategies, but little in the way of controlled clinical trials. Nonetheless, something of a consensus has emerged regarding the potential value of psychotherapeutic interventions for some patients, especially those with mild retardation. There also is general agreement that these areas are in need of additional investigation.

Prout and Nowak-Drabik [85] conducted a meta-analysis of studies of psychotherapy with persons who have MR. Studies conducted during a 30-year-period were rated by an expert consensus panel and classified with regard to the nature of the research and outcome and effectiveness domains. The meta-analysis on a small number of the studies found a wide range of research designs, types of interventions, and participants. A moderate degree of change in outcome measures and moderate effectiveness in terms of benefit to clients with MR was noted. The authors concluded that psychotherapeutic interventions should be considered as part of overall treatment plans for persons with MR. However, no studies with children were reported. Furthermore, only the behavioral intervention studies reported contained sufficient data to

compute effect sizes, and this was obtained from only eight of 92 studies reviewed. Thus there is limited effectiveness data to support the use of various psychotherapeutic methods.

For all types of individual therapies with patients with MR certain modifications in approach are beneficial. It is important, for example, that an active therapeutic stance be employed, as well as the use of concrete and supportive interventions, and careful attention to the language abilities and developmental level of the patient in treatment. When these types of alterations are made, many patients with MR are able to understand the treatment process and obtain considerable benefit [86,87].

Along with the slow but steady resurgence of interest in individual psychotherapy, group psychotherapies have also been gaining popularity. Groups are a valuable venue to provide support and education as well as opportunities for interpretation and confrontation. Group settings have been used recently for the application of cognitive behavioral techniques, including rehearsal and role-play. These efforts seem particularly well-suited to tackle issues of social skill deficits in patients with mild and moderate intellectual disability.

Finally, the role of family therapy, though not widely investigated, remains an area of particular practical importance. Clinical experience suggests that the impact that a child, adolescent or adult with intellectual disabilities has upon their family of origin is enormous, and vice versa. Many of the developmental difficulties encountered in 'normal' families are *writ large* in those with members who have developmental delays. Issues of independence and separation, or the inability to obtain these, can be wrenchingly difficult and have an impact on parents, patients, and siblings alike. Consequently, the range of family therapy techniques is an essential component of comprehensive treatment. Education and support for families is essential. So too is attention to the dynamics of family relationships and a recognition of the widespread impact on family structures that developmental disabilities pose.

The Child Psychiatrist as Consultant

As Tredgold noted 50 years ago [1], knowledge of MR, its causes, its manifestations, and its treatment had already become extensive. In the intervening half century, the rate of growth in our understanding of developmental disabilities has been remarkable. As a result of advances in such diverse fields as molecular biology, pharmacology, and psychology, clinicians are increasingly able to make a difference in the lives of patients with intellectual disability and those of their families.

Along with these advances has come a steadily expanding role for the child psychiatrist. The therapeutic nihilism long associated with psychiatric diagnosis and treatment of patients with MR has given way to a clear understanding of the important role such consultation must play in the careful identification and management of mental retardation syndromes and their associated behavioral phenotypes, in the recognition and treatment of comorbid psychiatric disorders, and the astute use of medications to augment behavioral, psychotherapeutic, and ecological treatments. The multidisciplinary approach to patients with MR is the state of the art, and the child psychiatrist is an essential member of that team.

References

1. Tredgold AF: *A Textbook of mental deficiency (amentia)*, 7th ed. Baltimore: Williams and Wilkins, 1947:vii.

2. American Association On Mental Retardation: *Mental Retardation: Definition, Classification, and Systems of Support*, 9th ed. Washington DC: American Association on Mental Retardation, 1992.

3. World Health Organization: In: World Health Organization, ed. *The ICD-10 Classification of Mental and Behavioural Disorders: Clinical Descriptions and Diagnostic Guidelines*. Geneva: World Health Organization, 1992.

4. American Psychiatric Association: *Diagnostic and Statistical Manual of Mental Disorders,* Fourth Edition TR. Washington DC: American Psychiatric Association, Washington, 2000.

5. Yeargin-Allsopp M, Boyle C: Overview: The epidemiology of neurodevelopmental disorders. *Mental Retard Develop Disabilities Res Rev* 2002; **8**:113–116.

6. Esquirol E: *Mental Maladies. A Treatise on Insanity.* Translated by Hunt EK. Philadelphia: Lea and Blanchard, 1845.

7. Fitzherbert A: De natura brevium. In: Kirman B, Bicknell J, eds. *Mental Handicap.* Edinburgh: Churchill Livingstone, 1975.

8. Swinburne H: Testaments. In: Kirman B, Bicknell J, eds. *Mental Handicap.* Edinburgh: Churchill Livingstone, 1975.

9. Sparrow SS, Balla DA, Cicchetti DV: *Vineland Adaptive Behavior Scales.* Circle Pines, MN: American Guidance Service, 1984.

10. Nihira K, Leland H, Lambert N: *AAMR Adaptive Behavior Scales.* Austin, TX: Pro-Ed, 1993.

11. Matthews CG, Reitan RM: Comparisons of abstraction ability in retardates and in patients with cerebral lesions. *Am J Mental Defic* 1961; **23**:63–66.

12. Trites RL: Neuropsychological variables and mental retardation. *Psychiatric Clin North Am* 1986; **9**:723–731.

13. Reitan RM, Wolfson D: The Halstead–Reitan Neuropsychological Test Battery and REHABIT: A model for integrating evaluation and remediation of cognitive impairment. *Cognitive Rehabil* 1988; **6**:10–17.

14. Wishart JG: Cognitive abilities in children with Down syndrome: Developmental instability and motivational deficits. In: Epstein CJ, Hassold T, Lott IT, L. Nadel L, Patterson G, eds. *Etiology and Pathogenesis of Down Syndrome.* NY: Wiley-Liss, 1995.

15. Carr J: *Down's Syndrome: Children Growing Up.* Cambridge: Cambridge University Press, 1995.

16. Fishler K, Koch R: Mental development in Down syndrome mosaicism. *Am J Mental Retard* 1991; **96**: 345–351.

17. Pulsifer MB: The neuropsychology of mental retardation. *J Int Neuropsycholog Soc* 1996; **2**:159–176.

18. Roeleveld N, Zielhuis GA, Gabreels F: The prevalence of mental retardation: A critical review of recent literature. *Develop Med Child Neurol* 1997; **39**:125–132.

19. Starza-Smith A: Recent trends in prevalence studies of children with severe mental retardation. *Disability, Handicap, Society* 1989; **4**:177–195.

20. Leonard H, Wen X: The epidemiology of mental retardation: Challenges and opportunities in the new millennium. *Mental Retard Develop Disab Res Rev* 2002; **8**:117–135.

21. Drews CD, Yeargin-Allsopp M, Decoufle P, *et al.*: Variation in the influence of selected sociodemographic risk factors for mental retardation. *Am J Public Health* 1995; **85**:329–334.

22. Croen LA, Grether JK, Selvin S: The epidemiology of mental retardation of unknown cause. *Pediatrics* 2001; **107**:E86.

23. King BH, State MW: Mental retardation. In: Klykylo W, Kay J, Rube D, eds. *Clinical Child Psychiatry*. Philadelphia: WB Saunders Co, 1998.

24. McKusick VA: *Mendelian Inheritance in Man. A Catalog of Human Genes and Genetic Disorders*, 12th ed. Baltimore, MD: Johns Hopkins University Press, 1998. http://www.ncbi.nlm.nih.gov/omim/

25. Kessler S, Moos RH: Behavioral aspects of chromosomal disorders. In: Creger WP, Coggins CH, Hancock EW, eds. *Annu Rev Med.* 1973; **24**:89–102.

26. Dykens EM: Measuring behavioral phenotypes: Provocations from the 'new genetics'. *Am J Ment Retardation* 1995, **99**:522–532.

27. Penrose LS: *The Biology of Mental Defect.* London: Sidgwick and Jackson, Limited, 1963.

28. Dykens EM: Annotation: Psychopathology in children with intellectual disability. *J Child Psychol Psychiatry* 2000; **41**(4):407–417.

29. Royal College of Psychiatrists: *DC-LD (Diagnostic Criteria for Psychiatric Disorders for Use with Adults with Learning Disabilities/Mental Retardation).* London: Gaskell, 2001.

30. Reid AH: Psychiatric disorders in mentally handicapped children: A clinical and follow-up study. *J Ment Def Res* 1980; **24**:287–298.

31. Bailey NM, Andrews TM: Diagnostic criteria for psychiatric disorders for use with adults with learning disabilities/mental retardation (DC-LD) and the diagnosis of anxiety disorders: A review. *J Intellectual Disability Res* 2003; **47**(suppl 1):50–61.

32. Esbensen AJ, Rojahn J, Aman MG, Ruedrich S: Reliability and validity of an assessment instrument for anxiety, depression, and mood among individuals with mental retardation. *J Autism Develop Disord* 2003; **33**:6.

33. King BH: Self-injury by people with mental retardation: A compulsive behavior hypothesis. *Am J Ment Retardation* 1993; **98**:93–112.

34. Gravestock S: Diagnosis and classification of eating disorders in adults with intellectual disability: The Diagnostic Criteria for Psyciatric Disorders for Use with Adults with Learning Disabilities/Mental Retardation (DC-LD) approach. *J Autism Develop Disord* 2003; **47**(suppl 1):72–83.

35. Menolascino FJ: Down's syndrome: Clinical and psychiatric findings in an institutionalized sample. In: Menolascino FJ, ed. *Psychiatric Approaches to Mental Retardation*. New York: Basic Books, 1970.

36. Reid AH: Psychoses in adult mental defectives: II. Schizophrenic and paranoid psychoses. *Br J Psychiatry* 1972; **120**:213–218.

37. Wright EC: The presentation of mental illness in mentally retarded adults. *Br J Psychiatry* 1982; **141**:496–502.

38. Sovner R: Limiting factors in the use of DSM-III criteria with mentally ill/mentally retarded persons. *Psychopharmacol Bull* 1986; **22**:1055–1059.

39. Reid AH: Psychoses in adult mental defectives: I. Manic depressive psychosis. *Br J Psychiatry* 1972; **120**:205–212.

40. Smiley E, Cooper SA: Intellectual disabilities, depressive episode, diagnostic criteria and Diagnostic Criteria for Psychiatric Disorders for Use with Adults with Learning Disabilities/Mental Retardation (DC-LD). *J Intellectual Disability Res* 2003; **47**(Suppl 1):62–71.

41. Baumeister AA: Origins and control of stereotyped movements. In: Meyers CE ed. *Quality of Life in Severely and Profoundly Mentally Retarded People: Research Foundations for Improvement*. Washington, DC: American Association on Mental Deficiency, 1978:353–384.

42. Rogers D, Karki C, Bartlett C, Pocock P: The motor disorders of mental handicap: An overlap with the motor disorders of severe psychiatric illness. *Br J Psychiatry* 1991; **158**:97.

43. Rush AJ, Frances A, eds. Expert Consensus Guideline Series: Treatment of psychiatric and behavioral problems in mental retardation. *Am J Ment Retard* 2000; **105**:159–226.

44. O'Brien G: The classification of problem behaviour in Diagnostic Criteria for Psychiatric Disorders for Use with Adults with Learning Disabilities/Mental Retardation (DC-LD). *J Intellectual Disability Res* 2003; **47**(Suppl 1):32–37.

45. Szymanski L, King BH: Practice parameters for the assessment and treatment of children, adolescents, and adults with mental retardation and comorbid mental disorders. American Academy of Child and Adolescent Psychiatry Working Group on Quality Issues. *J Am Acad Child Adolesc Psychiatry* 1999; **38**(12 Suppl):5S–31S.

46. Didden R, Duker PC, Korzilius H: Meta-analytic study on treatment effectiveness for problem behaviors with individuals who have mental retardation. *Am J Mental Retard* 1997; **101**:387–399.

47. National Institutes of Health: Consensus development conference statement: Treatment of destructive behaviors in persons with developmental disabilities. *J Autism Develop Disord* 1989; **20**:403.

48. Carr EG, Horner RH, Turnbull AP, Marquis JG, Magito McLaughlin D, McAtee ML, Smith CE, Anderson Ryan K, Ruef MB, Doolabh A: *Positive Behavior Support for People with Developmental Disabilities: A Research Synthesis*. Washington, DC: American Association on Mental Retardation Monograph Series, 1999.

49. Aman MG, Singh NN: Patterns of drug use, methodological considerations, measurement techniques, and future trends. In: Aman MG, Singh NN, eds. *Psychopharmacology of the Developmental Disabilities*. New York: Springer-Verlag 1988.

50. Baumeister AA, Todd ME, Sevin JA: Efficacy and specificity of pharmacological therapies for behavioral disorders in persons with mental retardation. *Clin Neuropharmacol* 1993; **16**:271.

51. Spreat S, Conroy JW, Jones JC: Use of psychotropic medication in Oklahoma: A statewide survey. *Am J Ment Retard* 1997; **102**:80–85.

52. Aman MG, Marks RE, Turbott SH, Wilsher CP, Merry SN: Clinical effects of methylphenidate and thioridazine in intellectually sub-average children. *J Am Acad Child Adolesc Psychiatry* 1991; **30**:246.

53. Handen BL, Breaux AM, Janosky J, McAuliffe S, Feldman H, Gosling A: Effects and noneffects of methylphenidate in children with mental retardation and ADHD. *J Am Acad Child Adolesc Psychiatry* 1992; **31**:455.

54. Handen BL, Breaux AM, Janosky J, McAuliffe S, Feldman H, Gosling A: Adverse side effects of methylphenidate among mentally retarded children with ADHD. *J Am Acad Child Adolesc Psychiatry* 1992; **30**:241.

55. Santosh PJ, Baird G: Psychopharmacotherapy in children and adults with intellectual disability. *Lancet* 1999; **354**:231–240.

56. Turgay A, Binder C, Snyder R, Fisman S: Long-term safety and efficacy of risperidone for the treatment of disruptive behavior disorders in children with subaverage IQs. *Pediatrics* 2002; **110**(3):e34.

57. Aman MG, De Smedt G, Derivan A, Lyons B, Findling RL: Risperidone Disruptive Behavior Study Group. Double-blind, placebo-controlled study of risperidone for the treatment of disruptive behaviors in children with subaverage intelligence. *Am J Psychiatry* 2002; **159**(8): 1337–1346.

58. Aman MG, Teehan CJ, White AJ, Turbott SH, Vaithianathan C: Haloperidol treatment with chronically medicated residents: Dose effects on clinical behavior and reinforcement contingencies. *Am J Mental Retard* 1989; **93**:452.

59. Sandman CA, Barron JL, Coleman H: An orally administered opiate blocker, naltrexone, attenuates self injurious behavior. *Am J Mental Retard* 1990; **95**:93.

60. Barrett RP, Feinstein C, Hole WT: Effects of naloxone and naltrexone on self-injury: A double blind, placebo controlled analysis. *Am J Mental Retard* 1989; **93**:644.

61. Benjamin S, Seek A, Tresise L, Price E, Gagnon M: Case study: Paradoxical response to naltrexone treatment of self-injurious behavior. *J Am Acad Child Adolesc Psychiatry* 1995; **34**:238.

62. Willemsen-Swinkels SHN, Buitelaar JK, Nijhof GJ, van Engeland H: Failure of naltrexone hydrochloride to reduce self-injurious and autistic behavior in mentally retarded adults: Double-blind placebo-controlled studies. *Arch Gen Psychiatry* 1995; **52**:766.

63. Gordon CT, State RC, Nelson JE, Hamburger SD, Rapoport JL: A double-blind comparison of clomipramine, desipramine, and placebo in the treatment of autistic disorder. *Arch Gen Psychiatry* 1993; **50**(6): 441–447.

64. Lewis MH, Bodfish JW, Powell SB, Parker DE, Golden RN: Clomipramine treatment for self-injurious behavior of individuals with mental retardation: A double-blind

comparison with placebo. *Am J Ment Retardation* 1996; **100**:654–665.

65. Markowitz PI: Effects of fluoxetine on self-injurious behavior in the developmentally disabled: A preliminary study. *J Clin Psychopharmacol* 1992; **12**:27.

66. Troisi A, Vicario E, Nuccelelli F, Clani N, Pasini A: Effects of fluoxetine on aggressive behavior of adult inpatients with mental retardation and epilepsy. *Pharmacopsychiatry* 1995; **28**:73.

67. Branford D, Bhaumik S, Naik B: Selective serotonin reuptake inhibitors for the treatment of perseverative and maladaptive behaviours of people with intellectual disability. *J Intellectual Disability Res* 1998; **42**(4):301–306.

68. Racusin R, Kovner-Kline K, King BH: Selective serotonin reuptake inhibitors in intellectual disability. *Mental Retard Develop Disab Res Rev* 1999; **5**:264–269.

69. Bregman JD: Current developments in the understanding of mental retardation part II: Psychopathology. *J Am Acad Child Adolesc Psychiatry* 1991; **30**:861.

70. Yudofsky SC, Silver JM, Hales RM: Treatment of aggressive disorders. In: Schatzberg AF, Nemeroff CB, eds. *Textbook of Psychopharmacology*. Washington, DC: American Psychiatric Press, 1995.

71. Ratey J, Sovner R, Parks A, Rogentine K: Buspirone treatment of aggression and anxiety in mentally retarded patients: A multiple baseline, placebo lead-in study. *J Clin Psychiatry* 1991; **52**:159.

72. King BH, Davanzo P: Buspirone treatment of aggression and self-injury in autistic and nonautistic persons with severe mental retardation. *Dev Brain Dysfunct* 1996; **9**:22–31.

73. Osman OT, Losche EL: Self-injurious behavior in the developmentally disabled: Pharmacologic treatment. *Psychopharmacol Bull* 1992; **28**:439.

74. Aman MG, White AJ, Vaithianathan C, Teehan CJ: Preliminary study of imipramine in profoundly retarded residents. *J Autism Devel Disord* 1986; **16**:263.

75. Lobaugh NJ, Karaskov V, Rombough V, Rovet J, Bryson S, Greenbaum R, Haslam RH, Koren G: Piracetam therapy does not enhance cognitive functioning in children with down syndrome. *Arch Pediatr Adolesc Med* 2001; **155**(4):442–448.

76. Department of Developmental Services. *Changes in the Population of Persons with Autism and Pervasive Developmental Disorders in California's Developmental Services System: 1987 through 1998. Report to the Legislature, March 1, 1999.* http://www.dds.ca.gov

77. Kavale K, Forness SR: *Efficacy of Special Education and Related Services.* Washington, DC: American Association on Mental Retardation, 1999.

78. Conners FA: Reading instruction for students with moderate mental retardation: A review and analysis of research. *Am J Mental Retard* 1992; **96**:577–597.

79. Buckley S: Teaching children with Down syndrome to read and write. In: Nadel L, Rosenthal D, eds. *Down Syndrome: Living and Learning in the Community*. New York: Wiley-Liss, 1995:158–169.

80. Johansson I: Teaching pre-reading skills to disabled children. *J Intellectual Disability Res* 1993; **37**:413–417.

81. O'Connor RE, Notari-Syverson A, Vadasy P: First-grade effects of teacher-led phonological activities in kindergarten for children with mild disabilities: a follow-up study. *Learning Disabil Res Prac* 1998; **13**:43–52.

82. Katims D: Literacy instructions for people with mental retardation: Historical highlights and contemporary analysis. *Educ Train Mental Retard Develop Disabil* 2000; **35**:3–15.

83. Stavrakaki C, Klein J: Psychotherapies with the mentally retarded. *Psychiatric Clin North Am* 1986; **9**:733.

84. Dagnan D, Chadwick P: Cognitive-behavior therapy for people with learning disabilities: Assessment and intervention. In: Kroese BS, Dagnan D, Loumidis K, eds. *Cognitive Behavior Therapy for People with Learning Disabilities* London: Routledge, 1997:110–123.

85. Prout HT, Nowak-Drabik KM: Psychotherapy with persons who have mental retardation: An evaluation of effectiveness. *Am J Mental Retard* 2003; **108**:82–93.

86. Hurley AD: Individual pscyhotherapy with mentally retarded individuals: A review and call for research. *Res Dev Disabil* 1989; **10**:261.

87. Nezu CM, Nezu AM: Outpatient psychotherapy for adults with mental retardation and concomitant psychopathology: Research and clinical imperatives. *J Consult Clin Psychol* 1994; **62**:34.

23

Tics and Tourette's Disorder

Barbara J. Coffey, Rachel Shechter

Introduction

Tics are stereotyped, rapid, recurring motor movements or vocalizations that are nonrhythmic, involuntary, and sudden in onset [1]. Tic disorders include transient tic disorder, chronic motor tic disorder, chronic vocal tic disorder, and Tourette's disorder [1]. Transient tic disorder, which can include both motor and vocal symptoms, is the most common of the tic disorders; the prevalence is estimated as up to 20% of children [2]. Chronic tic disorders are clinically important conditions that have gained increasing recognition in recent years; Tourette's disorder (TD), also known as Tourette's syndrome, is the most complex of the chronic tic disorders. Tourette disorder is characterized by multiple, waxing and waning, motor and vocal tics with onset in childhood.

A recent community-based study reported that about 3% of school-age children meet criteria for TD. Thought to be life-long, limited and somewhat contradictory information exists on the longitudinal course of TD. Recent studies suggest that while tics may often persist into adulthood, tic severity often declines significantly in adolescence. The past two decades have been marked by significant progress in the understanding of the clinical phenomenology, epidemiology, and psychiatric comorbidity of TD.

Comorbidity with psychiatric disorders such as attention deficit hyperactivity disorder (ADHD) and obsessive–compulsive disorder (OCD) is common in clinically referred individuals [3–8]. In addition, mood disorders, non-OCD anxiety disorders such as separation anxiety disorder, and generalized anxiety disorders are not uncommon [3].

The past decade has been marked by significant progress in the understanding of the etiology, genetics, and epidemiology of tic disorders. Treatment studies proliferated, focusing initially on the use of neuroleptic agents, and alternatives such as the alpha 2-adrenergic agonists clonidine and guanfacine [9–11]. Recent imaging studies have expanded the understanding of the neuroanatomy of the disorder [12–18]. Treatment studies have expanded to include the atypical neuroleptics and most recently, targeted combined pharmacotherapy. Nevertheless, TD and tic disorders continue to pose many challenges, especially in the areas of pathophysiology, genetics, developmental neuroscience, psychopathology, and treatment.

Classification and Clinical Phenomenology

Tics typically involve one muscle or a group of muscles and may be characterized by their anatomical location, number, frequency, duration, and complexity [19]. They can be classified as simple (involving one muscle or sound), or complex (slower, more purposeful movements involving multiple muscle groups or multiple sounds). Examples of simple motor tics are eye blinking, shoulder shrugging and head turning, and complex motor tics are touching objects, jumping, or rotating. Examples of simple vocal tics are throat clearing, coughing and sniffing; complex vocal tics include repeating syllables, phrases or echolalia (repeating others' words) (Table 23.1).

According to the *Diagnostic and Statistical Manual, Revised Version IV-TR* [1], tic disorders can be classified as transient (i.e., duration of at least four weeks but less than one year) or chronic (i.e., duration greater than one year).

Stress and excitement can exacerbate tics. Tics are experienced as irresistible, but can be suppressed for varying periods of time [20–23]. Many patients with TD characterize their tics as a voluntary response to an uncomfortable feeling that precedes them. These feelings, or premonitory sensations, have been

Clinical Child Psychiatry, Second Edition. Edited by W.M. Klykylo and J.L. Kay
© 2005 John Wiley & Sons Ltd.

Table 23.1 Some examples of tics.

Motor		Vocal	
Simple	Complex	Simple	Complex
Eye blinking	Touching objects or self	Throat clearing	Syllables or words
Nose twitching	Squatting or jumping	Coughing	Phrases
Shoulder shrugging	Hand gestures	Sniffing	Swearing, grunting

Table 23.2 Diagnostic features of Tourette's disorder.[a]

(A) Both multiple motor and one or more vocal tics have been present at some time during the illness, although not necessarily concurrently
(B) The tics occur many times a day (usually in bouts), nearly every day or intermittently throughout a period of more than one year, and during this period there was never a tic-free period of more than three consecutive months
(C) The onset is before 18 years
(D) The disturbance is not due to the direct physiological effects of a substance (e.g., stimulants) or a general medical condition (e.g., Huntington disease or postviral encephalitis)

[a] *DSM-IV-TR*. Reprinted with permission from the Diagnostic and Statistical Manual of Mental Disorders. Copyright, the American Psychiatric Association, 2000.

described by the majority of TD patients; these sensations can be localized or general, and physical or mental in nature [20,21,24,25].

Clinical Course

The typical course of TD is characterized by the onset of facial, head, or neck tics at about age six or seven years, followed by a rostral–caudal progression of motor tics over several years (Table 23.2). Vocal tics typically start at age eight or nine years; more complex tics often begin later, as do obsessive–compulsive symptoms at about age 11 or 12 years [26–29]. As many as half of clinically referred TD patients may show signs of ADHD, such as hyperactivity, impulsivity and distractibility, prior to the onset of tics [23,26,30,31]. Tics tend to stabilize over time, and some patients have lengthy periods during which most or all manifestations diminish or remit. Recent studies indicate that tic severity improves significantly in most patients by early- to mid-adolescence [27,32,33].

Table 23.3 Diagnostic features of chronic motor or vocal tic disorder.[a]

(A) Single or multiple motor or vocal tics (i.e., sudden, rapid, recurrent nonrhythmic, stereotyped motor movements or vocalizations) but not both, are present at some time during the illness
(B) The tics occur many times a day, nearly every day, or intermittently throughout a period more than one year, and during this period there was never a tic-free period of more than three consecutive months
(C) The disturbance causes marked distress or significant impairment in social, occupational, or other important areas of functioning
(D) The onset is before 18 years
(E) The disturbance is not due to the direct physiological effects of a substance (e.g., stimulants) or a general medical condition (e.g., Huntington's disease or postviral encephalitis)
(F) Criteria have never been met for Tourette's disorder

[a] *DSM-IV-TR*. Reprinted with permission from the Diagnostic and Statistical Manual of Mental Disorders. Copyright by the American Psychiatric Association, 2000.

Chronic motor and vocal tic disorders usually have a similar natural history and are considered closely related conditions or variants of TD [22,23] (Table 23.3, Table 23.4).

Epidemiology

Prevalence estimates for TD vary. As in all population-based studies, results may be influenced by a variety of factors, including the criteria used for diagnosis, the methods of sampling and inquiry, the sex and age distributions in the study population, or the size of the sample. Lifetime rate estimates vary from 1 to 10 per

Table 23.4 Diagnostic features of transient tic disorder.[a]

(A) Single or multiple motor and/or vocal tics (i.e., sudden, rapid, recurrent, nonrhythmic, stereotyped motor movements or vocalizations)

(B) The tics occur many times a day, nearly every day for at least four weeks, but for no longer than 12 consecutive months

(C) The disturbance causes marked distress or significant impairment in social, occupational, or other important areas of functioning

(D) The onset is before 18 years

(E) The disturbance is not due to the direct physiological effects of a substance (e.g., stimulants) or a general medical condition (e.g., Huntington disease or postviral encephalitis)

(F) Criteria have never been met for Tourette's disorder or chronic motor or vocal tic disorder

---

[a] *DSM-IV-TR*. Reprinted with permission from the Diagnostic and Statistical Manual of Mental Disorders. Copyright by the American Psychiatric Association, 2000.

thousand, and a common prevalence figure for individuals meeting criteria for TD is one per 200 for the full spectrum of chronic tic disorders. A population based epidemiological study of lifetime prevalence of TD in Israel yielded a point prevalence of 4.3 ± 1.2 (mean ± SE) per 10 000 in 16 and 17 year olds [22,34,35]. More recently, prevalence rates have been estimated to be as high as 4% in community-based study when all tic disorders are included [36] and 3% in a survey of middle school youth in the UK [37]. Kurlan and colleagues found rates of TD as high as 7% in special education classes in a school-based community survey, and about 4% in regular classrooms [2].

Studies in both children and adults suggest that males are at least three to four times more likely than females to manifest TD [38].

Psychiatric Comorbidity

The scientific relationship between TD and frequently observed psychiatric comorbid disorders has not yet been disentangled. Obsessive–compulsive symptoms, developmentally inappropriate motoric hyperactivity and inattention, anxiety, and aggressive dyscontrol frequently have been described in association with TD [4,6,8,27,39–42]. Motor, vocal, behavioral, cognitive, and emotional dysfunction may represent manifesta-

tions of an underlying central disinhibition problem [12,43].

Developmentally inappropriate hyperactivity, inattention, and impulsivity are also problematic for many TD patients. Some investigators have reported that 50%–75% of TD patients also meet criteria for ADHD [4,38,44–46]. The nature of the scientific relationship between ADHD and TD is not firmly established.

There appears to be a bidirectional relationship between TD and OCD in most patient cohorts [47–51]. Between 20% and 40% of TD patients have been reported to meet full criteria for OCD, and up to 90% have been reported to have subthreshold symptoms such as repetitive counting, touching or symmetry needs. Family studies indicate that OCD is found at a higher rate in close relatives than in controls which further supports this finding [49–54].

In addition to OCD, mood and anxiety disorders have been described in clinically referred TD patients, including major depression, bipolar disorder, separation anxiety disorder, panic disorder, simple and social phobias [3,8,51,55]. Furthermore, a substantial minority of youth with TD evaluated in clinical settings may meet criteria for intermittent explosive disorder manifest by rage attacks [39]. Whether these dysregulated emotions are primary (i.e., related to the underlying pathophysiology of TD) or secondary to the demoralization and/or impairment related to having the chronic illness remains to be clarified.

Genetic Findings

Genetic data have derived historically from family pedigree and twin studies. Tourette's disorder, chronic tic disorders, and OCD cluster in families. Twin studies have shown a high concordance rate for tic disorders among monozygotic (MZ) pairs (ranging from about 50% to 90%) in contrast to a relatively low rate among dizygotic twins (often around 20%) [56]. Other studies have shown that first-degree relatives of TD patients have a higher percentage of TD, chronic tics, and OCD than normal controls [49,52,56]. Historically, genetic analyses were thought to be consistent with an autosomal dominant mode (with incomplete penetrance) of inheritance [49,52,54]; some investigators argued that a semidominant, semirecessive pattern could also exist [57–59]. However, older studies have been confounded by relatively high rates of bilineality [60,61].

More recently investigators have proposed a major gene locus in combination with other genes and/or environmental factors. To date, no unique locus has been specifically identified for TD. A systematic genome scan with 76 affected sibling pair families with 110 sib-pairs demonstrated that 4q and 8p regions were regions of interest, with lod scores of 2.38 and 2.09 respectively. In addition, four other regions including on chromosome 1, 10, 13 and 19 had lod scores greater than one.

Etiology and Pathophysiology

The etiology and pathophysiology of TD and other tic disorders are unknown. Considerable data accumulated during the past decade from neuroanatomical and neurochemical studies of TD point to a diffuse process in the brain involving corticostriatothalami-cortical pathways in the basal ganglia, striatum, and frontal lobes [12,62]. Several neurotransmitters and neuromodulators have been implicated, including dopamine, serotonin, and endogenous opioids [13,14,63–78]. Although a specific animal model has not been identified, some parallels may exist with horses that display spontaneous motor tics accompanied by vocalizations as crib biting [79] and dogs with acral lick syndrome [80].

Neuroimaging studies employing cerebral blood flow and energy (glucose) metabolism parameters [e.g., positron emission tomography (PET) and single photon emission tomography (SPECT)] suggest altered activity (increased or decreased and at times unilaterally) in various areas of brain (e.g., frontal and orbital cortex, striatum, putamen) in TD patients compared to controls or across brain regions within TD patients [15–17,72,81,82]. Magnetic resonance imaging studies have indicated volume or asymmetry abnormalities in caudate or lenticular nuclei in subjects with TD compared to controls. Volumetric magnetic resonance spectroscopy studies have shown a loss of the normal asymmetry of the basal ganglia [83–85]. A study in MZ twins concordant for TD but discordant for severity demonstrated abnormalities in D2 receptors in the caudate area in the more severely afflicted twin [18]. In 10 pairs of MZ twins, the right caudate was smaller in the more severely afflicted individuals, supporting evidence for the role of environmental components [86].

Pediatric Autoimmune Neuropsychiatric Disorders Associated with Streptococcus

Swedo and colleagues have described a putative sub-group of children with TD and OCD with hypothetical antecedent Group A Beta Hemolytic *Streptococcus* (GABHS) infection who have symptom onset and/or exacerbation precipitated by *Streptococcus* infection (pediatric autoimmune disorders associated with streptococcus or PANDAS) [87]. They describe specific diagnostic criteria for PANDAS, including prepubertal onset, sudden, explosive onset and/or exacerbations and remissions, and a temporal relationship with symptoms and GABHS [88,89]. A double-blind, placebo crossover study of prophylactic oral penicillin to attempt to reduce recurrences of PANDAS failed to show any differences between drug and placebo [90]. A multisite, prospective case – control (PANDAS and control subjects) 24-month epidemiological study currently underway seeks to clarify the putative relationship between *Streptococcus* and tic exacerbations in both groups [91].

Differential Diagnosis

Differential diagnosis of TD and other tic disorders can be challenging. Diagnosis is made on clinical grounds, primarily based on characteristic historical features and examination. No specific laboratory tests are confirmatory. Many patients will suppress their symptoms during the initial office visit; the diagnosis can still be made provisionally (Table 23.5).

Diagnostic hallmarks of tic disorders include their waxing and waning natural history, onset in childhood or adolescence, and repetitive, rapid, nonrhythmic, and involuntary features.

Other movement disorders to be differentiated from TD include: (1) Sydenham's chorea, a neurological complication of streptococcal infection in which choreiform, writhing, and truncal movements are observed; (2) Huntington disease, an autosomal dominant disorder presenting with chorea and dementia and with an onset typically in the fourth or fifth decade; and (3) Parkinson disease, typically a late life disorder, characterized by flat facies, gait disturbance, rigidity, cogwheeling, and 'pill rolling' resting tremor; and (4) PANDAS. In psychiatric settings, patients who have been exposed to neuroleptics are at risk for neuroleptic-related dyskinesias, including tardive and withdrawal dyskinesias. Dyskinesias can also be seen in TD patients secondary to their neuroleptic therapy, but may be easily overlooked [92,93].

Clinical Evaluation

A comprehensive, detailed history with observations derived from multiple sources is the cornerstone of the clinical evaluation of patients with tic disorders.

Since TD is a diagnosis made primarily on the basis of its unique history and on tics observed during the examination, reliable sources of information are essen-

Table 23.5 Differential diagnosis of movement disorders.

Descriptive terms	Observable movement pattern(s)
Akathisia	Motor restlessness (an unpleasant need to move), usually in the lower extremities
Athetosis	Slow, writhing movements, usually in the hands and fingers
Ballismus	Large amplitude, jerking, shaking, flinging
Chorea	Irregular, spasmodic, usually limbs or face
Dyskinesia	Choreiform or dystonic, stereotyped and not suppressible
Dystonia	Sustained, tonic contraction that progresses to abnormal postures
Myoclonus	Sudden, brief, clonic, shock-like jerks or spasms, usually involving the limbs
Periodic movements of sleep	Periodic dorsiflexion of the foot and flexion of the knee, occurring during sleep
Stereotypy	Repetitive, usually meaningless, gestures, habits, or automatisms

tial. This is particularly important, because in many patients tics may be suppressed during the initial examinations.

Historical inquiry should include detailed medical and developmental information, medication history (including substances of abuse or recreation), educational and occupational data, social and interpersonal history, and a thorough family pedigree covering at least three generations. A careful, descriptive, longitudinal assessment of the movement disorder is important. The physical examination should include height, weight, presence or absence of dysmorphic features, posture, gait, reflexes, and a systematic rating of current abnormal movements. The Abnormal Involuntary Movement Scale (AIMS) is a systematic assessment procedure (and rating form) that can be adapted for use with children. Videotaped standardized interviews and evaluation procedures are used in some research studies; these could also be used in the clinical setting. However, absence of observed tics on initial examination does not preclude the diagnosis of a tic disorder.

Psychiatric evaluation should include a formal assessment of the behavioral and emotional problems known to clinically cluster with TD, including OCD, ADHD, other anxiety disorders, mood disorders and manifestations of impaired or dysregulated affect (e.g., impulsivity, aggressivity). The use of structured interviews, such as the Diagnostic Interview Schedule for Children (DISC) or the Children's Schedule for Affective Disorders and Schizophrenia (K-SADS) or other structured rating instruments can improve classification and the assessment of comorbidity [94,95]. Since rating instruments can provide quantifiable baseline data, such as frequency and intensity of tics, these data can also be used to measure treatment response. Standardized rating scales developed specifically for the

TD population have improved diagnostic reliability in research studies and can also be helpful in clinical care. The Yale-Global Tic Severity Scale (Y-GTSS) [96] and the Tourette Syndrome Symptom List (TSSL) [97] rate tics, compulsions, and other associated features. Specific rating scales for OCD (the Children's Yale-Brown Obsessive-Compulsive Scale or C-YBOCS) [98,99] and ADHD (Iowa Parent and Teacher Conners or SNAP) [100–102] can also be utilized.

Auxiliary data from outside sources is essential. Pediatric and medical records may document developmental and medical history, adequacy of medication trials and responses, hospitalization(s), or laboratory findings. A review of school records is advised for children, as many TD patients manifest their difficulties while in school settings. Report cards can document academic performance; direct phone contact with teachers may provide data about attentional functioning and social and emotional competencies. Neuropsychological or speech and language testing may be indicated for patients with impairments in school or occupational functioning. Identified areas of strength and weakness are subsequently conveyed to appropriate personnel for inclusion into educational or vocational planning.

Treatment

General Guidelines

At the present time, pharmacotherapy remains the cornerstone of effective treatment for tic disorders. Treatment goals should be to relieve symptoms or achieve symptom control, support adaptive functioning and strengths, and enhance developmental progress.

Self-esteem at all times should be supported, as most patients with tic disorders will have at least some sense of personal and emotional vulnerability. Early on in the diagnostic process, education as to phenomenology and natural history of TD is essential.

Clarification that the patient's symptoms are not voluntary in most situations eases psychological burdens for both patients and families. This is especially important since families observe that tics, at times, can be suppressed. Struggles over whether the symptoms are tics or 'negative behavior' are pointless and should be curtailed; a more practical goal involves personal management of, and responsibility for, symptoms and behavior, regardless of their origin.

Containment is another cornerstone of treatment. Even with use of effective medication(s), it is rare for tics to remit completely. Use of a 'tic room' or a 'time out' area provides an opportunity to contain problematic tics or compulsions and to 'de-stimulate.' Since emotional conflicts and stress frequently increase symptom intensity and frequency, time-limited withdrawal from stressful situations can be beneficial.

Specific Medications

The decision to treat tic and/or comorbid symptoms should be based on a comprehensive evaluation. Patients with symptoms that significantly interfere with adaptation to family, school, or work life, peer relationships, or developmental progress should be treated. Patients who suffer significant emotional distress or inadvertently cause significant distress to key persons in their lives may also be candidates for treatment, even when symptoms are relatively mild. Most patients with very mild symptoms need only monitoring, education, guidance, and support. Moderate to severe symptoms usually should be treated aggressively.

The clinical work-up before initiating any treatment should include a complete physical examination and neurological screening, psychiatric evaluation, vital signs, an AIMS screening, basic laboratory screening (including a complete blood count with differential, urinalysis, and a blood chemistry screen including liver and thyroid tests, fasting blood glucose, and metabolic screen including cholesterol and triglycerides), and an electrocardiogram (EKG).

Medication should be initiated at the lowest possible dose and dosage increments should be gradual in general. Most maximum doses will be low (compared to dosages needed for other indications for these same medications) in TD patients. When possible, a single medication (monotherapy) should be used initially. At times more than one agent will need to be prescribed simultaneously (targeted combined pharmacotherapy) when monotherapy has not been efficacious, or has resulted in limiting side effects.

Determining an adequate duration for a medication trial for patients with tics can be quite challenging, since the natural history of TD involves the waxing and waning of symptoms over time. A one-month baseline observation period before treatment is initiated is recommended, if feasible. In general, it is best to wait at least several weeks after changing a dose before making any conclusions about therapeutic response. External stressors must be taken into account at all times as potential determinants of increased symptomatology during medication trials.

Alpha Adrenergic Agonists

The alpha-adrenergic agents are recommended as first-line treatment for most patients with mild-moderate TD. Clonidine, an alpha 2-adrenergic (presynaptic) agonist, has been used for nearly 20 years for the treatment of TD [10,103,104]. Given in low doses, it is postulated that presynaptic noradrenergic effects mediate the observed clinical improvement in motor and vocal tics. In addition, clonidine also reduces the disinhibition, impulsivity, inattention, and hyperactivity often present in young TD patients.

Clonidine should generally be started at 0.025 mg daily to b.i.d. for children and increased by 0.025 mg every 1–2 weeks. Prepubertal patients will generally need t.i.d. to q.i.d. dosing. Adolescents or adults can be started on 0.05 mg daily and increased by 0.05 mg increments to b.i.d. dosing. The total daily dose typically is 0.05 mg to 0.45 mg (i.e., up to 8.0 μg/kg). Side effects commonly seen include sedation, headaches, or stomachaches. Sedation, the most common and sometimes limiting side effect, usually abates over several weeks; when it does not, dosage reduction may be helpful. Hypotensive effects are minimal in this dosage range, but blood pressure, pulse and EKG should be monitored at baseline and follow-up visits.

Guanfacine, an alternative alpha 2-adrenergic agonist, may also be efficacious for hyperactivity, impulsivity, and tics [11,105]. Prepubertal patients are typically started on 0.25 mg daily and increased by 0.25 mg increments given twice daily; older patients and adults are typically started on 0.5 mg daily and increased by 0.5 mg increments to about 3.0 mg daily.

Neuroleptic Agents

Since the late 1960s when haloperidol was first introduced as a treatment for TD patients, haloperidol (Haldol) and (Orap) have been the only Food and Drugs Administration (FDA) labeled, formally approved agents for treatment of TD [93,106–119].

Table 23.6 Pharmacotherapies for TD and tic disorders.

Class/medication	Typical range (mg)	Starting dose (mg)	Maximum dose (mg)[a]	Common side effects
Neuroleptics				
Haloperidol	0.25–5.0	0.25–0.5	5.0	Sedation, weight gain, dysphoria, extrapyramidal effects
Pimozide	1.0–10	0.5–1.0	15–20	Sedation, weight gain, EKG changes
Risperidone	1.0–3.0	0.25–0.5	4–6	Weight gain, sedation
Aripiprazole	2.5–15	1.25–2.5	20	Akathisia, sedation, agitation
Partial α2-adrenergic agonists				
Clonidine	0.05–0.45	0.025–0.05	0.45	Sedation, headaches, insomnia, stomach aches, hypotension
Guanfacine	1.0–3.0	0.25–0.5	3–4	Sedation, headaches, hypotension
Tricyclic antidepressants				
Desipramine	25–300	10–25	250–300	Sedation, dry mouth, weight gain, tachycardia, prolongation QTc
Clomipramine	50–200	10–25	250–300	Sedation, dry mouth, weight gain, tachycardia, prolongation QTc
SSRIs[b]				
Fluoxetine	5.0–40	2.5–10	60–80	Insomnia, anxiety, weight loss, headaches, gastrointestinal distress, sexual dysfunction; suicidality
Sertraline	25–200	12.5–25	200–300	Insomnia, activation, gastrointestinal distress, sexual dysfunction; suicidality
Paroxetine	10–40	5–10	50–60	As above
Fluvoxamine	50–300	12.5–25	300	As above
Citalopram	5–40	2.5–5	60	As above
Escitalopram	2.5–20	2.5	20	As above

[a] These are usual maximum doses for adults. [b] These medications have been found to be effective in patients with OCD.

These medications block D2 (dopamine) receptors in the basal ganglia, and thus reduce tics. These medications are generally effective in tic reduction; however, considerable variation exists in clinicians' and patients' thresholds for neuroleptic use. The decision to use a neuroleptic may be guided by both symptom severity and quality of life concerns. In general, neuroleptic agents are usually not recommended for tics that are mild.

The newer, atypical neuroleptics are recommended as first line treatment when a neuroleptic is indicated for moderate to severe tics. These agents, which block both D2 dopamine and serotonin receptors, have the potential advantage of less extrapyramidal side effects. Risperdone (Risperdal) has been found to be efficacious for tics. Doses are typically in the 1–3 mg range [108,120]. Additional studies of the atypicals in TD have included ziprasidone (Geodon) and olanzapine (Zyprexa) [121].

Aripiprazole, a novel atypical neuroleptic with partial agonist–antagonist effects on the dopamine and serotonin system, may be useful in some patients who have not responded to more established treatments. The author and her colleague (Budman) have conducted a systematic, open trial of aripiprazole in 22 youth with TD with and without explosive outbursts. Preliminary results indicated that aripiprazole is effective in reducing both tics and explosive outbursts at low–moderate doses (range 5–40 mg; mean 11.5 mg). Tics improved in 20 of the 22 subjects, and explosive outbursts improved in all 13 of the subjects who were treated for rage.

In this open series, aripiprazole was also reasonably well tolerated. Most common side effects were initial sedation, which diminished over time, and mild extrapyramidal side effects, such as akathisia and mild agitation. In only two subjects was aripiprazole ineffective for tics and/or explosive outbursts.

Neuroleptics should be initiated at the lowest possible doses and then increased very gradually. Risperidone is typically started at 0.125–0.25 mg daily to b.i.d. and titrated upward to about 1–2 mg daily in prepubertal children; adolescents are typically started on 0.25 mg daily to b.i.d. For haloperidol, children are typically started at 0.125–0.25 mg daily to b.i.d. and increased by 0.125–0.25 mg increments weekly or biweekly. Adults are usually started on 0.5 mg, with weekly or biweekly increases of 0.5 mg. Pimozide is an alternative D2-blocking agent, which may cause fewer side effects than haloperidol. However, because pimozide also has calcium channel blocking properties, normal cardiac function (ascertained from cardiac assessment and an EKG) is a prerequisite to its use. Approximately half as potent as haloperidol, pimozide should be started at 0.5–1.0 mg for children, and at about 1.0 mg for adolescents or adults. Most patients will require less than 10 mg daily.

Common side effects of neuroleptics include weight gain, sedation, muscle cramps and stiffness. Dosage reduction or switching to an alternative drug is the best way to address these side effects. Fortunately, extrapyramidal side effects (EPS) do not appear to be common sequelae from neuroleptic use at usual dosages in tic disorder patients; nevertheless, clinicians should be alert to the possibility of these reactions and consider appropriate interventions (e.g., anti-Parkinson agents, dosage reduction) on a case-by-case basis. Extrapyramidal side effects may be less common with the atypical agents than with the typicals. Tardive dyskinesia, while probably not common, has been described in patients with TD and may be difficult to differentiate from tics [92].

Weight gain is likely with both typical and atypical neuroleptics, but the risk appears to be greater with use of the atypical agents such as olanzapine and risperidone. The possibility of weight gain should be addressed proactively in all youth who are candidates for neuroleptics. Education regarding the need for a healthy diet and regular exercise at the outset of treatment is helpful; at times nutritional consultation may be indicated.

Selective Serotonin Reuptake Inhibitors (SSRIs)
Serotonergic agents such as fluoxetine, fluvoxamine and sertraline represent alternative pharmacotherapy for some of the target symptoms seen in TD [122,123]. Since many TD patients have obsessions or compulsions, and neuroleptics and the alpha 2-agonists do not effectively alter these specific symptoms, the SSRIs may be beneficial. In addition, complex motor tics such as repetitive squatting and touching may be very similar to compulsive rituals. Fluoxetine has received the most study in TD, but efficacy likely is relatively comparable among agents. Choice typically rests with consideration of the side effects profiles of the agents.

When obsessions or compulsions are of moderate to severe intensity or impair adaptive functioning, SSRIs are potentially indicated. Fluoxetine typically is started at 2.5–5.0 mg daily for children and at 5.0–10 mg for adolescents or adults. Dosage ranges are not well established for children and adolescents. It appears that most children will respond to 10–20 mg daily; adults may require 20–80 mg daily. Fluoxetine in combination with a neuroleptic can be useful for both tics and obsessive–compulsive symptoms; neuroleptic dosages may require reduction or adjustment because of the oxidative enzyme inhibiting properties of fluoxetine. Common side effects include activation, insomnia, headaches, anorexia, and weight loss.

Clomipramine should be started at 10–25 mg for children and 25–50 mg for adolescents or adults. Total dosage ranges are typically 100–300 mg daily; blood levels may be obtained, but at present no therapeutic range has been established. Common side effects are those seen typically with other tricyclic antidepressants, including sedation, dry mouth, constipation, blurring of vision, weight gain and EKG changes.

Sertraline, fluvoxamine, citalopram and escitalopram may also be beneficial, but experience with them is still limited. There is more data available on the use of clomipramine in OCD, but the side effects may be more problematic [124]. These may represent alternatives for patients who experience limiting side effects on fluoxetine.

Tricyclic Antidepressants
Some studies of desipramine have suggested potential efficacy for the treatment of tics in patients with comorbid ADHD [125–127]. Dosages are not established, but may parallel doses used in ADHD without tics. Careful cardiovascular monitoring must take place, including blood pressure, pulse and baseline and follow-up EKGs.

Benzodiazepines
Another class of medications that may hold some promise is the benzodiazepines (e.g., clonazepam). Some studies suggest a reduction in tics independent of anxiolytic effects [128]. This effect may also reflect a reduction in anxiety that, in turn, could reduce tic

frequency. In addition, benzodiazepines can be used to treat the comorbid anxiety symptomatology or panic attacks that can also occur in TD patients. Dosages are not established, but are often quite low (0.125 mg daily to b.i.d.). Side effects of particular concern in the juvenile population are sedation, cognitive impairment and disinhibition.

Stimulants

There has been a controversy in the past decade about the role of stimulants in TD; however, recent studies have demonstrated that some TD patients with significant ADHD may be candidates for methylphenidate when no other treatments have been effective [129,130]. Behavior improved and tics did not worsen at moderate dosages of 0.1–0.5 mg/kg. A recent randomized controlled study of clonidine and methylphenidate in ADHD and chronic tics reported that the combination, and each drug, was more effective than placebo in reducing both tics and ADHD symptoms. Increase in tics did not occur in the methylphenidate group to any extent more significantly than in the placebo group [131]. Side effects include insomnia, appetite suppression, and weight loss.

Nonstimulant ADHD Treatment

Atomoxetine

Atomoxetine (Strattera), a selective norepinephrine inhibitor, was recently approved for treatment of ADHD in children, adolescents and adults. It has also been studied in youth with ADHD and chronic tics. It is dosed based on body weight, and titrated typically from starting dose 0.5 mg/kg/day to 1–1.5 mg/kg/day. Therapeutic response, unlike stimulants, takes a few weeks. Side effects include headache, nausea, fatigue and stomachaches.

Other Alternatives

Many other medications have been used in TD patients. Opioid antagonists (e.g., naltrexone) may be an alternative for those patients with self-injurious behaviors [68–70,77,132]. Dosage range for naltrexone may be approximately 25–75 mg/day. Nicotine, both in gum and in the transdermal form has also been studied in TD [133–135]. Pergolide, a dopamine agonist, was found to be more effective than placebo in a randomized controlled trial in 24 youth with TD [136]. Botulinum toxins injected into the muscles of tics involved have been used in several studies [137,138]. In retrospective case studies of 24 patients with TD, mecamy-

lamine, a nicotine antagonist, in doses of 2.5 mg daily, reduced tics severity and improved irritability and mood [139,140]. However, in a double-blind, controlled trial in 61 subjects with TD at doses up to 7.5 mg daily, mecamylamine was found to be no more effective than placebo [141].

Baclofen, a GABAergic muscle relaxant, has been studied in one large open-label and one controlled trial [142,143]. In the open-label trial, at mean dose of 30 mg/day (range 10–80 mg/day), tics improved significantly [142]. In the controlled trial, there was no difference between drug and placebo in total tic score, but baclofen was superior to placebo with regard to tic related impairment on the YGTSS [143].

More recently, the author and her colleague (Gabbay) are conducting a controlled trial of Omega-3-fatty acids derived from fish oil in 40 youth with TD. Although the trial is ongoing, there appear to be no major problems with safety or tolerability. The dosing schedule is flexible, starting at 500 mg daily and titrating upward by clinical response to a maximum of 6000 mg.

Targeted combined pharmacotherapy, or the specific combination of two or more medications at one time, has evolved as a treatment option. Ideally, this approach should be utilized only after adequate trials of monotherapy have failed. However, many patients with TD also have comorbid ADHD or OCD, and often both, and frequently monotherapy addresses one problem but not the remaining disorders. Judicious use of SSRIs plus neuroleptics for TD and comorbid OCD is one example of this approach; in some patients with OCD and tics this approach may be more effective than monotherapy [144]. Another example is the combination of methylphenidate and clonidine to target tics and ADHD symptoms [131].

Surgical Treatment

Stereotaxic neurosurgical techniques have been used in a few cases of severely impaired adults [145]. Deep brain stimulation has been used in at least one case of an adult with intractable symptoms. However, given the significant medical risks for these procedures, there is no indication for use of these techniques in youth at this time.

Psychoeducational Approaches

Education of patients and their families is essential. Patients frequently experience relief at the time of diagnosis, as do many parents and families. There should be ongoing opportunities for discussion of patients' questions and concerns. Referral to the national Tourette Syndrome Association (TSA) or to local chapters of the TSA is an excellent way to maintain continuing education and support.

Behavioral Therapies

Behavioral paradigms are indicated for a number of difficulties in tic disorder patients. Simple behavioral approaches can be used with the majority of TD patients to 'de-stimulate' and contain the symptoms. Specific paradigms are indicated for obsessions, compulsions, and possibly some complex motor tics. Relaxation techniques, such as deep breathing, guided imagery, and use of relaxation tapes, can be useful for the anxious or stressed TD patient. Habit reversal, using competing response to oppose motor tics, may have utility in the treatment of tic disorders. Opposing muscles are contracted following the urge to have a tic. This competing response theoretically prevents the emergence of the tic [146]. Tic substitution (substituting a more socially tolerable tic for a less socially tolerable one) can be useful. Contingency management should emphasize positive reinforcement and avoid increased guilt or anxiety. Massed negative practice (i.e., self-imposed forceful repetition of the tic) for a period of time (with intervals for rest) is beneficial for some patients. The ensuing tiredness theoretically produces a decrease in tic frequency. About half of the published studies on massed negative practice have found this technique to be beneficial [147].

Psychotherapy

Individual, group, and family therapies are supportive adjuncts to pharmacotherapy. Individual supportive therapy is indicated for patients having difficulty adjusting to the disorder, to their peers or family, or with school or occupational functioning. It is particularly useful when there is evidence of moderate stress or anxiety or another comorbid psychiatric disorder responsive to this form of psychotherapy (e.g., mild depression). It can help to restore or maintain self-esteem and promote mastery and coping.

Family work or therapy is extremely useful in dealing with the many complex interpersonal and family issues that arise for children with TD. At a minimum, both parents should be seen at least once as part of the initial evaluation. Ideally, family members can be sources of support and nurturance. Ongoing family therapy is indicated when family development (i.e., growth and maturation) has slowed or halted because of the focus on the patient with the tic disorder. It may also help with maladaptive reactions from

or to siblings, or with specific symptoms that are affecting the entire family.

Group therapy is another important adjunct. Support and education for parents and family members of patients with TD can be found through the national TSA, which has created a well-organized network of state and community support groups. Informal, unstructured activity can be arranged through local TSA chapters. Formal, structured support is also possible through social skills groups.

School and Occupational Interventions

Learning problems and classroom difficulties occur commonly in tic disorder patients. Specific developmental disorders and ADHD- or OCD-related symptoms may interfere with academic performance.

Clinicians should be available to provide consultation, guidance, and education to teachers or employers of patients with tic disorders. Useful special educational interventions include creating moderate, task-oriented structure in the classroom, preferential seating, one-to-one support, or individualized educational or work plans. Flexibility is a key element in educational and occupational intervention. To promote tic control, there may be a need for optional 'time outs' from class or work settings. Time limits may have to be extended or eliminated for exams. Some patients also may benefit from writing aides, such as silent typewriters and computers. Silent typewriters allow patients with handwriting difficulties to take notes in class without disturbing others. Adaptive, as contrasted to regular, physical education can be particularly helpful for children with TD. This form of physical education can be arranged through special education departments in local schools. Programs can be tailored to each child's needs, strengths, and weaknesses.

Specific workplace interventions include structured tasks, organization of tasks into smaller units, flexible time limits, and ample physical space.

Summary

Tourette's disorder is a complex neuropsychiatric disorder with a heterogeneous phenotype characterized by core disinhibition mediated by the corticostriatothalamicortical tracts. Tourette's disorder is genetically determined in most cases. There is a growing appreciation and understanding of the role of psychiatric comorbidity in the diverse clinical presentation. Treatment strategies should be multimodal in nature, and include pharmacotherapy and, where indicated, behavior, individual and family intervention and educational monitoring. Future investigation is needed to better understand the phenomenology, developmental psychopathology, and treatment. Until then, TD remains as its 'character equivocal, cause unknown, and treatment problematical.'

References

1. American Psychiatric Association: *Diagnostic and Statistical Manual of Mental Disorders DSM-IV-TR.* Washington DC: APA Press, 2000.

2. Kurlan R, McDermott MP, Deeley C, Como PG, Brower C, Eapen S, *et al.*: Prevalence of tics in schoolchildren and association with placement in special education. *Neurology* 2001; **57**(8):1383–1388.

3. Coffey B, Biederman J, Spencer T, Geller D, Faraone S, Bellordre C: Informativeness of structured diagnostic interviews in the identification of Tourette's disorder in referred youth. *J Nervous Mental Dis* 2000; **188**:583–588.

4. Comings DE, Comings BG: A controlled study of Tourette syndrome. I. Attention-deficit disorder, learning disorders, and school problems. *Am J Hum Genet* 1987; **41**(5):701–741.

5. Comings DE, Comings BG: A controlled study of Tourette syndrome. II. Conduct. *Am J Hum Genet* 1987; **41**(5):742–760.

6. Comings DE, Comings BG: A controlled study of Tourette syndrome. IV. Obsessions, compulsions, and schizoid behaviors. *Am J Hum Genet* 1987; **41**(5):782–803.

7. Comings DE, Comings BG: Tourette's syndrome and attention deficit disorder with hyperactivity. *Arch Gen Psychiatry* 1987; **44**(11):1023–1026.

8. Robertson MM, Channon S, Baker J, Flynn D: The psychopathology of Gilles de la Tourette's syndrome: A controlled study. *Br J Psychiatry* 1993; **162**:114–117.

9. Leckman JF, Cohen DJ, Detlor J, Young JG, Harcherik D, Shaywitz BA: Clonidine in the treatment of Tourette syndrome: A review of data. *Adv Neurol* 1982; **35**:391–401.

10. Leckman JF, Hardin MT, Riddle MA, Stevenson J, Ort SI, Cohen DJ: Clonidine treatment of Gilles de la Tourette's syndrome. *Arch Gen Psychiatry* 1991; **48**(4):324–328.

11. Scahill L, Chappell, P, Kim Y, Schultz R, Katsovich I, Shepherd E, Arnsten A, Cohen D, Leckman J: A placebo controlled study of guanfacine in the treatment of children with tic disorders and attention deficit hyperactivity disorder. *Am J Psychiatry* 2001; **158**:1067–1074.

12. Leckman JF, Pauls DL, Peterson BS, Riddle MA, Anderson GM, Cohen DJ: Pathogenesis of Tourette syndrome. Clues from the clinical phenotype and natural history. *Adv Neurol* 1992; **58**:15–24.

13. Singer HS: Neurochemical analysis of postmortem cortical and striatal brain tissue in patients with Tourette syndrome. *Adv Neurol* 1992; **58**:135–144.

14. Singer HS, Hahn IH, Moran TH: Abnormal dopamine uptake sites in postmortem striatum from patients with Tourette's syndrome. *Ann Neurol* 1991; **30**(4):558–562.

15. Singer HS, Wong DF, Brown JE, Brandt J, Krafft L, Shaya E, *et al.*: Positron emission tomography evaluation of dopamine D-2 receptors in adults with Tourette syndrome. *Adv Neurol* 1992; **58**:233–239.

16. Singer HS, Reiss AL, Brown JE, Aylward EH, Shih B, Chee E, *et al.*: Volumetric MRI changes in basal ganglia of children with Tourette's syndrome. *Neurology* 1993; **43**(5):950–956.

17. Stoetter B, Braun AR, Randolph C, Gernert J, Carson RE, Herscovitch P, *et al.*: Functional neuroanatomy of Tourette syndrome. Limbic-motor interactions studied with FDG PET. *Adv Neurol* 1992; **58**:213–226.

18. Wolf SS, Jones DW, Knable MB, Gorey JG, Lee KS, Hyde TM, *et al.*: Tourette syndrome: Prediction of phenotypic variation in monozygotic twins by caudate nucleus D2 receptor binding. *Science* 1996; **273**(5279):1225–1227.

19. Shapiro A, Shapiro E: Proposed nosology, criteria, and differential diagnosis. In: Shapiro A, Shapiro E, Young JG, Feinberg T, eds. *Gilles de la Tourette Syndrome.* New York: Raven Press, 1988:343–380.

20. Lang A: Patient perception of tics and other movement disorders. *Neurology* 1991; **41**(2Pt1):223–228.

21. Leckman JF, Walker DE, Cohen DJ: Premonitory urges in Tourette's syndrome. *Am J Psychiatry* 1993; **150**(1):98–102.

22. Shapiro A. Epidemiology. In: Shapiro A, Shapiro E, Young JG, Feinberg T, eds. *Gilles de la Tourette Syndrome.* New York: Raven Press, 1988:45–60.

23. Shapiro A: Signs, symptoms and clinical course. In: Shapiro A, Shapiro E, Feinberg T, Young JG, eds. *Gilles de la Tourette Syndrome.* 1988:169–193.

24. Cohen AJ, Leckman JF: Sensory phenomena associated with Gilles de la Tourette's syndrome. *J Clin Psychiatry* 1992; **53**(9):319–323.

25. Miguel EC, Coffey BJ, Baer L, Savage CR, Rauch SL, Jenike MA: Phenomenology of intentional repetitive behaviors in obsessive-compulsive disorder and Tourette's disorder. *J Clin Psychiatry* 1995; **56**(6):246–255.

26. Bruun RD, Budman CL: The natural history of Tourette syndrome. *Adv Neurol* 1992; **58**:1–6.

27. Coffey BJ, Biederman J, Geller D, Frazier J, Spencer T, Doyle R, *et al.*: Reexamining tic persistence and tic-associated impairment in Tourette's disorder: Findings from a naturalistic follow-up study. *J Nervous Mental Dis* 2004; **192**(11):776–780.

28. Jankovic J: Tourette's syndrome. *New Engl J Med* 2001; **345**(16):1184–1192.

29. Luo F, Leckman JF, Katsovich L, Findley D, Grantz H, Tucker DM, *et al.*: Prospective longitudinal study of children with tic disorders and/or obsessive-compulsive disorder: Relationship of symptom exacerbations to newly acquired streptococcal infections. *Pediatrics* 2004; **113**(6).

30. Bruun RD, Shapiro AK, Shapiro E, Sweet R, Wayne H, Solomon GE, *et al.*: A follow-up of 78 patients with Gilles de la Tourette's syndrome. *Am J Psychiatry* 1976; **133**(8):944–947.

31. de Groot C, Bornstein R, Spetie L, Burriss BA: The course of tics in tourette's syndrome: A 5-year follow-up study. *Ann Clin Psychiatry* 1994; **6**(4):227–233.

32. Kerbeshian J, Burd L, Klug M: Comorbid Tourette's disorder and bipolar disorder: An etiologic perspective. *Am J Psychiatry* 1995; **152**(11):1646–1651.

33. Leckman J, Zhang H, Vitale A, Lahnin F, Lynch K, Bond C, et al.: Course of tic severity: The first two decades. *Pediatrics* 1998, submitted.

34. Apter A, Pauls DL, Bleich A, Zohar AH, Kron S, Ratzoni G, et al.: An epidemiologic study of Gilles de la Tourette's syndrome in Israel. *Arch Gen Psychiatry* 1993; **50**(9):734–738.

35. Apter A, Pauls DL, Bleich A, Zohar AH, Kron S, Ratzoni G, et al.: A population-based epidemiological study of Tourette syndrome among adolescents in Israel. *Adv Neurol* 1992; **58**:61–65.

36. Costello EJ, Angold A, Burns BJ, Stangl DK, Tweed DL, Erkanli A, et al.: The Great Smoky Mountains Study of Youth. Goals, design, methods, and the prevalence of DSM-III-R disorders. *Arch Gen Psychiatry* 1996; **53**(12):1129–1136.

37. Mason A, Banerjee S, Eapen V, Zeitlin H, Robertson MM: The prevalence of Tourette syndrome in a mainstream school population. *Dev Med Child Neurol* 1998; **40**(5):292–296.

38. Shapiro AK, Shapiro ES, Young JG, Feinberg TE: Patient characteristics. In: Shapiro AK, Shapiro, ES, Young JG, Feinberg TE, eds. *Gilles de la Tourette Syndrome.* New York: Raven Press; 1988:61–126.

39. Budman CL, Bruun RD, Park KS, Lesser M, Olson M: Explosive outbursts in children with Tourette's Disorder. *J Am Acad Child Adolesc Psychiatry* 2000; **39**(10):1270–1276.

40. Comings DE, Comings BG: A controlled study of Tourette Syndrome, V: Depression and mania. *Am J Hum Genet* 1987; 41:804–821.

41. Comings DE, Comings BG: A controlled study of Tourette syndrome. III. Phobias and panic attacks. *Am J Hum Genet* 1987; **41**(5):761–781.

42. Erenberg G, Cruse RP, Rothner AD: The natural history of Tourette syndrome: A follow-up study. *Ann Neurol* 1987; **22**(3):383–385.

43. Cohen DJ, Leckman JF: Developmental psychopathology and neurobiology of Tourette's syndrome. *J Am Acad Child Adolesc Psychiatry* 1994; **33**(1):2–15.

44. Comings D: ADHD in Tourette Syndrome. In: Comings D, ed. *Tourette Syndrome and Human Behavior.* Duarte, California: Hope Press, 1990:99–104.

45. Shapiro A, Shapiro E, Young J, Feinberg T: Psychology, psychopathology, and neuropsychology. In: Shapiro A, Shapiro E, Young J, Feinberg T, eds. *Gilles de la Tourette Syndrome,* 2nd ed. New York: Raven Press, 1988:195–252.

46. Spencer T, Biederman J, Harding M, Wilens T, Faraone S: The relationship between Tic disorders and Tourette's Syndrome revisited. *J Am Acad Child Adolesc Psychiatry* 1995; **34**(9):1133–1139.

47. Grad LR, Pelcovitz D, Olson M, Matthews M, Grad GJ: Obsessive-compulsive symptomatology in children with Tourette's syndrome. *J Am Acad Child Adolesc Psychiatry* 1987; **26**(1):69–73.

48. Leonard HL, Swedo SE, Rapoport JL, Rickler KC, Topol D, Lee S, et al.: Tourette syndrome and obsessive-compulsive disorder. *Adv Neurol* 1992; **58**:83–93.

49. Pauls DL: The genetics of obsessive compulsive disorder and Gilles de la Tourette's syndrome. *Psychiatric Clin North Am* 1992; **15**(4):759–766.

50. Pauls DL, Hurst CR, Kruger SD, Leckman JF, Kidd KK, Cohen DJ: Gilles de la Tourette's syndrome and attention deficit disorder with hyperactivity. Evidence against a genetic relationship. *Arch Gen Psychiatry* 1986; **43**(12):1177–1179.

51. Pitman RK, Green RC, Jenike MA, Mesulam MM: Clinical comparison of Tourette's disorder and obsessive-compulsive disorder. *Am J Psychiatry* 1987; **144**(9):1166–1171.

52. Pauls DL: Issues in genetic linkage studies of Tourette syndrome. Phenotypic spectrum and genetic model parameters. *Adv Neurol* 1992; **58**:151–157.

53. Pauls DL, Pakstis AJ, Kurlan R, Kidd KK, Leckman JF, Cohen DJ, et al.: Segregation and linkage analyses of Tourette's syndrome and related disorders. *J Am Acad Child Adolesc Psychiatry* 1990; **29**(2):195–203.

54. Pauls DL, Raymond CL, Stevenson JM, Leckman JF: A family study of Gilles de la Tourette's syndrome. *Am J Hum Genet* 1991; **48**(1):154–163.

55. Coffey B, Frazier J, Chen S: Comorbidity, Tourette syndrome, and anxiety disorders. *Adv Neurol* 1992; **58**:95–104.

56. Pauls DL, Leckman JF: The inheritance of Gilles de la Tourette's syndrome and associated behaviors. Evidence for autosomal dominant transmission. *New Engl J Med* 1986; **315**(16):993–997.

57. Comings DE, Comings BG: Alternative hypotheses on the inheritance of Tourette syndrome. *Adv Neurol* 1992; **58**:189–199.

58. Comings DE, Muhleman D, Dietz G, Dino M, LeGro R, Gade R: Association between Tourette's syndrome and homozygosity at the dopamine D3 receptor gene. *Lancet* 1993; **341**(8849):3.

59. Comings DE, Comings BG: A controlled family history study of Tourette's syndrome, I: Attention-deficit hyperactivity disorder and learning disorders. *J Clin Psychiatry* 1990; **51**(7):275–280.

60. Lichter DG, Dmochowski J, Jackson LA, Trinidad KS: Influence of family history on clinical expression of Tourette's syndrome. *Neurology* 1999; **52**(2):308–316.

61. Kurlan R, Eapen V, Stern J, McDermott MP, Robertson MM: Bilineal transmission in Tourette's syndrome families. *Neurology* 1994; **44**(12):2336–2342.

62. Cohen DJ, Friedhoff AJ, Leckman JF, Chase TN: Tourette syndrome. Extending basic research to clinical care. *Adv Neurol* 1992; **58**:341–362.

63. Anderson GM, Pollak ES, Chatterjee D, Leckman JF, Riddle MA, Cohen DJ: Brain monoamines and amino acids in Gilles de la Tourette's syndrome: A preliminary study of subcortical regions. *Arch Gen Psychiatry* 1992; **49**(7):584–586.

64. Bornstein RA, Baker GB: Urinary amines in Tourette's syndrome patients with and without phenylethylamine abnormality. *Psychiatry Res* 1990; **31**(3):279–286.

65. Bornstein RA, Baker GB: Urinary indoleamines in Tourette syndrome patients with obsessive-compulsive characteristics. *Psychiatry Res* 1992; **41**(3):267–274.

66. Bornstein RA, Baker GB, Carroll A, King G, Ashton S: Phenylethylamine metabolism in Tourette's syndrome. *J Neuropsychiatry Clin Neurosci* 1990; **2**(4):408–412.

67. Braun AR, Stoetter B, Randolph C, Hsiao JK, Vladar K, Gernert J, et al.: The functional neuroanatomy of Tourette's syndrome: An FDG-PET study. I. Regional

changes in cerebral glucose metabolism differentiating patients and controls. *Neuropsychopharmacology* 1993; **9**(4):277–291.

68. Chappell PB, Leckman JF, Riddle MA, Anderson GM, Listwack SJ, Ort SI, et al.: Neuroendocrine and behavioral effects of naloxone in Tourette syndrome. *Adv Neurol* 1992; **58**:253–262.

69. Chappell PB: Sequential use of opioid antagonists and agonists in Tourette's syndrome. *Lancet* 1994; **343** (8897):5.

70. Chappell PB, Leckman JF, Scahill LD, Hardin MT, Anderson G, Cohen DJ: Neuroendocrine and behavioral effects of the selective kappa agonist spiradoline in Tourette's syndrome: A pilot study. *Psychiatry Res* 1993; **47**(3):267–280.

71. Cohen DJ, Shaywitz BA, Young JG, Carbonari CM, Nathanson JA, Lieberman D, et al.: Central biogenic amine metabolism in children with the syndrome of chronic multiple tics of Gilles de la Tourette: Norepinephrine, serotonin, and dopamine. *J Am Acad Child Psychiatry* 1979; **18**(2):320–341.

72. Demeter S: Structural imaging in Tourette syndrome. *Adv Neurol* 1992; **58**:201–206.

73. Gillman MA, Sandyk R: The endogenous opioid system in Gille dela Tourette syndrome: A review. *Med Hypotheses* 1986; **19**(4):371–378.

74. Leckman JF, Riddle MA, Berrettini WH, Anderson GM, Hardin M, Chappell P, et al.: Elevated CSF dynorphin A [1–8] in Tourette's syndrome. *Life Sci* 1988; **43**(24):2015–2023.

75. Riddle MA, Leckman JF, Anderson GM, Ort SI, Hardin MT, Stevenson J, et al.: Plasma MHPG: Within- and across-day stability in children and adults with Tourette's syndrome. *Biol Psychiatry* 1988; **24**(4): 391–398.

76. Sandyk R: The opioid-noradrenergic link in Gilles de la Tourette's syndrome. *Clin Pharm* 1985; **4**(5): September–October.

77. Sandyk R, Bamford CR: Opioid-serotoninergic dysregulation in the pathophysiology of Tourette's syndrome. *Funct Neurol* 1988; **3**(2):225–235.

78. Singer HS, Butler IJ, Tune LE, Seifert W, Jr., Coyle JT: Dopaminergic dsyfunction in Tourette syndrome. *Ann Neurol* 1982; **12**(4):361–366.

79. Dodman NH, Shuster L, Court MH, Dixon R: Investigation into the use of narcotic antagonists in the treatment of stereotypic behavior pattern (crib-biting) in the horse. *Am J Veterin Res* 1987; **48**:311–319.

80. Dodman NH, Shuster L, White SD, Court MH, Parker D, Dixon R: Use of narcotic anatgonists to modify stereotypic self-licking, self-chewing, and scratching behavior in dogs. *J Am Veterin Assoc* 1988; **193**: 815–819.

81. Riddle MA, Rasmusson AM, Woods SW, Hoffer PB: SPECT imaging of cerebral blood flow in Tourette syndrome. *Adv Neurol* 1992; **58**:207–211.

82. Sieg KG, Buckingham D, Gaffney GR, Preston DF, Sieg KG: Tc-99m HMPAO SPECT brain imaging of Gilles de la Tourette's syndrome. *Clin Nucl Med* 1993; **18**(3).

83. Peterson B, Riddle MA, Cohen DJ, Katz LD, Smith JC, Hardin MT, et al.: Reduced basal ganglia volumes in Tourette's syndrome using three-dimensional reconstruction techniques from magnetic resonance images. *Neurology* 1993; **43**(5):941–949.

84. Peterson BS, Leckman JF, Tucker D, Scahill L, Staib L, Zhang H, et al.: Preliminary findings of antistreptococcal antibody titers and basal ganglia volumes in tic, obsessive-compulsive, and attention deficit/hyperactivity disorders. *Arch Gen Psychiatry* 2000; **57**(4): 364–372.

85. Singer HS, Reiss AL, Brown JE, Aylward EH, Shih B, Chee E, et al.: Volumetric MRI changes in basal ganglia of children with Tourette's syndrome. *Neurology* 1993; **43**(5):950–956.

86. Hyde TM, Stacey ME, Coppola R, Handel SF, Rickler KC, Weinberger DR: Cerebral morphometric abnormalities in Tourette's syndrome: A quantitative MRI study of monozygotic twins. *Neurology* 1995; **45**(6): 1176–1182.

87. Swedo SE, Leonard HL, Garvey M, Mittleman B, Allen AJ, Perlmutter S, et al.: Pediatric autoimmune neuropsychiatric disorders associated with streptococcal infections: Clinical description of the first 50 cases. *Am J Psychiatry* 1998; **155**(2):264–271.

88. Kiessling L, Marcotte A, Culpepper L: Antineural antibodies in movement disorders. *Pediatrics* 1993; **92**:39–43.

89. Allen AJ, Leonard H, Swedo S: Case study: A new infection-triggered, autoimmune subtype of pediatric OCD and Tourette's syndrome. *J Am Acad Child Adolesc Psychiatry* 1995; **34**(3):307–311.

90. Garvey MA, Perlmutter SJ, Allen AJ, Hamburger S, Lougee L, Leonard HL, et al.: A pilot study of penicillin prophylaxis for neuropsychiatric exacerbations triggered by streptococcal infections. *Biol Psychiatry* 1999; **45**(12):1564–1571.

91. Kurlan R: The PANDAS hypothesis: Losing its bite? *Move Disord* 2004; **19**(4):371–374.

92. Silva A, Magee, H, Friedhoff A: Persistent tardive dyskinesia and other neuroleptic related dyskinesias in Tourette's disorder. *J Am Acad Child Adolesc Psychiatry* 1993; **3**:137–144.

93. Bruun RD: Subtle and underrecognized side effects of neuroleptic treatment in children with Tourette's disorder. *Am J Psychiatry* 1988; **145**(5):621–624.

94. Robins LN, Helzer JE, Croughan J: *The National Institute of Mental Health (NIMH) Diagnostic Interview Schedule, Version III.* Rockville, Maryland: National Institute of Mental Health; 1981.

95. Orvaschel H, Puig-Antich J: *Schedule for Affective Disorders and Schizophrenia for School-Age Children: Epidemiologic 4th Version.* Ft. Lauderdale: Nova University, Center for Psychological Study, 1987.

96. Leckman JF, Riddle MA, Hardin MT, Ort SI, Swartz KL, Stevenson J, Cohen DJ: The Yale Global Tic Severity Scale: Initial testing of a clinician-rated scale of tic severity. *J Am Acad Child Adolesc Psychiatry* 1989; **28**:566–573.

97. Cohen D, Leckman J, Shaywitz B: The Tourette syndrome and other tics. In: Scaffer D, Ehrhardt AA, Greenhill LL, eds. *The Clinical Guide to Child Psychiatry.* New York: Free Press, 1985:3–28.

98. Goodman WK, Price LH, Rasmussen SA, et al.: The Yale-Brown Obsessive Compulsive Scale (YBOCS). Part I: Development, use and reliability. *Arch Gen Psych* 1989; **46**:1006–1011.

99. Goodman WK, Price LH, Rasmussen SA, Mazure C, Delgado P, Heninger GR, Charney DS: The Yale-

Brown Obsessive Compulsive Scale II. Validity. *Arch Gen Psychiatry* 1989; **46**:1012–1016.

100. Loney J, Milich R: Hyperactivity, inattention, and aggression in clinical practice. In: Routh DK, ed. *Advances in Behavioral Pediatrics.* Greenwich, Connecticut: JAI Press, 1982:113–147.

101. Pelham WE, Milich R, Murphy DA, Murphy HA: Normative data on the IOWA Conners teacher rating scale. *J Clin Child Psychol* 1989; **18**:259–262.

102. Swanson JM: *School Based Assessments and Interventions for ADD Students.* Irvine, California: K.C. Publishing, 1992.

103. Cohen DJ, Young JG, Nathanson JA, Shaywitz BA: Clonidine in Tourette's syndrome. *Lancet* 1979; **2**(8142):551–553.

104. Shapiro AK, Shapiro E, Eisenkraft GJ: Treatment of Gilles de la Tourette's syndrome with clonidine and neuroleptics. *Arch Gen Psychiatry* 1983; **40**(11):1235–1240.

105. Chappell P, Riddle M, Scahill L, Lynch K, Schultz R, Arnsten A, Leckman J, Cohen D: Guanfacine treatment of comorbid attention-deficit hyperactivity disorder and Tourette's Syndrome: Preliminary clinical experience. *J Am Acad Child Adolesc Psychiatry* 1995; **34**(9):1140–1146.

106. Boris M: Gilles de la Tourette's syndrome: Remission with haloperidol. *J Am Med Assoc* 1968; **205**(9):648–649.

107. Bruun RD: Gilles de la Tourette's syndrome: An overview of clinical experience. *J Am Acad Child Psychiatry* 1984; **23**(2):126–133.

108. Bruun R, Budman C: Risperidone as a treatment for Tourette's syndrome. *J Clin Psychiatry* 1996; **57**(1):29–32.

109. Cohen DJ, Riddle MA, Leckman JF: Pharmacotherapy of Tourette's syndrome and associated disorders. *Psychiatric Clin North Am* 1992; **15**(1):109–129.

110. Colvin CL, Tankanow RM: Pimozide: use in Tourette's syndrome. *Drug Intel Clin Pharm* 1985; **19**(6):421–424.

111. Goetz CG, Tanner CM, Klawans HL: Fluphenazine and multifocal tic disorders. *Arch Neurol* 1984; **41**(3):271–272.

112. Lombroso P, Scahill L, King R, Lynch K, Chappell P, Peterson B, et al.: Risperidone treatment of children and adolescents with chronic tic disorders: A preliminary report. *J Am Acad Child Adolesc Psychiatry* 1995; **34**(9):1147–1152.

113. Moldofsky H, Brown GM: Tics and serum prolactin response to pimozide in Tourette syndrome. *Adv Neurol* 1982; **35**:387–390.

114. Sallee FR, Sethuraman G, Rock CM: Effects of pimozide on cognition in children with Tourette syndrome: Interaction with comorbid attention deficit hyperactivity disorder. *Acta Psychiatrica Scandinavica* 1994; **90**:4–9.

115. Sandor P, Musisi S, Moldofsky H, Lang A: Tourette syndrome: A follow-up study. *J Clin Psychopharmacology* 1990; **10**(3):197–199.

116. Shapiro AK, Shapiro E: Treatment of Gilles de la Tourette's Syndrome with haloperidol. *Br J Psychiatry* 1968; **114**(508):345–350.

117. Shapiro AK, Shapiro E, Eisenkraft GJ: Treatment of Gilles de la Tourette syndrome with pimozide. *Am J Psychiatry* 1983; **140**(9):1183–1186.

118. Shapiro AK, Shapiro E, Fulop G: Pimozide treatment of tic and Tourette disorders. *Pediatrics* 1987; **79**(6):1032–1039.

119. Shapiro E, Shapiro AK, Fulop G, Hubbard M, Mandeli J, Nordlie J, et al.: Controlled study of haloperidol, pimozide and placebo for the treatment of Gilles de la Tourette's syndrome. *Arch Gen Psychiatry* 1989; **46**(8):722–730.

120. Lombroso P, Scahill, L, King R, Lynch K, Chappell P, Peterson B, McDougle C, Leckman J: Risperidone treatment of children and adolescents with chronic tic disorders: A preliminary report. *J Am Acad Child Adolesc Psychiatry* 1995; **34**(9):1147–1152.

121. Budman CL, Gayer A, Lesser M, Shi Q, Bruun RD: An open-label study of the treatment efficacy of olanzapine for Tourette's disorder. *J Clin Psychiatry* 2001; **62**(4):290–294.

122. Kurlan R, Como PG, Deeley C, McDermott M, McDermott MP: A pilot controlled study of fluoxetine for obsessive-compulsive symptoms in children with Tourette's syndrome. *Clin Neuropharmacol* 1993; **16**(2):167–172.

123. Riddle MA, Hardin MT, King R, Scahill L, Woolston JL: Fluoxetine treatment of children and adolescents with Tourette's and obsessive compulsive disorders: Preliminary clinical experience. *J Am Acad Child Adolesc Psychiatry* 1990; **29**(1):45–48.

124. Leonard H, Swedo S, Rapoport J: Treatment of childhood obsessive compulsive disorder with clomipramine and desmethylimipramine; A double blind crossover comparison. *Psychopharmacol Bul* 1988; **24**:93–95.

125. Riddle M, Hardin M, King R, Cho L, Woolston J, Leckman J: Desipramine treatment of boys with attention deficit disorder and tics: Preliminary clinical experience. *J Am Acad Child Adolesc Psychiatry* 1988; **27**:811–814.

126. Singer H, Brown J, Quaskey S, Rosenberg L, Mellits D, Denckla M: The treatment of attention-deficit hyperactivity disorder in Tourette's syndrome: A double blind placebo controlled study with Clonidine and Desipramine. *Pediatrics* 1995; **95**(1):74–81.

127. Spencer T, Biederman J, Kerman K, Steingard R, Wilens T: Desipramine treatment of children with attention deficit hyperactivity disorder and tic disorder or Tourette's syndrome. *J Am Acad Child Adolesc Psychiatry* 1993; **32**:354–360.

128. Gonce M, Barbeau, A: Seven cases of Gilles de la Tourette syndrome: Partial relief with clonazepam: A pilot study. *Can J Neurological Sci* 1977; **4**:279–283.

129. Gadow KD, Nolan EE, Sverd J: Methylphenidate in hyperactive boys with comorbid tic disorder: II. Short-term behavioral effects in school settings. *J Am Acad Child Adolesc Psychiatry* 1992; **31**(3):462–471.

130. Gadow KD, Sverd J: Stimulants for ADHD in child patients with Tourette's syndrome: The issue of relative risk. *J Develop Behav Pediatrics* 1990; **11**(5):269–271.

131. Tourette's Syndrome Study Group: Treatment of ADHD in children with tics: A randomized controlled trial. *Neurology* 2002; **58**(4):527–536.

132. Sandyk R: Naloxone abolishes obsessive-compulsive behavior in Tourette's syndrome. *Int J Neurosci* 1987; **35**(1–2):93–94.

133. McConville BJ, Fogelson MH, Norman M: Nicotine potentiation of haloperidol in reducing tic frequency

in Tourette's disorder. *Am J Psychiatry* 1991; **148**(6): 793–794.

134. McConville BJ, Sanberg PR, Fogelson MH, King J, Cirino P, Parker KW, *et al.*: The effects of nicotine plus haloperidol compared to nicotine only and placebo nicotine only in reducing tic severity and frequency in Tourette's disorder. *Biol Psychiatry* 1992; **31**(8):832–840.

135. Silver AA, Sanberg PR: Transdermal nicotine patch and potentiation of haloperidol in Tourette's syndrome. *Lancet* 1993; **342**(8864):17.

136. Gilbert DL, Dure L, Sethuraman G, Raab D, Lane J, Sallee FR: Tic reduction with pergolide in a randomized controlled trial in children. *Neurology* 2003; **60**(4): 606–611.

137. Jankovic J: Botulinum toxin in the treatment of dystonic tics. *Move Disord* 1994; **9**(3):347–349.

138. Scott BL, Jankovic J, Donovan DT: Botulinum toxin injection into vocal cord in the treatment of malignant coprolalia associated with Tourette's syndrome. *Move Disord* 1996; **11**(4):431–433.

139. Sanberg PR, Shytle RD, Silver AA: Treatment of Tourette's syndrome with mecamylamine. *Lancet* 1998; **352**(9129):705–706.

140. Silver AA, Shytle RD, Sanberg PR: Mecamylamine in Tourette's syndrome: A two-year retrospective case study. *J Child Adolesc Psychopharmacology* 2000; **10**(2): 59–68.

141. Silver AA, Shytle RD, Sheehan KH, Sheehan DV, Ramos A, Sanberg PR: Multicenter, double-blind, placebo-controlled study of mecamylamine monotherapy for Tourette's disorder. *J Am Acad Child Adolesc Psychiatry* 2001; **40**(9):1103–1110.

142. Awaad Y: Tics in Tourette syndrome: New treatment options. *J Child Neurol* 1999; **14**(5):316–319.

143. Singer HS, Wendlandt J, Krieger M, Giuliano J: Baclofen treatment in Tourette syndrome: A double-blind, placebo-controlled, crossover trial. *Neurology* 2001; **56**(5):599–604.

144. McDougle CJ, Goodman WK, Leckman JF, Lee NC, Heninger GR, Price LH: Haloperidol addition in fluvoxamine-refractory obsessive-compulsive disorder. A double-blind, placebo-controlled study in patients with and without tics. *Arch Gen Psychiatry* 1994; **51**(4): 302–308.

145. Babel TB, Warnke PC, Ostertag CB: Immediate and long term outcome after infrathalamic and thalamic lesioning for intractable Tourette's syndrome. *J Neurol Neurosurg Psychiatry* 2001; **70**(5):666–671.

146. Wilhelm S, Deckersbach T, Coffey BJ, Bohne A, Peterson AL, Baer L: Habit reversal versus supportive psychotherapy for Tourette's disorder: A randomized controlled trial. *Am J Psychiatry* 2003; **160**(6): 1175–1177.

147. Azrin N, Peterson A: Behavior therapy for Tourette's syndrome and Tic disorders. In: Cohen D, Bruun R, Leckman J, eds. *Tourette's Syndrome and Tic Disorders: Clinical Understanding and Treatment.* New York: John Wiley & Sons, 1988:237–576.

Section IV
Special Problems in Child and Adolescent Psychiatry

24

Psychotic Disorders

Michael T. Sorter

Introduction

The difficulties of the child or adolescent identified as suffering from childhood psychosis are frequently the most challenging the child and adolescent psychiatrist must manage, the most devastating for families and patients, and the most costly for society and communities [1]. These children demonstrate serious difficulties in all developmental lines. Although varied in their presentations, they struggle with simple adaptive functioning and suffer with cognitive, emotional, perceptual, and interpersonal difficulties.

In 1906, the term dementia praecoccissima was proposed by DeSanctis to identify a group of children with bizarre behavior, language abnormalities, social isolation, inappropriate affect, intellectual deficits, and developmental delays [2]. These children were likened to adults described by Kraeplin as having dementia praecox. Kraeplin later noted that some cases of dementia praecox began in childhood [3]. Following these early descriptions of children with multiple pervasive impairments, childhood psychosis was often equated with childhood-onset schizophrenia.

The diagnosis and classification of childhood and adolescent psychoses have been controversial. Both narrow and broad definitions have been applied to the diagnosis of schizophrenia in children, and the exact relationship between adult schizophrenia and childhood psychoses has been the center of debate. In the past, inclusive definitions were used such that children with autism and other forms of pervasive developmental disorders fell under the diagnosis of childhood schizophrenia. Psychiatrists such as Bender [4] and Fish [5] considered the presentations of children with pervasive developmental delays, such as difficulties in emotional and social functioning, intellectual deficits, disturbances in affect, social isolation, and bizarre behavior, to be similar to the difficulties seen in adult patients suffering with schizophrenia.

Kanner [6], Kolvin [7], and others challenged this inclusive definition and instead identified specific characteristics that appear to differentiate the child with autism from the child with schizophrenia. Kanner identified a group of children he regarded as distinct from those with childhood schizophrenia: these children were severely disturbed and demonstrated a powerful desire to be alone and to maintain 'sameness' [6]. Later work by Kolvin [7] and Rutter [8] suggested that childhood psychoses could be differentiated into separate groups, based on clinical characteristics, family history, and central nervous system (CNS) functioning. They described a group with very early onset that was characterized by a higher prevalence of mental retardation, seizures, electroencephalogram (EEG) abnormalities but that rarely developed hallucinations, delusions, or thought disorder. A group with later onset demonstrated more prominent hallucinations, delusions, thought disorder, and a family history of schizophrenia. This latter group was thought to resemble those patients diagnosed with schizophrenia in adulthood.

Data from these studies led to the classification of childhood psychoses in the *Diagnostic and Statistical Manual of Mental Disorders, 3rd ed.* (DSM-III) [9]. The separate diagnostic category of childhood schizophrenia was eliminated. Schizophrenia in childhood was defined using adult criteria, and separate criteria were used for infantile autism and childhood-onset pervasive developmental disorder. Subsequent research has reinforced the continuity and validity of diagnostic criteria between children and adults [10,11].

This trend to differentiate schizophrenia in childhood from the pervasive developmental disorders has continued. In the DSM-IV-TR, the current edition, the

Clinical Child Psychiatry, Second Edition. Edited by W.M. Klykylo and J.L. Kay
© 2005 John Wiley & Sons Ltd.

BOX A DSM-IV TR DIAGNOSTIC CRITERIA FOR SCHIZOPHRENIA

(A) *Characteristic symptoms:* two (or more) of the following, each present for a significant portion of time during a one-month period (or less if successfully treated):
   (i) delusions
   (ii) hallucinations
   (iii) disorganized speech (e.g., frequent derailment or incoherence)
   (iv) grossly disorganized or catatonic behavior
   (v) negative symptoms, i.e., affective flattening, alogia, or avolition
Note: only one Criterion A symptom is required if delusions are bizarre or hallucinations consist of a voice keeping up a running commentary on the person's behavior or thoughts, or two or more voices conversing with each other

(B) *Social/occupational dysfunction:* for a significant portion of the time since the onset of the disturbance, one or more major areas of functioning such as work, interpersonal relations, or self-care are markedly below the level achieved prior to the onset (or when the onset is in childhood or adolescence, failure to achieve expected level of interpersonal, academic, or occupational achievement)

(C) *Duration:* continuous signs of the disturbance persist for at least six months. This six-month period must include at least one month of symptoms (or less if successfully treated) that meet Criterion A (i.e., active-phase symptoms) and may include periods of prodromal or residual symptoms. During these prodromal or residual periods, the signs of the disturbance may be manifested by only negative symptoms or two or more symptoms listed in Criterion A present in an attenuated form (e.g., odd beliefs, unusual perceptual experiences)

(D) *Schizoaffective and mood disorder exclusion:* Schizoaffective disorder and mood disorder with psychotic features have been ruled out because either (1) no major depressive, manic, or mixed episodes have occurred concurrently with the active-phase symptoms; or (2) if mood episodes have occurred during active-phase symptoms, their total duration has been brief relative to the duration of the active and residual periods

(E) *Substance/general medical condition exclusion:* the disturbance is not due to the direct physiological effects of a substance (e.g., a drug of abuse, a medication) or a general medical condition

(F) *Relationship to a pervasive developmental disorder:* if there is a history of autistic disorder or another pervasive developmental disorder, the additional diagnosis of schizophrenia is made only if prominent delusions or hallucinations are also present for at least a month (or less if successfully treated).

Reprinted with permission from the Diagnostic and Statistical Manual of Mental Disorders, Copyright 2000. American Psychiatric Association.

---

same criteria used for the diagnosis of adult schizophrenia are applied to children, and the pervasive developmental disorders have been differentiated into several separate entities (Box A) [12]. These include autistic disorder, Asperger's disorder, childhood disintegrative disorder, and Rett disorder, all of which are marked by a symptom complex of difficulties in social relatedness, communication skills, and the presence of stereotyped behavior, interests, and activities [12].

Prevalence and Epidemiology

Owing to the changes in classification and our understanding of schizophrenia and childhood psychosis, studies using strict diagnostic criteria are limited. Research indicates that prepubertal-onset of schizophrenia is exceedingly rare but is somewhat more prevalent in individuals after they reach puberty [11].

Most studies examining the prepubertal rates of schizophrenia compare the prevalence of childhood schizophrenia with that of autism. Autism appears to be more prevalent than childhood schizophrenia [7]. Using DSM-III criteria, Burd and Kerbeshian found the prevalence of prepubertal schizophrenia to be approximately two cases per 100 000 [13]. Most studies indicate the male-to-female ratio of schizophrenic children to be from 1.5:1 to 2.5:1 [14,15].

The diagnosis of schizophrenia is much more frequently made in adolescents than in children, with the incidence rate in adolescents approaching that of adults [11]. Adolescent schizophrenia differs from childhood-onset schizophrenia in affecting males to females more equally [16]. In adult populations, the incidence of schizophrenia is the same between the sexes, with men having an earlier age of onset [17]. The peak ages of onset for the disorder range from 15 to 30 years [18], with a lifetime prevalence of about 1% and in adults an annual incidence of 0.2 to 0.4 per 1000 [19].

Clinical Description: Premorbid Functioning

Numerous studies have attempted to examine the children who later develop schizophrenia. Investigators have focused on high-risk populations such as the offspring of schizophrenic parents and have also conducted follow-up studies, which examine the past history and condition of patients diagnosed as schizophrenic and review past clinical records, school reports, and similar data to understand premorbid conditioning. Both types of studies have indicated that a variety of difficulties appear to be more prevalent in children who later develop schizophrenia, but no clear indicative pattern of symptoms or functioning was found [15,20,21]. These prospective high-risk and follow-back studies have implied numerous premorbid, vulnerabilities, including higher rates of abnormal physical and perceptual motor development [5], impaired attention and information processing, lower intelligence quotient (IQ), academic problems, delayed or disturbed language, excessive anxiety, social withdrawal, and isolation [20,22–27]. Childhood-onset cases appear to have higher rates of premorbid abnormalities [28].

McClellan [29], in a study comparing youth with early-onset psychotic disorders found that youth with schizophrenia had significantly higher rates of premorbid social withdrawal, global impairment and tended to have fewer friends than those with bipolar disorder or psychosis, not otherwise specified.

Symptoms of Schizophrenia

The onset of the disorder is usually insidious and is followed by a slow deterioration in functioning [7,30]. Acute-onset with no premorbid signs of disturbance and an acute exacerbation of symptoms in patients with insidious illness have also been described [7,14]. Symptoms of schizophrenia have been clustered into two sets. Positive symptoms include formal thought disorder, delusions, and hallucinations. Negative symptoms refer to paucity of thought and speech, flattened affect, and energy [18,31]. Both groups of symptoms are evident in early-onset schizophrenia.

Because of the previous lack of rigid diagnostic criteria for schizophrenia in childhood and adolescence, there is a paucity of studies that examine the exact nature of this thought disturbance. Some studies do indicate that auditory hallucinations, which are usually present in over 75% of patients, are the most common symptom presentation [15,32]. Auditory hallucinations may be persecutory in nature or may be command hallucinations, and they usually are simple rather than complex, often consisting of brief phrases or sentences [33]. In children, these auditory hallucinations may be a voice that is strange to them or one that is well known from family or frightening characters. The voices often tell the patient to do bad things or speak to them in a mean manner or curse. The voices may converse or make ongoing commentary about the child. Visual and somatic hallucinations are not rare but are less frequent than auditory hallucinations [32]. Visual hallucinations may be manifest as ghosts, threatening animals, or vague frightening entities [33].

Delusions appear to be common in children with schizophrenia, with prevalence rates from 50%–85% [7,32,34]. Delusions include a variety of presentations, such as persecutory thoughts, feelings of being tormented, somatic concerns, or grandiose perceptions or religious ideation. Delusional beliefs in young people are less likely to be organized systemic delusions than that commonly found in adults [35]. The emotional and cognitive developmental level may influence the expressed content of thought disturbance: younger children more frequently have disturbances regarding animals, ghosts, or monsters, whereas disturbances in adolescents more often have abstract themes, such as paranoia, mind control, that more closely resemble that found in adults [36].

Formal thought disorder may be difficult to assess in children, owing to a variety of other disorders first evident in childhood that may present with disorganized speech or behavior. Formal thought disorder may present as magical irrational thinking, tangentiality, illogicality, and a loosening of associations; occasionally, there may be sustained periods of incoherence [33]. Negative symptoms such as a low energy, apathy, social withdrawal, inattention, and flat affect may also be present [16,31].

Overall, the clinical picture of children with schizophrenia supports the observation that childhood-onset schizophrenia has the same manifestations as adolescent- and adult-onset schizophrenia [31,33].

Etiology

Schizophrenia is considered a neurodevelopmental disorder, with high rates of premorbid abnormalities that include neurological, cognitive, and social findings [31,37,38]. The etiology of schizophrenia remains unknown. Investigations have extended into several aspects of illness, including neurobiologic, genetic, psychologic processes, and environmental, family, and interpersonal dynamics.

Genetic Factors

Schizophrenia and schizophrenia spectrum disorder are found in higher rates in families of patients with schizophrenia. Adoptive and twin studies indicate that the risk is genetic [37,39]. There is a 10-fold increase in morbid risk for schizophrenia in the relatives of an affected first-degree family member [39,40]. Morbid risk increases to near 50% in offspring when both parents are affected [41]. Review of twin studies indicate a significant genetic component with higher concordance rate in monozygotic twins (50%) than dizygotic twins (17%) [39,42]. Estimates of the heritability of the disorder approached 80% [43,44]. Similarly, adoption studies have shown that the offspring of schizophrenic parents raised by nonschizophrenic adoptive parents demonstrate a much higher rate of schizophrenia than do the early-adopted offspring of nonschizophrenic biologic parents [45]. The prevalence of schizophrenia in the biologic offspring of schizophrenics who were later adopted did not differ significantly from that of offspring reared by a schizophrenic biologic parent [46]. Children born to nonschizophrenic biologic parents but adopted into a family in which a parent became psychotic tended not to develop schizophrenia [47].

Since the penetrance of schizophrenia found in twin studies of childhood-onset schizophrenia is much higher than that of adult-onset schizophrenia, it has been theorized that childhood-onset schizophrenia represents a more virulent form of illness, with more complete penetrance [48,49,109]. In a comparison of child-onset schizophrenia and adult-onset schizophrenia [50], parents of the patients of childhood-onset schizophrenia were found to have a morbid risk of schizophrenia spectrum disorders of nearly 25%. Parents of patients of adult-onset patients had a morbid risk of 11% while parents of comparison groups had a morbid risk of 1.5%. This may indicate a stronger familial association in childhood-onset schizophrenia. Schizophrenia studies indicate that the liability to schizophrenia is genetically mediated but not genetically determined and results from an interaction of genes and environment. Recent genome scan strategies have provided multiple chromosomal regions of interest that may contain one or more susceptibility genes for schizophrenia [39].

Neurobiological Deficits

There is no clear premorbid personality profile for children and adolescents who develop schizophrenia. Children who develop schizophrenia are more apt to have a premorbid history of social anxiety, withdrawal, academic difficulties, poor peer relationships, clingy withdrawn behavior, and suspiciousness [24]. There also may be a higher preponderance of deficits in language and communication functioning, causing early language to be delayed or disturbed [21,24,51,52]. It is unclear whether personality characteristics predispose patients to vulnerabilities associated with schizophrenia. Neurobiologic abnormalities in youth with schizophrenia indicate similar findings to the adult literature, and include smooth-pursuit eye movement, autonomic responsivity, and cognition [31].

The most consistent neuroimaging findings in adult-onset schizophrenia are the enlargement of the ventricular system [53] and overall reduction in cortical gray matter and brain volume [54]. Decreased volumes of multiple structures have also been indicated in adult schizophrenia. These include frontal lobes, amygdala, hippocampus, parahippocampus, thalamus, cingulate gyrus, superior temporal gyrus, and medial temporal lobe [37,53,55,56]. Patients with childhood-onset schizophrenia have similar findings in regard to smaller brain and enlarged lateral ventricles [57,58]. During adolescence patients with childhood-onset schizophrenia demonstrate progressive loss of cortical gray matter involving the frontal, parietal and temporal regions with loss slowing as they approach adult age [57,59]. Preliminary studies have also indicated alteration in brain white matter integrity in adolescents with early-onset schizophrenia similar to findings in adults with chronic schizophrenia [60].

Schizophrenia has been viewed as a neurodevelopmental disorder [37]. Psychosis emerges after many years of early structural brain changes [61]. The same patterns of structural abnormalities are found in first-degree family members [62] suggesting shared familial risk. Histological studies indicate abnormalities in neuronal migration, resulting in cellular disorganization, anomalous cortical development, and irregularities in laminar distribution of neurons [37,63]. The absence of glial reactions suggests that neuropathological changes are prenatal rather than postnatal [64]. Individuals with schizophrenia have significantly higher frequency of morphological brain abnormalities [53–55].

Psychology

Cognitive delays are commonly found in children with schizophrenia. Estimates of 10%–20% of patients with early-onset schizophrenia have borderline IQ or mental retardation [31,38]. The frequency of mental retardation may be significantly higher due to the exclusion of these patients from studies. Cognitive function deficits include lowered full-scale IQ, reduced information processing, sustained attention, memory and executive functioning, especially working memory and cognitive set shifting ability [26,49,65,66,109].

Family Factors

Numerous studies have investigated the families of patients with schizophrenia, but the majority were conducted prior to the use of strict diagnostic criteria. Most studies have examined aberrant communication patterns that were once believed to lead to schizophrenia. Communication deviances usually refer to a confusing and unclear communication style that precipitates a disruption in the focus of attention [67]. These communication deviances have been found to be more prevalent in parents of children with schizophrenia and schizotypal disorder than in parents of children with depressive disorders, and are thought to be more genetic traits than causal factors [68]. Other investigators have focused on the levels of expressed emotion, the harshness of criticism, and parents' excessive negative response to the child's negative or disruptive behavior. These patterns of interaction do negatively influence relapse rates [18,49]. Findings are inconclusive, and it remains unclear whether parent behavioral style promotes the child's pathology or is a response to it. Communication deviances in parents have been associated with a higher risk for adolescents to develop schizophrenia in adulthood [69]. High expressed emotion as evidenced by critical comments, hostility, or emotional overinvolvement has shown to be a robust predictor of relapse in adults with schizophrenia [70].

Environment

Low socioeconomic status has been associated with higher rates of schizophrenia [71]. It remains unclear, however, whether the lower socioeconomic level predisposes people to developing schizophrenia, is a result of the schizophrenic patient being unable to maintain the parent's socioeconomic level, or if the lower socioeconomic status is a result of underlying parental psychopathology [37]. Adverse life events such as the death of a parent or rejection of the child may be associated with the onset of a schizophrenic disorder. Little research has focused on environmental effects in childhood, and the effects are more thoroughly described in adult patients [72]. Relationship of socioeconomic status in child-onset schizophrenia remains unclear as most studies have had an inpatient bias and contra-

dictory results [31]. In adult studies of schizophrenia, diverse prevalence and incident rates have been reported among various cultural groups, but studies using strict criteria have indicated the incidence and clinical syndrome to be similar in a variety of cultural settings [19,37,73,74].

Assessment

To ensure adequate diagnostic evaluation and treatment planning, the proper assessment of a child or adolescent with psychosis requires an evaluation of all areas of functioning. The diagnostic process is often prolonged and usually requires multiple informants. Since the families are often under extreme stress from the child's illness and deterioration, early in the diagnostic evaluation, the clinician must be aware of the need to enhance the alliance with the family. Family members provide the majority of the data required for assessment and are the most important agents in the eventual care of the patient.

The evaluation of psychosis in children and adolescents requires a detailed history, including the age of onset, the nature of symptoms and their course, premorbid functioning, school and psychosocial adaptive skills, precipitants of trauma preceding the illness, and a biologic family history of psychiatric disorders. The family assessment must include current adaptive functioning and any specific family or cultural beliefs regarding psychiatric illness. Substance abuse history should investigate past patterns of use and its effects and also assess whether any intoxication or withdrawal syndrome is present. The developmental history must elucidate any deficits or delays in speech or language or in cognitive, sensory, and motor function. The medical history and review of systems must include any evidence of CNS insult or general medical conditions that may precipitate mental status changes.

A clinician conducting a mental status examination may require several sessions with the child. In the first encounter, the clinician must have special awareness of any fluctuations in the level of consciousness or impairments in orientation, since these may indicate delirium and organic processes requiring more immediate attention. Clinicians should evaluate any hallucinations, delusions, thought disorders, and the presence or absence of negative symptoms to assist in clarifying phenomenology. If prominent and significant in duration, mood disturbance may indicate affective disorder with secondary psychotic symptoms. An assessment of suicidal or homicidal ideation must be performed on initial contact and, if required, appropriate safeguards enacted.

A medical evaluation that includes a complete physical and neurologic examination is important to detect the presence of any physical disorders that might precipitate psychotic symptoms. Special attention must be paid to any abnormal neurologic history or functioning, the results of which may assist in determining if any special procedures or evaluation are required. Owing to the common occurrence of substance abuse and its propensity to cause psychotic symptoms, drug screening should be conducted on all patients.

Psychologic testing often helps to assess the nature and severity of impairment in patients with psychosis. Projective testing may help clinicians evaluate the severity and nature of psychotic thinking. Investigations into cognitive ability, educational achievement, and adaptive living skills often identify the strengths and weaknesses of an individual patient and initial directions for intervention.

Many well-researched and validated psychiatric interview schedules help assess psychotic symptoms and provide a systematic coverage of symptoms to ensure that all key symptom areas are probed [75]. Some of the schedules have an ease of use that allows them to be used in clinical work. Examples include the Schedule for Positive Symptoms (SAPS), which reviews hallucinations, delusions, bizarre behavior, and formal thought disorder, and the Schedule for Negative Symptoms that examines flat affect, anergy, avolition, asociality, and inattention [76]. The Kiddie PANNS is a modification of the Adult Positive and Negative Syndrome Scale [75,77].

Speech and language evaluations are often helpful, especially with young children for whom psychosis is suspected. Patients with communication difficulties may present with extremely disorganized speech that is suggestive of underlying psychosis or schizophrenia (for a summary of assessment procedures, see Table 24.1).

Differential Diagnosis

An organic etiology must be considered for all children and adolescents presenting with psychosis. Multiple substance-related disorders may present with psychotic symptomatology; substance intoxication from cocaine, amphetamines, hallucinogens, cannabis, phencyclidine, solvents, or alcohol; or withdrawal syndromes such as those from alcohol, barbiturates, benzodiazepines, and other sedatives. Both the frequency of a substance-related disorder that produces psychotic symptoms and the condition of comorbid substance abuse in a patient with schizophrenia underly the importance of initial and perhaps serial toxic screening. The associ-

Table 24.1 Assessment and evaluation.

History and development
 History of current difficulties
 Age of onset
 Course and nature of symptoms
 Premorbid functioning
 School and cognitive skills
 Psychosocial adaptive skills
 Precipitants
 History of trauma
 Family history of psychiatric disorders
 Family adaptive functioning
 Family and cultural beliefs concerning illness
 Substance use history
 Developmental history
 Communication/speech and language functioning

Mental status examination
 Level of consciousness and orientation
 Hallucinations and delusions
 Thought disorder and negative symptoms
 Affective symptoms
 Assessment of dangerous, impulsive activity
 Suicidality and homicidality

Psychologic evaluation
 Projective testing for evaluation of thought
  disturbance, hallucinations, etc.
 IQ and formal educational testing for assessment
  of achievement
 Assessment of adaptive skills
 Assessment of communication/speech and
  language

Medical and neurologic history and evaluation
 Physical examination for associated medical
  conditions
 Toxicology screen for evaluation of substance
  abuse
 Neurologic consultation, including EEG

Adapted from Volkmar FR: Childhood and adolescent psychosis: A review of the past 10 years. *J Am Acad Child Adolesc Psychiatry* 1996; **35**:843–851.

ated physical findings of many of the substance-use disorders and the persistence of symptoms seen in a primary psychotic illness often assist in differentiating these two disorders [78].

Other entities that must be excluded through careful medical and neurologic evaluation include metabolic disorders, heavy metal intoxication, CNS trauma, neoplasia, neurodegenerative disorders, seizure disorders, and delirium. Infectious diseases such as encephalitis and meningitis must be excluded, with special attention given to risk factors for human immunodeficiency virus (HIV) infection. HIV infection in adolescents is not uncommon [79], and the often chaotic, difficult backgrounds of these patients may be similar to those of patients most at risk for schizophrenia [80]. The high-risk behaviors of substance abuse and dangerous sexual activity are indicators for HIV testing.

Patients with schizophrenia and psychotic mood disorders often present with a wide variety of mood and psychotic symptoms [81]. Owing to similarities in presentation, patients later diagnosed with bipolar disorder are frequently previously misdiagnosed as having schizophrenia [82]. Bipolar disorder in adolescents is much like that in adults, although psychotic features appear to be more common in adolescents [83,84]. Early episodes may show many schizophrenic features such as bizarre delusions, hallucinations, paranoid ideation, and ideas of reference [83]. Younger children are more likely to present with irritability, emotional lability, and aggression, often with poor demarcation of discrete episodes [85]. Symptom overlap creates difficulties in diagnosis. In a study of youths with schizophrenia, bipolar disorder, and psychotic disorder not otherwise specified (NOS), no differences were found in measures of positive symptoms, behavioral difficulties or dysphoria. Measures of negative symptoms differentiated the patients with schizophrenia from the other two groups [81]. The presence of features such as grandiosity, euphoria, pronounced irritability, pressured speech, and hyperactivity may be indicators of the affective nature of the disorder. Due to the frequent overlay of affective and psychotic symptoms, schizoaffective disorder with its requirements for distinct mood and psychotic periods has been difficult to diagnose in a reliable, predictable method in youth [82]. Longitudinal reassessment is frequently required to confirm the accuracy of the diagnosis.

Patients with the pervasive developmental disorders characteristically present with severe deficits in language and social relatedness. Typically, they do not present with the characteristic symptoms of delusions and hallucinations. When delusions and hallucinations are present, however, they are usually temporary and not the predominant manifestation of the illness; they are also distinguished by their early age of onset and the absence of normal development [7]. It is possible that both illnesses may coexist, in which case the onset of the schizophrenia is significantly later than that of autism [31,78]. Asperger syndrome and childhood disintegrative disorder differ from autism in their absence of language deficits and in having a later onset, respectively. They also lack the pervasive hallucinations, delusions, and thought disorder characteristics of schizophrenia. Patients with significant communication disorders such as receptive and expressive language disorders are often difficult to assess, since the communication difficulties often resemble those of children with primary thought disorder. In younger children, normal fantasy and a distortion of communication through speech and language deficits exacerbate the task of proper diagnosis [86]. Prolonged, serial assessments are often required to determine the presence or absence of the hallucinations and delusions that are indicative of schizophrenia. The often illogical perseverative thoughts of the patient with obsessive–compulsive disorder (OCD) may resemble those of thought disorder seen in patients with psychotic illness. In severe cases of OCD, the perception that the obsessions are irrational may be intermittent or lacking, thus making it difficult to differentiate from true delusions. Patients with schizophrenia may have significant obsessive thoughts and compulsive behavior. The lack of hallucinations and delusions and more constricted nature of symptomatology of OCD frequently help to distinguish it from schizophrenia.

History of abuse or neglect in a child is often associated with reports of psychotic symptoms [87]. Investigations into children with psychotic disorder NOS reveal significant symptom overlap with schizophrenia, but have significantly higher rates of abuse histories and post-traumatic stress disorder (PTSD) [29]. Psychological trauma may produce dissociative phenomena similar to a psychotic state.

Patients with borderline and schizotypal personality disorders may exhibit symptoms of transient hallucinations and near delusional thinking [21]. They lack the delusions and formal thought disorder of patients with schizophrenia and show differences in relationship skills: the relationships of children with borderline personality disorders are chaotic and intense, whereas children with schizophrenia are often socially isolated and awkward [78].

Transient hallucinations may occur in preschool-age nonpsychotic children [88]. These hallucinations are often visual and tactile, frequently with onset at night, and are thought to be relatively benign. In young children, there may be magical thinking, fantasy figures, and a poor notion of adult rules of logic or reality. Their presentation may resemble those of a thought disorder, but it is the persistence of such symptoms into school age that is indicative of pathology [32,89]. Differential diagnosis is summarized in Table 24.2.

Table 24.2 Differential diagnosis of schizophrenia.

Autistic spectrum disorders
    Asperger's disorder
    Autistic disorder
    Childhood disintegrative disorder
    Pervasive developmental disorder (NOS)
	Differentiated by developmental history indicating deficits in social relatedness, activities, interest, and/or language. Hallucinations, delusions not the predominant manifestation

Psychosis associated with mood disorder
    Bipolar disorder
    Major depressive disorder
	In major depression and bipolar disorder, history of psychosis is associated with significant mood changes. Though not always reliable. Relative lack of negative symptoms may differentiate bipolar disorder from schizophrenia

Other psychotic disorders
    Psychotic disorder, NOS
    Schizoaffective disorder
	Schizophrenia associated with more prominent negative symptoms and less association with trauma than psychotic disorders, NOS. Diagnosis of schizoaffective disorder is poorly understood with unreliable predictability in children

Obsessive–compulsive disorder	In severe cases, obsessions and compulsions may be seen as irrational. OCD typically lacks the hallucinations and delusional characteristics of schizophrenia
Post-traumatic stress disorder dissociative disorder	Global impairment, negative symptoms, and chronic course more characteristic of schizophrenia

Personality disorders
    Schizotypal
    Schizoid
    Borderline
    Paranoid
	May have periods of transient hallucinations and delusions, but not the chronic course and differing pattern of relationships

Communication disorders	May present with disorganization in speech and communication that resemble formal thought disorder. Do not have typical hallucinations, delusions, or negative symptoms characteristic of schizophrenia
Substance-induced psychosis, and (amphetamines, cocaine, phencyclidine, marijuana, hallucinogens, alcohol, hallucinosis solvents, sedative withdrawal), toxic encephalopathy due to medications or toxins (corticosteroid, anticholinergics, heavy metals)	Clinical manifestations of acute, often transient psychosis, associated physical findings, toxic screening, and lack of negative symptomatology aid in differentiation from schizophrenia

Medical conditions
    Delirium
    Epilepsy
    CNS trauma or neoplasm
 	
Infectious diseases
    Human immunodeficiency virus infection
    Herpes encephalitis
    Neurosyphilis
    Encephalitis meningitis
    Neurodegenerative disease
    Metabolic disorders
	Comprehensive, medical, and neurological evaluation and monitoring required. Demands close attention to rule out medical emergency. Consider neuroimaging, EEG and laboratory assessment. Lack of blunted or flattened affect or presence of alterations in consciousness, disorientation, memory impairment, or other physical findings suggest psychosis secondary to medical condition or delirium

Treatment

The treatment of schizophrenia requires a comprehensive multimodal approach, with goals of decreasing the characteristic psychotic symptomatology, returning the child to more appropriate lines of development, and reintegrating the child into his or her home and community. Treatment requires a variety of medical, psychiatric, and community resources along with supportive and educational intervention by the family. Limited studies have been conducted on the efficacy of treatment for childhood- and adolescent-onset schizophrenia; treatment parameters result from these limited findings and extrapolation from adult studies [31,78].

Although there are numerous studies documenting the efficacy of neuroleptics in adults with schizophrenia, there are few parallel studies in adolescents and children. These latter studies do indicate, however, that the antipsychotic medications are superior to placebos in reducing symptoms of hallucinations and delusions [33,90]. However, many of these patients have had limited response and continued to demonstrate symptoms and had significant rates of adverse events. More recently, the atypical antipsychotics have been used in the treatment of children and adolescents with schizophrenia. In a randomized double-blind comparison study of clozapine and haloperidol, improvement in multiple assessments was found to be significantly greater with clozapine than haloperidol [91,92]. In open-label studies examining adolescents and younger children, clozapine has been found to improve the positive and negative symptoms of schizophrenia, with the most frequent adverse events, including drowsiness, weight gain, nonspecific changes in EEG, and hypersalivation [93,94]. The weight gain in an open trial of Clozapine in adolescents found a mean weight gain of 7 kg in six weeks – a faster increase than that found in adults [93]. Open-label studies of risperidone have indicated improvement in both positive and negative symptoms in adolescents. Common side effects have included weight gain, sedation, and extrapyramidal symptoms (EPS) [92,95–97]. Olanzapine in initial open–label trials produced equivocal results regarding improvement in both positive and negative symptoms [97]. More recent investigation has demonstrated improvement in positive and negative symptom scores. However, treatment was characterized by increased appetite and sedation as the most common adverse events [92,98]. Quetiapine has also been found in open-label trials to be effective in the treatment of adolescents with psychotic disorders [99]. An open-label extension trial demonstrated adolescents with psy-

choses that quetiapine was well tolerated long-term, with sustained symptom improvement [100]. The choice of a specific agent is guided by the patient's history of response and the clinician's judgment of how a specific agent's side effects will best interact with a particular patient's presentation.

Because of the long-term side effects that result from using antipsychotics, careful practice parameters must be followed. As in all areas of treating this disorder, the clinician should extensively educate the family about the potential side effects and benefits of these agents. The informed consent of the guardian and, if appropriate, the patient should be obtained. A baseline physical and the use of structured evaluations such as the Abnormal Involuntary Movement Scale are necessary to document the presence or absence of any abnormal movements [101]. Careful monitoring and frequent reevaluation are required to detect potential side effects of medication, such as extrapyramidal side effects, excessive sedation, cognitive blunting, tardive dyskinesia, and neuroleptic malignant syndrome. Atypical antipsychotics, because of their unique side effect profiles, including sedation, weight gain, prolactin elevation, and hematologic changes, require ongoing monitoring of height, weight, body mass index, and as required review of hematologic and serum chemistry values, along with glucose, prolactin, and thyroid hormones, and baseline ECG [102].

Psychosocial treatments must address the needs of the individual rather than the specific diagnosis of schizophrenia. All environmental and psychologic factors that may complicate recovery must be explored. The treatment plan must be well integrated and the intervention adapted to the developmental level of the child. Prospective investigations of this population are limited, and most treatment recommendations stem from data gathered in studies of adults. Supportive psychotherapy may benefit some children with schizophrenia [103]. Intensive traditional insight-oriented psychotherapies have not been clearly demonstrated as helpful and are usually not recommended in the acute phases of the illness [31,78].

In adult studies, the combination of psychoeducational family treatment, medication therapy, and social skills training has decreased relapse rates [104]. These recommendations have been extended to children and adolescents [31,78]. The initial focus of therapy is to support the patient and family during acute crisis and to provide information. Using a psychoeducational approach, the causes for schizophrenia and its prognosis, symptoms, and effects on development are shared with the family and the patient. Supportive and cognitive behavioral strategies are used to improve adaptive functioning. The adult literature gives strong support for improving neurocognition and processing speed with the use of cognitive enhancement therapy [105]. Individual and group interventions focus on improving conflict resolution, social skills, problem solving, and the activities of daily living. The clinician must work to establish a stable therapeutic relationship with the patient and his or her family. The family usually remains the strongest advocate for these children, and the clinician acts as their guide in negotiating the obstacles of obtaining the extensive care their children require. Intervention with families is primarily psychoeducational, but supportive therapy can be required to help families manage the grief and loss that are experienced with their child's illness. Advocacy and educational groups are also beneficial, since they may reduce the sense of stigma and isolation experienced by families.

Children and adolescents with schizophrenia typically struggle in a standard classroom setting: ongoing work with the school is required. Typically, special education is required to maintain the child in an educational facility and to address developmental and learning problems. Frequently, the psychiatrist must conduct ongoing consultation with contact people at the school, since they are often unfamiliar with the difficulties of such students and are ill-equipped to manage all their needs.

During the acute phase of the illness, psychiatric hospitalizations may be required. Once initial stabilization in the hospital is complete, transfer to a day or partial hospital program may ease the transition to the home or community environment. Community services can help in maintaining the patient outside the hospital. Case management, in-home therapeutic care, therapeutic recreation, and vocational rehabilitation may be offered by community mental health programs and are frequently required to meet the long-term needs of these patients.

Outcome

There are few data on the course of childhood schizophrenia, and most studies do not use the current restrictive criteria. Eggers reviewed the outcomes of 57 children with an onset of schizophrenia prior to age 14 years [36,106]. Low IQ and poor premorbid functioning were associated with poor outcome. The least reliable predictor of outcome was the onset of the illness early in life (i.e., before age 10 years). Of the 57 patients studied, approximately 25% were described as in remission, 25% improved, and 50% showing severe deficits. In a follow-up study, Werry and colleagues reported a

more severe course, with higher rates of early death from suicide or accidents and low levels of gainful employment or education [82]. Many patients (90%) continued to receive neuroleptics, and the majority exhibited severe levels of impairment [82]. Asarnow reported similar outcome figures to those seen in Eggers' study [36], but with higher rates of remission and better outcome [49,107]. In this study, however, there were high rates of multiple rehospitalizations and placement in residential treatment centers, often due to disruptive, out-of-control behaviors [49,107].

Predictors of poor outcome appear to be poor premorbid adjustment, nonacute insidious onset, and early age of onset; better outcomes are associated with the presence of affective symptoms, acute and older age of onset, and better premorbid adjustment [108,109].

CASE STUDY

Tom, age eight years, was initially brought to the Emergency Department by his mother after he was found in the street kicking moving cars. The mother reported that he had had increasing difficulties getting along with children at school and intermittently would complain about a 'ghost's hand' hitting him. She reported that he would frequently turn his head and yell, 'stop the devil!' Tom reported that he felt 'devils' were hitting him in the head. They would push him in the back and yell bad things at him. He reported that he saw the devil in cars passing his house and that he went out to kick the cars to make the devil leave his house.

On examination, Tom would stare blankly, interrupted by yelling at the spirits to go away and leave him alone. On later evaluations, he was found in a panic, screaming and rubbing his stomach. He later described that a ghost's hand had entered his mouth and he could see it coming out of his stomach with his bowels in the hand of the ghost. He reported wanting to die because he was 'bad.'

Tom's school reported that he was at the bottom of his class but was not a behavior problem. Over the past year, they had noted a deterioration in his performance, marked by his frequently not completing work and staring blankly at the floor or at other members of the class. They had not previously observed him demonstrating overtly delusional behavior or hallucinations.

The family history revealed that his maternal grandfather was diagnosed with schizophrenia and that Tom's mother had mild mental retardation. The mother rarely left the house and frequently deteriorated to a state in which she needed assistance from her children to care for the home.

Tom was placed in the hospital, where medical evaluation failed to reveal a cause for his mental status changes. The use of antipsychotic medication haloperidol coupled with propranolol to treat severe akathisia decreased the intensity of the auditory, visual, and tactile hallucinations.

After hospitalization, Tom was placed in a more tightly structured special education setting. A case manager was assigned to assist in administering medication and ensuring compliance with appointments. Psychologic testing revealed a full-scale IQ of 79 and marked impairments in adaptive functioning. At the five-year follow-up, Tom had remained out of the hospital but continued to believe that the devil hit him and lived outside his home. He rarely left his home, except for school and a therapeutic day camp. He continued to demonstrate paranoid delusions, tangential thinking, and blunted affect. Multiple attempts were made to decrease his haloperidol dosage and substitute an atypical antipsychotic. The addition of the atypical helped decrease some of his negative symptoms, but reduction of his baseline haloperidol dose precipitated re-emergence of hallucinations and delusions.

References

1. McGuire T: Measuring the economic costs of schizophrenia. *Schizophr Bull* 1990; **17**:375–388.
2. DeSanctis S: Sopra alcune varieta della demenzi precoce. *Rev Sper D Fen Med Leg* 1906; **32**:141–165.
3. Kraeplin E: *Dementia Pecos and Paraphernalia.* Barclay RM, trans. Edinburgh: Livingstone, 1919.
4. Bender L: Childhood schizophrenia. *Am J Orthopsychiatry* 1947; **17**:40–56.
5. Fish B: Neurobiologic antecedents of schizophrenia in children: Evidence for an inherited, congenital neurointegrative defect. *Arch Gen Psychiatry* 1977; **34**:1297–1313.
6. Kanner L: Autistic disturbances of affective contact. *Nerv Child* 1943; **2**:217–250.
7. Kolvin I: Studies in childhood psychoses: I. Diagnostic criteria and classification. *Br J Psychiatry* 1971; **118**:381–384.
8. Rutter M, Lockyer L: A five- to fifteen-year follow-up study of infantile psychosis: I. Description of sample. *Br J Psychiatry* 1967; **113**:1169–1182.
9. American Psychiatric Association: *Diagnostic and Statistical Manual of Mental Disorders.* Third edition. Washington, DC: American Psychiatric Association, 1980.
10. Beitchman JH: Childhood schizophrenia: A review and comparison with adult-onset schizophrenia. *Psych Clin N Am* 1985; **8**;793–814.
11. Werry JS: Child and adolescent (early-onset) schizophrenia: A review in light of DSM-IIIR. *J Autism Develop Disord* 1992; **22**:601–624.
12. American Psychiatric Association: *Diagnostic and Statistical Manual of Mental Disorders DSM-IV-TR.* Fourth edition. Washington, DC: American Psychiatric Association, 2000.
13. Burd L, Kerbeshian J: A North Dakota prevalence study of schizophrenia presenting in childhood. *J Am Acad Child Adolesc Psychiatry* 1987; **26**:347–350.
14. Green WH, Campbell M, Hardesty AS, *et al.*: A comparison of schizophrenic and autistic children. *J Am Acad Child Adolesc Psychiatry* 1984; **23**:399–409.
15. Russel AT, Bott L, Sarnmons C: The phenomenology of schizophrenia occurring in childhood. *J Am Acad Child Adolesc Psychiatry* 1989; **28**:399–407.
16. Remschmidt HE, Schulz E, Martin M, *et al.*: Childhood-onset schizophrenia: History of the concept and recent studies. *Schizophr Bull* 1994; **20**:727–745.
17. Murray RM, Van Os J: Predictors of outcome in schizophrenia. *J Clin Psychopharmacol* 1998; **18**(suppl 1):2S–4S.
18. American Psychiatric Association: Practice guideline for the treatment of patients with schizophrenia. *Am J Psychiatry* 1997; **154**(Suppl. 4):1–63.
19. Jablensky A: The 100-year epidemiology of schizophrenia. *Schizophr Res* 1997; **28**:111–125.
20. Cantor S: *Childhood Schizophrenia.* New York: Guilford, 1988.
21. King RA, Noshpitz JD: *Pathways of Growth: Essentials of Child Psychiatry, Vol. II: Psychopathology.* New York: John Wiley & Sons, 1991.
22. Cornblatt BA, Erlenrneyer-Kirnling L: Global attentional deviance as a marker of risk for schizophrenia: Specificity and predictive validity. *J Abnorm Psychol* 1985; **94**:470–486.
23. Green WH, Deutsch SI: Biological studies of schizophrenia with childhood onset. In: deutsch SI, ed. *Application of Basic Neuroscience to Child Psychiatry.* New York: Plenum Medical, 1990:217–229.
24. Watkins JM, Asarnow RF, Tanguay PE: Symptom development in childhood onset schizophrenia. *J Child Psychol Psychiatry* 1988; **29**:865–878.
25. Schaeffer JL, Ross RG: Childhood-onset schizophrenia: Premorbid and prodromal diagnostic and treatment histories. *J Am Acad Child Adolesc Psychiatry* 2002; **41**:538–545.

26. Lewis R: Should cognitive deficit be a diagnostic criterion for schizophrenia? *Rev Psychiatr Neurosci* 2004; **29**(2):102–113.

27. Isohanni M, Jones PB, *et al.*: Early developmental milestones in adult schizophrenia and other psychoses. A 31-year follow-up of the Northern Finland 1966 birth cohort. *Schizophrenia Res* 2001; **52**:1–19.

28. Alaghband-Rad J, McKenna K, Gordon CT *et al.*: Childhood-onset schizophrenia: The severity of premorbid course. *J Am Acad Child Adolesc Psychiatry* 1995; **34**:1273–1283.

29. McClellan J, Breiger D, McCurry C, Hlastala S: Premorbid functioning in early-onset psychotic disorders. *J Am Acad Child Adolesc Psychiatry* 2003; **42**:6.

30. Asarnow JR, Ben-Meir S: Children with schizophrenia spectrum and depressive disorders: A comparative study of onset patterns, premorbid adjustment, and severity of dysfunction. *J Child Psychol Psychiatry* 1988; **29**:477–488.

31. Practice Parameter for the Assessment and Treatment of Children and Adolescents With Schizophrenia. *J Am Acad Child Adolesc Psychiatry* 2001; **40**(7).

32. Volkmar FR: Childhood and adolescent psychosis: A review of the past 10 years. *J Am Acad Child Adolesc Psychiatry* 1996; **35**:843–851.

33. Spencer EK, Campbell M: Children with schizophrenia: Diagnosis, phenomenology, and pharmacotherapy. *Schizophr Bull* 1994; **20**:713–725.

34. Volkmar FR, Cohen DJ, Hoshino Y, *et al.*: Phenomenology and classification of the childhood psychoses. *Psychol Med* 1988; **18**:191–201.

35. Russell AT: The clinical presentation of childhood-onset schizophrenia. *Schizophr Bull* 1994; **20**:631–646.

36. Eggers C: Course and prognosis in childhood schizophrenia. *J Autism Childhood Schizophr* 1978; **8**:21–36.

37. Mueser KT and McGurk SR: Schizophrenia. *Lancet*, 2004; **363**:2063–2072.

38. McClellan J, McCurry C: Neurocognitive pathways in the development of schizophrenia. *Semin Clin Neuropsychiatry* 1998; **3**:320–332.

39. Riley B: Linkage studies of schizophrenia. *Neurotoxicity Res* 2004, **6**(1):17–34.

40. Kendler KS, Diehl SRT: The genetics of schizophrenia, a current, genetic-epidemiologic perspective. *Schizophr Bull* 1993; **19**:261–285.

41. McGuffin P, Own MJ, Farmer AE: Genetic basis of schizophrenia. *Lancet* 1995; **346**:678–682.

42. Cardno AG, Gottesman II: Twin studies of schizophrenia, from bow-and-arrow concordances to Star Wars Mx and functional genomics. *Am J Med Genet* 2000; **97**:12–17.

43. Cardno A, Marshall E, Coid B, *et al.*: Heritability estimates for psychotic disorders: The Maudsley twin psychosis series. *Arch Gen Psychiatry* 1999; **56**:162–168.

44. Farmer AE, McGuffin P, Gottesman II: Twin concordance for DSM-III schizophrenia. Scrutinizing the validity of the definition. *Arch Gen Psychiatr* 1987; **44**:634–640.

45. Lowing PA, Mirsky AF, Pereira R: The inheritance of schizophrenic spectrum disorders: A reanalysis of the Danish adoptee study data. *Am J Psychiatry* 1983; **140**:1167–1171.

46. Higgins J: Effects of child rearing by schizophrenic mothers: A follow-up. *J Psychiatr Res* 1976; **13**:1–9.

47. Wender PH, Rosenthal D, Kety SS, *et al.*: Crossfostering: A research strategy for clarifying the role of genetic and experimental factors in the etiology of schizophrenia. *Arch Gen Psychiatry* 1974; **30**:121–128.

48. Rosenthal D: *Genetic Theory and Abnormal Behavior.* New York: McGraw-Hill, 1970.

49. Asarnow JF: Childhood-onset schizophrenia. *J Child Psychol Psychiatry* 1994; **35**:1345–1371.

50. Nicolson R, Brookner BF, *et al.*: Parental schizophrenia spectrum disorders in childhood-onset and adult-onset schizophrenia. *Am J Psychiatry*, 2003; **160**(3):490–495.

51. Baltaxe CAM, Simmons JQ III: Speech and language disorders in children and adolescents with schizophrenia. *Schizophr Bull* 1995; **21**:677–692.

52. Caplan R: Communication deficits in children with schizophrenia spectrum disorders. *Schizophr Bull* 1994; **20**:671–674.

53. Wright IC, Rabe-Hesketh S, Woodruff PWR, *et al.*: Meta-analysis of regional brain volumes in schizophrenia. *Am J Psychiatry* 2000; **157**:16–25.

54. Andreasen NC, Flashman L, Flaum M, *et al.*: Regional brain abnormalities in schizophrenia measured with magnetic resonance imaging. *JAMA* 1994; **272**:1763–1769.

55. Byne W, Buchsbaum MS, Mattiace LA, *et al.*: Postmortem assessment of thalamic nuclear volumes in subjects with schizophrenia. *Am J Psychiatry* 2002; **159**:59–65.

56. Lawrie SM, Abukmeil SS: Brain abnormality in schizophrenia: A systematic and quantitative review of volumetric magnetic resonance imaging studies. *Br J Psychiatry* 1998; **172**:110–120.

57. Gogtay N, Giedd J, Rapoport JL: Brain development in healthy, hyperactive, and psychotic children. *Arch Neurol* 2002; **59**:1244–1248.

58. Sowell ER, Levitt J, *et al.*: Brain abnormalities in early-onset schizophrenia spectrum disorder observed with statistical parametric mapping of structural magnetic resonance images. *Am J Psychiatry* 2000; **157**:1475–1484.

59. Sporn AL, Greenstein DK, *et al.*: Progressive brain volume loss during adolescence in childhood-onset schizophrenia. *Am J Psychiatry* 2003; **160**(12):2181–2189.

60. Kumra S, Ashtari M, *et al.*: Reduced frontal white matter integrity in early-onset schizophrenia: A preliminary study. *Biol Psychiatry* 2004; **55**(12):1138–1145.

61. Allin M, Murray R: Schizophrenia: A neurodevelopmental or neurodegenerative disorder? *Curr Opin Psychiatry* 2002; **15**:9–15.

62. McDonald C, Grech, A, Toulopoulou T, *et al.*: Brain volumes in familial and non-familial schizophrenic probands and their unaffected relatives. *Am J Med Genet Neuropsych Genet* 2002; **114**:616–625.

63. Akbarian S, Vinuela A, Kim JJ, Potkin SG, Bunney WEJ, Jones EG: Distorted distribution of nicotinamindse-adenine dinucleotide phosphate-diaphorase neurons in temporal lobe of schizophrenics implies anomalous cortical development. *Arch Gen Psychiatry* 1993; **50**:178.

64. Weinberger DR, Marenco S: Schizophrenia as a neurodevelopmental disorder. In: Hirsch SR, Weinberger DR, eds. *Schizophrenia*, 2nd ed. Oxford: Blackwell Publishing, 2003:326–348.

65. Asarnow RF, Sherman T: Studies of visual information processing in schizophrenic children. *Child Dev* 1984; **55**:249–261.

66. Asarnow R, Granholm E, Sherman T: Span of apprehension in schizophrenia. In: Steinhauer SR, Gruzelier JH, Zugin J, eds. *Handbook of Schizophrenia, Vol. 5: Neuropsychology, Psychophysiology, and Information Processing.* Amsterdam: Elsevier Science Publishing Co., 1991:335–370.

67. Singer MT, Wynne LC: Thought disorder and family relations of schizophrenics. IV. Results and implications. *Arch Gen Psychiatry* 1965; **12**:201–209.

68. Asarnow JR, Goldstein MJ, Ben-Meir S: Parental communication deviance in childhood onset schizophrenia spectrum and depressive disorders. *J Child Psychol Psychiatry* 1988; **29**:825–838.

69. Goldstein MJ: The UCLA high risk project. *Schizophr Bull* 1987; **13**:505–514.

70. Butzlaff, RL, Hooley JM: Expressed emotion and psychiatric relapse: A meta-analysis. *Arch Gen Psychiatry* 1998; **55**:547–552.

71. Bruce MLK, Takeuchi DT, Leaf PJ: Poverty and psychiatric status: Longitudinal evidence from the New Haven epidemiologic catchment area study. *Arch Gen Psychiatry* 1991; **48**:470–474.

72. Rabkin JG: Stressful life events in schizophrenia: A review of the research literature. *Psychol Bull* 1980; **87**:408–425.

73. US Institute of Medicine: *Neurological, Psychiatric, and Developmental Disorders: Meeting the Challenges in the Developing World.* Washington, DC: National Academy of Sciences, 2001.

74. Jablensky A. Sartorius N, Emberg G, Anker M, Korten A, Cooper JE: Schizophrenia: Manifestations, incidence, and course in different cultures – a World Health Organization ten-country study. *Psychol Med Monograph Suppl* 1992; **20**:1–97.

75. Reimherr JP, McClellan JM: Diagnostic challenges in children and adolescents with psychotic disorders. *J Clin Psychiatry* 2004; **65**(Suppl 6):5–11.

76. Andreasen NC, Olsen S: Negative v positive schizophrenia: Definition and validation. *Arch Gen Psychiatry* 1982; **39**:789–794.

77. Fields JH, Grochowski S, Lindenmayer JP, *et al.*: The assessment of affective disorders in children and adolescents by semistructured interview: Test-retest reliability of the schedule for affective disorders and schizophrenia for school-age children, present episode version. *Arch Gen Psychiatry* 1985; **42**:696–702.

78. McClellan JM, Werry JS: Practice parameters for the assessment and treatment of children and adolescents with schizophrenia. *J Am Acad Child Adolesc Psychiatry* 1994; **33**:616–635.

79. American Academy of Pediatrics Task Force on Pediatric AIDS: Adolescents and human immuno deficiency virus infection: The role of the pediatrician in prevention and intervention. *Pediatrics* 1993; **92**:626–630.

80. *Report of the Presidential Commission on the Human Immunodeficiency Virus Epidemic.* Washington, DC: Government Printing Office, June 1988.

81. McClellan J, McCurry C, Speltz ML, *et al.*: Symptom factors in early-onset psychotic disorders. *J Am Acad Child Adolesc Psychiatry* 2002; **41**:791–798.

82. Werry JS, McClellan JM, Chard L: Childhood and adolescent schizophrenia, bipolar and schizoaffective disorders: A clinical and outcome study. *J Am Acad Child Adolesc Psychiatry* 1991; **30**:457–465.

83. Ballenger JC, ReusVI, Post RM: The 'atypical' clinical picture of adolescent mania. *Am J Psychiatry* 1982; **139**:602–606.

84. Rosen LN, Rosenthal NE, Van Dusen PH, *et al.*: Age at onset and number of psychotic symptoms in bipolar I and schizoaffective disorder. *Am J Psychiatry* 1983; **140**:1523–1524.

85. Carlson GA: Bipolar affective disorders in childhood and adolescence. In: Cantwell DP, Carlson GA, eds. *Affective Disorders in Childhood and Adolescence: An Update.* New York: Spectrum Publications, 1983.

86. Baker L, Cantwell DP: Disorders of language, speech, and communication. In: *Child and Adolescent Psychiatry: A Comprehensive Textbook*, Lewis M, ed. Baltimore: Williams & Wilkins, 1991:516–521.

87. Famularo R, Kinscherff R, Fenton T: Psychiatric diagnoses of maltreated children: Preliminary findings. *J Am Acad Child Adolesc Psychiatry* 1992; **31**:863–867.

88. Rothstein A: Hallucinatory phenomena in childhood: A critique of the literature. *J Am Acad Child Adolesc Psychiatry* 1981; **20**:623–635.

89. Caplan R: Thought disorder in childhood. *J Am Acad Child Adolesc Psychiatry* 1994; **33**:605–615.

90. Kydd RR, Werry IS: Schizophrenia in children under 16 years. *J Autism Dev Disord* 1982; **12**:343–357.

91. Kumra S, Frazier JA, Jacobsen LK, *et al.*: Childhood-onset schizophrenia: A double-blind clozapine-haloperidol comparison. *Arch Gen Psychiatry* 1996; **53**:1090–1097.

92. Findling RL, McNamara NK: Atypical antipsychotics in the treatment of children and adolescents: Clinical applications. *J Clin Psychiatry* 2004; **65**(Suppl 6):30–44.

93. Frazier JA, Gordon CT, McKenna K, *et al.*: An open trial of clozapine in 11 adolescents with childhood-onset schizophrenia. *J Am Acad Child Adolesc Psychiatry* 1994; **33**:658–663.

94. Turetz M, Mozes T, Toren P, *et al.*: An open trial of clozapine in neuroleptic-resistant childhood-onset schizophrenia. *Br J Psychiatry* 1997; **170**:507–510.

95 Armenteros JL, Whitaker AH, Welikson M, *et al.*: Risperidone in adolescents with schizophrenia: An open pilot study. *J Am Acad Child Adolesc Psychiatry* 1997; **36**:694–700.

96. Grcevich SJ, Findling RL, Rowane WA, *et al.*: Risperidone in the treatment of children and adolescents with schizophrenia: A retrospective study. *J Child Adolesc Psychopharmacol* 1996; **6**:251–257.

97. Kumra S, Jacobsen LK, Lenane M, *et al.*: Childhood-onset schizophrenia: An open label study of olanzapine in adolescents. *J Am Acad Child Adolesc Psychiatry* 1998; **37**:377–385.

98. Findling RL, McNamara NK, Youngstrom EA, *et al.*: A prospective, open-label trial of olanzapine in adolescents with schizophrenia. *J Am Acad Child Adolesc Psychiatry* 2003; **42**:170–175.

99. Shaw JA, Lewis JE, Pascal S, *et al.*: A study of Quetiapine: Efficacy and tolerability in psychotic adolescents. *J Child Adolesc Psychopharmacol* 2001; **11**:415–424.

100. McConville B, Carrero L, Sweitzer D, *et al.*: Long-term safety, tolerability, and clinical efficacy of Quetiapine in adolescents: An open-label extension trial. *J Child Adolesc Psychopharmacol* 2003; **12**:73–280.

101. National Institute of Mental Health: Abnormal Involuntary Movement Scale. *Psychopharmacol Bull* 1985; **18**:515–541.

102. McConville BJ, Sorter MT: Treatment challenges and safety considerations for antipsychotic use in children and adolescents with psychoses. *J Clin Psychiatry* 2004; **65**(Suppl 6):20–29.

103. Cantor S, Kestenbaum C: Psychotherapy with schizophrenic children. *J Am Acad Child Adolesc Psychiatry* 1986; **25**:623–630.

104. Asarnow, JR, Tompson MC, McGrath EP: Annotation: Childhood-onset schizophrenia: clinical and treatment issues. *J Child Psychol Psychiatry* 2004; **45**(2):180–194.

105. Hogarty, GE, *et al.*: Cognitive enhancement therapy for schizophrenia: Effects of a 2-year randomized trial on cognition and behavior. *Arch Gen Psychiatry* 2004; **61**:866–876.

106. Eggers C: Schizoaffective disorders in childhood: A follow-up study. *J Autism Dev Disord* 1989; **19**:327–342.

107. Asarnow JR, Tompson MC: Childhood onset schizophrenia: A follow-up study. *Eur J Child Adolesc Psychiatry* 1999; **8**:9–12.

108. Werry JS, McClellan JM: Predicting outcome in child and adolescent (early onset) schizophrenia and bipolar disorder. *J Am Acad Child Adolesc Psychiatry* 1992; **31**:147–150.

109. Zeitlin H: The natural history of psychiatric disorder in children. *Inst Psychiatry Maudsley Monogr* 1986; vol 29.

25

Neuropsychological Assessment and the Neurologically Impaired Child

Scott D. Grewe, Keith Owen Yeates

Introduction

This is an exciting time as it relates to our under-standing of brain–behavior relationships in children. Indeed, researchers have not only provided fascinating insights into the workings of the developing central nervous system [1,2] but also increasingly clarified the behavioral and cognitive sequelae associated with the various medical conditions that affect its functioning [3,4]. A number of factors are responsible for our increased ability to articulate the nature of and relationship between developing neuropsychological organization in children and deficits in functioning. These include both advances in neuroscience research [5,6] and increased survival rates for children suffering neurological trauma [7,8]. For example, the death rate for children with brain tumors decreased from 1/100 000 to 0.7/100 000 between 1975 and 2001, while five-year survival improved from rates in the 50s during the early 1970s to the high 70s in the late 1990s [9].

The purpose of this chapter is to introduce neuropsychology and neuropsychological assessment of children, with a focus on neurologically impaired children. Thus, we begin with a brief historic overview of the concept of neurologic impairment and neuropsychological assessment in children, and delineate the role of a neuropsychologist in diagnosis and assessment. Next, we offer a set of conceptual principles for neuropsychological assessment, review its related methods and procedures, and describe the differences in purpose and scope of evaluations conducted by school psychologists, clinical child psychologists, and neuropsychologists. After that, we review the neuropsychological outcomes associated with several of the more common childhood neurological disorders. Finally, we examine a neuropsychological management

approach and related intervention techniques used to help neurologically impaired children compensate for their difficulties.

Historical Overview

The field of child neuropsychology has been influenced by a variety of related disciplines. Indeed, child neuropsychological assessment has involved not only the downward extension of the methods of adult neuropsychological assessment [10], but also advances in child psychiatry, clinical child psychology, developmental psychology, developmental pediatrics, and pediatric neurology. The history of child neuropsychological assessment can be divided into three eras.

The first era developed as an outgrowth of early research on brain-injured soldiers in Europe during World War I. These severely brain-damaged individuals were described as stimulus bound (e.g., lacking in cognitive spontaneity and flexibility), perseverative, concrete, and emotionally labile. The application of these findings led to inferences about cognitive and emotional characteristics of intact adults and, later, of children.

Brain damage became an explanation for behavioral and educational problems in children following the epidemic of Von Economo's encephalitis in 1918. These postencephalitic children were described as antisocial, irritable, impulsive, and hyperkinetic. Additionally, other professionals working with mentally retarded children observed in their subjects many of the behaviors common to the brain-injured soldiers from World War I, and inferred underlying brain damage. Thus, the cardinal features of brain injury were originally elucidated as hyperkinesis, impulsivity, distractibility,

Clinical Child Psychiatry, Second Edition. Edited by W.M. Klykylo and J.L. Kay

emotional lability, and perseveration. This clinical picture became widely construed as *prima facie* evidence of brain injury.

However, the advances of this era were limited by the anecdotal nature of clinical reports. Additionally, considerable professional resistance existed regarding attempts to correlate behavior with specific brain regions. Indeed, such luminaries as Henry Head [11] argued that these and similar approaches were little more than revised phrenology, an argument that was not totally unfounded.

The second era of child neuropsychological assessment began around the time of World War II with the collaborative efforts of Strauss, Lehtinen, and Werner. They introduced experimental techniques for studying the behavior of children with purported brain injuries, and coined the term 'minimal brain injury' to describe the cluster of behaviors they believed were characteristic of brain-injured children [12,13]. Their work was very influential, and resulted in the popularity of the notion of 'minimal brain dysfunction' in the conceptualization of learning disorders [14]. One of the major shortcomings of this second era, though, was the often made but unwarranted assumption that the presence of cognitive or behavioral deficits in children without any known injury was indicative of brain dysfunction.

Interestingly, modern neuroimaging technology and advances in cognitive neurosciences have made feasible the third, and current, era of child neuropsychology. This era has involved a more sophisticated approach to the study of brain–behavior relationships in children with neurological disease, as well as in those with other systemic medical illnesses, developmental disorders, psychiatric disorders, and normal developmental status [15,16]. Moreover, it has seen the establishment of journals specifically focused in child and/or pediatric neuropsychology.

The transition to the most recent era of child neuropsychology also has been driven by attempts to ground child neuropsychological assessment in broader conceptual models [17–19], which help facilitate our understanding of neurobehavioral development through research and clinical practice. The goal of neuropsychological assessment, therefore, is not simply to document the presence of cognitive or behavioral deficits and their possible association with known or suspected brain damage. Rather, the goal is ultimately to enhance children's present and future adaptation by describing their cognitive, behavioral, and social functioning, relating their functioning to biological, developmental, and contextual variables, and anticipating typical developmental 'stress points' and providing recommendations and interventions to insure children meet these developmental demands.

What is a Neuropsychologist?

Much as child neuropsychological assessment went through a period of development, so has the general profession of neuropsychology. Indeed, although such as individuals as Paul Broca, Carl Wernicke, John Hughlings Jackson, Henry Head, and Kurt Goldstein were laying the foundation for neuropsychology in the nineteenth century, it was not until the mid-twentieth century that the term 'neuropsychology' began appearing in the professional literature [20,21]. Currently, most neuropsychologists are licensed psychologists who have earned a doctorate in psychology. For many neuropsychologists, the bulk of their specialized training occurs during a two-year postdoctoral fellowship. Indeed, recent guidelines [22] support postdoctoral training as an entry-level educational requirement for all new graduates. Following postdoctoral training, more advanced Diplomate status can be achieved through a board-certification process, although not all practicing neuropsychologists are board-certified.

The specialty of neuropsychology includes individuals functioning in various capacities within clinical, research, and academic settings. Additionally, within this broader field are those who share an interest in facilitating the adaptive outcomes of children with genetic, medical, environmental, behavioral, and social problems; namely, the child, or pediatric, neuropsychologist.

General Principles

Neuropsychological assessment of children is based on various models that have conceptual foundations and knowledge bases cogently articulated by Bernstein and Waber [17], Taylor and Fletcher [18], Rourke and his colleagues [19], and Yeates and Taylor [23]. These various assessment models highlight and stress different aspects and units of analysis in their respective approaches. However, the application of these knowledge bases is consistently grounded in understanding brain–behavior relationships across the developmental spectrum, all for the primary purpose of enhancing children's adaptation.

Adaptation

The primary focus of assessment is to promote the current and future adaptation of the child, rather than simply to document the presence or location of brain damage or dysfunction. Adaptation results from the interactions of children and their environments or contexts. Failures in adaptation, such as academic or behavioral difficulties, are usually the presenting problems that bring children to the attention of neuropsychologists. In this respect, neuropsychological assessment is optimally useful when it helps to explain those difficulties and facilitates successful future outcomes. Indeed, the goals of assessment extend beyond facilitating learning and behavior in the present to include promoting future adaptation to the demands of adult life.

Brain and Behavior

The second principle is that insight into children's adaptation can be gained through an analysis of brain–behavior relationships. Advances in the neurosciences over the past several decades have yielded clearer understandings of the relationships between brain and behavior. Old notions regarding the localization of functions have been replaced by more dynamic models involving the interaction of multiple brain regions [24–26]. Although most of these models concern adults, recent advances in functional neuroimaging and related techniques are providing opportunities to determine if similar models apply to children. Future research should, therefore, eventually yield major advances in our understanding of the brain–behavior relationships in children.

Context

The third principle is that environmental contexts are influential in constraining and determining behavior, and, subsequently, affecting brain functioning. Indeed, the brain does not function in isolation. Thus, a neuropsychological assessment must carefully examine the influences of environmental or contextual variables on a child's behavior. The reasons for examining these factors are to assess the nature of environmental and situational demands being placed on the child and assist in the process of explaining a child's adaptive difficulties. In this regard, neuropsychological assessment is designed not only to measure a child's specific cognitive, behavioral, and social skills, but also to determine how a child applies those skills in particular environments. Examining children's cognitive and behavioral profiles and how their profiles match the contextual demands of their environments allows the neuropsychologist to highlight the developmental risks facing children and make informed recommendations for intervention [17].

Development

The final guiding principle is that assessment involves the measurement of change, or development, across multiple levels of analysis. Developmental neuroscience has highlighted the multiple processes that characterize brain development (e.g., cell differentiation and migration, synaptogenesis, dendritic arborization and pruning, myelinization), and the timing of those processes [27]. Although less research has been conducted concerning developmental changes in children's environments, there is, nevertheless, a continuity and predictability to the environments of most children in our society [28].

Consequently, neuropsychological assessment of children requires closely scrutinizing the developmental changes that occur in brain, behavior, and context, because the interplay of these variables determines ultimate adaptational outcomes. Indeed, failures in adaptation often reflect a clash between different timetables (e.g., biological and environmental) that result in a lack of fit between children and the contexts within which they function.

Methods of Assessment

The four general principles outlined above serve as the foundation for specific methods used by many child neuropsychologists. Neuropsychological assessment is usually equated with the administration of a battery of tests. However, in practice, neuropsychologists draw on multiple sources of information, rather than relying solely on the results of psychological tests. The most common combination of methods involves the collection of relevant historic information, focused behavioral observations, and psychological testing. Together, they permit a comprehensive examination of neuropsychological functioning.

History

The collection of a thorough history is a critical component in any neuropsychological assessment and its importance cannot be overstated. Indeed, a thorough history helps in the process of clarifying the nature, onset, and source of a child's presenting problems.

Birth and Developmental History
Collection of information regarding a child's early development usually begins with the mother's pregnancy and extends to the acquisition of developmental milestones. This information is useful in identifying early risk factors and indicators of anomalous

Table 25.1 Perinatal risk factors.

Risk factor	Associated outcomes
Maternal age (<17 years)	General cognitive and motor deficits
Maternal cigarette consumption	Developmental delays, learning disabilities
Maternal alcohol consumption	Fetal alcohol syndrome/effects (FAS/FAE)
Maternal cocaine and/or methamphetamine use	Developmental delays, attention and executive function deficits
Maternal stress during pregnancy	Developmental and behavioral difficulties
Viral infections	Mental retardation, learning disabilities
Hypoxic events	Cerebral palsy, cognitive deficits
Extremely low, very low and low birth weight (ELBW, VLBW, LBW)	Graded IQ and neuropsychological function improvement with increasing birth weight
Peri and intraventricular hemorrhage (PVH/IVH)	Motor, perceptual, cognitive deficits

Table 25.2 Commonly used medications and their potential neuropsychological side effects.

Medication	Associated adverse effects
Stimulants (dextroamphetatime, methylphenidate, pemoline, amphetamine compounds)	Lowered seizure threshold, potential worsening of tics
Antipsychotics (clozapine, haloperidol, loxapine, thioridazine, thiothixene, olanzapine, risperidone)	Cognitive slowing from sedation, memory and attention difficulties
Anxiolytics (benzodiazepine class)	Learning-related memory difficulties
Anticonvulsants (phenobarbital, phenytoin primodine, valproate), especially polytherapy	Inattention, motor and cognitive slowing, memory deficits

development. Indeed, the presence of early risk factors or developmental anomalies helps makes a case for a primary biological rather than environmental basis for a child's failures in adaptation (Table 25.1).

Perinatal risk factors are of particular importance, because maternal illness during pregnancy, exposure to teratogens during gestation, complications during delivery, and early environmental deficiencies can affect later neuropsychological functioning.

The early development of the child also deserves attention, including language skills, gross- and fine-motor skills, attentional and behavioral functions, social interactions, eating and sleeping patterns, and development of hand preference, as delays in these domains are often precursors of later learning and behavior problems [29].

Medical History
A child's medical history often contains predictors of neuropsychological dysfunction, the most obvious being a documented brain abnormality or injury. Indeed, closed-head injuries during childhood can compromise cognitive and behavioral functions, and seizure disorders are frequently associated with neuropsychological deficits.

Another critical piece of medical information is whether the child is taking any medications. All medications have the potential to affect a child's neuropsychological functioning, including their performance on tests of cognitive skills. However, those that are especially likely to do so are certain anticonvulsant, stimulant, and psychotropic medications [30–32] (Table 25.2).

Family and Social History
Genetic variation, although intrinsically linked with environment in the eventual expression of any inherent biological risk, plays an important role in the etiology of learning problems. Consequently, information about a family's history of academic difficulties, psychiatric disorders, and neurologic illness helps indicate a potential biological foundation for later neuropsychological deficits [33].

A review of family history must also examine socioeconomic factors. Parental education and occupation help gauge the stimulation and learning opportunities that a child has received which, in turn, help predict later childhood intellectual competence [34]. Indeed, socioeconomic disadvantage is one of the primary risk factors for mental retardation [35].

Information regarding a child's social history is also informative. Questions regarding peer relationships and friendships are important in neuropsychological assessment because poor peer relationships in some cases suggest nonverbal learning problems [36]. In other instances, problems with peer relationships may signal psychological stress and poor self-esteem related to academic difficulties.

Educational History

A complete school history includes information about a child's current grade placement, any grade repetitions or special education involvement, and school placement changes. Information about school history is typically elicited from parents or guardians, although school personnel are often contacted to validate parent reports and to obtain additional descriptions of a child's academic and behavioral difficulties at school. More specifically, teachers and other school personnel can provide information on a child's ability to meet educational and social demands and how the child compares to peers.

For children who have been evaluated for or received special educational services in the past, the timing of those services provides insights about the nature of the underlying learning problems [28]. In addition, the results of prior testing can be compared to the child's current test performance, providing evidence of change or stability in neuropsychological functioning.

Details of prior and current educational interventions, often delineated in Individualized Education Programs (IEP) through formal special education or Section 504 Plans, are also valuable. They help to characterize not only the academic demands a child is expected to meet, but also the amount and type of support that has been provided. If prior services have been ineffective, information about other resources is needed to make practical recommendations.

Behavioral Observations

Behavioral observations of the child are a second source of information for the neuropsychologist, and an area that often does not receive the attention it deserves. Observations are important, not only in interpreting the results of neuropsychological testing, but also because they provide a more naturalistic measure of social, communicative, problem-solving, and sensorimotor skills. Behavioral domains to which neuropsychologists routinely attend include mood and affect; thought processes; motivation and cooperation; social interaction and pragmatics; attention and activity level; response style; speech, language, and communication; sensory and motor skills; and physical appearance.

The first two domains listed can enormously affect the entire assessment process. If children are upset, they are likely to be less motivated and cooperative. While lack of cooperation does not automatically invalidate the results of an assessment, it must be taken into account in interpreting findings. Even subtle disturbances in motivation or cooperation are noteworthy. Indeed, the child who is compliant and follows directions, but is generally unenthused and does not initiate many actions spontaneously, may be demonstrating 'frontal' symptomatology (e.g., flattened affect, poor self-initiation of behavior, impaired planning/problem solving) [37]. Conversely, a lack of enthusiasm or outright resistance to testing may suggest anxiety and avoidance characteristic of children with learning disabilities when they are presented with school-like tasks [38].

Observations of social interactions are also useful. A child who is antagonistic with parents but more appropriate with the examiner may not be managed very effectively at home. Conversely, a child who is consistently oppositional may be experiencing a more generalized behavioral disturbance. Similarly, a child who is appropriate with his or her parents and other adults, but is socially awkward or even inappropriate with the examiner and peers, may have a more subtle learning problem [39].

The capacity to regulate attention and activity level deserves close observation. Indeed, observations of inattention and motor disinhibition during an evaluation provide important information regarding children's capacity to modulate their behavior under performance demands.

Similarly, a child's response style provides a wealth of information regarding potential neuropsychological deficits. Qualitatively different errors (e.g., naming difficulties, retrieval problems, perseveration), for instance, have been associated with different types of brain dysfunction [40]. In general, the rate and organization of responses provide insight about a child's cognitive deficits and use of compensatory strategies (Table 25.3).

Speech, language, and communication skills also deserve close observation. Language disturbances are

Table 25.3 Response errors and potential attributions to brain regions.

Response error	Associated brain region
Perseveration, reduced verbal and nonverbal fluency, motor programming and problem-solving deficits	Dorsolateral prefrontal cortex
Confabulation, social disinhibition, impulsivity, emotional lability	Orbitofrontal cortex
Decreased spontaneity, stimulus-boundedness, apathy	Medial frontal cortex

presumed to cause many failures in acquisition of basic academic skills, such as reading and writing. Thus, neuropsychologists monitor numerous aspects of children's speech and language skills, including spontaneous conversation, language comprehension and expression, and the occurrence of more pathognomonic errors, such as anomia and paraphasia.

Nonverbal aspects of communication are also important to observe. These typically include pragmatics (e.g., reciprocity, topic maintenance, and supposition), discourse skills, and appreciation of paralinguistic features such as intonation, prosody, gesture, and facial expression. Difficulties in these areas provide qualitative information about behavioral and communicative regulation, which often mirror reports from other sources about social interactions.

Disturbances in sensory and motor functioning are also noteworthy because they may interfere with the standardized administration of psychological tests, and because of the asserted but not consistently proven association between neurological 'soft signs' and cognitive functioning [41]. Moreover, asymmetries in sensory and motor functions can often assist with the lateralization and localization of brain dysfunction and, thereby, provide support for the notion that a child's difficulties have a primary neurological basis.

The final category of observation is physical appearance. Some physical anomalies are indicative of genetic syndromes, which may be associated with specific neuropsychological profiles [42,43]. However, dress and hygiene also deserve consideration, because deviation from the 'norm' can suggest mild neuropsychological deficits, such as poor social awareness or adaptive behavior deficits.

Psychological Testing

Psychological testing is the third source of information about the child, and the one most often equated with neuropsychological assessment. Animated and contentious debate continues regarding the merits of standardized test batteries versus more flexible approaches to assessment. However, most child neuropsychologists administer a variety of tests that sample numerous cognitive domains. The administration of a comprehensive group of tests provides an accurate portrayal of a child's overall profile of functioning in the domains of general cognitive ability, verbal abilities, nonverbal abilities, learning and memory, attentional and executive functions, sensory and motor functions, academic skills, behavioral and emotional adjustment, and adaptive behavior.

As discussed earlier, these domains are assessed through review of a child's relevant history and through behavioral observations, as well as by formal testing. In the following sections, we give examples of measures, and briefly examine the rationale and limitations of measurement, in each domain.

General Cognitive Ability

General cognitive ability is typically assessed using intelligence tests. Intelligence tests are standardized measures that assess a variety of cognitive skills and provide an estimate of a child's overall cognitive functioning. However, intelligence tests are not, as is often suggested, measures of innate learning potential. Indeed, intelligence tests fail to measure many important skills, and were designed primarily to predict academic achievement. Thus, intelligence tests are only one, albeit significant, piece of a neuropsychological assessment (Table 25.4).

Verbal Abilities

The field of neuropsychology owes much to the early researchers of aphasia and other acquired language disorders. Indeed, when testing verbal abilities, neuropsychologists commonly draw from aphasia batteries. Tests of verbal abilities are relevant for neuropsychological assessment because language skills are significant contributors to academic success and social competence. As with intelligence tests, however, performance on language measures often reflects skills in addition to those for which the procedures were designed. Indeed, many of the tests routinely employed

Table 25.4 Commonly used intelligence tests.

Bayley Scales of Infant Development-Second Edition (BSID-II)	Commonly used preschool measure
Das Naglieri Cognitive Assessment System (CAS)	
Differential Ability Scales (DAS)	Preschool and school-aged versions
Kaufman Adolescent and Adult Intelligence Test (KAIT)	
Kaufman Assessment Battery for Children-Second Edition (KABC-II)	
Kaufman Brief Intelligence Test (KBIT)	Screening measure
Mullen Scales of Early Learning	Commonly used preschool measure
Stanford–Binet Intelligence Scales: Fifth Edition (SB-V)	Commonly used school-aged measure
Wechsler Preschool and Primary Scales of Intelligence-Third Edition (WPPSI-III)	Commonly used preschool measure
Wechsler Intelligence Scale for Children-Fourth Edition (WISC-IV)	Most widely used test for school-age children
Wechsler Adult Intelligence Scale-Third Edition (WAIS-III)	Most widely used test for adults
Wechsler Abbreviated Scale of Intelligence (WASI)	Screening measure

Table 25.5 Commonly used verbal tests.

Boston Naming Test	Core aphasia screening measure
Clinical Evaluation of Language Fundamentals Preschool-Second Edition (CELF Preschool-2)	Comprehensive preschool measure
Clinical Evaluation of Language Fundamentals-Fourth Edition (CELF-4)	Comprehensive school-age measure
Comprehensive Test of Phonological Processing (CTOPP)	Helpful adjunct when assessing for dyslexia
Expressive One-Word Picture Vocabulary Test and Receptive One-Word Picture Vocabulary Test	
Halstead–Wepman Aphasia Screening Test	
NEPSY	Assesses receptive and expressive domains
Peabody Picture Vocabulary Test-Third Edition (PPVT-III)	Commonly used receptive language screener
Preschool Language Scale-Fourth Edition (PLS-4)	Comprehensive preschool measure
Rapid Automatized Naming Test Sentence Repetition Test	Helpful adjunct when assessing for dyslexia
Token Test for Children	
Word Fluency Test	Commonly used measure of retrieval

by neuropsychologists are not 'pure' measures of any one skill or ability; rather, they are typically multi-factorial. Consequently, the interpretation of language test performance must take into account performance in other domains (Table 25.5).

Nonverbal Abilities

Tests of nonverbal abilities typically fall into two categories, those that draw on visuoperceptual abilities, and those that demand constructional skills and, hence, motor control and planning. Assessment of nonverbal skills is important because nonverbal deficits are often associated with poor performance in certain academic skills, particularly arithmetic, as well as with a heightened risk for psychosocial maladjust-

ment. In addition, nonverbal deficits are particularly common in children with acquired neurological insults, suggesting that nonverbal skills are especially vulnerable to brain damage in children. As with language tests, however, most tests of nonverbal abilities also draw on other skills. Consequently, test interpretation, again, requires an appreciation for a child's overall neuropsychological profile (Table 25.6).

Learning and Memory

Learning and memory difficulties are a frequent cause of referral to child neuropsychologists. However, despite the importance of learning and memory for children's adaptation, and especially their school performance, it is only recently that there have been instru-

Table 25.6 Commonly used nonverbal tests.

Benton Facial Recognition Test	
Clock Drawing	Measures planning and organization skills
Developmental Test of Visual-Motor Integration (VMI)	Commonly used constructional test
Hooper Visual Organization Test	
Judgment of Line Orientation Test	
Motor-Free Visual Perception Test-Revised (MVPT-R)	
NEPSY	Assesses visual perceptual and constructional skills
Rey-Osterrieth Complex Figure (ROCF)	Measures constructional, planning and organizational skills
Test of Nonverbal Intelligence-Third Edition (TONI-3)	
VMI-Visual Test and Motor Test	
Wide Range Assessment of Visual Motor Abilities (WRAVMA)	Comprehensive measure of visual perceptual and constructional skills

Table 25.7 Commonly used learning and memory tests.

Benton Visual Retention Test	
California Verbal Learning Test-Children's Version (CVLT-C)	Commonly used measure of verbal learning and memory
California Verbal Learning Test-Second Edition (CVLT-II)	Adult version of the CVLT
Children's Memory Scale (CMS)	Comprehensive measure of verbal/nonverbal memory
NEPSY	Screening of verbal and nonverbal memory
Rey-Osterrieth Complex Figure (ROCF)	Measure of nonverbal memory
Test of Memory and Learning (TOMAL)	Comprehensive measure of verbal and nonverbal memory
Verbal Selective Reminding Test (VSRT)	Commonly used measure of verbal learning and memory
Wechsler Memory Scale-Third Edition (WMS-III)	Comprehensive adult measure of verbal/nonverbal memory
Wide Range Assessment of Learning and Memory-Second Edition (WRAML2)	Comprehensive measure of verbal/nonverbal memory

ments available for assessing these skills. Performance on tests of memory and learning, however, is multiply determined. Performance on tests of verbal memory, for example, is affected by children's language abilities and attentional functions. A further limitation of measurement in this domain is that current tests of children's learning and memory do not necessarily reflect recent advances in the neuroscience of memory [44–46] (Table 25.7).

Attentional and Executive Functions

From a neuropsychological perspective, attention is a multidimensional construct that overlaps with 'executive' functions. Neuropsychological assessment of attention, therefore, usually involves evaluation of numerous aspects, such as sustained, selective, and divided attention; working memory, or the ability to internalize verbal and nonverbal task sequencing; the ability to shift set; and cognitive efficiency.

Attention problems are one of the more common reasons for referral to a child neuropsychologist, and are central to the diagnosis of attention deficit hyperactivity disorder. Unfortunately, the relationship between formal tests of attention and the attentional behaviors about which parents and teachers complain is modest at best [47]. Nevertheless, because attentional functioning moderates performance on many psychological tests, it will remain an important component of neuropsychological assessment.

Executive functions are those involved in the planning, organization, regulation, and monitoring of goal-directed behavior [37,48,49], and play a critical role in determining a child's adaptive functioning. Indeed, executive function deficits are a hallmark

Table 25.8 Commonly used attention and executive function tests.

Behavior Rating Inventory of Executive Function (BRIEF)	Parent, teacher, and self forms
Cancellation Tests	Measure of visual attention
Category Test	Commonly used measure of reasoning
Children's Paced Auditory Serial Attention Test (CHIPASAT)	
Consonant Trigrams	
Contingency Naming Test	
Delis-Kaplan Executive Function System (D-KEFS)	Comprehensive measure for children and adults
Fluency Tests	
Gordon Diagnostic System	Computerized measure of inhibition and attention
Matching Familiar Figures Test	
Rey-Osterrieth Complex Figure (ROCF)	Measure of planning and organization
Stroop-Color Word Test	
Test of Everyday Attention for Children (TEA-Ch)	Comprehensive measure of attentional functions
Test of Variables of Attention (TOVA)	Computerized measure of inhibition and attention
Tower of Hanoi	Measure of planning and problem solving
Tower of London	Measure of planning and problem solving
Trail Making Test	Measure of visuomotor scanning and psychomotor speed
Wisconsin Card Sorting Test (WCST)	Commonly used measure of problem solving

of the child who demonstrates neuropsychological impairment, whether as a result of focal brain dysfunction or in association with developmental learning disorders.

Although considerable research and theorizing has been devoted to clarifying the construct of executive function in children and to assessing its various dimensions, the exact nature of executive function remains uncertain [49–51]. This is due, in part, to the uncritical assumption that all skills subsumed under the executive function rubric are mediated by frontal brain systems, as well as to the paucity of studies examining the ecological validity of purported measures of executive function [52] (Table 25.8).

Sensory and Motor Functions

Tests of sensory and motor functions usually involve standardized versions of various components of the traditional neurological examination. Relevant sensory skills include sensory suppression, finger localization, graphesthesia, stereognosis, and left–right orientation, while those in the motor domain relate to speed and dexterity. In addition, tests of oculomotor control, motor overflow, alternating and repetitive movements, and other related skills are often used to assess 'soft' neurological status.

Tests of sensory and motor functions are useful because they are sensitive to acute and chronic neuro-

logical disorders and can provide confirmatory evidence for localized brain dysfunction. Tests of sensory and motor functions also may help to predict learning problems in younger children and to differentiate older children with different types of learning disorders [53]. Unfortunately, especially for young children and those with significant behavioral/emotional difficulties, the assessment of sensory and motor functions is often compromised by lapses in attention or motivation, and the results of sensory and motor testing do not always carry obvious implications for treatment (Table 25.9).

Academic Skills

Academic underachievement is one of the most common reasons for a child to be referred for neuropsychological assessment. Hence, testing of academic skills is typically critical in understanding a child's academic functioning. Indeed, academic skill assessment offers information about the nature and severity of underachievement, provides evidence of specific learning disabilities, is often used to determine whether a child is eligible for special education services, and is helpful in developing specific treatment approaches. However, achievement tests also suffer from the same multifactorial issues as many of the cognitive tests. Thus, knowledge of the specific demands of any given achievement test is required to accurately

Table 25.9 Commonly used sensorimotor tests.

Sensory-Perceptual Examination	Commonly used series of measures for children and adults
Finger Sequencing	
Finger Tapping Test	Measure of simple motor speed
Fist-Edge-Palm Test	
Grip Strength Test	
Grooved Pegboard	Measure of motor speed and coordination
Hand Pronation-Supination Test	
Lateral Dominance Examination	
Purdue Pegboard	
Timed Motor Examination	Commonly used series of motor tests for 5–10 year olds

Table 25.10 Commonly used academic achievement tests.

Bracken Basic Concept Scale-Revised (BBCS-R)	Measure of academic readiness for preschoolers
Kaufman Tests of Education Achievement-Second Edition (KTEA-II)	Comprehensive measure of academic skills
Key Math-Revised	
Nelson-Denny Reading Test (NDRT)	
Peabody Individual Achievement Test-Revised (PIAT-R)	Comprehensive measure of academic skills
Wechsler Individual Achievement Test-Second Edition (WIAT-II)	Comprehensive measure of academic skills
Wide Range Achievement Test-Revision 3 (WRAT-3)	Commonly used academic screener
Woodcock-Johnson Tests of Achievement-Third Edition (WJ-III)	Comprehensive measure of academic skills
Woodcock Reading Mastery Test-Revised (WRMT-R)	

interpret a child's performance beyond a standard score or grade equivalent (Table 25.10).

Behavioral and Emotional Adjustment, and Adaptive Behavior

Children referred for neuropsychological assessment often demonstrate psychological distress, inappropriate behavior, or other deficits in adaptive functioning. The central goal of neuropsychological assessment is to promote overall adaptation, so assessment of behavioral and emotional adjustment, as well as of adaptive functioning, is crucial. Awareness of deficits in adjustment and adaptive behavior can help identify a mismatch between children's neuropsychological profiles and their environmental demands (Table 25.11).

However, relationships between neuropsychological skills and adjustment problems or deficits in adaptive behavior are not always straightforward. Indeed, some premorbid behavioral characteristics (i.e., impulsivity, aggression, attention-seeking behavior) actually increase the risk of mild brain injury and associated neuropsychological deficits [54], and other behavioral difficulties or adaptive deficits may be a direct manifestation of a specific neuropsychological deficit [55].

Types of Assessment Compared

School psychologists, clinical psychologists, and child neuropsychologists employ similar measures when evaluating behavior – that is, they use psychological and other tests to examine how a child is functioning in comparison to his or her age-mates. Thus, any of these providers could use an intelligence test, academic achievement test, or test of a child's behavioral and emotional adjustment. Despite this overlap in instrumentation, the services offered by each discipline are quite different.

Assessments conducted by school psychologists typically address eligibility for special education or other school-related services and focus on evaluating a

Table 25.11 Commonly used behavioral/emotional adjustment and adaptive behavior tests.

ADHD Rating Scale-IV	Symptom checklist
Behavior Assessment System for Children-Second Edition (BASC-2)	Comprehensive measure with parent, teacher, and self-report versions
Child Behavior Checklist (CBC)	Commonly used parent screener
Child Depression Inventory (CDI)	
Conners' Rating Scales-Revised (CRS-R)	
Personality Inventory for Children-Second Edition (PIC-2)	Comprehensive, parent completed measure
Personality Inventory for Youth (PIY)	Comprehensive, self-report measure
Minnesota Multiphasic Personality Inventory-Second Edition (MMPI-2)	Comprehensive, self-report measure for adults
Minnesota Multiphasic Personality Inventory-Adolescent (MMPI-A)	Comprehensive, self-report measure for adolescents
Scales of Independent Behavior-Revised (SIB-R)	Comprehensive measure of adaptive behavior
Teacher Report Form (TRF)	Commonly used teacher screener
Vineland Adaptive Behavior Scales (VABS)	Comprehensive measure of adaptive behavior
Youth Self-Report (YSR)	Commonly used self-report screener

child's functioning in relationship to academic expectations and success. Assessments conducted by clinical psychologists often focus on the psychological/emotional functioning of the child, though they can examine almost any aspect of the child's cognitive or behavioral status. However, school and clinical psychological assessments generally emphasize skills, functions, or psychological processes, without explicitly referencing brain structures or mechanisms.

In contrast, since one focus of a *neuro*psychological assessment is to examine the integrity of the brain, these assessments comprehensively examine neurocognitive and neurobehavioral functioning, in addition to psychosocial adjustment and academic achievement. By definition, knowledge about brain–behavior relationships informs neuropsychological assessments. Whether an assessment is neuropsychological in nature is *not* determined by the use of traditional 'neuropsychological' tests. Rather, an assessment becomes neuropsychological when a properly trained child neuropsychologist invokes the developmental brain–behavior knowledge base, particularly as it relates to the child's context or environment, to evaluate, diagnose, and intervene with a particular child.

Childhood Neurological Disorders

The previous section delineated the various domains relevant to child neuropsychological assessment, the psychological tests used to assess them, and the differences among three types of child assessment. The relevant research provides a solid overview of the typical cognitive and behavioral sequelae associated with various neurological disorders in children, and the following section highlights the neuropsychological outcomes associated with three of the more common, and commonly researched, neurological disorders.

Head Injury

Head injuries are a leading cause of death and disability in children and adolescents. Although estimates of the rate of such injuries vary from study to study, the average incidence across studies is approximately 180/100 000 [56]. However, most researchers agree that the precise estimate depends on the type and severity of the injury, in part because many children with milder head injuries and no obvious sequelae often do not received medical attention. Moreover, children sustain traumatic brain injuries in various ways including bicycle accidents, sports-related injuries, motor vehicle accidents, falls, and child abuse, some of which may decrease the likelihood of the children receiving medical care.

Children sustain head injuries in a number of settings, with rates varying according to the chronological age of the child. Infants, toddlers, and young children sustain their head injuries primarily through falls, pedestrian versus motor vehicle accidents, bicycle versus motor vehicle accidents, and child abuse. By late childhood and adolescence, the leading causes of head injuries include motor vehicle and sports-related accidents. Motor vehicle-related injuries are often the most severe and account for a high proportion of fatal injuries among pediatric cases.

Neuropsychological Outcomes in Head Injury

The neuropsychological outcomes of head injuries in children vary greatly. Among the most important variables in determining outcome, however, are the nature and severity of the injury, the age and premorbid functioning of the child who sustains the injury, and the environmental context to which the child returns after the injury [57,58].

In general, children who sustain head injuries demonstrate deficits in overall IQ [59,60], and the magnitude of the decline is closely related to the severity of the injury. Although these children typically demonstrate significant recovery over time, their performance continues to be impaired relative to premorbid levels, particularly for children who sustain moderate to severe injuries. Long-term deficits are especially common on nonverbal subtests, presumably because they are novel and require speeded, motor performance. However, recent research indicates that performance on verbal subtests, which has traditionally been considered resistant to disruption because it involves retrieval of previously acquired knowledge and has minimal motor demands, is also likely to be impacted [61] (Table 25.12).

Table 25.12 Neuropsychological outcome in closed head injury.

Declines in measured intelligence, particularly in nonverbal domains and with increased injury severity

Subtle but pervasive language deficits, including pragmatics and discourse

Significant nonverbal deficits, especially on timed tasks and those with substantial organizational demands

Attention problems, particularly regarding response modulation and reaction time

Pervasive memory deficits, particularly regarding explicit memory and with increased injury severity

Generalized executive dysfunction

Academic difficulties, typically including grade retention and/or special education involvement

Behavior and personality changes (e.g., increased irritability, impulsivity, aggression, and hyperactivity), and difficulties in personal/social adaptation

---

Overt aphasic disorders are less common in children posthead injury, but more subtle difficulties do occur. Indeed, long-term deficits have been identified in such areas as object identification and description, sentence repetition, comprehension, and verbal fluency [62]. Additionally, deficits in language pragmatics and discourse are commonly observed [63]. In contrast, long-term deficits in nonverbal skills are relatively frequent, and the deficits are especially pronounced on timed tasks involving fine motor skills but also extend to those tasks with substantial organizational demands [64].

Attention problems are common for children following head injury. Indeed, although there are very few studies that have comprehensively assessed attention based on current theoretical models, those that have been completed tend to show deficits on measures of continuous performance. Moreover, these deficits tend to reflect poor response modulation and slowed reaction time [57].

Memory deficits are also quite common in children following head injury, and the magnitude of the observed deficits is dependent upon the severity of the injury [65]. Many studies have identified deficits in verbal and nonverbal memory, using learning, selective reminding, recall, and recognition formats. Additionally, recent studies have also addressed the question of differences between explicit and implicit memory, indicating that implicit memory is much more resistant to disruption [66–68].

Deficits in executive functions are nearly ubiquitous following head injury in children. Unfortunately, research in this area has been less common, in part, because measurement of complex reasoning and problem-solving skills is more difficult. However, recent research has demonstrated difficulties in planning, problem solving, verbal fluency, concept formation, cognitive flexibility, and organization [69,70].

Given the numerous cognitive difficulties outlined above, it is not surprising that children who sustain head injuries often experience academic difficulties. Interestingly, although academic skills often initially return to premorbid levels, subsequent performance frequently suffers, with growing discrepancies between the children with head injuries and their peers. Indeed, the vast majority of children who sustain a severe brain injury either fails a grade or qualifies for special education services by two years postinjury [71]. However, it is unclear whether the placement in special education services results from academic skills deficits or from behavioral disturbance and overall neuropsychological functioning [72].

Behavioral difficulties are a final area of difficulty for children who sustain head injuries. Posthead injury behavioral problems include changes in temperament, increased irritability, impulsivity, aggression, and hyperactivity, as well as difficulties in personal/social adaptation. Behavioral changes may occur even in cases of minor and mild head injury, but these tend to be transient and short-lived, although the insensitive nature of typical rating scales may account for some of the apparent lack of persistent symptomatology [73]. In general, severely head injured children are at the greatest risk for long-term problems in social adjustment [74].

The behavioral difficulties demonstrated by children who sustain head injuries are not attributed exclusively to injury-related factors, though. Indeed, these children must also cope with significant psychological stress resulting from acute and potentially permanent changes in function, reactions of family members, and subsequent changes in family interaction patterns [58]. Additionally, the type of behavioral difficulties may differ according to the child's age at the time of injury and at subsequent times in the future. Just as age-related factors influence the expression of cognitive difficulties following head injuries in children, they also affect the expression of behavioral difficulties.

In general, outcome research following head injury suggests that children who sustain mild head injuries typically return to or approach premorbid levels of functioning. In contrast, children who sustain moderate-to-severe head injuries generally suffer significant, long-term cognitive and behavioral sequelae. Specifically, these children are at increased risk for overall intellectual difficulties, as well as nonverbal, memory, and executive function deficits. Behavioral changes are also common, and may be exacerbated depending on the nature of the injury, premorbid characteristics, and social–environmental supports.

Epilepsy

Epilepsy refers to the recurrent convulsive or nonconvulsive seizures caused by local or generalized epileptogenic discharges in the brain. The prevalence of epilepsy in the pediatric population has been estimated between 4.3 and 9.3 per 1000 [75]. Seizures in infancy and childhood differ in many respects from those in adulthood. Most importantly, they occur far more frequently in individuals under the age of 15 years than in adults, and are considered by some experts to be a 'disorder of childhood' differing in type and etiology from the adult disorders. Indeed, at least 75% of all

individuals with epilepsy develop their initial symptoms before the age of 20 years [75].

Although trauma has been suggested as the primary identified cause of epilepsy, a full compliment of pre-, peri-, and postnatal disorders have also been considered. Moreover, an underlying etiology for epilepsy is identified in only 30% of the cases [75], and includes structural brain anomalies, metabolic derangement, birth anoxia, cerebrovascular insults, and central nervous system infections and/or neoplasms.

Neuropsychological Outcomes in Epilepsy

Many factors influence the outcome of children with epilepsy, including the etiology of seizure activity, age of onset, degree of seizure control, and associated neurological abnormalities. Consequently, adaptive difficulties in cognitive and behavioral domains are often encountered in children with epilepsy.

In general, the distribution of IQ scores in children with epilepsy is similar to that found in the general pediatric population. Although some epileptic syndromes are associated with poorer cognitive outcomes (i.e., Lennox–Gastaut, West syndrome), most children with epilepsy perform within the average range of intelligence and do not differ from their siblings. Additionally, when IQ declines have been observed, medication toxicity has often been implicated [76] (Table 25.13).

Although children with epilepsy typically have average levels of intellectual functioning, specific cognitive deficits may be present. Indeed, research findings consistently suggest a disruption of attentional functions in children with epilepsy [75]. Language skills have been identified as areas of difficulty, particularly when there are concomitant academic difficulties. Memory deficits have also been reported, but not as consistently as disruption of attentional functions.

Table 25.13 Neuropsychological outcome in epilepsy.

Attention problems
Language deficits, particularly when concomitant academic difficulties are present
Inconsistent verbal and nonverbal memory deficits, generally related to lateralization of seizure activity
Academic difficulties, commonly including grade retention and/or special education involvement
Behavioral and adjustment difficulties (e.g., low self-esteem, depression and anxiety, and external locus of control), resulting from neurological and psychosocial sources

More specifically, verbal and nonverbal memory deficits have been documented depending on the lateralized nature of the seizure activity [77], although other researchers [78] have failed to demonstrate seizure focus-specific cognitive dysfunction.

Academic achievement difficulties are common in children with epilepsy. Indeed, children with epilepsy are twice as likely as are their peers to repeat a grade or qualify for special education services [79,80]. Moreover, Dodrill [81] reported that adults whose seizures continued from childhood experienced lowered educational and occupational outcomes.

Specific academic difficulties do not appear to be associated with seizure focus, however. Indeed, when academic skills are examined, difficulties have been observed in all general skill areas. The etiology of these difficulties has been difficult to determine, but appears to relate more to socioeconomic and cultural variables than to seizure-specific factors [82].

Behavioral difficulties are also present in many children with epilepsy. Indeed, children with epilepsy have higher rates of psychiatric difficulties than do children in the general population or those with chronic illness [83]. Both neurological and psychosocial factors appear to contribute to the increased risk for psychological difficulties. However, most authorities agree that behavioral difficulties result from brain dysfunction. Indeed, behavioral and emotional difficulties appear to be closely linked to cognitive deficits [78,84].

Some studies have suggested that children with focal EEG abnormalities and temporal lobe epilepsy demonstrate a higher rate of psychiatric disorder. However, the preponderance of research provides negligible, empirical support for a specific behavioral syndrome, personality disorder, or increased aggression in individuals with temporal lobe epilepsy [85].

In general, children with epilepsy are prone to lower self-esteem, increased episodes of depression and anxiety, and an external locus of control. These difficulties appear to stem from the confluence of several factors including underlying brain impairment, increased seizure frequency, and psychosocial sources. Additionally, family variables, sociocultural attitudes, and level of knowledge about epilepsy are critical determinants of overall psychological functioning [75].

When considering the cognitive and behavioral difficulties experienced by children with epilepsy, consideration must be given to the impact of anti-epileptic drug (AED) treatment. Although the effects of AEDs have been difficult to isolate, they seem to exert their affect on attention and concentration, memory functions, processing and motor speed, and behavioral and emotional regulation.

Carbamazepine has been associated with few cognitive side effects. Indeed, although carbamazepine in moderate dosage has been found to affect memory functions [86], it seems to have minimal effects on sustained attention [87]. Valproate also appears to have minimal cognitive side effects, although effects may be significantly associated with dose level. Additionally, the fewest behavioral side effects have been noted with carbamazepine and valproate.

Phenytoin appears to have the most detrimental cognitive side effects of the AEDs. Indeed, phenytoin may result in a progressive encephalopathy with deterioration of intellectual function, particularly in children with already poor intellectual functions or neurological abnormalities [86]. Interestingly, phenytoin does not appear to have significant behavioral side effects [88].

Studies of phenobarbital have been equivocal in terms of cognitive side effects. Short-term memory difficulties have been reported when comparing phenobarbital to valproate [89]. In contrast, phenobarbital has consistently been associated with behavioral side effects such as hyperactivity, irritability, and sleep disturbances. Indeed, phenobarbital appears to exacerbate existing behavioral problems, particularly in children with lowered cognitive functions [75].

One consistent finding concerning AED effects is the negative impact of polytherapy compared to monotherapy on cognition and behavior [90], effects that appear to be independent of drug type. Specifically, monotherapy in children has been associated with improvements in both cognitive and behavioral functions [91]. However, consideration must also be given to the possibility that children who are on more than AED have more intractable seizures and/or underlying brain pathology.

In general, AEDs may result in cognitive and behavioral side effects that are exacerbated by higher serum levels and by polypharmacy. However, a child's response to AEDs is highly individualistic and established therapeutic ranges may not insure maximum seizure control and minimum side effects.

Hydrocephalus and Myelomeningocele

Hydrocephalus involves an imbalance in the production and absorption of cerebrospinal fluid. When normal pathways are interrupted or impaired, a progressive accumulation of fluid results, which exerts pressure on surrounding brain structures. Hydrocephalus is often associated with myelodysplasias, which refer to any of several malformations of the spinal cord and meninges. Myelodysplasias can range from reasonably benign pilonidal cysts to severe cases of spina bifida cystica. Myelomeningocele is one type of spina bifida cystica, and occurs with a frequency ranging from one to five per 1000 live births [92].

Neuropsychological Outcomes in Hydrocephalus and Myelomeningocele

Many factors influence the outcome of children with hydrocephalus and myelomeningocele, including the etiology of the hydrocephalus, duration, severity, timing of initiation of treatment, shunt complications, and associated neurological abnormalities. Consequently, adaptive difficulties in cognitive and behavioral domains are often encountered by children with hydrocephalus.

In general, children with hydrocephalus, particularly those with concomitant motor difficulties, have lower overall IQ scores than their peers, although the bulk of this lowered score is accounted for by nonverbal difficulties. However, research conclusions reflect group results and, as suggested above, the simple presence of hydrocephalus does not predict an individual child's intellectual performance [93], and the performance of such children is actually more variable than that observed in their peers [94].

While frank language disorders are relatively uncommon in children with hydrocephalus (i.e., problems with syntax, lexicon, and phonology), the literature contains many references to clinical descriptions of 'cocktail party' speech. However, this phenomenon of superficial and perseverative social speech patterns is more commonly seen in children with below average intellectual abilities. More typically, children with hydrocephalus show deficits reflecting difficulties with higher-order inferential language, inference, and discourse [95], which appear to be relatively independent of overall level of cognitive ability.

In addition to having problems with tasks found in nonverbal sections of intelligence tests, children with hydrocephalus may have particular difficulty with tasks involving visuoperceptual and constructional skills. Not surprisingly, there seems to be an association between intelligence and perceptual motor skills, with lower IQ scores associated with lower scores on visuomotor tasks. Recent research suggests that these difficulties are associated with not only the speed and motor demands but also the perceptual and organizational demands of such tasks [96].

Relatively few studies have specifically addressed memory functioning of children with hydrocephalus, despite the knowledge that an enlarging ventricular system may directly affect structures and pathways that subserve encoding and retrieval of information. Moreover, the handful of studies available has yielded equivocal findings regarding verbal and nonverbal memory deficits [97–99]. This is due, in part, to the multiple cognitive demands necessary to perform well on memory tasks. Indeed, children with hydrocephalus often have difficulty on verbal memory tasks because of the language demands, while perceptual, constructional, and organizational demands can interfere with performance on nonverbal memory tasks. In general, however, when difficulties are observed, they reflect problems with learning, organization of stimuli, and subsequent retrieval [100]; although recent research suggests that the discrepancy between intact implicit memory and impaired explicit memory is critical to understand memory functioning in children with congenital brain disorders [67].

Attentional and executive functions in children with hydrocephalus have been relatively unexamined. However, parents of children with shunted hydrocephalus commonly report problems pertaining to attention difficulties, distractibility, and concentration [100], as well as generalized executive dysfunction [101]. Moreover, more severe medical involvement is associated with more impairment of attentional functions [102]. These difficulties are similar to those found in children diagnosed with an attention deficit/hyperactivity disorder of the predominantly inattentive type.

Motor dysfunction is common in children with hydrocephalus, and this dysfunction typically affects fine- and gross-motor abilities. Fine-motor problems may be expressed as difficulties with copying, handwriting, writing speed, or in fine-motor coordination, speed, and dexterity, while gross-motor difficulties are often expressed in poor standing balance and gait abnormalities, independent of the level of spinal lesion in myelomeningocele. It is not surprising, therefore, that performance on cognitive measures that depend on visuomotor skills or on motor speed is frequently impaired in children with hydrocephalus [97].

Academic skills in children with hydrocephalus have been poorly researched. The few studies completed show a general pattern favoring basic language-based over mathematics skills. More specifically, word reading and decoding, as well as spelling skills, are typically intact, but reading comprehension, written expression and mathematics skills are much more deficient [103].

The behavioral difficulties experienced by children with hydrocephalus have also been poorly chronicled. However, the completed studies suggest that the adjustment problems displayed by children with hydro-cephalus are generally not as severe as those displayed by children referred for mental health services. Indeed, the majority of children with hydrocephalus are rela-tively well adjusted, at least according to parent ratings [104].

Although children with spina bifida do not display an extremely high rate of psychopathology or behav-ior problems, they are vulnerable to more subtle adjustment problems, such as declines in self-esteem. Indeed, research to date has shown that children with hydrocephalus are prone to symptoms of depression and anxiety [100,105] and disruptive behavior prob-lems, although treatment, family, and social–environ-mental factors are also contributory factors in the adjustment of these children, particularly during ado-lescence [106].

Hydrocephalus, with or without associated myelodysplasias, places a child at risk for a number of cognitive and behavioral difficulties. Cognitive deficits are most apparent in nonverbal, memory, and sensori-motor domains. However, higher-level language skills, as well as various aspects of attention and executive function, are also susceptible to disruption. Addition-ally, various behavioral and emotional difficulties are common in children with hydrocephalus. Indeed, lim-itations in functions and issues regarding body integrity and self-esteem are ever-present stresses for children with hydrocephalus.

Neuropsychological Management

As can be seen from the preceding section, there is not a clear cognitive or behavioral phenotype for the neurologically impaired child. Indeed, neurologically impaired children demonstrate neuropsychological deficits consistent with the nature of their injury or disorder, which are further influenced by numerous factors, including the etiology, injury or disorder sever-ity, age at onset, rapidity and efficacy of treatment, and associated medical complications. However, using the conceptual framework elucidated earlier, it is possible to develop a coherent management strategy that addresses the various cognitive, behavioral, and social difficulties of these children. Indeed, from that con-ceptual framework, the historical assumption that neurologically impaired children suffer from 'organic' difficulties that are not amenable to therapeutic inter-vention is unjustified.

The first step in the management process is to evalu-ate the relevant history, behavioral observations, and test results with reference to levels and patterns of performance. The second step involves determining relevant *diagnostic behavioral clusters* [17], which are groups of findings that, although not necessarily content- or domain-specific, are consistent with our knowledge of brain function in children and the nature of cognitive–behavioral relationships across develop-ment. For instance, delays in language acquisition, relative deficits in language and reading tests, configu-rational approaches on constructional tasks, and right-sided sensorimotor deficits, within the context of otherwise normal functioning, might be construed as left hemisphere implicating, without assuming that there is any focal brain lesion or dysfunction. Thus, diagnos-tic behavioral clusters are defined in terms of presumed neural substrates, but are not assumed to reflect under-lying brain damage (Table 25.14).

Treatment recommendations follow logically from this approach, with particular attention to risks for future difficulties, given an individual child's neu-ropsychological profile. However, the assessment of risks faced by a specific child takes into account not only the child's neuropsychological profile, but also the particular characteristics of the child's environment, including home, school, and community [107]. In other

Table 25.14 Common diagnostic behavioral clusters.

Diagnostic behavioral cluster	Neuropsychological assessment results
Left-hemisphere cluster	Delays in language acquisition, deficits on language and reading tests, right-sided sensorimotor deficits, configurational approach on constructional tasks, otherwise normal functioning
Right-hemisphere cluster	Relative nonverbal deficits, part-oriented approach on constructional tasks, left-sided sensorimotor deficits, arithmetic deficits, social pragmatics and skills deficits
Frontal brain regions cluster	Behavioral dysregulation, expressive language and constructional deficits, problem-solving deficits, poor abstract reasoning, motor deficits

words, recommendations for management arise from the integration of historical information, behavioral observations, and test results in light of the four general principles outlined earlier. Recommendations typically focus on remediating the child's weaknesses, promoting compensatory strategies, or modifying the environmental demands affecting the child. Consequently, interventions to address a child's specific neuropsychological profile are employed across a number of settings.

Educational interventions are paramount because of the impact of academic attainment on future outcomes. Although only limited empirical support exists for specific educational interventions, there is support for several general principles that can guide the development of an effective educational program. These principles typically address context- and content-specific issues, and relate to maximizing direct instructional time, providing structure and direction in the instructional process, individualizing instruction and teaching to mastery, promoting generalization and transfer of learning across settings, providing incentives contingent on performance, and teaching to all deficits [108].

In general, the more instruction children receive the better they achieve. Thus, children should be provided with as much instruction as possible, and classroom activities should be organized to maximize instructional time. Instructional time must not only be increased, though, but also be structured and directed for the child. Step-by-step and repeated presentations, modeling, and concrete aides are often helpful regardless of the content domain being taught.

The application of such instructional techniques must be individualized to a specific child's needs. More specifically, instructional techniques should be applied with reference to a child's particular pattern of neuropsychological strengths and weaknesses. To accomplish this, instruction often needs to occur in one-to-one or small-group settings.

Interventions must also stress generalization and transfer of learning to new settings and subjects. Indeed, helping such children with generalization and 'brainstorming' of alternative solutions and approaches is often a critical component of their intervention plan. In turn, reinforcements and consequences that are tied directly and logically to academic subjects are useful in keeping such children motivated and in promoting progress.

The final general principle stresses the need to teach to all areas of deficit. More specifically, specialized educational programs must address as many of a child's difficulties as possible. Remedial programs emphasize development of basic academic skills, tutorial programs provide assistance in learning regular curriculum content, and compensatory approaches teach children how to manage or adapt to the curriculum independently.

This last principle raises two issues about treatment strategies for children with neurological impairments. The first issue, cognitive remediation or rehabilitation, typically arises in the context of acutely brain-injured individuals. In general, research findings have not supported the notion that cognitive rehabilitation across groups of brain-injured subjects can result in restoration of cognitive functions to their preinjury status. However, there is support for interventions that teach compensatory skills to individuals [109–111], an approach consistent with the conceptual framework espoused throughout this chapter. The second issue, sensory integration therapy, arises most commonly in the context of children with various developmental or learning difficulties. Research findings continue to identify sensory integration therapy as not only an unproved, but also ineffective, remedial treatment for learning disabilities and other disorders [112–114].

Obviously, incorporating various academic interventions and modifications into a regular educational classroom may be difficult. Fortunately, special education services are available for children with neuropsychological impairments, assuming their difficulties are having an adverse academic affect and require specially designed instruction. There are several different categories in the special education system; the names of the specific categories vary from state to state but effectively are the same. Additionally, there exists a continuum of services ranging from tutorial assistance in the regular education classroom to full-time special education placement in a separate school or facility. Debate persists regarding the optimal provision of special education services (i.e., 'inclusion' programs in the regular education classroom versus 'pull-out' programs in separate classrooms), as federal law mandates children are to receive a free and appropriate public education in the least restrictive setting possible, often resulting in a trend toward more regular classroom and less special classroom education. However, the primary benefit of special education services for neurologically impaired children is the requirement of an IEP that makes explicit the interventions to be utilized in instruction and how the efficacy of those interventions will be determined.

A Section 504 Plan, which is a regular education approach, is another education vehicle to provide academic accommodations for such children. This approach is often utilized when a specific child's difficulties are not felt to require the intensity or specificity of intervention generally associated with formal special education. However, the vast majority of Section 504 Plans are vague and loosely structured, often limiting their effectiveness for such children.

Social interventions are also imperative, considering the psychosocial risk factors for neurologically impaired children. These interventions are typically focused on specific child difficulties, as well as relevant family issues. Behavior management interventions are the most common approaches, and allow for consistency between different environments (i.e., home and school). Indeed, such children typically benefit from classrooms and home environments that incorporate clear, brief, and more visible and external modes of presentation of behavioral requirements than is required for their peers. Consequences must also be more swift, immediate, frequent, and consistent than is necessary for their peers. Similarly, more frequently changing or rotating reinforcers or rewards helps maintain their salience and reward generating qualities. Finally, incentives or motivators must be present (i.e., 'rewarding early and often') before punishment can be implemented, because such children typically respond less robustly to response–cost measures or time-out if the availability of reinforcement is relatively low. Indeed, such children typically behave least appropriately in settings in which the opportunity for reinforcement is low or when the reinforcement–consequence ratio weighs heavily in the direction of consequences.

In many cases, neurologically impaired children present with psychosocial difficulties resulting from numerous factors. Moreover, family members of neurologically impaired children often suffer significant grief and loss as they confront the reality of adaptive changes in their child, and as they navigate the ongoing recovery and/or developmental process [115,116]. Consequently, individual, group, and family therapy are important because they help individuals and families become more active participants in their ongoing adjustment. These approaches also help family members become appropriate in their expectations, as well as become active advocates for their child.

Psychopharmacological medications are another worthy intervention. However, such interventions with neurologically impaired children have been woefully underinvestigated. The available research has often been methodologically poor in quality, making them difficult to interpret; single-case reports and non-blind trials do not yield sufficient information for informed psychopharmacological interventions. Moreover, these studies have suffered from numerous methodological

flaws including reporting bias, poor reliability of testing, retrospective and anecdotal reports, and the concurrent use of other psychotropic medications.

With these concerns in mind, several research models for assessing the efficacy of psychopharmacological interventions have been proposed, and seem to share several common features. These include the use of placebo controls and double-blind methodology, randomization of dose order across subjects, inclusion of multiple assessment measures, collection of assessment data when medication effects are most prominent, and evaluation of side effects during medication and nonmedication conditions [117]. Additionally, Phelps and her colleagues provided a model approach for collaborative medication management, which details assessment of behavioral and emotional problems, identification of treatment goals, selection of empirically supported interventions, assessment of readiness for change, development and interpretation of medication-monitoring protocols, and coordination of the intervention team [118]. Such an approach would allow the comprehensive evaluation of medication effects on relevant symptomatology, while minimizing side effects on cognitive and behavioral functioning.

A final area of intervention is the ongoing education of families of neurologically impaired children. Over the past few decades, numerous agencies and organizations have been established to advocate on behalf of children with cognitive, academic, and behavioral difficulties. Moreover, the resources provided by these organizations often help families identify and marshal the diverse resources highlighted above (Appendix 25.1).

Summary

The present chapter provided an overview of the neuropsychological assessment of children, focusing on children with various forms of neurologic impairment. The historical context of neuropsychological assessment in children bears consideration, as advances in related disciplines have spurred ongoing progress in the articulation of conceptual principles for neuropsychological assessment.

The model for child neuropsychological assessment espoused in this chapter considers adaptation, brain–behavior, context, and development to be dynamic factors that differentially influence any given child. Additionally, the relative importance of these factors changes over time, necessitating a developmental perspective to child neuropsychological assessment. Not surprisingly, child neuropsychological assessment has its roots in developmental neuroscience and develop-

Appendix 25.1 Advocacy organizations for children and their families.

Brain Injury Association of America	(800) 444-6443	www.biausa.org
The Spina Bifida Association of America	(800) 621-3141	www.sbaa.org
The Epilepsy Foundation of America	(800) 332-1000	www.epilepsyfoundation.org
Children and Adults with Attention Deficit/Hyperactivity Disorder (CHADD)	(301) 306-7070	www.chadd.org
The Learning Disabilities Association (LDA)	(412) 341-1515	www.ldanatl.org
LD Online		www.ldonline.org
International Dyslexia Association	(410) 296-0232	www.interdys.org
National Information Center for Handicapped Children and Youth (NICHCY)	(800) 695-0285	www.nichcy.org

mental psychology. Consequently, contributions from those disciplines will forge clearer pictures of brain–behavior relationships in children and set the stage for clearer determinations of the ecological validity of neuropsychological assessment across adaptive areas [119,120].

As stated previously, there is no phenotype for neurologically impaired children, largely because of the multitude of factors that influence outcome. However an outcome algorithm recently offered by Maureen Dennis considers *congnitive phenotype*, or neurobehavioral outcome, an expression of the *biological risk* associated with the medical condition, moderated by the child's *development*; by the *time since onset* of the condition; and by the *reserve* available within the child, family, school and community, and may help in characterizing the unique influence of these various factors [121]. Head injuries, seizure disorders, and hydrocephalus are only three of the neurological conditions common in children. However, they serve to highlight the various cognitive and behavioral deficits associated with neurological impairment, and also make the case for considering specific injury- and disorder-related variables in the neuropsychological management of neurologically impaired children.

When neuropsychological management is viewed from the aforementioned contextual model, intervention techniques are logical extensions of specific diagnostic behavioral clusters. Indeed, they are developed with respect to the specific neuropsychological profile of a child, as well as with attention to relevant environmental demands, all in the context of development. In the future, however, clinicians and researchers will need to consider more closely the factors that influence success and failure of specific interventions. Examination of these factors will allow a more precise determination of their efficacy, as well as facilitate the application of interventions across groups of neurologically impaired children.

References

1. Schwaab DF: Relation between maturation of neurotransmitter systems in the human brain and psychosocial disorders. In: Rutter M, Casaer P, eds. *Biological Risk Factors for Psychosocial Disorders.* Cambridge, UK: Cambridge University Press, 1991:50–66.
2. Bjorklund A, Hokfelt T, Tohyama M: *Handbook of Chemical Neuroanatomy.* Holland: Elsevier Science Publishers, 1992.
3. Anderson V, Bond L, Catroppa C, Grimwood K, Keird E, Nolan T: Childhood bacterial meningitis: Impact of age at illness and acute medical complications on long term outcome. *J Int Neuropsycholog Soc* 1997; 3:147–158.
4. Barnes MA, Dennis M: Discourse after early-onset hydrocephalus: Core deficits in children of average intelligence. *Brain Lang* 1999; **61**:309–334.
5. Molfese D: Electrophysiological responses obtained during infancy and their relation to later language development: Further findings. In: Tramontana MG, Hooper SR, eds. *Advances in Child Neuropsychology,* Vol. 3. New York: Springer-Verlag, 1995.
6. Bigler E: Advances in brain imaging with children and adolescents. In: Tramontana MG, Hooper SR, eds. *Advances in Child Neuropsychology,* Vol. 3. New York: Springer-Verlag, 1995.
7. Berkowitz GS, Papiernik E: Epidemiology of preterm birth. *Epidemiol Rev* 1993; **15**(2):414–443.
8. Kraus JF: Epidemiological features of brain in children: Occurrence, children at risk, causes and manner of injury, severity, and outcomes. In: Broman SH, Michel ME, eds. *Traumatic Head Injury in Children.* New York: Oxford University Press, 1995:22–39.
9. National Cancer Institute (NCI): *Childhood Brain Tumor. CancerNet: PDQ Treatment Statements for Physicians.* http://www.cancernet.nci.nih.gov
10. Benton AL: Foreword. In: Yeates KO, Ris MD, Taylor HG, eds. *Pediatric Neuropsychology: Research, Theory, and Practice.* New York: Guilford Press, 2000:XV.
11. Head H: *Aphasia and Kindred Disorders of Speech.* New York: Macmillan, 1926.
12. Strauss AA, Lehtinen L: *Psychopathology and Education of the Brain-Injured Child.* New York: Grune and Stratton, 1947.
13. Strauss AA, Werner H: The mental organization of the brain-injured mentally defective child. *Am J Psychiatry* 1941; **97**:1194–1203.

14. Taylor HG: MBD: Meaning and misconceptions. *J Clin Neuropsychol* 1983; **5**:271–287.

15. Dennis M: Childhood medical disorders and cognitive impairment: Biological risk, time, development, and reserve. In: Yeates KO, Ris MD, Taylor HG, eds. *Pediatric Neuropsychology: Research, Theory, and Practice.* New York: Guilford Press, 2000:3–24.

16. Dennis M, Barnes M: Developmental aspects of neuropsychology: Childhood. In: Zaidel D, ed. *Handbook of Perception and Cognition.* New York: Academic Press, 1994:219–246.

17. Bernstein JH, Waber DP: Developmental neuropsychological assessment: The systemic approach. In: Boulton AA, Baker GB, Hiscock M; eds. *Neuromethods: Vol. 17, Neuropsychology.* New York: Humana Press, 1990:311–371.

18. Taylor HG, Fletcher JM: Neuropsychological assessment of children. In: Goldstein G, Hersen M, eds. *Handbook of Psychological Assessment*, 2nd ed. New York: Pergamon Press, 1990.

19. Rourke BP, Bakker DJ, Fisk JL, Strang JD: *Child Neuropsychology: An Introduction to Theory, Research, and Clinical Practice.* New York: Guilford Press, 1983.

20. Hebb DO: *The Organization of Behavior: A Neuropsychological Theory.* New York: John Wiley & Sons, 1949.

21. Kluver H: *Behavior Mechanisms in Monkey.* Chicago: The University of Chicago Press, 1957.

22. Hannay HJ, Bieliauskas L, Crosson BA, Hammeke TA, Hamsher KdeS, Koffler S, eds. Proceedings of the Houston Conference on Specialty Education and Training in Clinical Neuropsychology. *Arch Clin Neuropsychol* 1998; **13**:157–250.

23. Yeates KO, Taylor HG: Neuropsychological assessment of older children. In: Goldstein G, Nussbaum P, Beers SR, eds. *Handbook of Human Brain Function: Vol III, Neuropsychology.* New York: Plenum Press, 1998:35–61.

24. Cummings JL: Frontal-subcortical circuits and human behavior. *Arch Neurol* 1993; **50**:873–880.

25. Middleton FA, Strick PL: Revised neuroanatomy of frontal-subcortical circuits. In: Lichter DG, Cummings JL, eds. *Frontal-Subcortical Circuits in Psychiatric and Neurological Disorders.* New York: Guilford Press, 2001:44–58.

26. Derryberry D, Tucker DM: Neural mechanisms of emotion. *J Clin Consult Psychol* 1992; **60**:329–338.

27. Nowakowski RS: Basic concepts of CNS development. *Child Dev* 1987; **58**:568–595.

28. Holmes JM: Natural histories in learning disabilities: Neuropsychological difference/environmental demand. In: Ceci SJ, ed. *Handbook of Cognitive, Social, and Neuropsychological Aspects of Learning Disabilities.* Hillsdale, NJ: Lawrence Erlbaum Associates, 1987:303–319.

29. Satz P, Taylor HG, Friel J, Fletcher JM: Some developmental and predictive precursors of reading disabilities: A six year follow-up. In: Benson AL, Pearl D, eds. *Dyslexia: An Appraisal of Current Knowledge.* New York: Oxford University Press, 1978:313–347.

30. Williams J, Sharp GB: Epilepsy. In: Yeates KO, Ris MD, Taylor HG: eds. *Pediatric Neuropsychology: Research, Theory, and Practice.* New York: Guilford Press, 2000:47–73.

31. Brown RT, Dreelin E, Dingle AD: Neuropsychological effects of stimulant medication on children's learning and behavior. In: Reynolds CR, Fletcher-Janzen E, eds.

Handbook of Clinical Child Neuropsychology, 2nd ed. New York: Plenum Press, 1997.

32. Cepeda ML: Nonstimulant psychotropic medication: Desired effects and cognitive/behavioral adverse effects. In: Reynolds CR, Fletcher-Janzen E, eds. *Handbook of Clinical Child Neuropsychology*, 2nd ed. New York: Plenum Press, 1989.

33. Rutter M, Silberg JL, O'Connor TG. Simonoff E: Genetics and child psychiatry: II. Empirical research findings. *J Child Psychol Psychiatry* 1999; **40**:19–55.

34. Yeates KO, MacPhee D, Campbell FA, Ramey CT: Maternal IQ and home environment as determinants of early childhood intellectual competence: A developmental analysis. *Dev Psychol* 1983; **19**:731–739.

35. Duyme M, Dumaret AC, Tomkiewicz S: How can we boost IQs of 'dull children'? A late adoption study. *Proc Natl Acad Sci USA* 1999; **96**:(15):8790–8794.

36. Rourke BP: Introduction: The NLD syndrome and the white matter model. In: Rourke BP, ed. *The Syndrome of Nonverbal Learning Disabilities: Neurodevelopmental Manifestations.* New York: Guilford Press, 1995:1–26.

37. Goldberg E: *The Executive Brain.* New York: Oxford University Press, 2002.

38. Spreen O: The relationship between learning disability, emotional disorders, and neuropsychology: Some results and observations. *J Clin Exp Neuropsychol* 1989, **11**:117.

39. Rourke BP, Tsatsanis KD: Nonverbal learning disabilities and asperger syndrome. In: Klin A, Volkmar FR, Sparrow SS: eds. *Asperger Syndrome.* New York: Guilford Press, 2000.

40. Kaplan E: A process approach to neuropsychological assessment. In: Boll T, Bryant BK, eds. *Clinical Neuropsychology and Brain Function: Research, Measurement, and Practice.* Washington, DC: American Psychological Association, 1988:125–168.

41. Shaffer D, O'Connor PA, Shafer SQ, Prupis S: Neurological 'soft signs': Their origins and significance. In: Rutter M, ed. *Developmental Neuropsychiatry.* New York: Guilford Press, 1983:144–163.

42. White BJ: The Turner syndrome: Origin, cytogenetic variants, and factors influencing the phenotype. In: Broman SH, Grafman J, eds. *Atypical Cognitive Deficits in Developmental Disorders: Implications for Brain Function.* Hillsdale, NJ: Erlbaum, 1994:183–195.

43. Fuerst KB, Dool CB, Rourke BP: Velocardiofacial syndrome. In: Rourke BP, ed. *The Syndrome of Nonverbal Learning Disabilities: Neurodevelopmental Manifestations.* New York: Guilford Press, 1995:119–137.

44. Nelson CA: The ontogeny of human memory: A cognitive neuroscience perspective. *Dev Psychol* 1995, **31**:723–738.

45. Butters N, Delis DC: Clinical assessment of memory disorders in amnesia and dementia. *Annu Rev Psychol* 1995; **46**:493–523.

46. Cowan NC, Hulme C: *The Development of Memory in Childhood.* Hove East Sussex, UK: Psychology Press, 1997.

47. Barkley RA: The ecological validity of laboratory and analogue assessment methods of ADHD symptoms. *J Abnorm Child Psychol* 1991; **19**:149–178.

48. Denckla MB: Measurement of executive function. In: Lyon GR, ed. *Frames of Reference for the Assessment*

of Learning Disabilities. Baltimore: Paul H. Brookes Publishing, 1994:117–142.

49. Stuss DT, Benson DF: *The Frontal Lobes.* New York: Raven Press, 1986.

50. Lezak M: *Neuropsychological Assessment,* 3rd ed. New York: Oxford University Press, 1995.

51. Nigg JT: On inhibition/disinhibition in developmental psychopathology: Views from cognitive and personality psychology and a working inhibition taxonomy. *Psycholog Bull* 2000; **126**:220–246.

52. Archibald S, Kerns KA: Identification and description of new tests of executive functioning in children. *Child Neuropsychol* 1999; **5**(2):115–129.

53. Casey JE, Rourke BP: Disorders of somatosensory perception in children. In: Rapin LI, Segalowitz SJ, eds. *Handbook of Neuropsychology (Vol. 6): Child Neuropsychology.* Amsterdam: Elsevier Science Publishers, 1992:477–494.

54. Rutter M, Chadwick O, Shaffer D: Head injury. In: Rutter M, ed. *Developmental Neuropsychiatry.* New York: Guilford Press, 1983:83–111.

55. Rourke BP, Fuerst DR: *Learning Disabilities and Psychosocial Functioning.* New York: Guilford Press, 1991.

56. Kraus JF: Epidemiological features of brain injury in children: Occurrence, children at risk, causes and manner of injury, severity, and outcomes. In: Broman SH, Michel ME, eds. *Traumatic Head Injury in Children.* New York: Oxford University Press, 1995:55–69.

57. Yeates KO: Closed-head injury. In: Yeates KO, Ris MD, Taylor HG, eds. *Pediatric Neuropsychology: Research, Theory, and Practice.* New York: Guilford Press, 2000:92–116.

58. Taylor HG, Yeates KO, Wade SL, Drotar D, Stancin T, Burant C: Bidirectional child-family influences on outcome of traumatic brain injury in children. *J Int Neuropsycholog Soc* 2001; **7**:755–767.

59. Ewing-Cobbs L, Iovino I, Fletcher JM, *et al.*: Academic achievement following traumatic brain injury in children and adolescents. *J Clin Exp Neuropsychol* 1991; **13**:93.

60. Baron IS, Fennell EB, Voeller EB: *Pediatric Neuropsychology in the Medical Setting.* New York: Oxford University Press, 1995.

61. Yeates KO, Taylor HG, Wade SL, Drotar D, Stancin T, Minich N: A prospective study of short- and long-term neuropsychological outcomes after traumatic brain injury in children. *Neuropsychology* 2002; **16**:514–523.

62. Ewing-Cobbs L, Levin HS, Eisenberg HM, Fletcher JM: Language functions following closed-head injury in children and adolescents. *J Clin Exp Neuropsychol* 1987; **9**:575–592.

63. Chapman SB: Discourse as an outcome measure in pediatric head-injured populations. In: Broman SH, Michel ME, eds. *Traumatic Head Injury in Children.* New York: Oxford University Press, 1995: 95–116.

64. Taylor HG, Yeates KO, Wade SL, Drotar D, Klein SK, Stancin T: Influences in first-year recovery from traumatic brain injury in children. *Neuropsychology* 1999; **13**:76–89.

65. Donders J: Memory functioning after traumatic brain injury in children. *Brain Inj* 1993; **7**:431–437.

66. Yeates KO, Blumenstein E, Patterson CM, Delis DC: Verbal learning and memory following pediatric

closed-head injury. *J Int Neuropsycholog Soc* 1995; **1**: 78–87.

67. Yeates KO, Enrile BG: (submitted for publication) Implicit memory in children with congenital and acquired brain disorder.

68. Vakil E, Jaffe R, Eluze S, Groswasser Z, Aberbuch S: Word recall versus reading speed: Evidence of preserved priming in head-injured patients. *Brain Cog* 1996; **31**:75–89.

69. Levin HS, Ewing-Cobbs L, Eisenberg HM: Neurobehavioral outcome of pediatric closed-head injury. In: Broman SH, Michel ME, eds. *Traumatic Head Injury in Children.* New York: Oxford University Press, 1995:70–94.

70. Mangeot S, Armstrong K, Colvin AN, Yeates KO, Taylor HG: Long-term executive function deficits in children with traumatic brain injuries: Assessment using the Behavior Rating Inventory of Executive Function (BRIEF). *Child Neuropsychol* 2002; **8**:271–284.

71. Miller LJ, Donders J: Prediction of educational outcome after pediatric traumatic brain injury. *Rehab Psychol* 2003; **48**:237–241.

72. Kinsella G, Prior M, Sawyer M, Murtagh D, Eisenmajer R, Anderson V, Bryan D, Klug G: Neuropsychological deficit and academic performance in children and adolescents following traumatic brain injury. *J Pediatr Psychol* 1995; **20**:753–767.

73. Yeates KO, Luria J, Bartkowski H, Rusin J, Martin L, Bigler ED: Post-concussive symptoms in children with mild closed-head injuries. *J Head Trauma Rehab* 1999; **14**:337–350.

74. Shaffer D: Behavioral sequelae of serious head injury in children and adolescents: The British studies. In: Broman SH, Michel ME, eds. *Traumatic Head Injury in Children.* New York: Oxford University Press, 1995: 55–69.

75. Williams J, Sharp GB: The neuropsychology of childhood epilepsy. In: Yeates KO, Ris MD, Taylor HG: eds. *Pediatric Neuropsychology: Research, Theory, and Practice.* New York: Guilford Press, 2000.

76. Corbett JA, Trimble MR, Nichol TC: Behavioral and cognitive impairments in children with epilepsy: The long-term effects of anticonvulsant therapy. *J Am Acad Child Psychiatry* 1985; **24**:17–23.

77. Cohen M: Auditory/verbal and visual/spatial memory in children with complex partial epilepsy of temporal origin. *Brain Cog* 1992; **20**:315–326.

78. Camfield PR, Gates R, Ronen G, *et al.*: Comparison of cognitive ability, personality profile, and school success in epileptic children with pure right versus left temporal lobe EEG foci. *Ann Neurol* 1984, **15**:122–126.

79. Dodson WE: Epilepsy and IQ. In: Dodson WE, Pellock JM, eds. *Pediatric Epilepsy: Diagnosis and Therapy.* New York: Demos, 1993:373–385.

80. Farwell JR, Dodrill CB, Batzel LW: Neuropsychological abilities of children with epilepsy. *Epilepsia* 1985; **26**:395–400.

81. Dodrill CB: Neuropsychological aspects of epilepsy. *Psychiatric Clin North Am* 1992; **15**:383–394.

82. Mitchell WG, Chavez JM, Lee H, Guzman BL: Academic underachievement in children with epilepsy. *J Child Neurol* 1991; **6**:65–72.

83. Kim WJ: Psychiatric aspects of epileptic children and adolescents. *J Am Acad Child Adolesc Psychiatry* 1991; **30**:874–886.

84. Fiordelli E, Beghi E, Boglium G, Crespi V: Epilepsy and psychiatric disturbance: A cross-sectional study. *Br J Psychiatry* 1993; **163**:446–450.

85. Mungas DM: Behavioral syndromes in epilepsy: A multivariate, empirical approach. In: Bennett TL, ed. *The Neuropsychology of Epilepsy.* New York: Plenum Press, 1992:139–180.

86. Forsythe I, Butler R, Berg I, McQuire R: Cognitive impairment in new cases of epilepsy randomly assigned to carbamazepine, phenytoin, and sodium valproate. *Dev Med Child Neurol* 1991; **33**:524–534.

87. Hara H, Fukuyama Y: Sustained attention during the interictal period of mentally normal children with epilepsy or febrile convulsions, and the influences of anticonvulsants and seizures on attention. *Jpn J Psychiatry Neurol* 1989; **43**:411–416.

88. Dodrill CB: Behavioral effects of antiepileptic drugs. *Adv Neurol* 1991; **55**:213–224.

89. Vining EPG, Mellits ED, Dorsen MM, *et al.*: Psychologic and behavioral effects of antiepileptic drugs in children: A double-blind comparison between phenobarbital and valproic acid. *Pediatrics* 1987; **80**:165–174.

90. Aldenkamp AP, Alpherts WCJ, Blennow G, *et al.*: Withdrawal of antiepileptic medication in children–effects on cognitive function: The multicenter Homfrid study. *Neurology* 1993; **43**:41–50.

91. Trimble MR, Cull C: Children of school age: The influence of antiepileptic drugs on behavior and intellect. *Epilepsia* 1988; **29**:515–519.

92. Fishman MA: *Pediatric Neurology.* Orlando, FL: Grune & Stratton, 1986.

93. Fletcher JM, Dennis M, Northrup H: Hydrocephalus. In: Yeates KO, Ris MD, Taylor HG. eds. *Pediatric Neuropsychology: Research, Theory, and Practice.* New York: Guilford Press, 2000.

94. Brookshire BL, Fletcher JM, Bohan TP, Landry SH, Davidson KC, Francis DJ: Verbal and nonverbal skill discrepancies in children with hydrocephalus: A five-year longitudinal follow-up. *J Pediatric Psychol* 1995; **20**:785–800.

95. Dennis M, Jacennik B, Barnes MA: The content of narrative discourse in children and adolescents after early onset hydrocephalus and in normally developing age peers. *Brain Lang* 1994; **46**:129–165.

96. Yeates KO, Loss N, Colvin AN, Enrile BG: Do children with myelomeningocele and hydrocephalus display nonverbal learning disabilities? An empirical approach to classification. *J Int Neuropsycholog Soc* 2003; **9**:653–662.

97. Wills KE: Neuropsychological functioning in children with spina bifida and/or hydrocephalus. *J Clin Child Psychol* 1993; **22**:247–265.

98. Yeates KO, Enrile B, Loss N, Blumenstein E, Delis DC: Verbal learning and memory in children with myelomeningocele. *J Pediatric Psychol* 1995; **20**:801–812.

99. Prigatano GP, Zeiner HK, Pollay M, Kaplan RJ: Neuropsychological functioning in children with shunted uncomplicated hydrocephalus. *Child's Brain* 1983; **10**:112–120.

100. Yeates KO, Fletcher JM, Dennis M: (in press). Spina bifida and hydrocephalus. In: Morgan JE, Ricker JH, eds. *Comprehensive Textbook of Clinical Neuropsychology.* Lisse, The Netherlands: Swets & Zeitlinger.

101. Mahone EM, Zabel TA, Levey E, Verda M, Kinsman S: Parent and self-report ratings of executive function in adolescents with myelomeningocele and hydrocephalus. *Child Neuropsychol* 2002; **8**:258–270.

102. Loss N, Yeates KO, Enrile B: Attention in children with myelomeningocele. *Child Neuropsychol* 1998; **4**:7–20.

103. Barnes MA, Dennis M: Reading in children and adolescents after early hydrocephalus and in normally developing age peers: Phonological analysis, word recognition, word comprehension, and passage comprehension skill. *J Pediatric Psychol* 1992; **17**:445–465.

104. Donders J, Rourke BP, Canady AI: Emotional adjustment of children with hydrocephalus and their parents. *J Child Neurol* 1992; **7**:375–380.

105. Fletcher JM, Brookshire BL, Bohan TP, Brandt ME, Davidson KC: Early hydrocephalus. In: Rourke BP, ed. *Syndrome of Nonverbal Disabilities: Neurodevelopmental Manifestations.* New York: Guilford Press, 1995: 206–238.

106. Holler KA, Fennell EB, Crosson B, Boggs SR, Mickle JP: Neuropsychological and adaptive functioning in younger versus older children shunted for early hydrocephalus. *Child Neuropsychol* 1995; **1**:63–73.

107. Rourke BP, Fisk JL, Strang JD: *Neuropsychological Assessment of Children: A Treatment-Oriented Approach.* New York: Guilford Press, 1986.

108. Taylor HG: Learning disabilities. In: Mash EJ, Terdal LG, eds. *Behavioral Assessment of Childhood Disorders,* 2nd ed. New York: Guilford Press, 1988:402–450.

109. Semrud-Clikeman M: *Traumatic Brain Injury in Children and Adolescents: Assessment and Intervention.* New York: Guilford Press, 2001.

110. Ben-Yishay Y, Prigatano G: Cognitive remediation. In: Rosenthal M, Griffith ER, Bond MR, Miller JD, eds. *Rehabilitation of the Adult and Child with Traumatic Brain Injury,* 2nd ed. Philadelphia: F. A. Davis Company, 1990:93–409).

111. Braga LW, de Paz AC: Neuropsychological pediatric rehabilitation. In: Christensen A, Uzzell BP, eds. *International Handbook of Neuropsychological Rehabilitation.* Dordrecht, Netherlands: Kluwer Academic Publishers, 2000:283–295.

112. Hoehn TP, Baumeister AA: A critique of the application of sensory integration therapy to children with learning disabilities. *J Learn Disabil* 1994; **27**:338–350.

113. Dawson G, Watling R: Interventions to facilitate auditory, visual, and motor integration in autism: A review of the evidence. *J Autism Develop Disord* 2000; **30**:415–421.

114. Rotenberg NA: Both sides of the story. *Am J Occ Ther* 1999; **53**:405–406.

115. Thompson RJ, Gustafson KE: *Adaptation to Chronic Childhood Illness.* Washington, DC: American Psychological Association, 1996.

116. Scorgie K, Wilgosh L, McDonald L: Stress and coping in families of children with disabilities: An examination of recent literature. *Develop Disab Bull* 1998; **26**:22–42.

117. DuPaul GJ, Kyle KE: Pediatric pharmacology and psychopharmacology. In: Roberts MC, ed. *Handbook of Pediatric Psychology,* 2nd ed. New York: Guilford Press, 1995:741–758.

118. Phelps L, Brown RT, Power TJ: *Pediatric Psychopharmacology: Combining Medical and Psychosocial Inter-*

ventions. Washington, DC: American Psychological Association, 2002.

119. Sbordone RJ, Long CJ, eds. *Ecological Validity of Neuropsychological Testing.* Delray Beach, FL: St. Lucie Press, 1995.

120. Silver CH: Ecological validation of neuropsychological assessment in childhood traumatic brain injury. *J Head Trauma Rehab* 2000; **15**:973–988.

121. Dennis M: Childhood medical disorders and cognitive impairment: Biological risk, time, development, and reserve. In: Yeates KO, Ris MD, Taylor HG, eds. *Pediatric Neuropsychology: Research, Theory, and Practice.* New York: Guilford Press, 2000:3–22.

26

The Somatoform Disorders

David Ray DeMaso, Pamela J. Beasley

Overview

It is well known that medical diseases and symptoms are not simply caused by physical conditions, but can also be influenced by a child's emotions, thoughts, and environment. Somatization describes a process in which a child and family seek medical help for symptoms which are misattributed to physical disease [1,2]. In this process, somatoform disorders represent the severe end of a continuum which includes unexplained 'functional' symptoms in the middle and everyday aches and pains at the other end [3]. There is much evidence to suggest that somatization is quite common in children and adolescents [2–4]. Pediatricians have long recognized unexplained physical symptoms as frequent and problematic in their practices [4–6].

Recurrent unexplained physical symptoms in children and adolescents generally fall into four symptom clusters: cardiovascular, gastrointestinal, pain/weakness, and pseudoneurological [7]. Large community samples have found that youngsters commonly report recurrent complaints of headache, abdominal pain, and limb pain as well as fatigue and gastrointestinal symptoms [2,4]. Somatization can also be polysymptomatic with multiple somatic complaints in one patient [7]. Physical symptom reporting increases across childhood into adolescence with females more likely to report symptoms [3]. While many physical complaints represent transient symptoms that are resolved with the pediatrician, there are some youngsters whose symptoms become disabling and functionally impairing as well as resulting in increased health care utilization [2,8–11].

The somatoform disorders are a group of emotional disorders characterized in DSM-IV-TR [11] by the production of physical symptoms with no demonstrable general medical condition that can account for the symptoms. The patient with combinations of physical and psychiatric symptoms represents a complex and challenging dilemma to even the most astute clinician. A wide differential must be considered as well as the frequent comorbidity of general medical conditions and other psychiatric disorders. This chapter presents these disorders in the order most often faced by child and adolescent psychiatrists when consulted by pediatricians in a pediatric teaching hospital (Table 26.1). The aim is to provide a practical understanding and approach to pediatric patients presenting with unexplained physical complaints.

PAIN DISORDERS

Jake is a nine-year-old boy who was admitted to the Medical Service to evaluate recurrent abdominal pain of five-months duration. A thorough work-up had failed to reveal a medical etiology for his chronic pain and nausea, so a psychiatric referral was made. On examination, Jake presented as a temperamentally anxious boy who was under a great deal of pressure to excel academically by his professional parents. He met full DSM-IV-TR criteria for an anxiety disorder. A comprehensive treatment program including cognitive behavioral techniques to reduce his anxiety, guidance for his parents, and ongoing medical follow-up resulted in a rapid reduction in Alex's symptoms of abdominal pain.

Definition

Pain of sufficient severity to warrant clinical attention is the primary DSM-IV-TR criteria for a pain disorder [11]. Psychological factors are deemed to play an

Clinical Child Psychiatry, Second Edition. Edited by W.M. Klykylo and J.L. Kay
© 2005 John Wiley & Sons Ltd.

Table 26.1 DSM-IV-TR somatoform disorders in order of frequency of psychiatric consultation in a pediatric teaching hospital.

Pain disorder
Conversion disorder
Undifferentiated somatoform disorder
Somatization disorder
Body dysmorphic disorder

---

important role in the onset, severity, exacerbation, or maintenance of the pain. The pain is not intentionally produced or feigned, nor can the pain be better accounted for by another psychiatric disorder. In addition, the pain must cause clinically significant distress or impairment in social, school, or home functioning.

Pain disorders are divided into two DSM-IV-TR subtypes: (1) pain disorders associated with psychological factors, in which emotional factors alone are judged to play a major role; and (2) pain disorders associated with psychological factors and a general medical condition, in which both together are deemed to have important roles in the onset, severity, exacerbation, or maintenance of the pain [11]. Each subtype is further classified as either acute (duration <six months) or chronic (duration >six months). Pain that is entirely related to a general medical condition is not considered a psychiatric disorder and is coded on DSM-IV-TR's Axis III.

Recurrent abdominal pain is a particularly common pediatric pain syndrome. Besides falling within the DSM-IV-TR criteria above, it is commonly defined as three or more pain episodes severe enough to affect the child's activities over a period longer than three months [3]. There is generally complete recovery between episodes. This pain syndrome is strongly associated with anxiety and depressive symptoms, anxious temperaments, and other pain syndromes (i.e., headache, limb pain, or chest pain) as well as other somatic symptoms (i.e., fatigue, dizziness, weakness, and numbness) [12]. While it is generally acknowledged that by far the most common etiology is unknown and likely functional in origin [3], there is increasing thought that recurrent abdominal pain and anxiety disorders may share a common risk factor or are different aspects of a singular causal process [12].

Epidemiology

Recurrent complaints of pediatric pain appear quite common. Headaches, recurrent abdominal pain, limb pain, and chest pain have been reported in prevalence rates ranging from 7% to 30% in both community and clinical samples [4,7]. The prevalence of pediatric pain disorders as defined by DSM-IV-TR remains to be documented in the literature.

Etiology

Psychological Theories

Psychodynamic theory holds that the defense mechanism of conversion underlies medically unexplained pain. Conversion refers to the transformation of repressed affect related to psychic conflict from the emotional realm to the physical one. The pain is viewed as symbolically representing unconscious conflicts. The symptom of pain can serve the unconscious goal of removing the individual from a conflictual situation as well as representing an unconscious form of self-punishment for unacceptable feelings [13,14].

The concept of a 'pain-prone patient or disorder' postulates that there are individuals with histories of childhood abuse or neglect who develop pain which is related to underlying feelings of guilt, depression, aggression, or loss [15,16]. Engel proposed that the experience of childhood abuse led to internalization of pain, association of pain with badness, and subsequent use of pain to alleviate feelings of guilt related to aggressive impulses toward the parent [15].

Biologic Factors

There are no unifying biologic explanations for pain disorders. The neurobiological components of pain involve complex interactions between ascending and descending pain pathways within the central and peripheral nervous systems. Endorphins and biogenic amine neurotransmitters such as serotonin and norepinephrine play important modulating roles in descending analgesic tracts. Drugs such as antidepressants that potentiate the central effects of biogenic amines have been useful in producing analgesia by increasing their concentrations in these descending pathways. Studies have shown that the concentrations of serotonin and endorphin metabolites are reduced in the spinal fluid of patients with chronic pain [17,18].

Chronic pain often causes decreased mobility and poor posture that may result in the development of pathological changes such as osteoporosis, contractures, myofibrositis, circulatory, and respiratory disturbances. These conditions often lead to stimulation of peripheral afferent fibers, which creates a 'vicious cycle of progressive deterioration' [17].

Learning Theory

Classical and operant conditioning can lead to the perpetuation of pain-related behaviors long after the initial noxious stimulus has been removed. Classical conditioning results from the repeated pairing of a neutral or conditioned stimulus with an unconditioned stimulus that evokes a response such that the neutral stimulus eventually comes to evoke the response. For example, settings that have been associated with pain may alone trigger pain-related behavior.

Operant conditioning holds that behaviors, which are rewarded, will increase in strength or frequency, while behaviors, which are inhibited or punished, will decrease. Attention and sympathy from others, euphoric effects of pain medications, and/or decrease in responsibilities may reinforce pain-related behaviors. If these behaviors or responses are reinforced early on in the course of the pain disorder, then it is likely that these behaviors will continue even after removal of the original painful stimulus. Conversely, health-related behaviors will diminish as they are no longer subject to systematic reinforcement [17,19].

Family Systems

Somatic preoccupation, recurrent pain complaints, alcohol abuse, and psychiatric disorder are factors within families that have been found to be associated with pain disorders [20,21]. Social learning theory suggests that the pain symptoms are a result of 'modeling' or 'observational learning' within the family [20]. Minuchin (1975) described four specific family transactional patterns: enmeshment, overprotectiveness, rigidity, and lack of conflict resolution [22]. Focus on the child's illness allows for avoidance of conflict within the family, which can reinforce the child's illness behavior.

Sociocultural

Studies investigating the effects of ethnicity on pain tolerance and behavior have provided mixed results. For example, some empirical studies report that Irish and Anglo-Saxons have greater pain tolerance than individuals of southern Mediterranean ethnicity, while others have found no significant differences among ethnic groups [17].

Diagnosis

Clinical Interview

In all somatoform disorders, thorough psychiatric interviews of the patient and family should be performed. The psychiatrist aims to determine if there is a psychiatric disorder present in the patient or family, to evaluate if there are etiologic factors associated with the pain syndrome, and to assess if these problems are comorbid with a pain syndrome secondary to a physical disorder or exist independently and are etiologic to the pain syndrome [23].

Close attention should be paid to current and past psychosocial stressors, in particular noting whether pain seems to be situation-dependent or temporally related to a stressor. The history of prior episodes of pain in the patient as well as of pain syndromes in other family members should be obtained [23–25].

Physical Examination

The symptoms are neuroanatomically inconsistent with known pathways or are in significant excess of what would be expected from the physical findings. If physical findings are present they are secondary to pathological changes associated with immobilization.

Studies

There are no specific laboratory abnormalities associated with pain disorders. Infrared thermography may be helpful in identifying changes in temperature and vascular flow associated with certain disorders that can cause chronic pain [17].

The MMPI has been used in the diagnostic evaluation of adults with chronic pain, and typically reveals elevations in the hypochondriasis and hysteria scales. The Personality Inventory for Children has been used for similar diagnostic purposes; however its ability to differentiate between physical and conversion symptoms is in question [26].

Differential Diagnosis

General Medical Conditions

Every child and adolescent has a psychological reaction to experienced pain. The diagnosis of disorder is made when the response is out of proportion to the general medical condition and when deficits or impairment in emotional and behavioral functioning occur.

Important physical causes of pain that can be confused with psychogenic pain disorders include headache syndromes, myofascial pain, post-traumatic syndromes, neuropathy, or tumors. Reflex sympathetic dystrophy (or complex regional pain syndrome) is characterized by pain that spreads beyond the area of injury along a dermatomal pattern resulting in a regional area of involvement. The pain is often accompanied by autonomic dysfunction, edema, movement difficulties, and dystrophy. While not thought to be causative, psychosocial stressors generally accompany and may exacerbate these disorders.

Depressive and Anxiety Disorders

Pain and depression frequently occur together. Some researchers have suggested that pain disorder may be a variant of depression. Lesse coined the term 'masked depression' to refer to clinical presentations in which pain is the primary complaint. The potential demoralization and learned helplessness experienced with pain may to lead to depressive symptoms [13,27,28]. Pain disorders should only be diagnosed if the symptoms cannot be better accounted for by depressive disorders, or if the symptoms are in excess of those associated with depression.

Anxiety is also a common comorbid condition with pain disorders. In a comparison between children with and without recurrent abdominal pain disorders, anxiety disorders were found in 79% of those with pain compared to 11% in the control group [12]. Depression was found in 43% of those with pain versus 8% of the controls [12]. It was also noted that only a small minority of these children had depression alone while the majority of patients had either an anxiety disorder alone or a mixed anxiety depression presentation [12].

Other Somatoform Disorders

Pain symptoms commonly occur in somatization disorders. The latter is diagnosed usually in adulthood with a history of symptom development often beginning in adolescence. Conversion disorders are medically unexplained deficits in motor and sensory functioning often accompanied by pain symptoms. Conversion and pain symptoms commonly occur together in patients.

Factitious Disorder

These disorders are characterized by physical symptoms, which are intentionally produced or feigned in order to assume the sick role. These disorders of illness falsification are generally described in adults though some cases in older children and adolescents have been reported [29,30]. The most common conditions falsified or induced are fevers, ketoacidosis, purpura, and infections.

Factitious disorder by proxy (or Munchausen syndrome by proxy) is the production of symptoms in another person who is under the individual's care [11,29–31]. This syndrome is most often presented with preschool children as the patient [31]. The motivation for the perpetrator's behavior has been hypothesized to be a psychological need to assume a sick role or relationship with a caring physician. An index of suspicion in the context of poorly understood symptoms combined with a thorough history is needed by physicians to make the diagnosis.

Malingering

Malingering involves the intentional production or feigning of symptoms. The motivation for the behavior is the conscious goal of gaining or avoiding something in the environment, e.g., avoiding criminal prosecution or financial gain. Generally, this diagnosis is rarely seen in pediatrics though occasionally an older adolescent with conduct or antisocial traits may present with somatic symptoms.

Course

There has been little written about the course of pain disorder in children and adolescents. Follow-up studies with patients with recurrent abdominal pain found that 25%–50% continue to suffer abdominal discomfort in adulthood [4]. There is emerging evidence regarding a specific association between childhood abdominal pain and anxiety in young adulthood [32]. The course of illness has been related to associated psychopathology, duration of pain, and extent of environmental reinforcement.

CONVERSION DISORDERS

Julie was a previously physically healthy 14-year-old girl who developed the inability to walk over a period of one month. Repeated physical examinations were normal as were X-rays of her legs. Consultation with specialists from orthopedics and neurology found normal examinations. The presenting symptoms were not explained by a general medical condition. A psychiatric consultation was requested. A psychiatric interview with Julie and her parents revealed a premorbidly emotionally healthy girl with a tendency to have frequent somatic complaints. Significant losses in this same time period included the separation of her parents along with the death of a close maternal grandmother. Her grandmother had been unable to walk for the last six months of her life due to complications of diabetes mellitus. The prior history of somatic complaints, temporally-related family stresses, and symptom model combined with symptoms unexplained by a general medical condition supported the diagnosis of a conversion disorder.

Definition

In DSM-IV-TR conversion disorders are characterized by one or more symptoms affecting voluntary motor or sensory function that suggest a neurological or other general medical condition [11]. Psychological factors are judged to be associated with the symptom because conflicts or stressors precede the initiation or exacerbation of the symptom. The symptom is not intentionally produced or feigned. After appropriate investigation, the symptom cannot be fully explained by a medical condition, by the direct effects of a substance, or as a culturally sanctioned behavior or experience. The disorder causes clinically significant distress or impairment in psychological functioning. A conversion disorder is not diagnosed when symptoms are limited to pain alone.

Conversion symptoms usually occur suddenly and temporarily. Typical sensory losses include blindness, deafness, loss of touch, pain sensation, and diplopia. Motor symptoms include paralysis, ataxia, aphonia, dysphagia, and urinary retention along with alterations in consciousness to produce seizures and unconsciousness. Pseudoseizures, unexplained falls, and fainting are the most common abnormalities, followed by gait and sensory deficits [4].

Epidemiology

The incidence of childhood conversion disorders varies among studies because of different patient populations and diagnostic criteria. In most studies the incidence varies between 0.5%–10% [33]. It is three times more common in adolescents than children and rarely occurs under age five years. Females predominate among adolescents with conversion disorders, while equal numbers of boys and girls are generally found in childhood.

Etiology

Psychological Theories
As in pain disorders, psychodynamic theory holds that the symptoms are the direct symbolic expression of an underlying psychological conflict. The unconscious conflict is 'converted' to a somatic symptom. Primary gain is obtained by keeping the conflict from consciousness and minimizing anxiety. The symptom can provide secondary gain by providing an escape from unwanted consequences or responsibilities. Some theorists hold that the symptoms do not necessarily have symbolic meaning, but may be related to more general unconscious conflicts involving dependency needs or performance anxiety [34].

Biological Factors
There is some evidence that conversion symptoms may be precipitated by excessive cortical arousal, which in turns triggers reactive inhibition signals at synapses in sensorimotor pathways by way of negative feedback relationships between the cerebral cortex and the brainstem reticular formation [17]. This is postulated to help explain the consistent relationship between stress events, reduction in anxiety, and symptom production. At present it is not thought that conversion disorders are genetically mediated conditions [3].

Learning Theory
A child may quickly learn the benefits of assuming the sick role and may be reluctant to give up the symptoms. Increased parental attention and avoidance of unpleasant school pressures may only further reinforce the symptom. Physical symptoms have been called a form of body language for children who have difficulty expressing emotions verbally [34]. Difficulties with disclosing sexual abuse or expressing anger toward parents are common communication problems, as well as high-achieving children who cannot admit they are under too much pressure.

Family Systems
Family systems play important roles in the initiation and maintenance of symptoms in the same manner as described earlier for pain disorders. Two broad patterns of disturbance among families of children with conversion disorders are common: anxious families preoccupied with disease and disorganized/chaotic families [35].

Sociocultural
Conversion disorder has been reported to be more common in rural areas, individuals of lower socioeconomic status, and in individuals less knowledgeable about medical and psychological concepts [11]. Spells or visions are common aspects of culturally sanctioned religious and healing rituals, while falling down with loss or alteration in consciousness is a feature in a variety of culture-specific syndromes. The form of symptom reflects local cultural ideas about acceptable and credible ways to express distress [11].

Diagnosis

Clinical Interview
A temporal relationship between psychological stress or conflict and the development of the conversion symptom is sought in thorough psychiatric interviews of the patient and family (Table 26.2). Prior history of conversion disorders or recurrent somatic complaints,

Table 26.2 Interview criteria important for diagnosis of a conversion disorder.

Psychological stress temporally related to symptom
Prior history of conversion symptoms
Prior history of recurrent somatic complaints
Dissociative and/or somatization disorders
Family stress and/or psychopathology
Symptom model

---

dissociative disorders, and somatization disorders are especially helpful in making the diagnosis [17]. Recent family stress, unresolved grief reactions, and family psychopathology occur at a higher frequency in children with conversion symptoms [36].

The presence of a symptom model (e.g., family member with similar deficits) is helpful in making the diagnosis. Patient with pseudoseizures have been found to have significant prior histories of trauma, especially sexual abuse [37]. On the other hand, la belle indifference and histrionic personality traits have not proven to be reliable diagnostic criteria in children and adolescents.

The diagnosis is not one of exclusion. If the consultant is unable to elicit any of the diagnostic criteria except for the motor or sensory symptoms, then the possibility of an underlying medical diagnosis should be reconsidered.

Physical Examination

The symptoms do not conform to known anatomical pathways and physiological mechanisms. If physical findings are present they may relate to either disuse atrophy or to sequelae of medical procedures.

Studies

There are no specific laboratory studies associated with conversion disorders. Video-EEG monitoring has been increasingly used to investigate seizure disorders. The lack of electrical evidence in the face of a seizure makes pseudoseizure or conversion disorder a likely diagnosis [34,38]. Drug-assisted interviews (e.g., amytal, pentothal, or methohexital) have been found to be useful in some children and adolescents [39]. The symptom can disappear transiently or even permanently following a drug-assisted interview. Psychological tests can be helpful in adding to the evidence for a conversion disorder though they cannot confirm a diagnosis [34].

Differential Diagnosis

General Medical Conditions

The major diagnostic concern is the exclusion of neurological or physical conditions. Migraine syndromes, temporal lobe epilepsy, and central nervous system tumors have presented difficult diagnostic dilemmas. Multiple sclerosis, myasthenia gravis, periodic paralysis, polymyositis, and other myopathies are important additional considerations. The psychiatrist must also be alert to the dual existence of a physical condition and a conversion disorder, e.g., seizures and pseudoseizures in the same patient.

Psychological Factors Affecting Medical Conditions

The essential DSM-IV-TR feature is the presence of one or more specific psychological or behavioral factors that adversely affect a general medical condition [11]. A mental disorder, personality traits, coping style, maladaptive health behaviors, or stress-related physiological responses are different psychological factors that can impact on a diagnosable general medical condition. This contrasts with conversion disorders where no medical condition exists to completely account for the symptoms produced.

Depressive and Anxiety Disorders

As stated earlier, depressive disorders can present with somatic symptoms in children and adolescents. Separation anxiety disorders can present with headaches, stomachaches, nausea, or vomiting at times of separation. Acute stress and post-traumatic stress disorders can present with symptoms suggestive of a conversion disorder. However, a conversion disorder should not be diagnosed if the symptoms are bettered accounted for by these disorders.

Somatoform Disorders

Conversion symptoms can occur in the course of a somatization disorder. The multiple symptom pattern of a somatization disorder contrasts with the mono-symptomatic and often time-limited presentations of conversion disorders. Pain disorder is diagnosed if the symptoms are limited to pain. Hypochondriasis usually begins in adulthood and is characterized by a preoccupation with having a serious disease. Body dysmorphic disorder does not involve motor or sensory deficits, but rather a preoccupation with defect in appearance.

Dissociative Disorders

These disorders share symptoms that may suggest neurological dysfunction and may occur in the same individual. Studies have suggested that reclassification of conversion seizures with the dissociative disorders should be considered [37]. Both diagnoses are made if conversion and dissociative symptoms appear in the same individual.

Malingering and Factitious Disorder

As described previously, these disorders involving the intentional or feigned production of symptoms are important in the differential for any somatoform disorder.

Course

Conversion symptoms typically occur suddenly and are of short duration. Pediatricians are most likely to see transient reactions while psychiatric consultation occurs in more difficult cases. Symptoms may become chronic or recurrent, especially when the precipitating stress is persistent or repetitive, when there is associated significant psychopathology, or when the symptom has significant secondary gain [17]. Patients with pseudoseizures are more likely to have recurrences than are patients with paralysis or aphonia [40,41].

Early studies reported high percentages of children and adolescents with an initial diagnosis of conversion disorder that were subsequently found to have a medical illness [13]. More recent samples have revealed a more modest risk (<10%) of faulty diagnosis in children and adolescents [4].

SOMATIZATION AND UNDIFFERENTIATED SOMATOFORM DISORDERS

Jill was a 16-year-old girl who had not felt well for over three years. She presented with symptoms of generalized weakness and fatigue. She had shown evidence for a 'strep throat' in the beginning of her illness but subsequent evaluations were normal. Additional medical work-ups by nearly a half dozen specialists found no general medical condition that could account for her symptoms. Prior to her symptoms, Jill was described as a remarkable girl with excellent grades as well as outstanding performances as a gymnast and violinist. She was noted to have good friendships though she was often viewed as intensely competitive. A conflicted relationship between her professional parents had improved at the same time that her symptoms had continued. Jill's mother had a long history of multiple somatic complaints involving multiple organ systems.

The long-standing unexplained somatic complaints and positive family history for recurrent somatic complaints, combined with the possible secondary gains of avoiding high expectations and lowering parental conflict supported the diagnosis of an undifferentiated somatoform disorder.

Definition

Somatization disorder is characterized by a chronic pattern of multiple clinically significant complaints [11]. These symptoms cannot be explained by any known physical condition. Each individual complaint is considered to be clinically significant if it results in medical treatment or causes impairment in functioning.

Each of the following DSM-IV-TR criteria [11] must have been met before age 30 years over a period of several years. There must be pain symptoms related to at least four different sites or functions. There must be a history of at least two gastrointestinal symptoms other than pain. A history of one sexual or reproductive symptom must have been present as well as one pseudoneurological symptom. These criteria are the latest modification of a disorder originally called Briquet's syndrome.

Obviously, the number of symptoms required over a several-year time period and the inclusion of criteria, which are appropriate only for postpubertal and/or sexually active patients, mitigate against the diagnosis in children. Children and adolescents are more likely to meet DSM-IV-TR criteria for an undifferentiated somatoform disorder with criteria requiring only one or more unexplained physical complaint/s, functional impairment, and a duration of six months. Symptoms of less than six months are coded in DSM-IV-TR as a somatoform disorder not otherwise specified.

Epidemiology

While somatic complaints in childhood and adolescence are common, the diagnosis of somatization disorder is rarely made before adulthood. Lifetime prevalence rates range from 0.2% to 2% among women and less than 0.2% among men [11,42]. Women have a five- to tenfold increase in the lifetime risk of the disorder compared to men [43]. In the majority of cases, the symptoms begin during adolescence. Low socioeconomic, occupational, and educational status are more common in this disorder [17].

The criteria for undifferentiated somatoform disorder in DSM-IV-TR are new so that the epidemiology is uncertain. However, child and adolescent 'somatic complaints syndromes' have been reported in studies with prevalence rates ranging from 4.5% to 15% [44–46].

Etiology

Psychological, Learning, Family System Theories
The psychodynamic, learning, and family system theories discussed earlier in relation to pain and conversion disorders influence the severity and frequency of the somatic symptoms.

Biologic Factors
Adoption studies have shown genetic factors may contribute to the development of this disorder [47,48]. Studies have also found evidence for a relationship with attention deficit hyperactivity disorder [49]. Somatization disorder is observed in 10%–20% of female first-degree relatives of probands with the disorder. Having a male or female relative with antisocial personality increases the risk for development of somatization disorder [11].

A 'hysterical' information processing pattern characterized by distractibility, difficulty distinguishing target and nontarget stimuli, and impaired verbal communication has been found in individuals with somatization disorder [17]. This pattern or deficit has been postulated to underlie the frequent physical complaints along with the vague and circumstantial processing of social and personal problems. This pattern has not been shown in child or adolescent patients.

Diagnosis

Clinical Interview
The key interview finding is a medical history involving recurrent unexplained physical complaints involving multiple systems. The four areas of recurrent symptoms are pain, gastrointestinal, sexual, and pseudoneurological complaints. There often is history of concurrent treatment from many physicians. Comorbid anxiety and depressive symptoms are common as well as conduct or substance-related disorders. On mental status examination, circumstantial, imprecise, and vague thinking may be prominent given the 'hysterical' information processing deficit described earlier.

In an undifferentiated somatoform disorder, a similar clinical picture is elicited though without the required symptom criteria. The most frequent complaints are chronic fatigue, anorexia, or gastrointestinal/genitourinary symptoms [11]. 'Neurasthenia' which is characterized by fatigue and weakness is classified in DSM-IV-TR as an undifferentiated somatoform dis-

order. This latter syndrome is historically quite similar to 'chronic fatigue syndrome' which has been a focus of attention over the past decade [50].

Physical Examination
As with conversion disorders, the symptoms do not conform to known physiological mechanisms. If physical signs are present they relate most often to the sequelae of medical procedures.

Studies
The absence of laboratory findings is characteristic. Psychological testing may be useful in understanding the individual though they cannot confirm a diagnosis. The Children's Somatization Inventory [51,52] has been used in some studies to identify children at risk. The measure is a list of 36 somatic symptoms derived from the DSM-III's somatization disorder criteria.

Differential Diagnosis

General Medical Conditions
The psychiatrist faces the challenge of identifying somatization disorder early in its course. Illnesses with vague and multiple somatic symptoms (e.g., acute intermittent porphyria, hypercalcemia, collagen vascular diseases, or multiple sclerosis) need to be ruled out.

Depressive and Anxiety Disorders
As noted previously, depressive disorders can be accompanied by multiple somatic complaints. Recurrent panic attacks and generalized anxiety disorder may be difficult to distinguish from somatization disorders. Symptoms associated with depressive and anxiety disorders encompass a broader range of complaints. In contrast, somatization disorders have a focused and primary concern with somatic complaints. Nevertheless, these disorders may be comorbid with somatization disorder.

Chronic Fatigue Syndrome
This syndrome is characterized by the onset of persistent or relapsing, debilitating fatigue often following an acute infection in a person that impairs daily activity for at least six months [50]. The fatigue cannot be explained by either medical or psychiatric illness though viral infections, immune dysfunction, and neuropsychologic problems are either inciting or perpetuating factors [50]. Additional symptoms may include muscle weakness, headaches, mild fever, painful adenopathy, and migratory arthralgia. Chronic fatigue syndrome can be a markedly impairing disorder in later childhood or adolescence [53,54].

Depression and anxiety-related symptoms are common in this syndrome. The syndrome is most likely a result of multiple etiologies of which one is an undifferentiated somatoform disorder.

Hypochondriasis

Hypochondriasis is a DSM-IV-TR somatoform disorder characterized by a preoccupation with fears of having, or the idea that one has, a serious disease based on a misinterpretation of one or more bodily signs or symptoms [11]. It is often associated with medical care dissatisfaction, deteriorating interpersonal relationships, and the risk of iatrogenic complications from excessive diagnostic procedures [3]. As a childhood symptom hypochondriasis can occur as described in this chapter's overview, but as a childhood disorder there is poor supporting literature [3,4]. This disorder develops far more commonly in adults.

Schizophrenia

Multiple somatic delusions need to be differentiated in some cases. Family history is important to illicit as there is no familial aggregation of the two disorders [17].

Malingering and Factitious Disorders

The additional presence of intentionally produced symptoms is not uncommon in somatization disorder. The majority of symptoms however are not consciously produced as in either malingering or factitious disorders.

Personality Disorders

The presence of personality disorders is very common as suggested by the frequently chaotic lifestyles in addition to the multiple somatic complaints [55]. Histrionic, borderline, and antisocial personality disorders have been most frequently associated in adults with somatization disorder [11].

Course

The course of somatization disorder is chronic, with fluctuation in the frequency and diversity of symptoms but without complete remission [56,57]. While there are few studies of children who meet the full criteria, nevertheless there are clusters of pediatric patients who experience multiple and troubling somatic complaints [58]. The diagnosis of these children would likely be consistent with DSM-IV-TR's criteria for an undifferentiated somatoform disorder.

The outcome for patients with recurrent somatic complaints is less positive when follow-up functional and psychiatric status is compared as opposed to the presence or absence of the original symptom [4]. Pseudoneurological symptoms may be especially predictive of later functional disability [4]. Chronic fatigue syndrome appears to be a nonprogressive disease with a general trend for improvement, if not complete recovery [50].

BODY DYSMORPHIC DISORDER

Alexa was a lovely 17-year-old girl who was seen in the hospital's Craniofacial Clinic due to concerns about wanting to remove a disfiguring facial scar. The plastic surgeon found the scar to be minimal or even nonexistent. The psychiatric consultant who worked in the clinic found Alexa to have a persistent and excessive concern that her scar was readily apparent to others.

Definition

Body dysmorphic disorder as characterized by DSM-IV-TR refers to a preoccupation with an imagined bodily defect or flaw in a normally appearing person [11]. If a physical anomaly is present, the concern and degree of distress exhibited by the individual is grossly out of proportion to the degree of the defect. This preoccupation causes significant distress and/or interferes with social or occupational functioning, is not better accounted for by another psychiatric disorder, and is not of psychotic proportions.

The intense preoccupation regarding a bodily defect may involve any part of the body, however it most often involves imagined or slight flaws of the face or head such as acne, scars, paleness/redness of complexion, thinning hair, facial asymmetry, or excessive facial hair. The preoccupation is frequently very distressing and difficult to resist. Associated behaviors, i.e., frequent mirror checking, questioning and reassurance seeking, or avoidance of photographs can be very time-consuming. Social avoidance, embarrassment, and ideas of reference are not uncommon.

Epidemiology

There has been little written about this disorder in the child literature, and what information does exist is in the form of case reports [59–64]. The onset seems to occur during adolescence with close to equal proportions of males and females [63–64]. Most patients are secretive about their symptoms and are reluctant to seek psychiatric treatment. Many of these patients have had consultations with surgeons and dermatologists. Reports in the literature suggest that patients wait a mean of six years before seeking psychiatric intervention [66].

Etiology

Psychological Theories

Psychodynamic theories have described the 'unconscious displacement of sexual or emotional conflict or feelings of inferiority, guilt, or poor self-image onto a body part.' [66]

Biological Factors

Many similarities exist between body dysmorphic and obsessive–compulsive disorders, and a link between the two disorders has been suggested [64,67–69].

Diagnosis

Clinical Interview

A high index of suspicion is needed as individuals with this disorder are generally embarrassed by their 'defect' and may be reluctant to discuss their concerns. Within the context of the interview, it can be difficult to distinguish between the 'overvalued idea' of body dysmorphic disorder and the fixed false belief of a delusional disorder. The patient has persistent and excessive concern that these 'defects' are readily apparent to others. Their impaired insight and judgment leads to a marked persistence in demanding inappropriate treatment [70].

Physical Examination

The physical examination does not conform to the bodily complaints.

Differential Diagnosis

Normal Appearance Concerns

Adolescence is a time of physical and emotional change, as well as a time when a great deal of attention is paid to appearance. As such, heightened concern about physical appearance is considered to be a normal part of adolescence. The disorder is differentiated by its greater distress and increased severity of symptoms.

Obsessive–Compulsive Disorder

Preoccupation with imagined bodily defect and their associated behaviors are similar to obsessions and compulsions. In obsessive–compulsive disorder the symptoms are not limited to concern about appearance.

Depressive Disorder

In depressive illnesses, mood congruent ruminations about physical appearance occur only during the episode of mood disturbance.

Anorexia Nervosa

There is intense preoccupation with fatness in anorexia nervosa. Individuals with body dysmorphic disorder do not demonstrate the dissatisfaction of generalized body image seen in eating disorders.

Gender Identity Disorder

In this disorder, the patient's preoccupation is related to feelings of discomfort with primary and secondary sexual characteristics.

Avoidant Personality Disorder/Social Phobia

Individuals may worry that actual defects in appearance may lead to embarrassment when with other people. The concerns are not as prominent, distressing, or time-consuming as in body dysmorphic disorder.

Course

The diagnosis may not be made for many years [66]. The onset may be abrupt or gradual. The patients generally present initially to specialists in dermatology or plastic surgery programs. Without treatment, body dysmorphic disorder is a chronic condition, which persists for years and perhaps decades. The body part(s) of concern may remain the same or shift over time.

Treatment of Somatoform Disorders

An Integrated Medical and Psychiatric Approach

The biological, psychiatric, and social dimensions need to be evaluated both separately and in relation to each other in all somatoform disorders [71]. Given the common 'diagnostic uncertainty' in these disorders with frequent dual medical/psychiatric diagnoses, a combined treatment program is strongly recommended. An integrated medical and psychiatric approach to somatoform illness sidesteps the organic versus psychiatric dilemma faced by the clinicians (Table 26.3) [33].

Treatment begins with the pediatric evaluation. These patients and family present the belief that there is a medical cause for their problem. Beginning with

Table 26.3 Psychiatry consultation in pediatric somatoform disorders – guidelines to an integrated medical and psychiatric approach.

Complete a psychiatric assessment
- Review histories, examinations, and studies by pediatrician and pediatric specialists
- Perform patient and family interviews
- Elicit diagnostic criteria
- Develop a developmental biopsychosocial formulation of the patient and family
- Facilitate a better understanding of experience by the patient and family

Convey developmental biopsychosocial formulation to pediatrician
- Remember somatoform illness is not a diagnosis by exclusion
- Remember symptoms can be in significant excess of what would be expected from the physical findings that are present
- Remember that physical findings may have accounted for early symptoms, but may no longer be the etiology for the current symptoms

Convene informing conference between pediatrician and family
- Convey integrated medical and psychiatric findings to family
- As family has medical model as their frame of reference, help reframe this understanding of symptoms into a developmental biopsychosocial formulation

Implement interventions in *both* medical and psychiatric domains
- Consider the following medical interventions
  - Set up ongoing pediatric follow-up appointments
  - Physical therapy or other face saving remedies may be added depending on symptoms
  - Psychopharmacology (assess for target symptoms for psychotropic medications)
- Consider the following psychiatric interventions
  - Individual psychotherapy (i.e., cognitive-behavioral intervention or other modalities)
  - Parent psychoeducation (i.e., advice, guidance, behavioral recommendations, etc.)
  - Family therapy
  - System intervention (i.e., school recommendations)
  - Consider extended evaluation (rather than treatment) in situation of diagnostic uncertainty

---

the pediatrician (or physician primarily responsible) the evaluation should include both medical and psychosocial histories. This integrated approach allows for the exploration of both physical and psychological factors, which may be contributing to the clinical presentation. In many cases, reassurance and suggestion from the pediatrician that the symptom will improve is helpful [34]. However, in more complicated cases psychiatric consultation and intervention is indicated.

Families of youngsters with somatoform disorders can be resistant to referral. The family can be told by the pediatrician that he or she is requesting a consultation as part of a full evaluation that includes all aspects of the child. The pediatrician can facilitate the referral and subsequent treatment recommendations by establishing communication with the psychiatrist prior to the actual referral. The pediatrician should not send the family away after a mental health referral, but rather communicate to the family that he or she will integrate the psychiatric results to obtain a more complete understanding of the child's symptomatology.

The psychiatrist should take a full history and mental status examination being alert to the areas highlighted in the previous clinical interview sections. This assessment should include both the patient and his parents (or caretakers). In addition, close attention during the interviews to the patient's and the family's 'narrative' or 'story' is important. This process of narration alone will frequently allow the family to better understand and gain perspective on their current experience. It will allow the psychiatrist the opportunity to later help the family 'make meaning' of their experience by understanding and using the 'family's own words.'

The formulation of the problem is crucial. Families come in believing that the symptom picture is due to a general medical condition. They have a narrow medical model view. This view of the problem needs to be reframed to a developmental biopsychosocial understanding. Once the psychiatric assessment is complete, the psychiatrist should begin by communicating this understanding to the pediatrician. In doing so, the psychiatrist should be alert to the frustration engendered in physicians by these patients, as they may not be felt to be 'deserving' of the sick role. Other reactions have included dismissing the patient as being 'hysterical' or pursuing the 'million dollar work-up' [14].

With acceptance of the formulation by the pediatrician, the next step is an 'informing conference' that includes both the physician and family. The psychiatrist may or may not attend this meeting depending on the comfort and expertise of the pediatrician. In a supportive and nonjudgmental manner, the pediatrician should present the patient and the family with both the medical and psychosocial findings. The family should be told that many important things have been discovered, e.g., 'We have good news we have ruled out a number of serious illness . . .' Statements such as 'We couldn't find anything . . . It's in your mind . . . The symptoms are not real . . .' should be avoided. Close attention to the 'family's words' allows them to be integrated into the biopsychosocial formulation, thereby facilitating family acceptance.

Following an acceptance of a new formulation of the problem, the pediatrician and psychiatrist together can facilitate the formation of an integrated medical and psychiatric team. This team supports both the pediatrician's ongoing monitoring and treatment for possible physical illness and the psychiatrist's interventions [13].

Management and Treatment

The pediatrician can provide ongoing follow-up while avoiding unnecessary medical investigations and procedures. The use of physical therapy with a graduated return to the child's usual activities is a helpful intervention for many patients. The pediatrician may initiate benign face-saving remedies, e.g., lotions, vitamins, slings, heating pads, etc., during acute phase [3].

Psychiatric treatment is directed toward understanding the child and family's dynamics and reasons for assuming the sick role. The goal is to help the child and family to develop a 'coping approach' [72]. Psychoeducation can be a first intervention that is directed at understanding and adhering to treatment regimens, clarifying when to worry about symptoms and when not to worry, enhancing communication with treating professionals, and using problem-solving coping techniques [3]. Potential interventions include individual, behavioral, cognitive, family, and pharmacologic therapies.

Children with high levels of 'psychological insight' can benefit from individual psychotherapy. Psychodynamic therapy may be helpful in identifying unconscious conflicts, which may be maintaining symptoms. Expression of feelings can be facilitated, and more adaptive coping mechanisms can be encouraged. Behavioral modification techniques are common interventions especially in families less psychologically minded [33]. The therapy should be aimed at reinforcing health-related behaviors and diminishing pain or physical complaints. Techniques such as hypnosis,

biofeedback, and relaxation training can be used to teach the patient the control he or she can have over certain physiological processes such as autonomic system activity [3]. Cognitive behavioral therapy can be helpful in identifying negative, maladaptive thoughts or emotions which can increase the degree of pain, suffering, and disability [73].

Family therapy and parent guidance are important components of any treatment program. Family therapy should explore ways in which the child's symptoms may serve to stabilize the system, i.e., focus on the symptoms allows for avoidance of conflict. The family should be discouraged from reinforcing the symptoms, and learn ways of providing positive reinforcement for improvement of functioning. The child should be assisted in abandoning the sick role through the encouragement of developmentally appropriate activities, which can lead to a sense of mastery.

It is not uncommon for families to remain resistant to psychiatric intervention. In these cases it is helpful for the psychiatrist to remain a consultant to the pediatrician, through advising alternative ways in which the physician can decrease reinforcement for the sick role as well as encouraging mobilization of the patient. The psychiatrist can also help advise regarding the need for social service intervention around possible parental neglect, i.e., seeking multiple unnecessary medical procedures.

Pharmacotherapy

There is little information in the literature pertaining to pharmacological treatment of somatoform disorders in the pediatric population. As has been noted previously, comorbid psychiatric disorders are common in somatizing patients as well as those meeting DSM-IV-TR criteria for a somatoform disorder. The target symptoms of mood and anxiety disorders may respond to pharmacotherapy. Clinical experience suggests that these disorders will respond to psychotherapy and medications even when somatization complicates the picture [3].

For chronic pain disorders, tricyclic and serotonergic antidepressants have been effective in adult populations [74–76]. While there is an extensive literature [77] on the use of analgesics for the treatment of acute pediatric pain, there are significant limitations in existing data for the use of these medications for childhood pain disorders. For instance, while 84% of 25 children with recurrent abdominal pain responded to a citalopram trial, the study is limited by its open-trial methodology and small sample size [78]. Clinical experience would suggest that the psychiatrist and pediatrician must be alert not to under-treat pain in the context of a presentation that has both psychological and physical contributing factors. Medication targeting the pain associated with the specific general medical condition should be an important consideration in an integrated medical and psychiatric intervention program. It is important for physicians to be alert to the use of analgesics to treat pain due to a general medical condition. Under-treated physical pain will only exacerbate any associated psychological factors, maintain functional disability, and undermine the treatment alliance.

The pediatric literature regarding the psychopharmacological treatment of body dysmorphic disorder is sparse, consisting of several case reports and small open clinical trials [61,64,67,68]. In these studies, the selective serotonin reuptake inhibitors were judged to be effective in treating body dysmorphic disorder as evidenced by reductions in preoccupation about appearance and improvement in functioning. Nevertheless, the most effective treatment strategy appears to be a combination of pharmacologic, behavioral, and family therapies [63,64].

Specifics for Undifferentiated Somatization Disorder

While the integrated medical and psychiatric approach is also applicable for somatization disorders, Cloninger (1994) described the particular importance of establishing the diagnosis along with developing a therapeutic alliance [17]. He noted the importance of explaining to patients about their disorder so that they can manage their own life more effectively. The number of doctors needs to be limited as well as the number of diagnostic evaluations and treatments. Treatment and attention should be directed toward personal and social problems rather than somatic complaints. Prescription medications need to be kept at a minimum. With comorbid anxiety or depressive disorders appropriate psychotropic medications can be considered. Firm limits on excessive or manipulative demands from the patient need to be maintained.

Finally, it should be remembered that cases identified in adolescence might represent the early presentation of somatization disorder. While there is no supporting research, aggressive intervention is indicated before establishment of an ingrained 'sick role.' Multimodal interventions including psychotherapy, cognitive behavioral methods, family therapy, and inpatient psychiatry admission have all been used in the treatment depending on the formulation of the problems in each individual case.

Conclusion

Unexplained somatic complaints in children and adolescents represent a significant challenge to the consulting psychiatrist and his pediatric colleagues. The economic costs of somatization are great, in terms of loss of patient and family productivity and the negative impact on health care costs and the delivery of services [3,4]. The continuity of these disorders from childhood through adulthood is in need of further study to help the early identification of those 'at risk' for chronic disabling illness. Clinical outcome studies are needed to assess impact of integrated medical and psychiatric treatment interventions in children and adolescents.

References

1. Murphy MR: Somatization: Embodying the problem. *BMJ* 1989; **298**:1331–1332.
2. Campo JV, Jansen-McWilliams L, Comer DM, Kelleher KJ: Somatization in pediatric primary care: Association with psychopathology, functional impairment, and use of services. *J Am Acad Child Adolesc Psychiatry* 1999; **38**:1093–1101.
3. Fritz GK, Fritsch S, Hagino O: Somatoform disorders in children and adolescents: A review of the past 10 years. *J Am Acad Child Adolesc Psychiatry* 1997; **36**:1329–1338.
4. Campo JV, Fritsch SL: Somatization in children and adolescents. *J Am Acad Child Adolesc Psychiatry* 1994; **33**:1223–1235.
5. Garralda ME, Bailey D: Psychosomatic aspects of children's consultation in primary care. *Arch Psychiatry Neurol Sci* 1987; **236**:319–322.
6. Garralda ME, Bailey D: Paediatric identification of psychological factors associated with general paediatric consultations. 1990; **34**:303–312.
7. Garber J, Walker LS, Zeman J: Somatization symptoms in a community sample of children and adolescents: Further validation of the children's somatization inventory. *Psychol Assess* 1991; **3**:588–595.
8. Belmaker E, Espinoza R, Pogrund R: Use of medical services by adolescents with non-specific somatic symptoms. *Int J Adolesc Med Health* 1985; **1**:150–156.
9. Robinson JO, Alverez JH, Dodge JA: Life events and family history of children with recurrent abdominal pain. *J Psychosom Res* 1990; **34**:171–181.
10. Livingston R: Children of people with somatization disorder. *J Am Acad Child Adolesc Psychiatry* 1993; **32**:536–544.
11. American Psychiatric Association: *Diagnostic and Statistical Manual of Mental Disorders (DSM-IV-TR)*, 4th ed. Text Revision. Washington: American Psychiatric Association, 2000.
12. Campo JV, Bridge J, Ehmann M, Altman S, Lucas A, Birmaher B, Di Lorenzo C, Iyengar S, Brent DA: Recurrent abdominal pain, anxiety, and depression in primary care. *Pediatrics* 2004; **113**:817–824.
13. Ramsay AR: The relationship of pathogenetic mechanisms to treatment in patients with pain. *Psychother Psychosom* 1984; **42**:69–79.

14. Stinnett JL: The functional somatic symptom. *Psych Clin N Am* 1987; **10**:19–33.

15. Engel GL: Psychogenic pain and the pain-prone patient. *Am J Med* 1959; **26**:899–918.

16. Roy R: Engel's pain-prone disorder patient: 25 years after. *Psychother Psychosom* 1985; **43**:126–135.

17. Cloninger CR: Somatoform and dissociative disorders. In: Winokur G, Clayton PJ, eds. *The Medical Basis of Psychiatry*, 2nd ed. Philadelphia: WB Saunders Co, 1994:169.

18. Kaufman DM: *Clinical Neurology for Psychiatrists*, 3rd ed. Philadelphia: WB Saunders, 1990:286.

19. Fordyce WE, Fowler RS, Lehmann JF, *et al.*: Operant conditioning in the treatment of chronic pain. *Arch Phys Med Rehab* 1973; **54**:399–408.

20. Jamison RN, Walker LS: Illness behavior in children of chronic pain patients. *Int J Psychiatry Med* 1992; **22**:329–342.

21. Mohamad SN, Weisz GM, Waring EM: The relationship of chronic pain to depression, marital adjustment, and family dynamics. *Pain* 1978; **5**:285–292.

22. Minuchin S, Baker L, Rosman BL, *et al.*: A conceptual model of psychosomatic illness in children. *Arch Gen Psychiatry* 1975; **32**:1031–1038.

23. Mufson MJ: Chronic pain syndrome: Integrating the medical and psychiatric evaluation and treatment. In: Branch WT, ed. *Office Practice of Medicine*, 3rd ed. Philadelphia: WB Saunders, 1994:1019–1027.

24. McGrath PJ: Annotation: Aspects of pain in children and adolescents. *J Child Psychol Psychiatry* 1995; **36**:717–730.

25. Jellinek MS, Herzog DB: Introduction to psychiatric consultation with children. In: Cassem NH, ed: *Massachusetts General Hospital Handbook of General Psychiatry*, 3rd ed. St. Louis: Mosby Year Book, 1991:131.

26. Pritchard CT, Ball JD, Culbert J: Using the Personality Inventory for Children to identify children with somatoform disorders: MMPI findings revisited. *J Pediatr Psychol* 1988; **13**:237–245.

27. Rubin EH, Zorumski CF, Guze SB: Somatoform disorders. In: Millo T, Klerman GL, eds. *Contemporary Directions in Psychopathology: Toward the DSM-IV.* New York: Guilford Press, 1986:520–533.

28. Davidson J, Krishnan R, France R: Neurovegetative symptoms in chronic pain and depression. *J Affect Disorders* 1985; **9**:213–218.

29. Schreier HA, Libow JA: *Hurting for Love Munchausen by Proxy Syndrome.* New York: Guilford Press, 1993.

30. Libow JA: Child and adolescent illness falsification. *Pediatrics* 2000; **105**:336–342.

31. Rosenberg DA: Web of deceit: A literature review of Munchausen by proxy syndrome. *Child Abuse Neglect* 1987; **11**:547–563.

32. Campo JV, Di Lorenzo C, Chiappetta L, Bridge J, Colburn KD, Gartner CJ, Gaffney P, Kocoshis S, Brent D: Adult outcomes of pediatric recurrent abdominal pain: Do they just grow out of it? *Pediatrics* 2001; 108:e1.

33. Woodbury MM, DeMaso DR, Goldman SJ: An integrated medical and psychiatric approach to conversion symptoms in a four-year-old. *J Am Acad Child Adolesc Psychiatry* 1992; **31**:1095–1097.

34. Nemzer ED: Somatoform disorders. In: Lewis M, ed. *Child and Adolescent Psychiatry A Comprehensive Textbook*. Baltimore: Williams & Wilkins, 1991:697.

35. Gratton-Smith P, Fairley M, Procopis P: Clinical features of conversion disorder. *Arch Dis Child* 1988; **63**:408–414.

36. Maloney MJ: Diagnosing hysterical conversion reactions in children. *J Pediatr* 1980; **97**:1016–1020.

37. Bowman ES, Markand ON: Psychodynamics and psychiatric diagnoses of pseudoseizure subjects. *Am J Psychiatry* 1996; **153**:57–63.

38. Kotagal P, Costa M, Wyllie E, Wolgamuth B: Paroxysmal nonepileptic events in children and adolescents. *Pediatrics* 2002; **110**(4):e46.

39. Weller EB, Weller RA, Fristad MA: Use of sodium amytal interviews in pre-pubertal children: Indications, procedure, and clinical utility. *J Am Acad Child Psychiatry* 1985; **24**:747–749.

40. Hafeiz HB: Hysterical conversion: A prognostic study. *Br J Psychiatry* 1980; **136**:548–551.

41. Weintraub MI: *Hysterical Conversion Reactions: A Clinical Guide to Diagnosis and Treatment.* New York: Spectrum, 1983.

42. Cloninger CR, Reich T, Guze SB: The multifactorial model of disease transmission: III. Familial relationship between sociopathy and hysteria (Briquet's syndrome). *Br J Psychiatry* 1975; **127**:11–22.

43. Cloninger CR, Martin RL, Guze SB, *et al.*: A prospective follow-up and family study of somatization in men and women. *Am J Psychiatry* 1986; **143**:873–878.

44. Achenbach TM, Conners CK, Quay HC, *et al.*: Replication of empirically derived syndromes as a basis for taxonomy of child/adolescent psychopathology. *J Abnorm Child Psychol* 1989; **17**:299–323.

45. Garrick T, Ostrov E, Offer D: Physical symptoms and self-image in a group of normal adolescents. *Psychosomatics* 1988; **29**:29:73–80.

46. Offord DR, Boyle MH, Szatmari P, *et al.*: Ontario Child Health Study: II. Six-month prevalence of disorder and rates of service utilization. *Arch Gen Psychiatry* 1987; **44**:832–836.

47. Bohman M, Cloninger CR, von Knorring A-L, *et al.*: An adoption study of somatoform disorders: III. Cross-fostering analysis and genetic relationship to alcoholism and criminality. *Arch Gen Psychiatry* 1984; **41**:872–878.

48. Cloninger CR, Sigvardsson S, von Knorring A-L, *et al.*: An adoption study of somatoform disorders: II Identification of two discrete somatoform disorders. *Arch Gen Psychiatry* 1984; **41**:863–871.

49. Morrison JR, Stewart MA: The psychiatric status of the legal families of adopted hyperactive children. *Arch Gen Psychiatry* 1973; **28**:888–891.

50. Dale JK, Straus SE: The chronic fatigue syndrome: Considerations relevant to children and adolescents. *Adv Pediatr Infect Dis* 1992; **7**:63–83.

51. Walker LS, Greene JW: Children with recurrent abdominal pain and their parents: More somatic complaints, anxiety and depression than other families? *J Pediatr Psychol* 1989; **14**:231–243.

52. Walker LS, Garber J, Greene JW: Somatization symptoms in pediatric abdominal pain patients: Relation to chronicity of abdominal pain and parent somatization. *J Abnorm Child Psychol* 1991; **19**:379–394.

53. Garralda ME, Rangel L: Chronic fatigue syndrome in children and adolescents. *J Child Psychol Psychiatry Allied Disciplines* 2002; **43**:169–176.

54. Garralda ME, Rangel L: Impairment and coping in children and adolescents with chronic fatigue syndrome:

A comparative study with other paediatric disorders. *J Child Psychol Psychiatry Allied Disciplines* 2004; **45**:543–552.

55. Bass C, Murphy M: Somatoform and personality disorders: Syndromal comorbidity and overlapping developmental pathways. *J Psychosom Res* 1995; **39**:403–427.

56. Guze SB, Perley MJ: Observations on the natural history of hysteria. *Am J Psychiatry* 1963; **119**:960–965.

57. Guze SB, Cloninger CR, Martin RL, *et al.*: A follow-up and family study of Briquet's syndrome. *Br J Psychiatry* 1986; **149**:17–23.

58. Kriechman AM: Siblings with somatoform disorders in childhood and adolescence. *J Am Acad Child Adolesc Psychiatry* 1987; **26**:226–231.

59. Thomas CS: Dysmorphophobia: A question of definition. *Br J Psychiatry* 1984; **144**:513–516.

60. Braddock LE: Dysmorphophobia in adolescence: A case report. *Br J Psychiatry* 1982; **140**:199–201.

61. El-khatib ME, Dickey TO: Sertraline for body dysmorphic disorder. *J Am Acad Child Adolesc Psychiatry* 1995; **34**:1404–1405.

62. Tanquary J, Lynch M, Masand P: Obsessive compulsive disorder in relation to body dysmorphic disorder. *Am J Psychiatry* 1992; **149**:1283–1284.

63. Phillips KA, Atala KD, Albetini RS: Case study: Body dysmorphic disorder in adolescents. *J Am Acad Child Adolesc Psychiatry* 1995; **34**:1216–1220.

64. Phillips KA, McElroy SL, Keck PE, *et al.*: Body dysmorphic disorder: 30 cases of imagined ugliness. *Am J Psychiatry* 1993; **150**:302–308.

65. Adreasen NC, Bardach J: Dysmorphophobia: Symptom or disease? *Am J Psychiatry* 1977; **134**:673–675.

66. Phillips KA: Body dysmorphic disorder: The distress of imagined ugliness. *Am J Psychiatry* 1991; **148**:1138–1149.

67. Hollander E, Cohen LJ, Simeon D: Body dysmorphic disorder. *Psych Ann* 1993; **23**:359–364.

68. Hollander E, Cohen LJ, Simeon D: Fluvoxamine treatment of body dysmorphic disorder. *J Clin Psychopharm* 1994; **14**:75–77.

69. Hollander E, Neville D, Frenkel M, *et al.*: Body dysmorphic disorder: Diagnostic issues and related disorders. *Psychosomatics* 1992; **33**:156–165.

70. Munro A, Stewart M: Body dysmorphic disorder and the DSM-IV: The demise of dysmorphophobia. *Can J Psychiatry* 1991; **36**:91–96.

71. Richtesmeier AJ, Aschkenasy JR: Psychological consultation and psychosomatic diagnosis. *Psychosomatics* 1988; **29**:338–341.

72. Schulman J: Use of a coping approach in the management of children with conversion reactions. *J Am Acad Child Adolesc Psychiatry* 1988; **27**:785–788.

73. Turner JA, Romano JM: Cognitive-behavioral therapy for chronic pain patients. In: Loeser JD, Egan KJ, eds. *Managing the Chronic Pain Patient.* New York: Raven Press, 1989:95104.

74. Ansari A: The efficacy of newer antidepressants in the treatment of chronic pain: A review of the current literature. *Harv Rev Psychiatry* 2000; **7**:257–277.

75. Carter GT, Sullivan MD: Antidepressants in pain management. *Curr Opn Investig Drugs* 2002; **3**:454–458.

76. Goldstein DJ, Lu Y, *et al.*: Effects of Duloxetine on painful physical symptoms associated with depression. *Psychosomatics* 2004; **45**:17–28.

77. Berde CB, Sethna NF: Analgesics for the treatment of pain in children. *New Engl J Med* 2002; **347**:1094–1103.

78. Campo JV, Perel J, Lucas A, Bridge J, Ehmann M, Kalas C, Monk K, Axelson D, Birmaher B, Ryan N, DiLorenzo C, Brent DA: Citalopram treatment of pediatric recurrent abdominal pain and comorbid internalizing disorders: An exploratory study. *J Am Acad Child Adolesc Psychiatry* 2004; **43**(10):1234–1242.

27

Sleep Disorders

Martin B. Scharf, Cyvia A. Scharf

Introduction

After the birth of our first child 24 years ago, I (M.B.S.) experienced a clinical awakening, when on the first night home from the hospital, my daughter wouldn't sleep or stop crying. The cacophonous screaming was upsetting us all and adding to our frustration. When Grandma awoke, came downstairs, and took the child, it was if the Marines had landed: Rosalyn instantly quieted and went to sleep.

Few things can disrupt a healthy family like a sleepless child. Sleep occupies the preponderance of the first few months of life and, but as human beings we intuitively know that it is important for growth, development, and good health. Disordered sleep can be an indication of other problems, both physiologic and psychologic, and can also contribute to and exacerbate medical and psychiatric conditions.

Unfortunately, most physicians, even those earning their degrees as recently as the early 1990s, have been exposed to less than two hours of didactic material regarding sleep throughout their medical training [1]. Although adult psychiatrists have a better appreciation for insomnia because of its ubiquity in their patients, little is generally taught regarding childhood sleep disorders. Our goal in this chapter is to familiarize the reader with the nuances of normal sleep and to provide insight into the array of childhood sleep disorders and their diagnosis, management, and treatment.

Normal Sleep

Normal sleep is characterized by recurring cycles of nonrapid eye movement (NREM) sleep followed by rapid eye movement (REM) sleep, each cycle lasting on average between 70 and 90 minutes in adults. NREM sleep is divided into four stages. *Stage 1* is the lightest stage and is generally a transient state; it is the stage associated with falling asleep and usually also occurs after body movements or arousals. Individuals can be easily awakened from stage 1 sleep and their eyes move slowly under the eyelids. Heart rate and breathing tend to slow down, and thought patterns are still associated with daytime activity. Individuals awakened from this stage of sleep often state that they were not sleeping and indicate an awareness of things occurring around them but indeed may even have been snoring. *Stage 2* is a deeper stage of sleep characterized by electroencephalogram (EEG) patterns known as *sleep spindles* and *K-complexes*. Eye movements are absent, and the heart rate continues to slow, as does respiration. Individuals awakened from this stage of sleep generally have little or no recall. *Stages 3 and 4* are the deepest stages of sleep, in which high-voltage slow waves are prominent EEG patterns. These stages include the slowest rates of breathing and heart activity and the highest frequency of night sweats. Recall is difficult to obtain from this sleep stage, in part because individuals are very slow to awaken.

In REM sleep, eyes move rapidly under the eyelids. Heart rate and breathing become irregular and more rapid. There is a loss of muscle tone that results in a generalized paralysis except for twitches of small peripheral muscles. Watching a dog or cat sleeping – seeing it twitch its paws, moves its whiskers, and make yelping noises – one can appreciate that even pets dream; we wonder what they think they are chasing. The paralysis observed in REM sleep seems to allow a safe expression of dream material by preventing people from acting out their dreams [2].

Newborn sleep is described as either quiet, active, or indeterminate. Quiet sleep consists of NREM sleep, but with marked differences from that of adults. NREM sleep is undifferentiated, and infants do not experience stage 1 to 4 sleep until sometime during their first year. Newborns also show no loss of muscle

Clinical Child Psychiatry, Second Edition. Edited by W.M. Klykylo and J.L. Kay
© 2005 John Wiley & Sons Ltd.

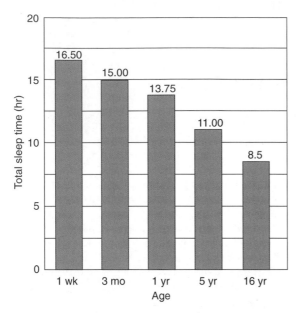

Figure 27.1 The development of sleep patterns, states, and stages. 0–3 months: longest sleep period less than four hours; sleep spindles develop at trace alternate pattern disappears; true slow waves with delta activity appear; sleep scoring consistent of three states – active (REM), quiet (NREM), indeterminate (ambiguous). 3–6 months: clear sleep cycles develop; sleep consolidated into four to five periods a day; two-thirds of sleep occurs at night; diurnal pattern begins to develop. 6 months: fewer daytime sleep periods; sleep gets progressively longer at night; longest sleep period now about seven hours. 5 years: sleeps 10–12 hours consisting chiefly of nighttime sleep and one daytime nap. The amount of sleep gradually decreases throughout childhood and adolescence until it reaches the average eight hours of sleep per night experienced by adults.

tone, and as a result, their REM sleep is more clear and is referred to as active sleep, because of the eye movements, grimacing and sucking activity, twitching and writhing body movements and the increased level of physiologic activity.

Newborn infants sleep approximately 16 hours per day in polyphasic, short bursts of 2–4 hours. REM or active sleep occupies the majority of total sleep time (Figure 27.1) [3–5]. Infants usually experience REM periods with the onset of sleep, unlike adults, whose *REM latency* (time from sleep onset to the first REM period) is 70 to 90 minutes [6]. Newborns' sleep time decreases over the course of the first year, and they

continue to nap regularly until the age of about two or three years. Between the ages of two and five years, sleep is consolidated and reduced to a 10-hour period, with most children giving up daytime naps between three and five years of age [7–10].

By the end of their third month, infants exhibit the four distinct stages of NREM sleep as well as regular patterns of REM and NREM sleep, with little or no indeterminate sleep. Sleep cycles that last approximately 40–60 minutes at this age will gradually lengthen to the levels of adolescence and adulthood. The longest sleep period now tends to occur at night, and most children sleep through the night by six months of age [7–10].

Sleep patterns at all ages alternate through cycles that are generally 90 minutes in length; 5%–10% of the night is spent in stage 1, 50% in stage 2, 20% in either stage 3 or 4 sleep, and a similar amount in REM sleep. Young children spend more time in *slow wave* (stages 3 and 4) sleep than do adults. The overall sleep cycle is shorter in children, averaging less than 60–70 minutes [7–10].

In children, slow wave sleep tends to occur with each sleep cycle. Children between two and five years of age usually obtain as much as two hours of slow wave sleep over the course of a night. This is particularly significant because the preponderance of the 24-hour total growth hormone is released during these stages of sleep. Indeed, when sleep is moved to a different time of the 24-hour day, the timing of growth hormone secretion changes accordingly [3,4].

As sleep cycles repeat throughout the night, REM sleep occupies a greater portion of each cycle, becoming as long as 40–60 minutes within the latter REM periods. Dreams occur in both REM and NREM sleep, but their characteristics are quite different. In NREM sleep, dream phenomena are concrete and more thought like; recall is less elaborate and tends to be related to activities that normally occur during the day. Dreams occurring in REM sleep are less logical, more elaborate, and are associated with emotional experiences [11–14].

Several theories exist regarding the function and purpose of dreams. Some researches have hypothesized that dreams play a role in information processing and learning; they may function to consolidate newly acquired information, thereby reconciling new information with existing memories [15,16]. The increased protein synthesis that occurs during REM sleep seems to support this view [17]: protein build-up in some synapses has been shown to strengthen those synapses, increasing their influence on postsynaptic neurons and cumulatively serving to reorganize the neural pathways

[18]. Crick and Mitchison have proposed that dreams may be important in unlearning faulty information and processing, making the subjective experience of dreaming merely a by-product of this 'waste removal' process [19].

Dreams in childhood tend to be shorter than those in adult life. The age of the child influences the subject matter: by about 12–18 months of age, the subject matter of children's dreams mirrors that of their waking fears [20]. Children's reports of their dreams are less elaborate, have less of a story line, and involve more intense imagery and emotion. It is possible that since sleep is so much deeper in children than in adults, the delay in coming to full alertness allows the dream content to escape recall, or alternatively, that the differences in recall are more apparent than real.

Dream recall is first described at approximately two years of age (Table 27.1). Children's dreams generally reflect emotionally significant events of the previous day. According to Golbin [20a], there are recognizable stages in the development of dreams. Children between three and five years of age have easily identifiable negative images, which are generally singular. By five years of age, their dreams become more complex and can symbolically reflect real situations such as family conflict. Children become active participants in their dreams, trying to run away, escape, or defend themselves. By seven or eight years of age, concrete images become rich, with some elaborate and bizarre situations.

Children can become heroes instead of simply victims and can experience pleasant sensations in their dreams. By 10–12 years of age, children often experience movements and other sensations in their dreams that can be indistinguishable from hallucinations; they can experience senses of smell, feel, and touch. By adolescence, dreams can become repetitive or continuous. One only remembers the dreams from which one awakens. Thus, when patients report frequent dreaming, they may be describing the last dream of the night from which they awoke or may also be providing an indication that frequent awakenings are occurring [20].

Sleep Hygiene

Sleep hygiene is a term used to describe the set of behaviors that influence a person's ability to initiate and maintain sleep. Good sleep hygiene can facilitate stable sleep patterns and prevent some behaviorally caused sleep disorders, whereas poor hygiene can serve to initiate or antagonize some sleep disorders. The exact behaviors of sleep hygiene may vary with a person's age, time constraints, and individual preferences, and they generally center on the themes of forming and adhering to a consistent prebedtime routine, maximizing comfort, and avoiding counterproductive habits.

Sleep Hygiene in Infants

Given the changes in sleep continuity that occur during infancy, optimal sleep hygiene behaviors vary even within this age group. Parents should generally not attempt to change the neonate's sleep patterns, because the highly fragmented nature of neonate sleep is a part of their natural development. Although it may be frustrating to parents at times, they can be reassured by the fact that severe sleep fragmentation typically does not last beyond the first 3–6 months. If an infant's sleep patterns must be modified to accommodate transient time constraints such as while traveling, it is typically more effective to facilitate the change by waking the child from sleep than attempting to force sleep at normally nonsleeping times. As the infant's sleep begins to consolidate, sleep hygiene can help facilitate the natural transition. In fact, this is a good time to start providing external cues that will help orient the child's sleep/wake patterns to adaptive cycle [21–23].

Routines

Routines serve to facilitate consistency in sleep patterns. Bedtimes and wake times should remain as constant as possible. When sleep begins to consolidate, an infant typically begins to respond to external cues that indicate when to sleep. It may be necessary at this time to supplement natural cues with parental cues. If, for example, an infant over six months of age tends to sleep more during the day than at night, it may be nec-

Table 27.1 The progression of dream content in children.

0-12 months	Shorter periods than adults; content unknown
12–18 months	Association with waking fears
2 years	Recall begins; content usually related to emotionally significant events of the previous day
3–5 years	Easily identifiable negative images
5 years	Increased complexity that may reflect reality
10–12 years	Experiences such as pleasure, smell, and touch
Adolescence	Content increasingly repetitive or continuous

essary to gradually shorten the daytime sleep period by waking the child early from his or her daytime sleep; this process should result in a lengthening of nocturnal sleep. Feedings and changings at night should be quiet, and it may help to reduce the amount of light during these times. It may also help to use loosely fitting clothing on the child at night, so that changing diapers involves less activity and stimulation [21–23].

Prior to evening bedtime, it is important to begin a bedtime ritual. Although the particular activities may vary among individuals, they should follow some guidelines. The bedtime ritual should involve activities that minimize physical activity and elicit a calming response that prepares the infant for sleep. Often, presleep rituals for infants involve parents giving them a warm bath; changing them into pajamas; reading, humming, or singing to them; changing their diapers; and feeding and burping them (not necessarily in that order.) At this point in development, the content of the reading or singing is not as important as the sound of the parent's voice and contact with the parent. The routine should remain constant from night to night: Repeating the same activities in succession at the same time each night provides additional cues that bedtime is approaching. After a good bedtime ritual, an infant should be more relaxed and mentally prepared to sleep [21–23].

Maximizing Comfort

Several steps can be taken to maximize an infant's comfort during sleep, which may help to eliminate some of the disruptions that can occur during nighttime awakenings. Although increasing comfort is helpful at any time, it is particularly appropriate if an infant experiences several nocturnal awakenings accompanied by fussing rather than a quiet return to sleep. Infants should be placed in bed awake but drowsy in a position that seems to be the most comfortable for them. It is not imperative that they be placed in a bed awake every night, however; allowing infants to fall asleep on their own while drowsy conveys to them a sense of self-ownership of the task of falling asleep. An infant may therefore be less likely to demand the attention of an adult during each nighttime arousal and may instead learn to fall back to sleep independently [21]. Making the crib itself more comfortable should also increase an infant's comfort. Parents may warm the sheets with a heating pad before placing the infant in bed (be sure to check the temperature by hand before placing the infant in bed). An article of the parent's clothing may also be placed securely in the crib to make the crib smell more familiar [22].

Nocturnal congestion may affect an infant's breathing and sleep, given their physical propensity for difficult breathing during sleep. Sleep position may have an effect on the infant's ease of breathing: slightly raising the head may reduce respiratory disturbance due to congestion [23]. Using a humidifier may also be beneficial, as might the use of an external nasal dilator (e.g., Breathe Right). In a pilot study conducted in our laboratory, we demonstrated a marked reduction in obstructive breathing events in infants suffering nasal congestion [93].

Avoiding Counterproductive Habits

Generally, these habits include anything that may interfere with the routines and comforts explained in the previous two sections. Some specifics include the following:

(1) Avoid permitting the child to dictate his or her sleep schedule after 3–6 months of age. Instead, actively provide cues that allow the child to adapt to the new sleep schedule.
(2) Avoid regularly sleeping with the child. Everyone's sleep is more disturbed from the extra movement of an additional person, and sleeping alone may reduce later separation anxiety [21,24].
(3) Avoid engaging in physically stimulating activity immediately prior to bedtime. This is most easily accomplished by planning a bedtime ritual and adhering to it.
(4) Avoid behaviors that make the child dependent on parents to fall asleep. Examples are consistently rocking the child to sleep or lying with the child until he or she is asleep. These behaviors become associated with falling asleep and can be counterproductive: because children associate parents and parental behavior as a necessary part of falling asleep, if they awake during the night, they may need the sleep onset associations to be back to sleep [21,24].

Sleep Hygiene in Older Children

As children learn to comprehend and use language, the process of sleep hygiene should evolve to incorporate these changes. Once children can understand language, it becomes easier for parents to understand their needs and for children to understand the parents' expectations.

Routines

These can become more stable once a child's sleep has consolidated. Bedtimes and wake times can be more regular and should continue to be enforced. Bedtime rituals continue to prepare a child's body and mind for sleep, but the activities change as the child becomes older. The bedtime ritual should be discussed with the child, and the length of time should be agreed on before the ritual is used. Examples of appropriate ritual activities at the age of five years include quiet play, preparing for bed (brushing teeth, changing into pajamas, etc.) reading stories in bed, and spending time quietly discussing the day's events. Most important at this age is that the child understands the progression of events. The child should know the order of activities and the time at which each activity should occur. This child should also be occasionally reminded of the planned progression throughout the ritual (e.g., 'Remember, it will be time to change into your pajamas in five minutes'.) Such reminders will help avert struggles over when to go to bed and will make bedtime a pleasurable experience for the child, rather than one of uncertainty [21]. The activities should not include physically active behavior and should instead provide a sense of closure for the day. A quiet time to talk about the day's events, for example, may provide the child a chance to voice concerns and worries, which may prevent extensive brooding and a lack of sleep after the ritual is completed [21,24].

Avoiding Counterproductive Habits

Children should not be allowed to stay up as they wish. Bedtime and wake time should be consistent and determined by the parent. Bedtime rituals are employed in part to make the parentally imposed bedtime more acceptable to the child. Children should not be allowed to routinely fall asleep in rooms other than their own bedrooms or in front of a television. If a child begins to get drowsy, he or she may go to bed early. Activities in a child's bedroom should be restricted to sleeping and bedtime rituals only, so that the child associates going to his or her bedroom with going to sleep.

Changing the child's environment after he or she has fallen asleep should be avoided. Examples of changes include moving the child to a different room or a parent leaving the room after the child has fallen asleep. Such changes may confuse the child when he or she next awakens and may make returning to sleep more difficult. These changes can be avoided by planning a bedtime ritual that places the child in his or her bedroom alone before initiating sleep.

Problems of Childhood Sleep

When sleep problems occur in children, they tend to evoke pain and discomfort in the family, often raising more concern by the parents than by the child. Disorders such a chronic bedwetting, sleepwalking, night terrors, and nightmares can affect children's opportunities to socialize and can ultimately affect their self-image and self-esteem. Circadian rhythm disturbances (which can cause difficulty in falling asleep) can result in severe daytime sleepiness, which affects school performance and self-image. In addition, sleep apnea, a condition most usually associated with middle age and older adults who are overweight, can occur in children, especially those with enlarged tonsils or nasal airway deformities. Recognizing how poor sleep can affect mood, daytime function, and overall development is an important responsibility of parents, physicians, and especially psychiatrists. Sleep laboratory evaluations are rarely necessary in children with a history of insomnia, sleepwalking, night terrors, or enuresis; however, when sleep apnea is suspected, home or laboratory recording is important. Often the polysomnogram can be preceded by an overnight oximetry screen. Our preference is to record children in their home environment whenever possible to minimize the anxiety of being away from home and to make the recording less 'hospital-like.'

Sleeplessness

Although the onset of adult-like insomnia in childhood is rare (and even more rarely diagnosed), social, environmental, psychologic, medical, and chronophysiologic factors can interfere with a child's normal pattern of sleep [25]. The importance of identifying and treating sleep disorders in childhood is underscored by the marked deficits in performance and intelligence tests demonstrated by children who are experiencing sleeping problems [25]. Children with sleeping problems may also be more likely to develop behavioral problems. One primary difference between the presentation of childhood and adult sleep disorders, however, is that it is typically the parents, not the patient, who have the complaints. Disordered sleep habits that keep the parents awake at night or influence the child's performance at school are more likely to be recognized than those that simply bring discomfort to the child (as might be more the case in adult insomnia) [21,24].

Childhood disruptions in sleep are often a source of serious frustration to parents, and they may trigger child abuse [26]. Therapy tends to focus on correcting the presenting complaint rather than determining the original cause. In most of these disorders, the child–parent interaction is a crucial part of the therapy, regardless of the underlying cause. Since children often respond differently to family authority figures, however, consulting a physician or a sleep specialist may be helpful.

CASE ONE

Recently, I (M.B.S.) saw a seven-year-old boy with a history of sleep difficulty. His parents were told that he might have attention deficit hyperactivity disorder (ADHD), but they resisted this diagnosis; to them, he just seemed extremely bright and inquisitive. By his bedtime at eight o'clock each evening, however, he would complain about his 'aching legs' and his fears and inability to sleep. He would usually end up in the parent's bed. The parents were becoming increasingly exhausted: Evan was wearing them out. When I saw Evan, he seemed extremely bright, albeit that at night he couldn't turn his mind off. I suggested that he take a hot bath two hours before bedtime and take 1 mg of melatonin 30 minutes before bedtime. He called the next morning to tell me he had slept well. On the second morning, he called to say he hadn't done well but admitted that the bath water hadn't been warm (the goal is to raise core body temperature; bath water needs to be warm enough to precipitate mild sweating within 15 minutes.) On the third morning, he again claimed success. I recommended a reduction in dose to half a tablet (0.5 mg). After a successful fourth night, I suggested putting the tablet in the bath water (placebo?). Success again. By the end of two weeks, he had given up this routine and was sleeping alone in his own bed. The ritual had reestablished sleep patterns, and he had no need for it again. The crystal baseball on my desk is a daily reminder of his parents' appreciation for the change in *their* lives.

A first major concern for 20% of parents is colic, which develops during the second or third week after birth [27]. Colic consists of extended spells of extreme fussiness, including inconsolable crying [28] and a hypertonic state characterized by clenched fists, twisting, writhing, batting, flapping, facial grimaces, and a sensitivity to light [29]. The exact cause of colic is unknown, but it may include immaturity of the central nervous system, a need to exercise the lungs [30], an allergy to cow's milk, pain from excess gas, and decreased progesterone levels [31]. Evidence suggests that colic may serve some adaptive purpose, but the negative impact on the parents' sleeping pattern and ability to cope with the child may have future deleterious effects.

Studies suggest that although colic itself usually subsides by four months of age, postcolic infants have a greater tendency toward disturbed sleep and are also more likely to develop a 'difficulty' temperament (Table 27.2). Weissbluth and colleagues reported that 76% of postcolic infants experiences problems with frequent nocturnal awakenings and generally show a shorter sleep duration [32]. Some postcolic infants are also very sensitive to changes in the sleep/wake schedule such as might occur during vacations or illnesses. Parental mismanagement of sleep patterns in postcolic infants has been implicated as a major source of later sleep problems. To avoid possible budding problems, parents should set and adhere to strict sleep/wake schedules immediately after colic has subsided. Unfortunately, the nurturing behavior and overresponsiveness learned by parents during the colic phase may antagonize the tendency toward problems caused by overstimulating children during the postcolic phase. The resulting child behaviors may include irregular sleep (settling problems and prolonged awakenings), crankiness, easy frustration, and impatience. In contrast, adherence to a sleep/wake schedule combined with good sleep hygiene can lead to a more positive infant mood, more flexible behavior, and a calmer expression of emotion [27–32].

Children typically 'settle' into mature sleeping patterns between the ages of 6 and 12 months [33]. Disturbed sleep may recur throughout early childhood, however. Reports on the prevalence of disordered sleep continue to range between approximately 25% and 33% until children reach school age [21,24]. One study of 60 children aged 15–48 months found that 42% had experienced some sleep problems [34]. Many of the earlier behavioral causes of troubled sleep surrounded a difficulty in navigating this transition into mature sleepiness patterns.

Sleep Onset-Association Disorder

Children, like adults, learn to associate certain environmental surroundings with sleep. Specific environmental cues (such as our bedrooms, our beds) alert us to the proper time and place to sleep. Even though we occasionally awaken during the night, these cues are available to reassure us that everything is as it should be and allow us to return to sleep often without the

Table 27.2 Medical associates of sleeplessness.

Colic	Inconsolable fussiness in late afternoon or evening, with manifestations such as clenched fists, twisting, writhing, batting, and facial grimaces
	Usually presents in the third or fourth week of life
	Usually subsides by three to four months of age
Sleep onset-association disorder	Child depends on specific caretaker behaviors (such as rocking) to initiate or reinitiate sleep
Feeding-related disorder	Child must feed on awakening to return to sleep
Limit-setting disorder	Failure by parents to exercise appropriate limits to child's behavior
Medical factors	Otitis media, gastroesophageal reflux, respiratory difficulties that may or may not meet the criteria for obstructive sleep apnea syndrome
Medication effects	All medications must be considered a possible cause, either by their intended effects, side effects, or withdrawal effects

awareness of having awakened. Anders and Keener [35] reported that even at two months of age, 50% of infants' nocturnal awakenings require no parental attention. A disorder arises in children, however, when they learn to associate sleep with environmental characteristics that are no longer available in subsequent nocturnal awakenings. If a child is consistently rocked to sleep, for example, the child begins to associate sleep with rocking and may have difficulty falling asleep without it. This becomes more of a problem for parents during nocturnal awakenings, because the child cannot return to sleep without active parental participation. Problematic activities include consistently moving the child after the onset of sleep or holding the child until he or she is asleep, because the child cannot reestablish these conditions without some assistance. The distinguishing feature of this particular problem is that once the 'required' conditions are reestablished, the onset of sleep occurs rapidly. Note that the problem lies not in abnormal awakenings but rather in an inability to return to sleep, which abnormally prolongs the awakenings.

The basic components of treatment for this type of disorder involve learning new associations with the onset of sleep that the child can establish without parental participation. A child must learn to go to sleep in his or her own bed alone. To facilitate this learning process, parents must remove themselves from the environment to the furthest extent possible. The child should be placed in the crib, and the parent should leave the room while the child is still awake. In the case of crying, parents should return to the room only after a predetermined period (usually no less than 15 minutes), and they should make only visual contact. This return allows the parent to show the child that he or she has not been abandoned but reaffirms that the

task of falling asleep is the child's own responsibility. The length of time between the initiating of crying and the parental response should be gradually increased. If the problem is properly diagnosed, this treatment will typically result in dramatic improvements within the first few days. Since the treatment depends on parental commitment, parents should be involved in deciding the appropriate schedule [21,24,36–39].

Feeding-Related Disorders

Although the nutritional need for nighttime feedings is gone by six months of age, such feedings may persist. Problems arise when the child associates feeding with sleep; the child must then feed to return to sleep, which results in an excessive intake of fluid. The resulting bladder distention causes frequent awakenings, producing a circular pattern of arousals followed by feeding. The child's diapers are typically soaked by morning. If this pattern of feeing persists, it may prevent the child from developing a mature sleep/wake cycle by reinforcing an altered circadian rhythm. Since the child no longer has a biologic need for nighttime feedings, treatment of this disorder consists of gradually decreasing and then ceasing feedings over 1–2 weeks [21,25,40,41].

Setting Parental Limits

As a child gets older, poor sleep may result from a lack of setting appropriate parental limits. Children presenting with this problem typically report no consistent bedtime routine. Parents may give in to a child's demands to read one more story or stay awake to watch a television program. The onset of sleep frequently occurs in atypical places such as in front of the television, resulting in poor sleep onset-associations. Parental inconsistency reinforces the child's attempts to make demands, eventually resulting in a nightly power struggle. Difficulties in setting limits may concurrently manifest in other areas of the parent–child relationship.

Treatment of this disorder focuses first on the parents. They should be educated about the use of bedtime rituals and the importance of being consistent and persistent in setting limits for their children. The creation of and adherence to a bedtime ritual that uses constant reminders to set expectations for the child can help turn bedtime into a positive experience for both parents and children. When the agreed on bedtime arrives, the child must go to bed without exception. It may be necessary at first to place barriers to keep the child in his or her bedroom, but this tactic must always be used in conjunction with proximal parent supervision.

It is important when establishing limits that parents distinguish legitimate nighttime fears from a child's attempt to stay awake by professing fears; treating legitimate nighttime fears by setting strict limits may result in serious emotional problems [21,24].

Medical or Organic Origins of Sleeplessness

Several medical conditions may result in childhood sleep difficulties. Younger children may experience an allergy to the cow's milk found in formula, resulting in frequent nocturnal awakenings and a shorter total sleep time than that of normal age cohorts [42]. Pain from otitis media is another reported source of younger childhood sleep disturbances [21]. Children with ADHD often report restlessness and frequent awakenings, although sleep latency and total sleep time are typically normal [43,44]. A number of studies of suggested that sleep disturbance in children can impact negatively on daytime function. It has been documented that sleepy children, unlike sleepy adults, can become hyperactive and show decreases in attention span and increases in activity level [45,46]. Studies involving experimental sleep restriction in children show resultant ADHD-like behavior and reduced cognitive performance [47,48]. Another study showed that 5–10-year-old boys diagnosed with ADHD were sleepier than controls [45]. This was confirmed in a study comparing Multiple Sleep Latency Tests (MSLT) in ADHD children to controls, suggesting that the attention deficits and hyperactivity may at least, in part, be due to insufficient or disordered nighttime sleep.

Picchietti has suggested that children with ADHD have a higher prevalence of periodic limb movement syndrome (PLMS) [52–55]. This is reasonable given the impact of PLMS on subsequent daytime function [56]. PLMS presents differently in children than in adults. Children with PLMS may have nonspecific symptoms like growing pains, restless sleep, complaints of insomnia and often many of these issues go unrecognized by parents of family members. In many cases the movements are just amusing and topics of discussion among family and friends but never meet the ears of the clinician.

Another disorder associated with PLMS is restless legs syndrome. In adults with restless legs, patients describe a sensory discomfort in their legs during periods of quiescence [56]. The majority of patients with restless legs also experience PLMS during sleep [56]. In children with restless legs the symptoms may manifest with 'growing pains' [49]. These are limb discomforts that do not meet the criteria for other diagnostic criteria, such as arthritis or other types of joint pathology. While the cause of 'growing pains' is unknown a recent review of the literature suggests that many children with growing pains meet the criteria for restless legs syndrome [50,51].

The Internal Restless Leg Syndrome Study Group have recently provided revised criteria for this diagnosis [56]:

(a) An urge to move the legs usually accompanied or caused by uncomfortable and unpleasant sensations in the legs. (Sometimes the urge to move is present without the uncomfortable sensations and sometimes the arms or other body parts are involved in addition to the legs).

(b) The urge to move or unpleasant sensations begin or worsen during periods of rest or inactivity such as lying or sitting.

(c) The urge to move or unpleasant sensations are partially or totally relieved by movement, such as walking or stretching, at least as long as the activity continues.

(d) The urge to move or unpleasant sensations are worse in the evening or night than during the day or only occur in the evening or night. (When symptoms are very severe, the worsening at night may not be noticeable but must have been previously present).

Many chronic conditions are also the cause of disrupted sleep, including migraine headaches, asthma, diabetes, gastroesophageal reflux, seizures, and neurologic deficits and disorders [24]. In most of these instances, therapy involves treatment medical problems and concurrently applying good sleep hygiene principles.

Medications

Medications may interfere with a child's ability to sleep. Paradoxically, sedating antihistamines may actually *cause* insomnia. Major sedatives, antihistamines, and short-acting benzodiazepines all have the potential for residual grogginess the next day, which may negate the effects of any improvements in sleep. Other medications, such as antibiotic preparations or non-prescription combination cold remedies, have also been noted to disturb sleep in children. If a medication is causing sleeplessness, it should be discontinued if possible. If discontinuation is not an option, the treatment should focus on examining the dosing regimen; changing the dose or the time the medication is taken may ameliorate the symptoms, as may changing to another drug of the same class [25].

Psychosocial Factors

A range of psychologic factors may also influence a child's quality of sleep. It is important to properly diagnose and address these issues to prevent their evolution into even more serious emotional disturbances. Childhood affective disorders tend to negatively affect sleep continuity. Children in a depressed mood frequently experience early morning awakenings, sleep onset problems, and more frequent nighttime arousals [57–60]. Maternal depression is also associated with sleep problems [25]. Emotional stressors such as family tension or grieving the death of a family member are associated with disrupted sleep. Five specific stressors have been found to be more prevalent in children with sleep disorders than in other children. These include: (1) an accident or illness in the family; (2) the unaccustomed absence of the mother during the day; (3) a depressed mood of the mother; (4) co-sleeping (i.e., sleeping with a parent); and (5) maternal attitude of ambivalence toward the child [21,25].

Nighttime fears and anxieties are a substantial psychologic contributor to sleep disruption. The experience of fears and anxieties is normal in children but can become problematic if quality sleep is prevented. Typical topics include issues the child is currently facing, such as sibling rivalry, a fear of death or separation from a parent, and anxieties about negotiating the socialization process. The greatest treatment for these fears, even if they become excessive, is often parental understanding. Setting strict limits is not advised for this particular problem, but a change in bedtime or in the bedtime ritual may help alleviate some of the fears. For example, if children experience a phase delay (i.e., their actual sleep schedule falls behind their expected sleep schedule; see next section) but are put to bed early, the resulting hours awake in bed before the onset of sleep may produce some imaginative fears. The revised bedtime ritual for a child with excessive nighttime fears should include those parental involvement and a gradual rather than abrupt withdrawal of the parent from the environment at bedtime [21,24,25].

Chronophysiologic Factors

The influence of circadian rhythm on the human sleep/wake cycle is first evident between six weeks and three months of age [61,62]. Infants' entrainment cues are initially related more to the their feeding schedule than to light/dark cues. As entrainment shifts to light/dark cues, individual differences in the chronologic distribution of circadian rhythms, or sleep phases, become apparent: some people are more active in the early morning, whereas others seem to prefer being active at night [63]. These differences are normal and become the source of sleep disturbance only when they conflict with a person's social, work, or school schedule. In childhood, problems may also arise if children's circadian rhythms conflict with their parents' schedule. Four basic problems associated with circadian rhythm may emerge: phase delay, phase advance, regular but inappropriate schedule, and irregular schedule (Table 27.3).

Phase delay occurs when a child's sleep schedule falls behind his or her expected sleep schedule [64–66]. A child with phase delay is physiologically ready for sleep later and naturally arises later than is expected or desired by the parents. Phase delay may result from the practice of going to bed later or from an inherited predisposition to sleep later. It occurs more in adolescents than in younger children and often begins after a summer of late bedtime and 'sleeping in.' Since the human circadian rhythm follows a 25-hour cycle without external cues, phase delay may occur quite easily [21,24,25]. The presenting complaint for phase delay is frequently insomnia associated with the onset of sleep or morning sluggishness [64–66]. These children struggle to achieve sleep at bedtime because they are not physiologically ready; as a result, they may lie in bed for hours or struggle with parents at bedtime. Mornings are difficulty for them, and they typically

Table 27.3 Chronophysiologic factors associated with sleep disorders.

Transition	From feeding cues to light/dark cues (infants only)
Constitutional factors	Owl versus lark (i.e., naturally more alert in the morning vs. evening)
Phase delay	Individual does not become sleepy until late; is difficult to awaken for school; exhibits no intrasleep problem
Phase advance	Individual becomes sleepy too early and awakens too early
Irregular schedule	Free-running life style with no regular sleep/wake schedule

Table 27.4 Treatment of sleep phase disorders.

Phase delay	Awaken the child progressively earlier
	Prevent excessive napping
	Consider augmentation with bright light
Phase advance	Keep the child awake progressively later
	Prevent compensatory napping
	Delay dinner

The initial treatment of both types of sleep phase disorders involves adjusting the child's bedtime to his or her current sleep phase.

sleep late whenever possible to 'catch up.' If forced to awaken before they are ready (e.g., for school), they may experience sleep deprivation.

Proper diagnosis of phase delay is best accomplished by keeping a sleep diary for 23 weeks, including both weekdays and weekends (vacations too, of possible). A clue to the diagnosis lies in weekend sleep behavior: often the children stay up and sleep in late and feel much better than during the week when they are getting up at a time inconsistent with their optimal arising time. Diaries typically show that sleep onset occurs at approximately at the same time regardless of bedtime (insomnia disappears on weekends or when the child is allowed to stay up later).

The treatment of phase delay should focus on accomplishing a phase advance that will synchronize the child's clock with his or her environment (Table 27.4). First, the child should be allowed to go to bed at the physiologically appropriate time (this effectively eliminates insomnia complaints). Next, the child should be awakened progressively earlier and prevented from taking excess naps. The resulting sleep deprivation will eventually function to advance the child's phase. In severe cases of phase delay, it may be more effective to allow the child's circadian clock to 'free run,' thereby delaying around the clock until it reaches the appropriate phase. Intense exposure to light at the appropriate times may facilitate the phase adjustment by providing additional external cues. When diagnosing symptoms as phase delay, it is impor-

tant to be aware of a problem with similar symptoms called motivational phase delay. A child with motivational phase delay has trouble waking in the mornings and going to sleep at night owing to school avoidance rather than a maladjusted biologic clock. Children with this disorder may feel ambivalent toward treatment programs that address the phase problems because they really want to be told that they cannot go to school. In these instances, the reason for avoidance should be the initial focus of treatment [67,68].

Phase advance results when children go to bed early and wake early. It is less common than phase delay [21,25]. Children with phase advance may feel sleepy before their regular bedtime, and they frequently experience early morning awakenings. Again, the symptoms are related to the child's physiologic readiness for sleep at a certain time. Often their entire schedule is advanced, including meals and naptimes as well as sleep onset and awakening. The symptoms may go unnoticed by parents if the child's schedule fits well with their own. Treatment involves adjusting the sleep/wake schedule to a later time by gradually (e.g., 30–60 minutes/day) adjusting the child's bedtime backward and allowing no extra napping during the day (see Table 27.4). Often it helps to delay dinner, making sure that the child is not eating an excessive number of snacks. Rest assured; despite the complaints, the child will not miss a meal but will likely stay awake longer to enjoy it. Since the human circadian rhythm naturally runs 25 hours, treating phase advance is typically easier than treating phase delay [21,25].

Children with irregular sleep/wake patterns have time cues that are either inconsistent or completely lacking [25]. Their lives are often characterized by a lack of routine and possibly social instability. They may eat meals at irregular times and receive no appropriate cues to help orient their sleep/wake patterns. Children experiencing this problem often live in homes with little structure, in which some type of family dysfunction may coexist. Treatment should focus on teaching the parents to provide the appropriate structure that allows their children to form a consistent sleep/wake schedule.

Some children may simply sleep less and apparently need less sleep than other children. These 'short sleepers' have less total sleep time but are otherwise normal, with no associated complaints. They may present with bedtime struggles or early awakenings.

Adolescence

Adolescence represents a gradual change from childhood to adulthood. As such, some emerging sleep problems of adolescence may reflect this transition. Adolescents, for example, are more likely to exhibit symptoms of adult-like insomnia or to adjust their sleep patterns to reflect a more adult-like total sleep time, even though they may still biologically need more sleep than adults. Adolescents frequently stay up later than children but must still wake early to attend school on time. This adjustment frequently results in sleep deprivation or phase delay. Adolescents as a group seem to exhibit several symptoms of disturbed sleep, including difficulty awakening, excessive daytime sleepiness, and irritability [69].

Parasomnias

Several seemingly different disorders are categorized as parasomnias [70]. These disorders include dramatic, sometimes bizarre symptoms and may cause distress for the observing parent. Treatments may work only temporarily, but the disorders often end with a spontaneous remission at the onset of puberty. Although the pathologic prevalence of parasomnias is unknown, most of the normal population occasionally experiences some of these symptoms, and the infrequent parasomnia event is generally not perceived to be problematic. Parasomnias are less frequently the cause of referral to a sleep-related specialist than are other sleep disorders, and they may be perceived as more normal in preadolescent children. Parasomnias may be considered more problematic in older children when they begin to curtail the child's participation in social events such as camps or sleepover. For the patients who are referred, it is important for the clinician to be able to recognize when therapeutic intervention is necessary; often the best therapy is to merely reassure the parents

Table 27.5 Common parasomnias in children and their treatment.

Sleepwalking and night terrors (pavor nocturnus)
  Occur primarily in slow wave sleep (stage 3 and 4)
    Most frequent in young children
    Usually outgrown by adolescence
    Can be precipitated by sleep deprivation or excessive fatigue
    Treatment: increased total nocturnal sleep time or late afternoon naps; benzodiazepine may help by lightening deep sleep
  Occur at any age, but most common during preadolescence
    Can be precipitated by traumatic events (even a frightening movie) or separation anxiety
    Treatment: reassurance and/or counseling usually helpful; recurring dreams may be extinguished by the daytime rehearsal of an acceptable ending

Sleep-related enuresis
  Primary enuresis in 90% of patients; secondary in 10%
  Family history of enuresis common
  Most children dry by the age of four years, but 10% of six-year-olds still wet
  Spontaneous dryness achieved at rate of 15% a year
  Treatment: behavioral approaches most helpful

that their child's behavior is normal and will most likely cause him or her no harm. The key to determining whether a given child's symptoms are normal or abnormal and in need of treatment lies in the frequency and persistence of events over time and, in some instances, the amount of danger or health risk that results from the events [21,24,25].

The most common parasomnias are sleepwalking, night terrors, nightmares, and sleep-related enuresis (Table 27.5). In 1968, Broughton proposed calling these for disorders *disorders of arousal*, since electrophysiologic features were common to each, including an arousal that most often occurs from slow wave sleep [71]. Other features of these disorders include frequent body movements during sleep, autonomic activation, automatic and sometimes repetitive motor activity, mental confusion and disorientation, and relative unresponsiveness to external stimuli. In most instances, there is generalized amnesia to the episode, with little recall of mental activity during the event. These features are seen most consistently in sleep-walking and sleep terror episodes.

Sleepwalking

Sleepwalking episodes are characterized by a flurry of motor behavior that typically originates during the deep slow wave sleep of the first third of the night [72]. It occurs most commonly in pubescent children and can persist into adulthood. Its pathogenesis is unknown, but physiologic and psychological stress can precipitate episodes. Although usually benign, serious injury and even death can result from the behavior. Episodes typically begin most commonly within the first 60 minutes after the onset of sleep. The individual sits up in bed and may perform a number of repetitive movements such as picking at the bed covers. Rarely, the individual performs behaviors that require complex motor function and cognitive ability, such as driving, talking on the telephone, or playing a musical instrument. Usually verbalization is rare unless a night terror is occurring. Individuals can hurt themselves during these episodes, for example, by stumbling or banging into furniture or by exiting open windows or climbing onto fire escapes. One of our patients was stopped just prior to exiting the back of a moving camper vehicle while sleepwalking. Occasionally, violent behavior can be a part of sleepwalking, although it is unusual for aggressive behavior to be directed toward specific individuals. Attempts at restraining the sleepwalker can be met with resistance and even a primitive level of ferocity, however [21,25,72,73]. The following case studies involve sleepwalking in which destructive behavior occurred.

CASE TWO

A young man began experiencing violent and destructive sleepwalking events – kicking in doors and walls and attacking anything in sight. He continued this behavior throughout his teenage years. In the episode that resulted in his referral to our sleep disorders center, his father attempted to restrain him. The child attacked his father with such ferocity that the father had to be hospitalized.

CASE THREE

A 14-year-old boy presented with a lengthy history of sleepwalking and night terrors that had begun with the divorce of his parents at the age of five years. His behavior during a recent episode was destructive, including breaking windows, walls, doors, and anything in his path. On two occasions he had thrown his mother across the room when she attempted to stop his sleepwalking. The events were controlled with a low dose of diazepam (Valium), but his compliance to the regimen was poor. At age 24 years, after spending 18 hours working, he attended a wine festival, where he stayed up until early morning and then fell asleep outside in a chair. The police later found him wandering through the woods screaming that someone was trying to kill him. When confronted, he had difficulty answering questions and pleaded to be allowed to sleep. The next day he was told that someone matching his description had attacked an elderly couple and beat them viciously. He claimed absolutely no recall of having participated in this event. The victims lived directly across from where he had been sleeping.

Fifteen to 30% of healthy children have at least one episode of sleepwalking. Two to 3% have more frequent episodes. Peak prevalence occurs at 12 years of age, and most children outgrow the behavior by 15 years of age. Less than 1% of adults exhibit sleepwalking. Some researchers have suggested a genetic component to the disorder, which a recessive mode of inheritance and incomplete penetrance. There is no evidence for racial or cultural differences, however. Sleep deprivation, excessive fatigue, sedatives, hypnotics, and even episodes of obstructive sleep apnea can precipitate sleepwalking. Sleepwalking in children is considered benign and is not usually associated with psychopathology [72].

Sleepwalking can be distinguished from psychogenic fugue in that the latter tends to occur in people with severe psychopathology and typically lasts for hours or days. REM behavior disorder, although similar to sleepwalking, tends to occur more in the elderly, rarely occurs in children, and is associated with more elaborate recall.

Treatment of sleepwalking involves securing the patients' bedroom to prevent injury and placing either an alarm or wind chime on the patient's door. Psychotherapy, relaxation therapy, and hypnosis all are reported to be equally effective. Benzodiazepines can be helpful, and we have obtained positive results with antidepressant therapy such as the use of desipramine [72,73].

Night Terrorrs

Night terrors, which are termed *pavor nocturnus* in children and *incubus* in adults, are characterized by a person's arousal within the first third of the night usually from deep (stage 3 or 4) sleep [74]. The episode may begin with a loud, piercing scream usually accompanied by an intense autonomic response and is followed by a sense of anxiety and panic. The sleep terrors can precipitate or be associated with sleepwalking events. The person typically sits up in bed, seems to be frightened, and may be sweating and experiencing rapid breathing and tachycardia. Heart rate changes can occur precipitously to rates as high as 160 beats per minute. Patients may be inconsolable until the intense agitation dissipates (usually within 15 minutes). There is little if any recall of dream imagery, although there may be a sense of doom or impending death. In adults, there have been reports of cursing with night terrors. Polysomnographs indicate events similar to those occurring with sleepwalking. The severity of the episodes is proportional to the duration of the preceding stage 3 or 4 sleep, and individuals with repetitive sleep terrors tend to show many brief awakenings from these stages of sleep [75].

One to 6% of pubescent children experience recurrent episodes of night terror. The peak prevalence occurs between five and seven years of age, and the prevalence in adults is less than 1%. There is no evidence for racial or cultural differences in the prevalence of sleep terrors, but there is an increased familial incidence, with up to 96% of individuals having at least one family member with the condition [21,25,75].

Night terrors can be precipitated by stress, fatigue, and febrile illness [76]. The disorder in adults more typically indicates some pathology and has been reported to occur as a symptom of post-traumatic stress disorder [64]. Benzodiazepines can be helpful in treating the condition, and very low doses of diazepam (2–5 mg) can reduce or ameliorate the condition; these doses can ultimately be given only on alternate nights. Imipramine has also been reported to be helpful. The disorder should be distinguished from dream anxiety attacks (nightmares), which tend to occur during REM sleep rather than deep sleep and are less likely to be associated with intense autonomic activity. Individuals experiencing dreaming anxiety attacks are usually awake and not amnesiac for the events [72,73].

Jactatio Capitis Nocturna

Nightmares, head banging, body rocking, and head rolling are rhythmic movement disorders termed *jactatio capitis nocturna*. Although they may persist into adulthood, these disorders are most prevalent in infants and children. They generally occur during the transition to sleep but can also appear later in the sleep cycle. They are not necessarily benign: injuries to the head or limbs can occur, especially with head banging. Head banging involves a rhythmic, forceful ramming of the head into a pillow or, less frequently, into a rigid surface such as a wall or a headboard. It typically occurs while the person is in a prone or supine position [77–80].

Body rocking is typically characterized by an individual positioned on hands and knees rocking his or her entire body in an anterior–posterior motion. When a child is in a crib, the body rocking may cause the crib to move all over the room and bang into the wall. These episodes tend to occur on a nightly basis and may last up to an hour. Head banging generally occurs in association with stressful situations, whereas body rocking typically occurs in conjunction with more pleasurable activities such as listening to music or getting ready for bed. Children rarely cry when exhibiting these behaviors, even when the movements are violent.

Polysomnographic studies show that *jactatio capitis nocturna* events occur primarily during wakefulness and in sleep stages 1 and 2. Head banging occurs in approximately 4% of children, typically with onset during the infant's first year at about 6–8 months of age; it rarely develops after 18 months of age. Head rolling activity has been reported to occur in 6% of healthy children. The prevalence of this disorder declines rapidly with age: although more than 50% of infants exhibit some form of this activity, less than 25% of two-year-olds less than 10% of four-year-olds exhibit this disorder. Head banging tends to occur more frequently in boys than in girls, but no gender differences have been noted for other rhythmic movements disorders. The behavior is more prevalent in individuals with mental retardation.

One explanation for the cause of bedtime rhythmic activity is that it is the child's attempt to reproduce his or her parents' cradling or rocking motions. Other hypotheses involve the rhythm of the mother's heartbeat or respiratory rhythm as a model for imitation. More recently, a model of self-stimulation has been suggested, in which rhythmic activity gives a rise to pleasurable sensations and reinforcement. Rhythmic body movements should be distinguished from seizure disorder or spasms nutans, which consists of fine head oscillations that are more commonly seen during wakefulness. In most cases, rhythmic movements disorders require no treatment other than providing reassurance to the family that injury is unlikely. When particularly violent activity occurs, however, such as in a child with mental retardation, more caution should be exercised; the use of extra padding and in some instances protective helmets may be needed to prevent injury. Some studies have shown that replacing the rhythmic activity with a frequency-matched metronome placed next to the bed at night can be helpful. Others have suggested allowing the opportunity for vigorous rocking in a rocking chair or a rocking horse before bedtime may reduce the behavior.

Enuresis

Childhood enuresis is ubiquitous. From earliest recorded history in primitive and civilized societies, enuresis has been a source of unhappiness and embarrassment. Shame and ridicule have often been used to deter bedwetting. Even today in our society, it is not unusual for patients to shame the enuretic child by hanging soiled bedsheets outside the child's window or by threatening to rub the child's face into wet clothing and sheets. Fortunately, these attitudes appear to be giving way to more enlightened approaches [81].

Enuresis is technically defined as an involuntary discharge of urine, but it is usually used to denote bedwetting in children old enough to have acquired control of the urinary bladder. The age at which complete bladder control is attained (usually 4–5 years) depends on developmental, social, and cultural factors, the personality of the child, the general emotional climate in the home, and parental attitudes toward toilet training. There are two distinct subgroups of enuresis: primary and secondary. In primary enuresis, the child has never been consistently dry for more than one or two weeks at a time. Primary enuresis generally involves developmental and maturational factors and a strong genetic component. Psychologic and medical factors usually play a minimal role in primary enuresis. In secondary enuresis, the child begins to wet again after an extended period of dryness. Psychologic and medical factors are usually a major cause of secondary enuresis. Studies have variously estimated that primary enuresis constitutes 67%–90% of all cases and secondary enuresis only 10%–33%.

It is generally agreed that between five and seven million people in the US have enuresis. The disorder affects all cultures, and boys are more likely than girls to be affected. Some studies have suggested that approximately 10% of all six-year-olds wet their beds and the spontaneous cure rate thereafter is about 15% per year. The current view is that enuresis does not ordinarily reflect any abnormality of sleep. Early studies suggested that enuresis was one of the disorders of arousal that occurred during sleep stages 3 and 4. We have concluded, however, that there is no unique correlation between slow sleep and enuretic episodes: the frequency of enuretic episodes in each stage of sleep is proportional to the amount of time spent in each stage. The predominance of episodes during slow wave sleep, therefore, appears to be related to the time of night at which this type of sleep occurs. Researchers have investigated the possibility that enuresis is directly correlated to dreaming, since bedwetters frequently describe dreams of wetting or being wet. Studies have shown that children who are awakened and given dry clothing immediately after micturition do not report any dreams of wetness. Those children who were not awakened after micturition, then, may have incorporated a sense of wetness into a subsequent dream and on awakening, may have believed that wetting actually occurred during a dream [81–83].

In sleep laboratory tests, people with enuresis recorded more frequent and intense contractions of the primary detrusor muscle – both spontaneous and evoked – as well as greater bladder pressure than control subjects [85,86]. In addition, non-REM sleep arousals were found to provoke primary bladder contractions in people with enuresis. Genetic factors may play a role in primary enuresis: a family history has been reported in 70% of enuretic children, which suggests that a maturation component may underlie the disorder [81,87,88].

The maturation of bladder function and control may be premature or delayed in people with enuresis. Studies have shown that these individuals experience more bladder irritation than do control subjects. This partially accounts for the smaller bladder capacity in children with enuresis: if their bladder is of normal size but their functional bladder capacity is smaller, they will have a decreased ability to tolerate a full bladder [87].

In patients with primary enuresis, emotional problems are usually a consequence of the disorder rather than any biologic factor. Although enuresis has gener-

Table 27.6 Key points in taking of history of enuresis.

Primary vs. secondary enuresis (has the patient every
   been dry)
Age
Current medications
Known ailments
Any signs of symptoms of obstructive sleep apnea
   syndrome (snoring, snorting, gasping)
Fluid intake pattern (quantity and time)

ally been described in the psychiatric literature as an expression of the need to regress and receive excessive attention and care – particularly following stresses such as the birth of a sibling or a family illness – such scenarios relate more significantly to secondary enuresis [81,82].

A causal factor often overlooked in both primary and secondary enuresis is sleep apnea. A study at Dartmouth College reported that in some instances the removal of tonsils to alleviate obstructed nocturnal breathing resulted in significant improvement or the resolution of enuresis [85].

The most important component of evaluating a child with enuresis is obtaining a clear history (Table 27.6). The evaluation should include a thorough general history with specific attention to the bedwetting, a physical examination, and urinalysis. A more complete urologic work-up is indicated only when the history of physical examination suggests a urologic disorder. Cystoscopy and intravenous pyelogram should be avoided unless there is a strong suspicion of urinary tract infection or blockage [81–83].

Most pediatricians tend to suggest a treatment approach of benign neglect: do nothing and allow nature to eventually solve the problem. This approach can lead to considerable frustration for parents and children, however. The use of behavior modification to treat enuresis is well established. Use of the bedwetting alarm has a demonstrated success rate of 60%–75%. Unfortunately, relapse just after conditioning is high, ranging from 35%–80%. However, the disorder can be treated quickly and permanently with subsequent reconditioning and reapplication of the alarm.

In recent years, we have instituted a comprehensive treatment program for childhood enuresis, combining some of the treatment paradigms described here. The program employs five methods: (1) bladder stretching exercises, (2) stream interruption, (3) counseling for motivation and responsibility, (4) visual sequencing, and (5) conditioning therapy. Each of these techniques

has been used by other practitioners to treat enuresis. For our program, however, the methods have been modified slightly and organized into a paradigm that also incorporates a current understanding of sleep physiology. Our method relies heavily on personal contact between the clinic and the patient, motivation by the clinicians, and the active involvement of the child and his or her parents.

The effective of this treatment program was evaluated in 100 children with primary enuresis. Children average 11.5 wet nights during the first two-week period and decreased to 4.3 wet nights at the end of 16 weeks. Ninety-one percent of the children entering the program showed significant improvement by the end of 30 weeks. Most of the individual approaches used in our treatment program have been reported in the literature to be effective on their own. Stream interruption and bladder-stretching exercises have been reported to ameliorate enuresis in up to 30% of patients, and 29% of people with enuresis have been reported to respond to motivation and responsibility counseling. As much as 65%–75% of children respond favorably to the use of conditioning alarms. These results suggest that enuresis should be considered a treatable condition whose resolution can be extremely gratifying for the patient, the family, and the clinician [81].

Obstructive Sleep Apnea

Obstructive sleep apnea syndrome is the most common form of apnea in childhood. In older children and adults, the main feature of the syndrome is loud snoring associated with gasping, snorting, and respiratory pauses. Sleep is often restless, and there may be concurrent nightmares and night terrors [1,89]. During the day, adults complain of excessive daytime fatigue and sleepiness. In children, the symptoms are more insidious, often being associated with increased irritability, a shortened attention span, and 'crabbiness.' There may be behavioral difficulties, morning headaches, obesity, a failure to thrive, or symptoms of cor pulmonale [90–92]. In children, the main causes of obstructive sleep apnea are hypertrophy of the tonsils and adenoids, craniofacial abnormalities such as micrognathia or retrognathia, abnormalities of the long soft palate, cleft palate repair, and macroglossia. This syndrome is common in patients with Down syndrome. In addition, obesity can contribute to obstructive sleep apnea, as can neuromuscular disorders such as the Arnold–Chiari malformation, syringobulbia, cerebral palsy, myotonic dystrophy, and bulbar poliomyelitis.

Whereas in adults the snoring is often interrupted by pauses, children with sleep apnea usually snore continuously. Nasal obstructions such as polyps, enlarged turbinates, and a deviated septum may cause sleep apnea and should be treated with antihistamines or topical preparations. Enlarged tonsils and adenoids should be removed. These treatments generally result in a resolution of all symptoms. Nasal continuous positive airway pressure is a treatment of choice for obstructive sleep apnea syndrome in adults and can be effective for children as well. Long-term compliance is questionable, however [24,25]. Another effective treatment for snoring and apnea in adults is a recently developed dental prosthesis that is worn like a boxer's mouthguard and stabilizes the jaw and tongue. Similar appliances can be fit for children and simply require patent nasal airway. We frequently recommend the use of an external nasal dilator (Breathe Right) in children who snore or have nasal obstruction. These can be quite effective, and the national exposure given to the use of these devices by athletes has aided their acceptance by children.

CASE FOUR

A two and a half-year-old boy presented with difficulty falling asleep and with an inability to maintain sleep for more than 50 minutes at a time without awakening and disturbing his parents. He was unwilling to sleep in his own bed and upon awakening in the morning was extremely cranky and exhibited what his parents referred to as 'energy sucking' behavior. The parents were exhausted and extremely frustrated. A neurological examination showed no significant abnormalities but some suspicious findings in the frontal EEG leads resulted in the child being placed on Tegretol. The Tegretol was somewhat helpful and decreased the number of nocturnal awakenings from 15–20 by half. After an afternoon nap the child seemed completely normal and calm. Examination of his nose and throat showed hypertrophic tonsils. He was a mouth breather and unable to maintain nasal airway patency. He had frequent upper airway infections and one could hear his tonsils vibrating while awake. During sleep his breathing was punctuated by sucking noises and snoring. The parents were informed that a 50-minute sleep cycle is not unusual for a child of this age but that he is likely to be experiencing obstructive sleep apnea. A polysomnogram confirmed this. A Breathe Right nasal strip was utilized to maintain nasal airway patency and he was provided with melatonin at bedtime. This improved his ability to fall and stay asleep and markedly reduced his 'energy sucking' behavior. However, his polysomnogram also revealed the presence of 15 apnea and hypopnea events per hour with oxygen desaturation levels reaching 79% of maximum – clear obstructive sleep apnea. Otolaryngologic evaluation resulted in the removal of his tonsils and adenoids and a dramatic improvement in his sleep and waking behavior.

In patients with obstructive sleep apnea, attempts at breathing are compromised by a collapsing airway. Patients with central sleep apnea, however, suffer from a lack of respiratory effort [24]. During sleep, respiration is controlled by a metabolic respiratory control system. A defect at any point in this system can contribute to central sleep apnea. The causes include encephalitis, cervical cordotomy, brain stem infarction, tumor, and bulbar poliomyelitis. Certain neuromuscular disorders such as neuromyopathy, myotonic dystrophy, muscular dystrophy, myasthenia gravis, diaphragmatic paralysis, and postpolio syndrome can also contribute to central sleep apnea. Finally, thoracic restrictive disorders such as kyphoscoliosis have also been associated with the condition. Patients with central sleep apnea exhibit normal voluntary respiration function during wakefulness but abnormal automatic control of ventilation. There is no response to hypocarbia during wakefulness or sleep, indicating that chemoreceptor abnormalities may be critical factors in this disorder. Patients also exhibit a blunted response to hypoxia and hypoventilation during sleep. Treatment for central sleep apnea can involve diaphragmatic pacing, mechanical ventilatory support, and negative pressure ventilation [24,25].

References

1. Rosen RC, Rosekind M, Rosevear C, *et al.*: Physician education in sleep and sleep disorders: A national survey of U.S. medical schools. *Sleep* 1993; **16**:249–254.
2. Hartmann E, Baekeland R, Zwilling G: Psychological differences between long and short sleepers. *Arch Gen Psychiatry* 1972; **26**:463–468.
3. Aserinsky E, Kleitman N: Regularly occurring periods of eye motility, and concomitant phenomena during sleep. *Science* 1953; **118**:273–274.

4. Carskadon MA, Dement WC: Normal human sleep: An overview. In: Kryger MH, Roth T, Dement WC, eds. *Principles and Practice of Sleep Medicine.* Philadelphia: WB Saunders; 1994:16–25.

5. Carskadon MA, Rechtschaffen A: Monitoring and staging human sleep. In: Kryger MH, Roth T, Dement WC, eds. *Principles and Practice of Sleep Medicine.* Philadelphia: WB Saunders; 1994:943–960.

6. Roffwarg HP, Muzio IN, Dement WC: Ontogenetic development of the human sleep-dream cycle. *Science* 1996; **152**:604–619.

7. Anders TF, Keener M: Developmental course of night-time sleep-wake patterns in fullterm and premature infants during the first year of life. I. *Sleep* 1985; **8**:173–192.

8. Anders TF, Keener MA, Kraemer H: Sleep-wake organization, neonatal assessment and development in premature infants during the first year of life. II. *Sleep* 1985; **8**:193–206.

9. Anders TF: Night-waking in infants during the first year of life. *Pediatrics* 1979; **63**:860–864.

10. Anders TF, Carskadon MA, Dement WC: Sleep and sleepiness in children and adolescents. *Pediatr Clin North Am* 1980; **17**:29–43.

11. Synder F: The phenomenology of dreaming. In: Madow L, Snow L, eds. *The Psychodynamic Implications of the Physiological Studies on Dreams.* Springfield, IL: Charles C. Thomas, 1970:124–151.

12. Foulkes D: Dream reports from different stages of sleep. *J Abnorm Psychol* 1962; **65**:14–28.

13. Foulkes D, Vogel G: Mental activity at sleep onset. *J Abnorm Psychol* 1965; **70**:231–243.

14. Dement W, Kleitman N: The relation of the eye movements during sleep to dream activity: An objective method for the study of dreaming. *J Exp Psychol* 1957; **53**:339–346.

15. Dewan EM: The P (programming) hypothesis for REMS. *Psychophysiology* 1968; **5**:365–366.

16. Greenberg R, Dewan E: Aphasia and dreaming: A test of the P-hypothesis. *Psychophysiology* 1968; **5**: 203–204.

17. Levental M, Susie V, Rusic M, Rakic L: Rapid eye-movement (REM) sleep deprivation: Effect on acid mucopolysaccharides in rat brain. *Arch Int Physiol Biochim* 1975; **83**:221–232.

18. Shashoua V: The role of extracellular proteins in learning and memory. *Am Sci* 1985; **73**:364–370.

19. Crick F, Mitchison G: The function of dream sleep. *Nature* 1983; **304**:111–114.

20. Foulkes D: Longitudinal studies of dreams in children. In: Masserman J, ed. *Science and Psychoanalysis,* 9th ed. New York: Grune & Stratton, 1971.

20a. Golbin AZ: *The World of Children's Sleep.* Salt Lake City, UT: Michaelis Medical Publishing Corp., 1994.

21. Ferber R: Sleeplessness in the child. In: Kryger MH, Roth T, Dement WC, eds. *Principles and Practices of Sleep Medicine.* Philadelphia: WB Saunders, 1989: 633–639.

22. Lansky V: *Getting Your Child to Sleep and Back to Sleep: Tips for Parents of Infants, Toddlers and Preschoolers.* Derphaven, MN: Bood Peddlers; 1991.

23. Ferber R: *Solve Your Child's Sleep Problems.* New York: Simon and Schuster, 1985.

24. Guilleminault C, ed.: *Sleep and Its Disorders in Children.* New York: Raven Press, 1987:243–252.

25. Sheldon SH, Spire JP, Levy HB: *Pediatrics Sleep Medicine.* Philadelphia: WB Saunders, 1992.

26. Bax MCO: Sleep disturbance in the young child. *Br Med J* 1980; **280**:1177–1179.

27. Weisbluth M: Sleep in the colicky infant. In: Guilleminault C, ed.: *Sleep and Its Disorders in Children.* New York: Raven Press, 1987:129–138.

28. Wessel MA, Cobb JC, Jackson EB, *et al.*: Paroxysmal fussing in infancy, sometimes called "colic." *Pediatrics* 1954; **14**:421–434.

29. Jorup S: Colonic hyperperistalisis in neurolabile infants: Studies in so-called dyspepsia in breast infants. *Acta Paediatr* 1952; **85**:1–92.

30. Darwin C: *The Expression of Emotions in Man and Animals.* London: Murray; 1889.

31. Weissbluth M, Green OC: Plasma progesterone concentrations in infants: Relation to infantile colic. *J Pediatr* 1983; **103**:935–936.

32. Weissbluth M, Davis AT, Poncher J: Night waking in 4- to 8-month-old infants. *J Pediatr* 1984; **104**:477–480.

33. Moore T, Vcko C: Night waking in early infancy: Part 1. *Arch Dis Child* 1957; **32**:333.

34. Kataria S, Swanson MS, Trevathan GE: Persistance of sleep disturbances in preschool children. *J Pediatr* 1987; **110**:642–646.

35. Anders TF, Keener M: Deveopmental course of night-time sleep-wake patterns in full-term and premature infants during the first year of life. I. *Sleep* 1985; **8**: 173–192.

36. Younger JB: The management of night waking in older infants. *Pediatr Nurs* 1982; **8**:155–158.

37. Jones DPH, Verdyn CM: Behavioral management of sleep problems. *Arch Dis Child* 1983; **58**:442–444.

38. Cuthbertson J, Schevill S: *Helping Your Child Sleep Through the Night.* Garden City, NY: Doubleday, 1985.

39. Van Tassel EB: The relative influences of child and environmental characteristics on sleep disturbances in the first and second years of life. *J Dev Behav Pediatr* 1985; **6**:81–86.

40. Ferber R, Boyle MP: Nocturnal fluid intake: A cause of, not treatment for, sleep disruption in infants and toddlers. *Sleep Res* 1983; **12**:243.

41. Anders TF: Night-waking in infants during the first year of life. *Pediatrics* 1979; **63**:86–864.

42. Kahn A, Mozin MJ, Casimir G, *et al.*: Allergy to cow's milk: A possible cause for chronic insomnia in infants. *Sleep Res* 1985; **14**:16.

43. Busby K, Firestone P, Pivik RT: Sleep patterns in hyperkinetic and normal children. *Sleep* 1981; **4**:366–383.

44. Greenhill L, Puig-Antich J, Goetz R, *et al.*: Sleep architecture and REM sleep measures in prepubertal children with attention-deficit disorder with hyperactivity. *Sleep* 1993; **6**:91–101.

45. Chervin RD, Dillon JE, Bassetti C, Ganoczy DA, Pituch KJ: Symptoms of sleep disorders, inattention, and hyperactivity in children. *Sleep* 1997; **20**:1185–1192.

46. Dahl RE, Holttum J, Trubnick L: A clinical picture of child and adolescent narcolepsy. *J Am Acad Child Adolesc Psychiatry* 1994; **33**:834–841.

47. Fallone G, Acebo C, Arnedt JT, Seifer R, Carskadon MA: Effects of acute sleep restriction on behavior, sustained attention, and response inhibition in children. *Percept Mot Skills* 2001; **93**:213–229.

48. Randazzo AC, Muehlbach MJ, Schweitzer PK, Walsh JK: Cognitive function following acute sleep restriction in children ages 10–14. *Sleep* 1998; **21**:861–868.

49. Ekbom KA: Growing pains and restless legs. *Acta Paediatr Scand* 1975; **64**:264–266.

50. Walters AS: Is there a subpopulation of children with growing pains who really have restless legs syndrome? A review of the literature. *Sleep Med* 2002; **52**:297–302.

51. Walters AS, Picchietti DL, Ehrenberg BL, Wagner ML: Restless legs syndrome in childhood and adolescence. *Pediatr Neurol* 1994; **11**:241–245.

52. Picchietti DL, Walters AS: Moderate to severe periodic limb movement disorder in childhood and adolescence. *Sleep* 1999; **22**:297–300.

53. Picchetti D, Walters A, Underwood D, *et al.*: Periodic limb movement disorder in attention-deficit hyperactivity disorder in children. *Sleep Res* 1997; **26**:469.

54. Picchietti DL, England SJ, Walters AS, Willis K, Verrico T: Periodic limb movement disorder and restless legs syndrome in children with attention-deficit hyperactivity disorder. *J Child Neurol* 1998; **13**:588–594.

55. Picchietti DL, Underwood DJ, Farris WA, *et al.*: Further studies on periodic limb movements disorder and restless legs syndrome in children with attention-deficit hyperactivity disorder. *Mov Disord* 1999; **14**:1000–10007.

56. Walters AS. Toward a better definition of the restless legs syndrome. The International Restless Legs Syndrome Study Group. *Mov Disord* 1995; **10**:634–642.

57. Kane J, Coble P, Conners K, Kupfer DJ: EEG sleep in a child with severe depression. *Am J Psychiatry* 1977; **134**:813–814.

58. Kupfer DJ, Coble P, Kane J, *et al.*: Imipramine and EEG sleep in children with depressive symptoms. *Psychopharmacology* 1979; **60**:117–123.

59. Puig-Antich J: Affective disorders in childhood: A review and perspective. *Psychiatr Clin North Am* 1980; **3**:403–424.

60. Young W, Knoles JB, MacLean AW, *et al.*: The sleep of childhood depressives: Comparison with age-matched controls. *Biol Psychiatry* 1982; **17**:1163–1168.

61. Coons S, Guilleminault C: Development of consolidated sleep and wakeful periods in relation to the day/night cycle in infancy. *Dev Med Child Neurol* 1984; **26**:169–176.

62. Anders TF: State and rhythmic processes. *J Am Child Psychiatry* 1978; **17**:401–420.

63. Horne JA, Ostberg O: Individual differences in human circadian rhythms. *Biol Psychol* 1979; **5**:179–190.

64. Weitzman ED, Czeisler CA, Coleman RM, *et al.*: Delayed sleep phase syndrome: A chronobiologic disorder with sleep onset insomnia. *Arch Gen Psychiatry* 1981; **38**:737–746.

65. Ferber R, Boyle MP: Delayed sleep phase syndrome versus motivated sleep phase delay in adolescents. *Sleep Res* 1983; **12**:239.

66. Loxoff B, Wolf AW, Davis NS: Sleep problems seen in pediatric practice. *Pediatrics* 1985; **75**:477–483.

67. Largo RH, Hunziker UA: A developmental approach to the management of children with sleep disturbances in the first three years of life. *Eur J Pediatr* 1984; **142**:170–173.

68. Czeisler CA, Richardson GS, Coleman RM, *et al.*: Chronotherapy: Resetting the circadian clocks of patients with delayed sleep phase insomnia. *Sleep* 1981; **4**:1–21.

69. Carskadon MA, Dement WC: Sleepiness in the normal adolescent. In: Guilleminualt C, ed. *Sleep and Its Dis-orders in Children.* New York: Raven Press; 1987:53–66.

70. Association of Sleep Disorders Centers' Sleep Disorders Classification Committee, Roffward HP, chair: Diagnostic classification of sleep and arousal disorders. *Sleep* 1979; **2**:1–137.

71. Broughton R: Sleep disorders: Disorders of arousal? *Science* 1968; **59**:1070–1078.

72. Kales A, Soldatos CR, Caldwell AB, *et al.*: Somnambulism: Clinical characteristics and personality patterns. *Arch Gen Psychiatry* 1980; **37**:1413–1417.

73. Ferber R: Sleep, sleeplessness, and sleep disruptions in infants and young children. *Ann Clin Res* 1985; **17**(5):227–237.

74. Kales A, Soldatos CR, Bixler ED, *et al.*: Hereditary factors in sleepwalk night terrors. *Br J Psychiatry* 1980; **137**:111.

75. Kales JD, Kales A, Soldatos CR, *et al.*: Night terrors: Clinical characteristics and personality patterns. *Arch Gen Psychiatry* 1980; **37**:1414–1417.

76. Kales JD, Kales A, Soldatos CR, *et al.*: Sleep walking and night terrors to febrile illness. *Am J Psychiatry* 1979: 136.

77. deLissovoy V: Head banging in early childhood: A study of incidence. *J Pediatr* 1961; **58**:803.

78. Kravitz H, Rosenthal V, Teplitz Z: A study of head-banging in infants and children. *Dis Nerv Syst* 1960; **21**:203.

79. Sallustro MA, Atwell CW: Body rocking, head banging, and head rolling in normal children. *J Pediatr* 1978; **93**:704.

80. Thorpy AJ, Glovinsky P: Jactatio capitis nocturne. In: Kryger M, Roth T, Dement WC, eds. *Principles and Practice of Sleep Medicine.* Philadelphia: WB Saunders; 1989:648–654.

81. Scharf MB: *Waking Up Dry: How to End Bedwetting Forever.* Cincinnati, OH: Writers Digest, 1986.

82. Agarwal A: Enuresis. *Am Fam Physician* 1982; **25**:203–207.

83. McLain LG: Childhood enuresis. *Curr Probl Pediatr* 1979; **9**(8):1–36.

84. Gerard MW: Enuresis: A study in etiology. *Am J Orthopsychiatry* 1933; **9**:48–58.

85. Welder DJ, Hauri PI: Nocturnal enrusis in children with upper airway obstructions. *Int J Pediatr Otorhinolaryngol* 1985; **9**:173–182.

86. Kales A, Scharf MB, Tan TL, Zweizig JR: Sleep laboratory studies on the effects of Tofranil, Valium and placebo on sleep stages and enuresis. *Psychophysiology* 1971; **7**:348.

87. Starfield B: Functional bladder capacity in enuretic and nonenuretic children. *J Pediatr* 1967; **70**:777–781.

88. Frary LG: Enuresis: A genetic study. *Am J Dis Child* 1935; **49**:557–578.

89. Rigatto H: Apnea. *Pediatr Clin North Am* 1982; **29**:1105–1116.

90. Guilleminault C, Korobkin R, Winkle R: A review of 50 children with obstructive sleep apnea syndrome. *Lung* 1981; **159**:275–287.

91. Carskadon MA, Harvey K, Dement WC, *et al.*: Respiration during sleep in children. *West J Med* 1978; **128**: 477–481.

92. Guilleminault C, Winkle R, Korobkin R, Simmons B: Children and nocturnal snoring: Evaluation of the effects of sleep related respiratory resistive load and daytime functioning. *Eur J Pediatr* 1982; **139**:165–171.

93 Scharf MB, Berkowitz DV, McDannolo MO, Stover R, Brannen DE, Reyna R: Effect of an external nasal dilator on sleep and breathing patterns in congested and noncongested newborns. *J of Pediatrics* 1996; **129**:804–808.

28

Loss: Divorce, Separation, and Bereavement

Jamie Snyder

Introduction

Almost every young person experiences loss of some type before they reach adulthood. It may be as common as a friend who moves away or the death of a pet. It may involve witnessing the violent death of a parent or sibling, the loss of innocence of a sexually or physically abused child, or the loss of an intact family in divorce. Children (defined in this chapter as people below the age of 18 years) of different developmental stages experience and cope with loss in different ways. Their response depends not only on the severity of the loss but also their age, support system, coping skills, and numerous other factors.

I discuss in some detail the specific losses of separation, divorce, and bereavement, the epidemiology and research in these areas, clinical diagnoses that may arise, and recommended treatment approaches.

Separation and Divorce

The US National Center for Health Statistics estimates that since 1975 more than one million children annually have been involved in a divorce [1]. In 2003, the US Census Bureau reported that more than 10 million children lived in single-parent households designated as resulting from divorce or separation [2]. As large numbers of children continue to grow up in disrupted families, it is important to consider the impact of divorce, both sociologically and individually: 'The higher incidence of divorce reflects and, in turn, influences the changing relationships between men and women [and] has significantly raised levels of anxiety' [3]. On an individual basis, divorce may exacerbate a pre-existing condition or be a causative agent in a new condition. For example, a child might present to a child psychiatry clinic with symptoms of a behavioral disturbance that began at the time he was told of a pending parental separation or divorce; similarly, a child with a previously stable condition (such as attention deficit hyperactivity disorder) might present with an intensification of symptoms.

Research

The impact of divorce on a child's development, once viewed as a short-lived crisis, has been recognized as a significant long-term stressor [3]. Many longitudinal studies of the long-term effects of divorce have been published within the last 10–20 years (Table 28.1). Kalter and Rembar found that a greater representation of divorced children presented to child and adolescent psychiatric clinics than did children of intact families [6]. *The Diagnostic and Statistical Manual of Mental Disorders*, Fourth edition, Text Revision (DSM-IV-TR) recognizes divorce (on Axis IV) as a problem that may affect the diagnosis, treatment, and prognosis of mental disorders [13].

Although many of the studies cited in Table 28.1 examine separation and divorce as part of the same process, one study elucidated the effect of geographic separation from a parent as a separate issue [14]. Since geographic separation alone is a only a small part of the potential impact of divorce, several studies have examined the loss of one parent as part of the divorce process and have attempted to delineate the effect of this variable alone. Geographic separation due to a military deployment may add some insight to this clinical presentation: children geographically separated from one parent (generally the father) experienced elevated self-reported symptom levels of depression, as

Table 28.1 Summary of representative research on the impact of divorce on children.

Investigators	Title	Sample and design	Variables assessed	Summary of findings
Guidubaldi and Perry [4]	Divorce and mental health sequelae for children: a 2-year follow-up of a nationwide sample	2-year follow-up of 110 (of 699) elementary school boys and in divorced and intact families. girls Average time since divorce was 6 years at follow-up	Academic functioning School behavior Peer acceptance Locus of control General mental health	Children from divorced families performed at levels below those of children of intact families; boys showed more negative effects than girls
Hetherington and colleagues [5]	Long-term effects of divorce and remarriage on the adjustment of children	6-year follow-up of 124 (of 144) middle-class families, including 60 divorced and 64 intact families; mean age of children at time of follow-up was 10.1 years	Behavioral observation of home adjustment Academic performance Teacher and peer evaluation	Divorce has more adverse effects for boys, whereas remarriage is more difficult for girls
Kalter and Rembar [6]	The significance of a child's age at the time of parental divorce	144 children of divorced families ranging between 7 and 17 years of age who presented for evaluation in a child psychiatry outpatient clinic	Level of family stress Social competence Locus of control Presenting complaints, overall degree of emotional adjustment based on clinical evaluation	When divorce occurs in a child's life it is unrelated to the overall level of adjustment, but associated with characteristic patterns of problems at different stages of development
Wallerstein and Kelly [7]	Surviving the break-up: how children and parents cope with divorce	60 middle-class families with 131 children 2 to 18 years of age who participated in divorce counseling at time of divorce and were evaluated again at 18 months postseparation and at 5 years postdivorce	Assessment of child's response to 'and experience' of divorce, parent–child relationships, and support systems outside the home (including school)	The initial decision to divorce is associated with acute distress, including anxiety, depression and anger at parents; preadolescent boys seem to have the most difficulty adjusting at home and school; 30% of children present as clinically depressed at their 5-year evaluation; good adjustment depends on the quality of life in the postdivorce family
Wallerstein [8]	Children of divorce: preliminary report of	40 young adults between 19 and 29 years of age who were	Clinical evaluation of young adults (continuation of the	Subjects continue to view divorce as a major

Author	Focus	Sample	Variables measured	Findings
		between 9 and 19, years of age at time of divorce	earlier study)	influence on their lives; most are committed to a lasting marriage, but women tend to fear repeating parents' mistakes
	a 10-year follow-up of older children and adolescents			
Fergusson, Horwood, and Lynskey [9]	Parental separation adolescent psychopathology, and problem behavior	15-year longitudinal study of 935 children	Exposure to parents' separation during childhood. Measurements of adolescent psychopathology and problem behaviors at 15 years old. Confounding factors	When confounding variables are accounted for, there remains a small but detectable increase for adolescent conduct disorder, mood disorder, and substance use disorders
Black and Pedro-Carroll [10]	Role of parent–child relationships in mediating the effects of marital disruption	Self-administered questionnaire from 288 college students, 60 of whom were children of divorce	Current and past levels of interparental conflict. Current affective quality of parent–child relationships. Present adjustment	Effects of interparental conflict mediate to parent–child relationships. For women, parental divorce affects adjustment indirectly (via disrupting father–daughter relationship)
Kurtz [11]	Psychosocial coping resources in elementary school-age children of divorce	61 children of divorce compared with a nondivorced control group matched for gender, age, and parents' education	Self-perception. Family environment. Beliefs about parents' divorce. Coping behaviors. Family demographics	Children of divorced parents have lower levels of self-efficacy, self-esteem and social support and a less effective coping style
Bolgar, Zweig-Frank and Paris [12]	Childhood antecedents of interpersonal problems in young adult children of divorce	605 students awaiting routine medical exam (125 from a separated or divorced family, 467 with parents still married) completing an inventory of interpersonal problems and a family demographic questionnaire	Family demographics. Level of current interpersonal problems. Level of preseparation hostility. Level of interference between parents on child's relationship with other parent. Frequency of contact with noncustodial parent	Young adult children of divorce experience more problems with submission and over-control. More interpersonal problems develop when mother never remarries, remarries numerous times, or in cases of high levels of parental discord

did the parent that was left behind [14]. Furthermore, these families reported higher levels of stress during the year prior to separation, compared with a control group who did not undergo separation. These differences held up even after applying statistical controls for such things as children's age and parent's military rank. Although the elevated levels of depression did not reach statistical significance, this was attributed to inadequate statistical power. Geographic separation infrequently provoked a pathological level of symptoms: only 6% of the studied children had symptoms severe enough to warrant treatment. A somewhat higher effect of separation on boys compared to girls and particularly among young boys was found. This may be because the great majority of the absent parents were fathers and as has been suggested in several studies, young boys may be more vulnerable to the loss of a male figure in the home [15]. There was also a correlation between the number and severity of symptoms in the studied child and symptoms in the parent left behind to care for the child/children. Findings did not suggest that the parent's distress caused the child's symptoms but that the functioning of the parent and child are closely intertwined.

Clinical Course

While most studies of divorce begin with the separation or legal divorce of the parents, one naturalistic study by Block and colleagues examined antecedent processes of 41 families participating in a 10-year study of personality and cognitive development of children. They found that by the time the marriage breaks down, many children have spent years in a conflict-ridden home, often feeling relatively unsupported or ill-tended by their parents [16]. Undercontrolled, impulsive behaviors described as characteristic of boys during and after the divorce seem continuous with their behavior over many years in the predivorce family. Behaviors identified by researchers and clinicians as acute and reactive to the stress of a separation, therefore, may well have existed long before the actual break-up. There may, of course, be an exacerbation of the behaviors at the time of the separation as well.

Block and colleagues also examined the nature of the preseparation and postseparation parent–child relationships. They documented the following [17]:

(1) long-term and very early disengagement of fathers;
(2) unreliable paternal behavior toward the sons;
(3) anger of both parents at their sons;
(4) more modulated responses by both parents to their daughters.

These findings contradict the common belief that disengagement and withdrawal by the father occur at the time of the divorce in response to the anger of the mother toward the father. This study did not explore the link between a troubled marital relationship and deteriorating parenting within the still-intact family, that is, whether disagreements regarding parenting were caused by or resulted from the marital problems [17].

Most studies report a childhood crisis at the time of the permanent separation and often at the time of the actual divorce decree, which is usually manifest as high emotional distress and severe behavioral problems. Table 28.2 summarizes the characteristic responses based on children's developmental stages.

Several long-term studies have identified a deterioration in parent–child relationships after the divorce, with both custodial and noncustodial parents, especially among boys. In Hetherington's studies three groups were examined: a nonremarried mother-custody group, a remarried mother–stepfather group, and a nondivorced group [23]. The target children were 30 sons and 30 daughters within these three groups. At the time of the legal divorce they were four years old. At the six-year follow-up, the divorced, nonremarried mother–son dyad showed more negative features than other parent–child dyads in the study, with the exception of the stepfather–daughter relationship in the newly remarried time frame. In contrast, nonremarried mother–daughter relationships differed little from the nondivorced mother–daughter dyad. In remarried families, boys were doing significantly better than girls by two years after remarriage. In the first two years after remarriage, mother–daughter conflict was high. The relationship of mothers and daughters improved over time but was overall more antagonistic and disruptive than other relationships. In instances in which the remarriage occurred before adolescence, boys were also very difficult initially, but by two years post remarriage were no more aggressive or noncompliant than boys in nondivorced families. Although both early adolescent boys and girls exhibited many behavioral problems two years after remarriage, stepfathers saw greater improvement among stepsons and greater involvement and warmth with them than with stepdaughters.

There seems to be a second peak of problems in late adolescence and early adulthood, when the young person begins to confront issues regarding love, commitment, and marriage. In the California children of divorce study, 10 years after their parents' divorce, young people 19–29 years old acknowledged their parents' divorce as the major formative experience of

Table 28.2 Summary of characteristic responses to divorce at different developmental stages.

Developmental stage	Cognitive understanding	Emotional and behavioral responses (0–2 years after divorce)	Long-term sequelae (2 years after divorce)
Preschool to kindergarten Infancy (0–2 years) Preschool (3–5 years)	**4–5-year olds** Understand divorce in terms of physical separation Perceive divorce as temporary Are confused by parents' positive and negative feelings about each other Understand divorce in linear terms and believe they can cause behavior of parents Are cognitively unable to separate parental motives from their own	**3–5-year-olds** Fear Regression Separation anxiety Macabre fantasy Bewilderment Replaceability–fear of own Fantasy denial Disruption or inhibition of play Increased aggression Inhibited aggression Guilt Emotional neediness [7]	**Separation or divorce occurring when child 0–2.5 years of age** Increased separation-related difficulties during latency Nonaggression with parents by both boys and girls Aggression with peers in elementary school-aged girls Nonaggression with peers and academic problems in adolescent boys [6] **Separation or divorce occurring when child 3–5 years of age** Increased subjective symptoms in elementary school boys Increased aggressive behavior with parents in adolescent boys and girls Increased academic problems in adolescent girls [6] Increased externalizing behavior in elementary school boys and girls who were aggressive as preschoolers [5]

Table 28.2 *Continued*

Developmental stage	Cognitive understanding	Emotional and behavioral responses (0–2 years after divorce)	Long-term sequelae (2 years after divorce)
Elementary school age Early (6–8 years) Late (9–12 years)	**6–8-year-olds** Understand the finality of divorce Appreciate psychologic and, physical effects of parental conflict Are unable to tolerate ambivalent feelings; usually blame one parent May interpret divorce egocentrically and believe their behavior affects parental decision **9–12-year-olds** Understand psychologic motives for divorce Appreciate each parent's perspective of divorce Less likely than younger children to blame themselves Believe cessation of conflict will be a benefit of divorce for themselves	**6–8-year-olds** Grief Fear leading to disorganization Feeling of deprivation Yearning for departed parent Inhibition of aggression at father Anger at custodial mother Fantasies of responsibility and reconciliation Conflicts in loyalty **9–12-year-olds** Initially superficially well defended Attempt mastery by activity and play Anger Shaken sense of identity Somatic symptoms Alignment withone parent Identity issues; environment important	**School-age children and early adolescents** Both girls and boys from divorced families emerge as performing more poorly on mental health measures than children from intact families [4] Boys' performance significantly worse than girls'; boys experience more behavior problems in school and at home [4,5] Girls living in single mother custody homes as well adjusted as girls living in intact homes 6 years after divorce [5] Girls living in remarriage families experience more difficulty adjusting than boys, who show good adjustment 2 years after remarriage [5] Father's absence seems to contribute more significantly to cognitive development in boys than in girls [19]

Adolescence
Early adolescence (12–14 yr)
Late adolescence (15–18 yr)

12–14-year-olds
Appreciate complexity of
  communication and can
  recognize incongruence,
  between verbal and nonverbal
  cues
Understand stability of
  personality characteristics
Express concern about parental
  intention and believe that
  negative responses result from
  malevolent motives

15–18-year-olds
Explain divorce in terms of
  parental incompatibility and
  feel it was a mature decision
Detach from parental conflict
  and focus on personal
  concerns [18,20]

13–18-year-olds
Change in parent–child relationships
Worry about sex and marriage
Mourning
Anger and aggression
Changing perceptions
Loyalty conflicts
Strategic withdrawal
Greater maturity and moral growth
  possible than in children of
  nondivorced parents
Changed responsibilities within
  the family

13–18-year-olds
Adolescent girls and young
  women appear to be vulnerable
  to problems with feminine
  self-esteem and heterosexual
  development [8,21,22]

their lives [3]. Many appeared to be troubled and underachieving. Many young women who had initially coped well became very frightened of failure. Almost all expressed significant anxiety regarding love, commitment, and marriage, fearing betrayal and abandonment. As a consequence, many young people either threw themselves counterphobically into short-term sexual relationships or avoided relationships altogether. Although most subjects reported being ideologically committed to the ideals of a lasting marriage, romantic love, and fidelity, they were terrified of repeating their parents' mistakes and inflicting their pain on their own future children. Early results from the 15-year follow-up found many of these subjects working hard to resolve issues around male–female relationships and a significant number entering psychotherapy.

Bereavement

According to the US Census Bureau in March 2003, 836 000 children (under 18 years of age) lived with a widowed parent [2]. This particular statistic includes only those children still living with one parent and does not account for those children who have lost both parents or whose parents were never married.

Bereavement, as defined in the DSM-IV-TR, consists of the reaction one has to the death of a loved one [13]. For purposes of clarity, the majority of the studies conducted on children and adolescents examine a young person's reaction to the death of a parent. Grief is mostly the *affect* that results from bereavement, such as mental suffering or distress over the affliction of loss, sorrow, or regret. Mourning is the psychological process begun by the loss of a loved one; grief is the parallel subjective state [39].

Research

It was once believed that bereavement was not possible in children because they lack mature personality structure [24]. Similarly, it was not until 1975 that a group of researchers concluded that depression can exist in children and adolescents [25]. Both of these views had an impact on many of the early studies of children undergoing various types of losses.

Many of the earlier studies of bereavement suffered from methodologic flaws:

(1) Retrospective studies examined the frequency of childhood loss in child and adult *patients* and were therefore prone to underestimate or overestimate the frequency of bereavement in a 'normal' population [26–29]. Moreover, they did not account for environmental variables such as the stability of the home environment prior to the loss or the response and adaptation of the remaining parent.

(2) Prospective studies followed bereaved and normal adolescents into adulthood [30–32]. These three studies examined the same group of adolescents but assessed them at different ages. The first two studies found a higher rate of involvement in the legal system (the first in 10th graders and the second when these same individuals were in their early 20s) compared to matched controls. The third study (with the individuals in their 30s) found no relationship between bereavement and criminal behavior but did find higher rates of serious medical illness and emotional distress. Limitations in these studies included the lack of information regarding the duration, frequency, and type of symptoms experienced by bereaved adolescents as well as the age of the child at bereavement, the cause of the parent's death, and the coping ability of the surviving parent.

(3) Studies of psychiatric patients are problematic because their sample sizes are low [24,33,34]. They focus on extreme reactions to grief and do not reflect normal grieving processes. In addition, the subjectivity of the ratings employed in these studies limits their general applicability.

(4) Studies of bereavement in normal children also examined few children and were thus limited by sample size [35–38]. Two studies used subjects from a kibbutz, which makes subsequent comparisons difficult with children in 'average' US families. Studies often relied more on teacher or parent reports than on information obtained directly from the child. Many researchers questioned the reliability of child informants, assuming that parents knew more about their children, were more reliable, and were easier to interview. It is more difficult to interview children, especially those of prepubertal age: establishing rapport is more difficult, and questions must be framed in an age-appropriate manner. But although parents accurately report overt signs and symptoms of behavioral changes in their children, they are frequently unaware of subjective symptoms such as sleep disturbance, anxiety, guilt, and suicidal thoughts [39]. Often the child tries to conceal such symptoms from the parent, especially if they perceive the parent as being under stress.

Studies conducted during the 1990s have tried to address some of the above questions. Weller and colleagues conducted a study on 38 nonreferred prepubertal children who had recently experienced the death of one but not both of their parents [40]. The comparison group consisted of 38 hospitalized, depressed children individually matched to each bereaved subject in age, sex, and socioeconomic level. Each child and their surviving parent was independently evaluated using the parent and child versions of the Diagnostic Interview for Children and Adolescents – child and parent versions (DICA-C/P). Family histories and other demographic data were also obtained. When using symptoms reported by both parents and children, 37% of the bereaved children met the DSM-III-R (Third Edition-Revised) criteria for a major depressive episode [41]. When parent-reported symptoms were used exclusively, this same statistic dropped to 8%. The factors associated with increased depressive symptoms were: (1) the mother as the surviving parent; (2) preexisting untreated psychiatric disorders in the child; (3) a family history of depression; and (4) high socioeconomic level.

Using this same sample, another study examined anxiety symptoms in bereaved children [42]. This study also included a control group of 19 normal children and added the Grief Interview to the DICA-C/P Although no bereaved children met the DSM-III-R criteria for an anxiety disorder, anxiety symptoms were reported in 55% of the bereaved children immediately after parental death and in 63% approximately eight weeks later. Anxiety typically focused around the fear of other family members dying. Despite this finding, bereaved children did not report significantly more anxiety symptoms during this eight-week period than did the comparison children, and they had significantly fewer symptoms than depressed children. Bereaved children with the most anxiety symptoms were also likely to have a depressive disorder. None of the following factors was significantly associated with increased anxiety: the age and sex of the child, the sex of surviving parent, the anticipation of death, and a family history of anxiety or depressive disorders. The major limitation of these studies, however, was the relatively small sample size and therefore the possibility of not finding a statistically significant difference when one actually exists.

One study compared 26 suicide-bereaved (SB) children with 332 children bereaved from paternal death not caused by suicide (NSB) in interviews conducted at 1, 6, 13, and 25 months after the death [52]. While in many ways these two groups were similar, several significant differences were found: (1) SB children experienced significantly more anger and shame six months after the death than the NSB group; (2) fewer

SB children were described as experiencing acceptance of the death at 6 and 13 months than their counterparts; (3) SB children were more likely to experience anxiety symptoms immediately and at one month after the death; and (4) SB children experienced significantly more depressive episodes in their lifetime, and more depressive symptoms at six months and at lifetime than the NSB children.

Clinical Course

Classic models of the grief process have emphasized different stages of grief, such as numbness, protest, despair, and detachment [43–45]. Although these models are descriptive, they can lead to oversimplification and are often unhelpful in conceptualizing treatment. More recently, the concept of tasks of grief has been used by several authors in understanding bereavement [34,46,47]. These tasks are time specific. Early tasks involve gaining an understanding of what has happened as well as guarding against the full emotional impact of the loss. Middle tasks include accepting and reworking the loss and coping with intense psychologic pain. Late tasks include consolidating the child's identity and resuming appropriate developmental progress. A timing model can be useful in guiding clinical work, so interventions can be planned according to which tasks the child is trying to master. It also promotes a more adaptive view of grief behaviors as related to certain goals, thereby providing a useful alternative to pathology-based models that identify individuals as stuck in grieving [48].

Early Tasks

Children struggling with the early tasks of grieving focus on understanding the fact that someone has died and the meaning of this. They are preoccupied with protecting themselves and their families. To understand death and its implications, children need information about what death is in general as well as information about the particular death at hand. Children listen carefully and watch others intently, ask questions, and act out conflicts through play. Gaps in their information are often filled by fantasy. Even with accurate information, however, they can rarely grasp events entirely, and they only gradually understand and integrate what they have been told. For preschool children particularly, there are cognitive limitations to how well they can understand death, which is why it is important to provide them with accurate information in age-appropriate language. This information is often the foundation for the child's struggle to understand the meaning of their loss [48].

Children must feel secure in their environment to accomplish the difficult tasks of grieving. They commonly fear that they too may die or that their families will disintegrate. Children and their families engage in denial, distortion, and emotional or physical isolation to protect themselves and avoid affective overstimulation. They put much of their energy into protecting other family members. Adults sometimes withhold information from their children about death in a misguided attempt to protect them [48].

Middle Tasks

Three main tasks characterize this stage: (1) accepting and emotionally acknowledging the reality of the loss; (2) reevaluating the relationship with the lost loved one; and (3) facing and learning to bear the psychologic pain that comes with the realization of the loss. These middle-phase tasks were described by Sigmund Freud as a process of detachment, but several studies of normal bereavement have found that an internal attachment to the lost loved one continues long after the death and may be a sign of health and recovery [46,49,50]. During this period children must deal with their ambivalence and guilt regarding their lost loved one and their anger at the deceased for abandoning them. Open acknowledgment of these difficult feelings may be very threatening to the children, since they fear losing their positive connection with their deceased loved one. Often these relationship issues are played out with the therapist, friends, or a transitional object or through fantasies about the dead person. Children often maintain a fantasy that the dead person is alive or will return. Although this reflects denial on the child's part, it may also serve an adaptive function, especially in the case of parental death; the child's fantasy allows a slow, step-by-step separation from the lost parent. Children may have a lower tolerance for psychologic pain and may need more time during this middle phase to approach the pain gradually, so as to not become overwhelmed. Preschool children who have not fully developed their ability to discern what is real and what is unreal may not fully accept the reality of a loved one's death until they are several years older [48].

Late Tasks

This stage involves a reorganization of children's sense of self and of significant relationships in their life. The children must develop a new identity that includes but is not limited to the experience of the loss and identifications with the deceased person. This new identity allows them to reengage in their environment. Children need to develop new relationships without an excessive fear of loss or constantly comparing the new relationship to that with the deceased. They must maintain an enduring internal relationship to the lost loved one. As with adults, they must resume the age-appropriate developmental tasks and activities that were interrupted by the emotional loss and must be able to tolerate the periodic return of their pain, typically at points of developmental transition, specific anniversaries, or holidays. Sometimes these anniversary reactions may occur years after the death, and children may not directly connect their current feelings with a loss that occurred some time ago. This may also be true of the surviving parents who perceive their children to have 'gotten over' their loss long ago. Conflicts may arise between different tasks in this later phase, such as the need for new relationships conflicting with the development of a strong internal attachment to the lost loved one. This can be especially problematic if a new member is added to the family, such as the birth of a new sibling after a sibling loss or a new stepparent after a parental loss. Significant limitations may arise if other members of the family have become arrested in the grieving process. For instance, a parent in a state of chronic, unresolved grief may heighten the child's sense of loyalty and thus make it difficult for the child to pursue new relationships outside the family [48].

Differential Diagnosis

Adjustment Disorder

The most likely symptoms that arise from any type of loss are typically compatible with an adjustment disorder (see Box A). This diagnosis can encompass both acute and chronic disturbances as well as numerous symptom presentations. The distinction between acute and chronic disturbances can be challenging to make in the instance of divorce, especially if divorce is considered a chronic stressor, as most of the longitudinal studies seem to show. Another confounding variable is the possibility that by the time of the divorce, the children have often spent years in a conflict-ridden home and that some of the behaviors often identified as reactive to the divorce may have been chronic prior to the break-up [17]. The clinical question then becomes, 'When is the termination of the stressor in the case of divorce?' The differential diagnoses of adjustment disorder include bereavement, major depression, anxiety disorders, and disruptive behavior disorders. In rare cases, a child who has experienced a loss might present with symptoms of post-traumatic stress disorder, acute stress disorder, or one of the somatoform disorders.

Bereavement

As previously mentioned, bereavement is the deprivation due to loss or death. Feelings of sadness, insomnia, poor appetite, and weight loss, although characteristic of a major depressive disorder, are only diagnosed as such in the context of bereavement if they persist for more than two months. The fact that children's expression of bereavement varies considerably in different cultural groups should be considered when making this diagnosis. See Table 28.3 for the DSM-IV-TR description of symptoms not considered 'normal' during bereavement. If any of these symptoms are exhibited, the diagnosis of bereavement may be complicated by a major depressive episode. In some cases bereavement may be complicated by an anxiety disorder, a disruptive behavior disorder, a post-traumatic stress disorder, or a somatoform disorder.

Major Depressive Episode

Any child who has suffered a significant loss may show some symptoms of depression. If the loss is due to the death of a person important to them, then the most appropriate initial diagnosis is bereavement. If the symptoms are severe enough (or persist long enough) to meet criteria for a major depressive episode, then this diagnosis could be given as well.

Symptoms of guilt and worthlessness or fatigue (which are both more common in depressed subjects) best discriminate bereaved from depressed subjects [40]. By relying on these two symptoms, a study reports, 74% of bereaved children and 82% of depressed children can be correctly identified. Even so, 21% of bereaved children endorse feelings of worthlessness and guilt. Although 61% of bereaved children in this study reported having suicidal ideation, none had actually attempted suicide. In contrast, 89% of depressed subjects reported having suicidal ideation and 42% had attempted suicide at least once [40]. Weller hypothesized that suicidal ideation in bereaved children represents a reunion fantasy rather than the devaluation of one's own life. This explanation was given by several subjects who reported suicidal ideation, and it may account for the lack of suicide attempts and the less frequent reports of worthlessness by the bereaved children (Table 28.4).

Children experiencing a divorce may also suffer a major depressive episode. One must primarily decide if their symptoms exceed those more characteristic of adjustment disorder with depressed mood or are severe and persistent enough to meet criteria for a major depressive episode. Consistent with the findings of the

Table 28.3 DSM-IV-TR diagnostic criteria for adjustment disorders.

(A) The development of emotional or behavioral symptoms in response to an identifiable stressor(s) occurring within three months of the onset of the stressor(s)

(B) These symptoms or behaviors are clinically significant as evidenced by either of the following:
   (1) marked distress that is in excess of what would be expected from exposure to the stressor
   (2) significant impairment in social or occupational (academic) functioning

(C) The stress-related disturbance does not meet the criteria for another specific Axis I disorder and is not merely an exacerbation of a preexisting Axis I or Axis II disorder

(D) The symptoms do not represent bereavement.

(E) Once the stressor (or its consequences) has terminated, the symptoms do not persist for more than an additional six months.

Specify if:

Acute: if the disturbance lasts less than six months

Chronic: if the disturbance lasts for six months or longer. By definition, symptoms cannot persist for more than six months after the termination of the stressor or its consequences. The chronic specifier therefore applies when the duration of the disturbance is longer than six months in response to a chronic stressor or to a stressor that has enduring consequences

Adjustment disorders are coded based on the subtype, which is selected according to the predominant symptoms. The specific stressor(s) can be specified on Axis IV:

309.0	With depressed mood
309.24	With anxiety
309.28	With mixed anxiety and depressed mood
309.3	With disturbance of conduct
309.4	With mixed disturbance of emotions and conduct
309.9	Unspecified

Table 28.4 Symptoms not characteristic of 'normal' grief.

1. Guilt about things other than actions taken or not taken by the survivor at the time of the death
2. Thoughts of death other than the survivor feeling that he or she would be better off dead or should have died with the deceased person
3. Morbid preoccupation with worthlessness
4. Marked psychomotor retardation
5. Prolonged and marked functional impairment
6. Hallucinatory experiences other than thinking that he or she hears the voice of, or transiently sees the image of, the deceased person

Reprinted with permission from the *Diagnostic and Statistical Manual of Mental Disorders*, 4th ed., Text Revision. Copyright 2000 American Psychiatric Association.

long-term effects of divorce, some consideration might need to be given to a diagnosis of dysthymia or chronic adjustment disorder if less severe symptoms persist.

Anxiety Disorders

Anxiety symptoms are commonplace when a child has experienced a loss. Typically there are concerns regarding further loss. For instance, children of divorce may be upset not only that a parent has moved out but that they may never see the parent again or that the parent will not love them anymore. A child who has lost a loved one through death often fears losing other loved ones, especially the surviving parent. Sometimes this results in separation anxiety. If symptoms are time limited and of expected intensity given the stressor, adjustment disorder with anxiety is the most appropriate diagnosis. If the symptoms persist for longer than six months, are more severe, or represent an exacerbation of a previously diagnosed anxiety disorder, then the appropriate specific anxiety disorder should be diagnosed.

Disruptive Behavior Disorders

Disruptive behaviors are a common response to loss in children. Young children are less able to express their feelings verbally and tend to act out or express emotional conflicts through disruptive behaviors. If children have lost a parent to death or divorce, their environment is also likely to be more chaotic, at least temporarily, until the remaining parent can optimize his or her coping skills and access the necessary support systems. Although some children respond to a chaotic environment by becoming caretakers (e.g., the pseudomature child in an alcoholic household), many more respond with disruptive behaviors. Even within a single family unit, often both styles of coping and their variations are present. The pseudomature caretaker may actually need as much help as the child with disruptive behavior, although the focus of treatment for the parent is likely to center on the disruptive child. In the case of recent loss from death or divorce, the diagnosis of a disruptive behavior disorder should be made only if an adjustment disorder diagnosis (with disturbance of conduct or with mixed disturbance of emotions and conduct) is no longer appropriate given the severity of symptoms or their chronicity.

Post-traumatic Stress Disorder and Acute Stress Disorder

These diagnoses are primarily applicable if a child witnessed the traumatic death of a loved one and is experiencing the specific constellation of symptoms characteristic of these disorders. If the extreme stressor is present but the symptoms do not meet diagnostic criteria for post-traumatic stress disorder or acute stress disorder, a diagnosis of adjustment disorder is still appropriate.

Somatoform Disorders

Children who have experienced a loss sometimes express their emotional pain with physical symptoms, especially if they come from a family that tends to be somatic. Their symptoms are often vague, center on abdominal complaints or headaches, or have numerous sites of origin. For example, a child might develop physical symptoms that keep him or her home from school after a parent's funeral. One recent study of persistently somatizing adult patients found that those who experienced the childhood loss of a parent had the poorest treatment outcome, whereas the group with recent loss (within the past two years) had the best treatment outcomes [51]. The first point of contact for children exhibiting somatoform disorders is usually their primary care physician. If the physician is aware of the recent loss or is astute enough to ask about recent stressors, the problem may be correctly identified and treated as a symptom of the child's emotional distress. Many primary care physicians give parents appropriate initial intervention strategies; if these are unsuccessful, however, physicians should refer the child to a psychiatry clinic for evaluation and possible treatment.

Treatment

As with any referral to a behavioral health practitioner, the treatment plan must be developed to meet the individual needs of a particular patient and his or her family. It must take into account the availability of various forms of treatment, the nature and severity of the presenting symptoms, the family's recognition of the symptoms as problematic, and the family's emotional and financial resources.

Family therapy is often the preferred treatment during the crisis immediately following a loss. Whether the loss is due to death or divorce, it is sure to have affected all family members. Many times there is an *identified patient*. The first task of the therapist, then, is to reframe the problem in terms of optimizing *family* functioning and engaging the family in treatment. If the remaining or custodial parent is so wrapped up in his or her own grieving process that little thought has been given to the needs of the child, the therapist may need to guide the parent to help the child. This is especially true in the case of younger children who lack the emotional resources to cope with the loss themselves but instead must depend on the structure provided by others. In certain situations parents may require a referral for their own individual therapy, particularly if they have features of a major depressive disorder.

Historically, psychodynamic individual therapy has been the treatment of choice for children and adolescents, especially if they continue to experience psychiatric symptoms or developmental inhibition years after the loss. Although this remains the ideal treatment, changes in our medical system have caused the emphasis to shift to short-term or group treatments. The increased emphasis on short-term treatments has led to a resurgence in cognitive behavioral therapy. This treatment focuses on helping children develop a realistic appraisal of their situation and modify their behavior accordingly, for example, through effective problem solving and communication skills. Support and therapy groups have become more available in recent years. Often schools conduct support groups for children of divorce, and in many communities, the hospice organization conducts groups for bereaved children and their families.

When the experience of loss is complicated by a major depressive episode or an anxiety disorder, some consideration should be given to the use of appropriate medication. In the case of a disruptive behavior disorder, medication should only be considered if there has been no response to therapy or if behavior is dangerous to the patient or others.

Conclusion

The dynamics of loss have been examined for many years, yet it was only during the 1990s that the effects of loss were effectively quantified. It has become clear that there are long-term effects from early loss, that approximately one-third of the cases of bereavement are complicated by major depression, and that divorce causes long-term relationship problems in approximately half of the affected individuals [3]. Little systematic research has been done to evaluate treatment modalities and their outcomes with regard to the issue of loss, however. One disturbing consequence is that public policy regarding custody issues changes every few years. To be successful advocates for children and adolescents then, we must address these challenges.

References

1. US National Center for Health Statistics of the United States: Vital statistics of the United States (annual), Monthly vital statistics report, and unpublished data.
2. US Bureau of the Census: Current Population Survey, 2003 Annual Social and Economic Supplement. Internet Release Date: September 15, 2004.
3. Wallerstein JS: The long-term effects of divorce on children: A review. *J Am Acad Child Adolesc Psychiatry* 1991; **30**(3):349–360.
4. Guidubaldi J, Perry JD: Divorce and mental health sequence for children: A two-year follow-up of a nation-wide sample. *J Child Psychiatry* 1985; **24**:531–537.
5. Hetherington EM, Cox M, Cox R: Long-term effects of divorce and remarriage on the adjustment of children. *J Child Psychiatry* 1985; **24**:518–530.
6. Kalter N, Rembar J: The significance of a child's age at the time of parental divorce. *Am J Orthopsychiatry* 1981; **51**:85–100.
7. Wallerstein JS, Kelly JB: *Surviving the Break-up.* New York: Basic Books, 1980.
8. Wallerstein JS: Children of divorce: Preliminary report of a ten-year follow-up of older children and adolescents. *J Am Acad Child Adolesc Psychiatry* 1985; **24**: 545–553.
9. Fergusson DM, Horwood LJ, Lynskey MT: Parental separation, adolescent psychopathology, and problem behaviors. *J Am Acad Child Adolesc Psychiatry* 1994; **33**(8):1122–1131.
10. Black AE, Pedro-Carroll J: Role of parent-child relationships in mediating the effects of marital disruption. *J Am Acad Child Adolesc Psychiatry* 1993; **32**(5): 1019–1027.
11. Kurtz L: Psychosocial coping resources in elementary school-age children of divorce. *Am J Orthopsychiatry* 1994; **64**(4):554–563.
12. Bolgar R, Zweig-Frank H, Paris J: Childhood antecedents of interpersonal problems in young adult children of divorce. *J Am Acad Child Adolesc Psychiatry* 1995; **34**(2):143–150.

13. American Psychiatric Association: *Diagnostic and Statistical Manual of Mental Disorders*, 4th ed., Text Revision. Washington, DC: American Psychiatric Association, 2000.
14. Jensen PS, Martin D, Watanabe H: Children's response to parental separation during Operation Desert Storm. *J Am Acad Child Adolesc Psychiatry* 1996; **35**(4): 433–441.
15. Blount BW, Curry A Jr., Lubin GI: Family separations in the military. *Mil Med* 1992; **157**:76–80.
16. Block JH, Block J, Gjerde PF: The personality of children prior to divorce. *Child Dev* 1986; **57**:827–840.
17. Block J, Block JH, Gjerde PF: Parental functioning and the home environment in families of divorce. *J Am Acad Child Adolesc Psychiatry* 1988; **27**:207–213.
18. Kurdek LA: Children's reasoning about parental divorce. In: Ashmore JRD, Brodzinsky PM, eds. *Thinking About the Family: Views of Parents and Children*. Hillsdale, NJ: Lawrence Erlbaum Associates Inc., 1986:233–276.
19. Radin R: The role of the father in cognitive, academic, and intellectual development. In: Lamb M, ed. *The Role of the Father in Child Development*. New York: John Wiley & Sons, 1985:237–276.
20. Neal JH: Children's understanding of their parents' divorce. In: Kurdeck LA, ed. *New Directions for Child Development, Vol 19. Children and Divorce*. San Francisco: Jossey-Bass, 1983:3–14.
21. Kalter N, Riemer B, Brickman A, Chen JW: Implications of parental divorce for female development. *J Am Acad Child Psychiatry* 1985; **24**:538–544.
22. Kalter N: Long-term effects of divorce on children: A developmental vulnerability model. *Am J Orthopsychiatry* 1987; **57**:587–599.
23. Hetherington EM: Coping with family transitions: Winners, losers, and survivors. *Child Dev* 1989; **60**:1–14.
24. Wolfenstein M: How is mourning possible? *Psychoanal Study Child* 1966; **21**:92–123.
25. Schulterbrandt JG, Raskin A: *Depression in Childhood: Diagnosis, Treatment, and Conceptual Models*. New York: Raven Press, 1977.
26. Barry H Jr., Lindeman E: Critical ages for maternal bereavement in psychoneuroses. *Psychosom Med* 1960; **22**:166–181.
27. Beck AT, Sethi BB, Tuthill RW: Childhood bereavement and adult depression. *Arch Gen Psychiatry* 1963; **9**: 295–302.
28. Caplan MG, Douglas UI: Influence of parental loss in children with depressed mood. *J Child Psychol Psychiatry* 1969; **10**:225–232.
29. Tennant C, Bebbington P, Hurry J: Parental death in childhood and risk of adult depressive disorder: A review. *Psychol Med* 1980; **10**:289–299.
30. Gregory I: Anterospective data following childhood loss of a parent: I. Delinquency and high school dropout. *Arch Gen Psychiatry* 1965; **13**:99–109.
31. Markuson T, Fulton R: Childhood bereavement and behavioral disorders: A critical review. *Omega* 1971; **2**: 107–117.
32. Bendickson R, Fulton R: Death and the child: An anterospective test of the childhood bereavement and later behavior disorder hypothesis. In: Fulton R, ed. *Death and Identity*. Bowie, MD: Charles Press, 1976.
33. Arthur B, Kemme ML: Bereavement in childhood. *J Child Psychol Psychiatry* 1964; **5**:37–49.
34. Furman E: *A Child's Parent Dies*. New Haven, CT: Yale University Press, 1974.
35. Kliman G: *Psychological Emergencies of Childhood*. New York: Grime & Stratton, 1968.
36. Lifshitz M, Berman D, Galili A, *et al.*: Bereaved children: The effect of mother's perception and social system organization on their short-range adjustment. *J Am Acad Child Adolesc Psychiatry* 1977; **16**:272–284.
37. Van Eerdewegh MM, Bieri MD, Parilla RH, *et al.*: The bereaved child. *Br J Psychiatry* 1982; **140**:23–29.
38. Elizur E, Kaffman M: Factors influencing the severity of childhood bereavement reactions. *Am J Orthopsychiatry* 1983; **53**:668–676.
39. Weller EB, Weller RA: Grief in children and adolescents. In: Garfinkel BD, Carlson GA, Weller EB, eds. *Psychiatric Disorders in Children and Adolescents*. Philadelphia: WB Saunders Co., 1990:37–47.
40. Weller RA, Weller EB, Fristad MA, *et al.*: Depression in recently bereaved prepubertal children. *Am J Psychiatry* 1991; **148**:536–540.
41. American Psychiatric Association: *Diagnostic and Statistical Manual of Mental Disorders*, 3rd ed., Revised. Washington, DC: American Psychiatric Association, 1994.
42. Sanchez L, Fristad M, Weller R, *et al.*: Anxiety in acutely bereaved prepubertal children. *Ann Clin Psychiatry* 1994; **6**(1):39–42.
43. Bowlby J: Grief and mourning in infancy and early childhood. *Psychoanal Study Child* 1960; **15**:952.
44. Bowlby J: Childhood mourning and its implications for psychiatry. *Am J Psychiatry* 1961; **118**:481–498.
45. Bowlby J: Pathological mourning and childhood mourning. *J Am Psychoanal Assoc* 1963; **11**:500–541.
46. Schuchter SR: *Dimensions of Grief. Adjusting to the Death of a Spouse*. San Francisco: Jossey-Bass, 1986.
47. Worden W: *Grief Counseling and Grief Therapy. A Handbook for the Mental Health Practitioner*. New York: Springer-Verlag, 1982.
48. Baker J, Sedney M, Gross E: Psychological tasks for bereaved children. *Am J Orthopsychiatry* 1992; **62**(1): 105–116.
49. Glick 10, Weiss RS, Parkes CM: *The First Year of Bereavement*. New York: Wiley-Interscience, 1974.
50. Silverman PR, Nickman S, Worden JW: Detachment revisited: The child's reconstruction of a dead parent. *Am J Orthopsychiatry* 1992; **62**(4):494–503.
51. Mallouh SK, Abbey SE, Gillies LA: The role of loss in treatment outcomes of persistent somatization. *Gen Hosp Psychiatry* 1995; **17**(3):187–191.
52. Cerel J, Fristad MA, Weller EB, Weller RA: Suicide-bereaved children and adolescents: A controlled longitudinal examination. *J Am Acad Child Adolesc Psychiatry* 1999; **38**(6):672–679.

29

Foster Care and Adoption

Jill D. McCarley, Christina G. Weston

Foster Care

Until the mid- to late-nineteenth century, the care of children who had no other means of provision other than state custody was frequently dismal. Children who lost both parents due to illness or war, were abandoned, or whose parents simply had no means to care for them usually resided in custodial institutions such as infirmaries and almshouses. These institutions were the catchall placement for the poor and infirm of all ages, therefore it was not uncommon for orphaned and abandoned children to reside with the severely mentally ill, the aged, or contagious.

The situation changed during the latter half of the nineteenth century, with the evolution of the orphanage. Here, an orphaned or abandoned youth could obtain adequate, if perhaps less than ideal, care. It was also during this same time that the concept of foster care evolved, furthered by the efforts of Charles Loring Brace, who began the movement of placing children from large custodial institutions to live with Midwestern farm families. And so was born the idea of foster care although among much controversy at the time [1]. Foster care in the US has become a system for placing children unable to live with their biological parents, with other families to live. These other families receive money to cover the cost of caring for these children. These children are considered to be in the custody of the county child welfare/children's services board.

Controversy then at its inception and still yet today, foster care is much beleaguered by debate both about its concept and implementation. Foster care has long been a source of public policy debate over the role of child welfare agencies in determining when to remove a child and more recently the ever increasing cost of paying of out-of-home placements and how to finance the additional services that these children often need. Current controversies are gay and lesbian foster care, custody relinquishment, multiple placements and healthcare delivery while in foster care. No matter the theoretical underpinnings of the current foster care system, there is no doubt that children in foster care face unique challenges, as do their guardians and health care providers.

Entry into Foster Care

The death of a child due to abuse or neglect occurs to approximately two of every 100 000 children in the US each year, and usually at the hands of adults who are responsible for their care [2]. Educators, health care providers, relatives and other concerned persons report their apprehensions about the well-being of a child to children's protective agencies, who in turn send out their case workers to investigate suspicions of abuse or neglect. During the course of the investigation, a case worker will have to make the difficult choice on whether or not to remove a child from the custody of his or her parent(s) in order to assure the child's safety and well-being.

The decision to remove a child from his or her home for placement into foster care is never an easy choice. Case workers for children's protective services often have to make the best possible selection out of what seems to be no truly good options. On one hand they know the decision to remove a child will bring about pain and conflict at the very least, on the other they are painfully aware of the risks involved in not being cautious.

Unfortunately, there is limited consensus on what criteria are used in determining when a child is to be

Clinical Child Psychiatry, Second Edition. Edited by W.M. Klykylo and J.L. Kay
© 2005 John Wiley & Sons Ltd.

removed and placed into foster care. As a result, there are wide variations in the rate of child removal among states, with California (highest rate of removal) being 16 times more likely than Alabama (lowest rate of removal) to remove a child from his or her home for suspected abuse or neglect. Multiple studies have suggested that the major determining factor in the decision to remove a child seems to be the socioeconomic status of the family involved [1]. As a result, a child entering foster care is much more likely to come from an impoverished background.

VIGNETTE ONE

Robert was brought to his doctor's appointment by his foster parent and caseworker from children's protective services. Robert, an 11-year-old boy, had been diagnosed three years previously with attention deficit hyperactivity disorder (ADHD) but had received only intermittent treatment since the diagnosis was made. He had been living in foster care for the three weeks after he and his brothers were found to be neglected by their biological mother, mostly due to her problems with substance dependence. Since the placement, Robert's behavior had become unmanageable and he had been suspended from school for fighting. The foster parent describes both impulsive behavior and irritability. Medical history is unknown, as is family history. Robert described having been on several stimulant medications in the past but was unable to remember dosages or how he responded to any specific one, stating, 'It doesn't matter, anyway. I'm going to act up until I get to go home.'

The above vignette, while fictitious, illustrates several issues that are, unfortunately, commonly encountered by pediatricians, family practice and emergency room physicians, as well as child and adolescent psychiatrists.

Delivery of health care to foster children is complicated by several factors, including but not limited to:

- unexpected entry of the child into the foster care system;
- lack of known medical or mental health history;
- increased risk of chronic health, mental health and developmental problems;

- lack of a central care coordinator;
- cost of care;
- multiple placements;
- severity of a child's social and psychological deficits.

Children who enter foster care frequently do so in an emergent basis. Victims of abuse or neglect are commonly taken from a chaotic environment, perhaps after normal business hours. This precipitous transition, while no doubt difficult for the child, also creates difficulties when medical or mental health care is required immediately upon entry into foster care or shortly thereafter. There may be confusion as to issues of consent or confidentiality that need to be addressed, therefore delaying nonemergent care. In addition, health care coverage may be unknown or not yet initiated which may make finding a provider challenging. As a result, a foster child may be taken to an emergency room for nonemergent health or mental health issues that could be better addressed in a routine visit with a primary care physician. Besides increasing the cost of medical care dramatically, the trip to the emergency room has the potential of making an already stressful event much more difficult for the child involved.

Lack of Health History

Many children enter foster care from chaotic environments, and as a result will not often have had the usual well-child examinations or routine screenings. What medical care has been obtained may not be clear, as records may reside in various clinics or are lost by parents. Also, the sudden transfer of the child into foster care may not allow for the prompt possession of what medical records do exist. Important information regarding allergies, immunizations, medications, or medical conditions may be unknown or at the very least delayed in finding their way to new providers via the agency. Unfortunately, this leaves the next provider in the dark, as well as the foster parents. Often, this necessitates the repetition of testing and/or subspecialty referrals that may have been unnecessary. In addition to a child's health history the family history of mental illness is important. Many psychiatric disorders can be difficult to diagnose in young children and the knowledge of the parent's history can help to validate the diagnosis.

Commonly, the early period of foster care is marked with much activity among agency representatives, and obtaining medical records may not be a high priority unless stressed by a physician. It is more likely that existing records can be much more easily obtained earlier rather than later in the course of foster care. By strongly encouraging that every effort is made to obtain any available records, providers can make a positive influence on the short and long-term care of a child.

Increased Probability of Chronic Health, Mental Health, and Developmental Problems

Children who enter foster care have much higher rates of chronic medical, mental, and developmental problems when compared to other children not in foster care. Many factors are thought to be related to this, including inadequate medical treatment or routine physical examinations and high rates of parental substance abuse.

Estimates for rates of emotional/behavioral problems range widely. Zima *et al.* in 2000 found that 27% of 302 children in foster care exhibited at least one behavioral problem within a level of clinical significance [3]. Another study found that 13% had also taken psychotropic medication within the past year [4]. Comparison of foster children to children receiving other types of governmental aid, such as Supplemental Security Income (a US federal program that provides income for adults and children with physical or psychiatric disabilities), found that youths in foster care were twice as likely to have a mental disorder [5].

In another study which used a national survey of children who had involvement with child welfare agencies revealed that almost half scored within the clinical range for problems on the Child Behavior Checklist. Of those, adolescents were more likely to score in the clinical range as compared to younger children, as were children placed in nonrelative foster care. On the other hand, while almost half of the children surveyed scored within the clinical range for emotional or behavioral difficulties, only 15.8% had obtained any mental health intervention within the year prior to the survey [6].

Perhaps connected to this increased rate of emotional and behavioral disorders is the significant amount of parental substance abuse. One source estimates that perhaps as many as 62% of children entering foster care had prenatal exposure to drugs or alcohol and/or have experienced postnatal environmental deficits due to parental substance abuse [7].

Another risk factor associated with emotional disorders in children is a history of prior abuse. To this end, it is important to realize that at least half of children in foster care have been victims of some form of abuse [8]. While not all children who have been abused will meet full criteria for post-traumatic stress disorder

(PTSD), a great many will and no doubt numerous others will display other sequelae related to the abuse experience.

Care Coordination

Medical care of children in foster care is also complicated by the lack of a central care coordinator. Under the best of circumstances, a child would have a defined primary care provider who, in concert with a guardian, would follow the care of a child for an extended period of time. Under this model, the primary provider would offer the usual basic care as well as arrange for subspecialty referral when required. Having a centralized locus of care also simplifies record keeping and minimizes duplication of services that may be unnecessary.

Coordination of care within the foster care system creates its own challenges. Aside from the concerns already mentioned, there frequently are the additional complications of consent and confidentiality. For instance, the guardian of a child in foster care may not have the legal power to consent for treatment. It is also common that the child welfare agency itself is required to consent for medical or psychiatric treatment of a child in its custody, sometimes creating another barrier to timely care as the appropriate paperwork and signatures are sought. There are also instances where the biological parent retains the right to consent or refuse treatment of his/her child even while the child resides in foster care.

Because of these issues and those previously discussed, medical providers need to be acutely aware of who has the power to consent for treatment and who has legal access to the child's medical information in each case. Once the legality and appropriateness of information sharing is established, good communication and distribution of data may aid in filling the gap left by not having a dedicated central care coordinator.

Multiple Placements

It is not uncommon for a child in foster care to have a series of different placements for various reasons. Occasionally, foster families experience a change in situation resulting in the child's return to the agency for placement with another family. A child may be reunited with his or her family briefly, then return to state custody. At times, a child's behavior itself may be so unmanageable as to precipitate a move to another foster family. Additionally, a child with mental, medical, or developmental challenges is more likely to have multiple placements.

These multiple moves and placements create special problems for children. Although data and controlled studies are limited, it seems that multiple placements for children in foster care have negative consequences that get expressed via the health care system. One study of Medicaid claims found that over 40% of children in foster care had had three or more placements within the past year [9]. The same study also indicated that multiple placements increased the probability of high mental health resource utilization.

VIGNETTE TWO

Seven-year-old twin boys present to a child and adolescent psychiatrist with their foster parents. They have been in foster care for the past two years and in this foster home for the past four months. This is their third foster home, chosen because these foster parents have had extra training to provide therapeutic foster care, as both boys have significant developmental delays as well as bipolar disorder. They have not had psychiatric treatment since the move into this foster home, but the parents present a thick packet of records from an assortment of previous providers. These records describe a lengthy history of partial responses to multiple medication trials and two previous hospitalizations for one of the boys due to his uncontrollable and occasionally dangerous behavior. The children are loud and boisterous during the evaluation, at times requiring physical separation while arguing over toys. The foster parents handle each situation calmly and offer expert redirection and positive reinforcement for good behavior. They smile warmly at the boys and indicate a strong commitment to 'hang on to these guys,' expressing a desire to eventually adopt them.

A provider when faced with situations similar to the above vignette may have to decide to 'start fresh' due to some of the unique situations that foster care introduces. Complicated medical and/or psychiatric histories, often incomplete or unclear, can be overwhelming. Multiple trials of medications in the past – sometimes inadequate in dosage or length of time attempted due to the movement of a foster child – may yield less than favorable results. This, combined with treatments attempted in the face of other, perhaps rather dramatic

changes in a child's social or academic environment clouds the picture of what may or may not have been effective. For these reasons, it is not necessarily wise to dismiss or disregard a prior treatment as a universal failure for a child. It is plausible that an option that failed or met with limited success may have a vastly different outcome when paired with a stable environment or other interventions.

A provider might feel a sense of dread when reviewing page after page of previous treatment failures for a particular child. However, when the commitment of the parent(s) is evident, that dread feeling conceivably could lead to hope when the stability of the home and positive regard for the child is present. These assets may just provide the child with the link that was previously missing for treatment to meet with success.

Grandparent/Kinship Care

There has been a dramatic increase in the number of grandparents raising their grandchildren in the US. Some are in kinship care while others are in the full custody of their grandparents. Kinship care refers to the practice of placing foster care children with family members rather than nonbiologically related foster parents. From 1990 to 1998 the number of custodial grandparents increased by 53% [10,11]. The structure of these homes with grandparents as head of household can be difficult to define. They can have both grandparents present, grandmother present or grandfather present. They can also have some of the parents present or no parents present. In their analysis of 1997 census data Casper and Bryson found that 6.7% of families with children were maintained by grandparents [10]. Thirty-five per cent were both grandparents, with some parents present; 17% were both grandparents, with no parents present; 29% were grandmother only with some parents present; 14% were grandmother only, with no parents present; and 6% were grandfather only. From 1990 to 1997 the highest increase among these groups was among grandfather only, 39%; both grandparents, with no parents present, 31%; grandmother only with no parents present, 27%. The very same factors that are contributing to increasing rates of foster care are creating custodial grandparents. Parental substance abuse, incarceration, teenage pregnancy, divorce, the rapid rise of single parenthood, and increasing rates of child abuse are all believed to be contributing to this trend.

The grandparents and children in these homes are more likely to suffer economic hardships. Children in a grandparent's household without a parent were twice as likely to be below the poverty level when compared with children living with both grandparents and a parent [10]. They were also twice as likely to be uninsured when they lived with their grandparent's household without a parent present, 36% vs. 15% of children living with grandparents in their parent's home. They were also more likely to be receiving public assistance. In custodial grandparent homes, significant health problems are found in both the grandparents and the grandchildren. The grandparents have been found to have high rates of depression, poor self-rated health, multiple chronic health problems and a decreased ability to perform activities of daily living [12,13]. The grandchildren raised by grandparents have higher rates of physical disabilities; hyperactivity, asthma, and poor sleeping and eating patterns [13,14].

In addition to health effects the children in grandparent-headed homes are more likely to have caregivers who haven't graduated from high school. They are also more likely to be younger, have an older nonworking head of household, live in the South, inner cities, and to be poor [9]. Over half of the children living in grandparent's homes are under six years old. When racial differences are examined, historically African–American grandmothers have acted as surrogate parents for their grandchildren more often than did white grandmothers [15]. In 2002, the largest ethnic group to live within their grandparents household was African–American children at 9% followed by 6% of Hispanic children, 4% of non-Hispanic white children and 3% of Asian children. Two-thirds of the African–American children living in their grandparents' household were with only one grandparent. All other ethnic groups were more likely to have both grandparents present.

This trend towards grandparents as parents of their grandchildren creates many psychosocial issues. As discussed above, many of these grandparents are less physically, emotionally and financially able to support their grandchildren. In cases where their grandchildren were removed due to their children's substance abuse, incarceration and/or abuse/neglect of the children they may have the added emotional guilt of having failed to raise the children successfully. They may feel pressure to raise their grandchildren better the second time around. They frequently are conflicted between helping their children or their grandchildren. As this trend has increased rapidly, there are several public policy implications. Some welfare reform rules designed for young parents unfairly punish retirement-age custodial grandparents for not working. Foster care advocates have recommended that parity should be established between kinship foster care homes and nonrelative foster care payment rates. Currently non-relative foster care homes receive higher reimbursement. Policies for securing adoption and guardianship can be made easier for grandparents to use.

With increasing trend towards grandparents raising their grandchildren, there has been an interest in creating support programs for these grandparents. In a small pilot program with separate grandparent and child groups, participants found the experience helpful [16]. The grandparents even went to great lengths to attend sessions that they found helpful. While this pilot study didn't quantify how much families improved it highlighted the need for longer groups and continued contact with social workers after an initial group, as the families found the social interaction and support helpful. It identifies ways to structure therapeutic interventions to grandparent-led families so they can be most beneficial.

Adoption

After World War II, adoption became more common and more widely accepted than it had been before. For the first time, a broad white middle-class consensus proclaimed adoption the 'best solution' to the 'problem' of pregnancy out of wedlock.

Barbara Melosh [17]

The face of adoption changed significantly over time. The above quote marks one milestone of change, when during 1945–1965 there was a shift to a more uniform practice surrounding adoption policies. Specifically, children were matched to parents ethnically and only upon a confidential basis. These 'closed' adoptions were the norm for many decades, where neither the child nor the biological parents knew the identity or whereabouts of the other. At times, even birth certificates were amended to reflect the identity of the adoptive parents. Children were often matched according to physical appearance and temperament, with the goal of affecting the equivalence of full kinship [17].

Starting in the 1980s, adoption agencies began to utilize the concept of 'open' adoption. The concept was that birth mothers who were ambivalent about giving up their children into anonymity forever might be more willing to grant adoption if they knew more about where and with whom their children were placed. The term open adoption has since come to mean a spectrum of contact, from yearly reports all the way to active, regular participation of the biological parent with the adoptive family. Some agencies even allow the birth mother to choose which family her child will eventually go to.

Not surprisingly, this change from closed to open adoption has caused much heated debate. Both sides present sound arguments. Proponents of open adoption argue that the secretive nature of closed adoption creates psychological difficulties linked with a veil of shame or guilt about unknown backgrounds. They contend that an individual has a basic right to know his or her own history. Proponents of open adoption also point out that it may be important for older children in foster care see their future adoptive parents welcomed into their current home by caretakers that they have grown to trust. In this way, it is less likely to be perceived by the child that he or she has been 'snatched away' by a caseworker to be delivered to the adoptive family. Also, when a child begins to have positive feelings for his or her new adoptive family, he or she may feel less conflicted about being unfaithful to the former caretakers or loving them less.

Opponents of open adoption cite that the biological parents' involvement may confuse children and disrupt relationships or bonding with the adoptive parent. Ideological positions aside, research seems to indicate that there is not typically enough contact between the biological parent and adoptive family to make much difference, for good or ill, upon the development of the child [17].

Nevertheless, there has been a movement among adopted adults to force open previously sealed documents about their own births and adoptions. This surge has been powerful enough to challenge state laws, establish adoption registries, and allow third-party delegates to read sealed adoption records. The drive of many adopted persons who take the time and effort to pursue these records likely mean that many others, if not most, struggle less obviously with the ramifications of not knowing their own histories. In addition, they may be conflicted by even having the desire to uncover their pasts, feeling guilt over 'betraying' the adoptive parents that they care deeply for.

Race, Age and Adoption

In the US, of the almost 550 000 children in foster care in 2001, 126 000 were awaiting adoption, and 50 000 were actually adopted from the public foster care system [18]. It is interesting to compare the race and age distribution of children awaiting adoption and those who were adopted (Table 29.1).

These numbers indicate that there is a racial as well as an age discrepancy between children awaiting adoption and those who are adopted. Most striking is the significant over-representation of Black, non-Hispanic children awaiting adoption.

Children aged 11–15 years are also at a disadvantage for successful adoption compared to younger children

Table 29.1 Race and age distribution of children who were adopted, and those awaiting adoption.

	Awaiting adoption (%)	Adopted (%)
Race		
Black, non-Hispanic	45	35
White, non-Hispanic	34	38
Hispanic	12	16
Age (years)		
1–5	32	46
6–10	32	39
11–15	28	16
16–18	4	2

Source: US Department of Health and Human Services, Administration for Children and Families, Administration on Children, Youth and Families, Children's Bureau: Preliminary FY 2001 Estimates as of March 2003.

who are available for adoption. Parents wishing to adopt are usually seeking younger children or infants, often working with the notion that a younger child is less likely to exhibit difficulties as they may have less of a 'bad' history and therefore less 'damage' was done. Also, future adoptive parents may view an older child with some degree of skepticism, perhaps wondering if something was wrong with the child to prevent earlier adoption.

Another striking factor in adoption from foster care is the length of time the process itself takes to occur. The mean number of months between termination of parental rights to adoption was 16 months, although 19% waited two years or more before adoption. However, 59% of those adopted were adopted by a foster parent. For those children who were awaiting adoption, the mean number of months in continuous foster care was 44. Yet almost half of all children awaiting adoption in 2001 had been in foster care for three years or more [18].

Understandably, children who are awaiting adoption from foster care may be quite conflicted about the possibility of adoption. Although parental rights may have been terminated, a great many children have difficulty accepting or understanding this fact and continue to express a hope to eventually return. Conversely, a child who is angry at his or her parents may openly express a desire to break all ties and see adoption as a way for this to occur. However, if this anger at parents remains unreckoned with, relationships with alternate parental figures may be compromised. Encouraging open, honest exploration of a child's feelings about adoption may smooth the transition.

VIGNETTE THREE

A four-year-old girl presents with her adoptive mother for evaluation. The mother expresses worry about her daughter's defiant behavior. The child often refuses to follow directions from her mother, frequently erupting into a tantrum which usually results in the child getting her way. This pattern of behavior occurs only with the mother, as the child's father and preschool teacher have described her as 'a little stubborn, but overall a good kid.' When questioned about relenting to the child's wishes, the mother rather sheepishly defends her parenting style, stating, 'Well, she had such bad luck before she came to us. What she went through was just awful and I want her to be happy.'

Adoptive and foster parents may have conflicting feelings about disciplining their children. On one hand, they realize that children need rules and consequences, yet may feel a need to 'make up' for the child's bad experiences prior to entering their home. In addition, they may also try to hasten or aid the bonding relationship of the child to them by being excessively permissive. While parents may know logically that no amount of 'Santa Cause' parenting will make up for the suffering the child endured, many parents experience a different affective state when disciplining their adopted child versus other children. As with any child, foster and adoptive children need firm rules and boundaries in order to meet developmental goals successfully. Stressing this to parents may relieve them of some of the guilt or anxiety they feel about disciplining their child.

Controversies in Foster Care/Adoption

Gay and Lesbian Foster/Adoptive Parents

As more children are placed in the out-of-home care system in the US, the available pool of prospective families has decreased. Case workers are frequently forced to seek out more nontraditional families to care for and adopt these children. Single parents, transracial families and most recently gay and lesbian couples are becoming options to meet the increased need. The placement of foster children with gay men and lesbians is controversial in some conservative parts of American society. Research on gay and lesbian biological families has found that they are just as capable at raising children as heterosexual parents. A common fear is that children raised by homosexual parents will have difficulty with gender identity, or are more likely to develop a homosexual sexual orientation. In fact these children have been found to develop appropriate gender roles and sexual orientation consistent with their biologic gender [19,20]. The only negative found in these children is that they are more likely to remember being teased by other peers about being gay or lesbian themselves. The teasing doesn't appear to affect their social adjustment when compared to that of children raised by heterosexual parents [19]. Few studies have examined the issues of lesbian and gay men raising foster and adoptive children. In a study of social work staff and homosexual foster and adoptive parents, Brooks and Goldberg made several findings that highlight the challenges in lesbian and gay placements. A bias towards extra scrutiny of prospective homosexual foster parents based only on their sexual orientation was found. Gay men and lesbians were more likely to accept children with special needs. A lack of clear, local and state social service policy on gay and lesbian placements made agency decisions difficult. In most states two individuals cannot jointly adopt a child if they are not legally married, leading most children to be adopted by one primary parent of a homosexual couple [21].

VIGNETTE FOUR

Gayle is a 14-year-old who came to her first appointment with her child and adolescent psychiatrist. She was brought by her new foster mother. She had been neglected in her birth family and removed three years ago after it was determined that her older brother had sexually abused her. She had been in several foster homes since her removal and had placements changed mainly due to her outbursts and anger towards older men. The most recent change came when her custody status changed and she became eligible for adoption. She moved to her current foster to adoptive home one week ago. Her foster parents are a lesbian couple in their mid-50s who are professionals. One parent has grown adult children biological children. Both the foster mom and child report that things are going well during the first week of placement. The child denies any difficulties with being placed with a lesbian home and replies that she tells her friends she has 'many moms.' Her foster mom discusses how they have prepared Gayle for possible teasing by her peers. Over the next several months of visits Gayle and her mothers continue to do well. Her outbursts decrease and she is becoming academically successful for the first time in her life. After the six-month-waiting period she is adopted by one of her foster mothers as allowed by state law.

This case illustrates a successful placement with a lesbian couple. It also illustrates the need for preparation of children for possible expressions of homophobia and discrimination based on their parents' sexual orientation. Since foster children may already feel different from children raised in biologic families, discussing sexual orientation as well in advance can prepare them for possible teasing.

Custody versus Care

For many parents of a child with a severe mental illness, they may have to make an agonizing choice to relinquish custody of their child in order to obtain adequate treatment for the child's mental illness. It is a choice far more common than once thought. A report of the General Accounting Office estimated that in 2001, over 12 700 children were placed in child welfare or juvenile justice agencies so as to procure treatment for mental disorders [22]. At the same time, the report cautions that this number is merely an approximation, as there is no formal tracking method for these placements and several states were unable to even provide estimates. A recent report in Virginia found that almost one in four children were in the foster care system to receive treatment for their emotional disturbances [23].

Families face this choice for several reasons. First, health insurance often does not cover, or has limited coverage, for mental health services, particularly those that require long-term treatments such as residential services. This often leaves a wide financial gap for families to fill. At the same time, care of the ill child may interfere significantly with the parent's ability to work in order to provide the coverage needed.

Other issues surround the availability of services. Mental health services for children are often in short supply, especially psychiatric services. Long waiting lists or distance to the service are commonplace. Even when resources happen to be available, children may not meet eligibility requirements for various agencies

or coordination between agencies is poor. As a result, parents stressed by the needs of their child and frustrated by the lack of, or access to, care may see giving up custody as the only chance their child has for obtaining proper care.

VIGNETTE FIVE

At an early age Joey's behavior was difficult for his mother to handle. His rages and violent actions threatened his own health and the health of his family. Trials of medication and outpatient counseling from 5–6 years old were unsuccessful in improving his behavior. At the age of six his mother and stepfather decided to give up custody to the local county children's services board so he could be placed in a residential treatment center. He was placed in a series of residential treatment centers, foster homes, and juvenile detention facilities over a period of several years. At one point he was sexually abused by a peer and then began to act out sexually. His mother remained involved in his treatment and he was able to visit with his family regularly throughout his care. After four years, Joey was returned to his mother and stepfather when the residential treatment center he was at closed its doors due to lack of funding. His problems remain and he is still has rage attacks and is violent and threatening to his family.

This case highlights some of the difficulties with treating severely mentally ill children. While giving up custody of a child is something parents would never want to do, some are forced to do so out of desperation when a child's behavior becomes dangerous. To do so is to take on terrible risks, however. Parents who relinquish custody may also lose control over what treatment their child receives or where he/she is sent. In order to regain custody, parents may have to appeal to a court for a ruling. Custody relinquishment can be seen as unfairly biasing poor, minority and single parent families as they are more likely to have to relinquish their children to obtain services. It can be harmful on a parent's self-esteem and perception of family in society. It can led to adversarial relationships between parents and agencies and further erode the relationship between parents and their children [24]. Sometimes, parents may lose track of their child altogether for a period of time.

The plight of these families has become more visible within the popular press, which may aid in prompting changes within the system of care delivery. Several states have either passed or are considering mental health parity laws, which would require insurance to provide equal coverage for mental health treatments on par with other medical coverage. In 1993, Oregon passed the Voluntary Child Placement Agreement (VCPA) to allow caregivers to voluntarily place their child in out-of-home care without giving up custody. Initially some parents had problems having their wages garnished adversarily for support of their children. In an evaluation of the first five years of the law it was discovered that VCPA children weren't easily identified and were hard to track. A lack of knowledge among caseworkers about the law was found, only 3% of caseworkers could identify which hypothetical cases could qualify for the program [25]. While a step in the right direction, these laws are still a long way from correcting the problems faced by families of children with severe mental illness.

Conclusion

Children who are in foster care or who have been adopted often face uncommon challenges, as do their families and providers. In particular, child and adolescent psychiatrists have a unique role in aiding these children and their adult caretakers. Though at times the complexities may seem daunting, the reward of seeing a child improve while in a new, stable environment is well worth the endeavor.

Acknowledgments

Special thanks to Lila Roberts, RN, for her invaluable insights as both a foster parent and mental health nurse.

References

1. Lindsey D: *The Welfare of Children.* New York, NY: Oxford University Press, 2004:12–13, 168–175.
2. National Adoption Information Clearinghouse (NAIC): *Child Abuse and Neglect Fatalities: Statistics and Interventions.* Washington, DC: Government Printing Office, 2004.
3. Zima B, *et al.*: Behavior problems, academic skill delays and school failure among school-aged children in foster care; their Relationships to placement characteristics. *J Child Fam Studies* 2000; **9**:87–103.
4. Zima B, *et al.*: Psychotropic medication use among children in foster care: Relationship to severe psychiatric disorders. *Am Public Health* 1999; **89**:1732–1735.
5. dosReis S, *et al.*: Mental health services for youths in foster care and disabled youths. *Am J Public Health* 2001; **91**:1094–1099.
6. Burns B, *et al.*: Mental health need and access to mental health services by youths involved with child welfare: A national survey. *J Am Acad Child Adolesc Psychiatry* 2004; **43**:960–969.
7. US General Accounting Office: *Foster Care: Health Needs of Many Young Children are Unknown and Unmet.* Washington, DC: Government Printing Office, 1995.
8. Finch SJ, Fanshel D: Testing the equality of discharge patterns in foster care. *Social Work Res Abstracts* 1985; **21**(3):3–10.
9. Rubin D, *et al.*: Placement stability and mental health costs for children in foster care. *Pediatrics* 2004; **113**: 1336–1341.
10. Casper LM, Bryson K: Co-resident grandparents and their grandchildren: Grandparent maintained families. (Technical Working Paper No. 26) 1998 Washington, DC: US Census Bureau. Population Division.
11. US Census Bureau: Children's Living Arrangements and Characteristics: March 2002. Washington, DC: US Government Printing Office, 2003.
12. Minkler M, Fuller-Thomson E: The health of grandparents raising grandchildren: Results of a national study. *Am Public Health* 1999; **89**:1384–1389.
13. Dowdell EB: Caregiver burden: Grandparents raising their high risk children. *J Psychosocial Nursing* 1995; **33**: 27–30.
14. Minkler M, Roe KM: Grandparents as surrogate parents. *Generations* 1996; **20**:34–38.
15. Thomas JL, Sperry L, Yarbrough MS: Grandparents as parents: Research findings and policy recommendations. *Child Psychiatry Hum Dev* 2000; **31**:3–22.
16. Dannison LL, Smith AB: Custodial grandparents community support program: Lessons learned. *Children Schools* 2003; **26**:87–95.
17. Carp W: *Adoption in America Historical Perspectives.* Ann Arbor, MI: University of Michigan Press, 2002: 218–219, 218–220.
18. US Dept of Health and Human Services: The AFCARS Report; preliminary FY 2001. Estimates as of March 2003. www.acf.hhs.gov/programs/cb
19. Tasker F, Golombok S: Adults raised as children in lesbian families. *Am J Orthopsychiatry* 1995; **65**:203–215.
20. Green R, *et al.*: Lesbian mothers and their children: A comparison with solo parent heterosexual mothers and their children. *Arch Sexual Behav* 1986; **15**:167–184.
21. Brooks D, Goldberg S: Gay and lesbian adoptive and foster care placements: Can they meet the needs of waiting children. *Social Work* 2001; **46**:147–157.
22. US General Accounting Office: Child Welfare and Juvenile Justice: Federal Agencies Could Play a Stronger Role in Helping States Reduce the Number of Children Placed Solely to Obtain Mental Health Services. April 2003, p14.
23. Bender E: State seeks solutions to foster care crisis. *Psychiatr News* 2005; **40**:8–56.
24. Friesen BJ, Giliberti M: Research in the service of policy change: The 'custody problem'. *J Emot Behav Disord* 2002; **11**:39–47.
25. Blankenship K, Pullmann M, Friesen BJ: Keeping Families Together: Implementation of an Oregon Law Abolishing the Custody Relinquishment Requirement. Portland, OR: Portland State University, Research & Training Center on Family Support and Children's Mental Health, 1999.

30

Child Psychiatry and the Law

Douglas Mossman

Introduction

The idea that the legal system should treat children differently from adults and afford them special rights and protections is a recent historical phenomenon, one that coincides with many other twentieth-century social developments that have altered Western societies' views of children and their preparation for citizenship. English common law traditionally regarded immaturity ('infancy') as a barrier to criminal prosecution, and children have long been barred from exercising many legal rights accorded to adults (e.g., voting). Yet it was only around 1900 that the US legal system began developing special courts for children in recognition of their distinct mental states and special developmental needs. At the time, most American children lived in rural areas. They often attended school sporadically, few finished high school, and most began full-time employment when they entered adolescence. Notions about the legal treatment of children that we now take for granted – that they are not the property of their parents, that they should attend school until adulthood, that they deserve special protection in employment settings, that society owes them protection from their parents' violence, and that special, 'juvenile' courts should handle their lawbreaking – reflect distinctly twentieth-century views about and expectations of children.

Practicing child forensic psychiatry forces the clinician to confront the ever-changing clinical, social, and legal issues that reflect Americans' seemingly constant reconfiguration of their work habits, family life, and communities. Although this chapter cannot provide an exhaustive treatment of a continually developing subject, it attempts to provide basic background information about the legal matters that child psychiatrists commonly encounter in their practices.

Legal Issues in the Treatment of Minors

Competence and Consent for Treatment

Competence is the legal capacity to perform a legal function, such getting married, writing a will, entering into a business contract, managing funds, or obtaining medical treatment. The law presumes that adults are competent for all such functions and that minors are incompetent. Although some 16-year-olds can understand and reason about medical information better than most adults, the law generally does not let adolescents give authorization for medical treatment. Before treating minors, clinicians usually must obtain express permission from the child's legal custodian (in intact families, either biological parent; otherwise, the child's custodial parent or legal guardian), an adult with the right to make the major decisions about a child's life.

Though there are exceptions to this general rule, most do not involve circumstances where minors are obtaining psychiatric care. Child psychiatrists should be aware of the exceptions, however, because fellow professionals may request their consultation on youths whose medical treatment was appropriately initiated without the legal custodian's consent, but whose receiving psychiatric treatment would require such consent.

Emergencies

One may assume consent for a minor's treatment in situations where delaying treatment to obtain the appropriate adult's permission would jeopardize the life or health of the child. Most states have statutes that specify what constitutes an emergency exception to the normal requirement for adult consent, and what efforts (if any) physicians must make to contact the legal

Clinical Child Psychiatry, Second Edition. Edited by W.M. Klykylo and J.L. Kay
© 2005 John Wiley & Sons Ltd.

custodian before beginning urgently needed treatment. Clinicians who work in emergency settings should be familiar with local laws that address this issue. They should also be aware that federal law [1] entitles every patient presenting to the emergency room of a hospital that receives federal funds to a medical screening examination, regardless of capacity to consent.

Psychiatrists should realize that there are circumstances in which emergency medical treatment may be rendered without an adult's consent, but in which a psychiatrist's interventions should await express permission from the legal custodian. For example, an adolescent brought to a hospital after an overdose may need medical treatment quickly to avert serious consequences. Once the child is stabilized, however, a psychiatric consultation to assess future suicide risk and any need for further treatment can usually wait until the appropriate adult has been contacted and has given permission for the evaluation.

Emancipated and Mature Minors

Children who are married, living independently, or supporting themselves and who can show that they can manage their own affairs may ask a court to recognize them as 'emancipated.' Emancipated minors are treated as adults for a variety of legal purposes, including consent to treatment. Because a child must petition a court to attain this status, clinicians rarely encounter patients who truly are emancipated. Interestingly, an adolescent mother generally may make medical treatment decisions for herself and her child(ren), but may or may not be regarded as legally competent to make other decisions. In many jurisdictions, 'mature minor' statutes recognize that adolescents, as they approach majority, can participate intelligently in medical treatment decisions although they are living at home and are financially dependent on adults. These statutes specify minimum ages and circumscribed clinical contexts (such as drug/alcohol dependence, need for brief mental health outpatient treatment, and obtaining contraceptives) in which teenagers may receive care without an adult's permission.

Children of Divorced Parents

When the need arises, a parent who has physical custody of a child generally may authorize treatment for an acute pediatric problem, even if the parent is not the child's legal custodian. If the treatment is elective, ongoing, and/or nonroutine, however (as is much psychiatric treatment), the clinician should obtain consent for treatment from the child's legal custodian [2]. When a divorced parent brings a child for nonemergency outpatient psychiatric care, the psychiatrist should make sure that the parent is the legal custodian; if not, the psychiatrist should await the custodial parent's express permission before initiating treatment. In some circumstances (e.g., where the psychiatrist wonders whether a noncustodial parent has kidnaped the child), the prudent psychiatrist may ask to see written proof of custody.

Reproductive Counseling and Abortion

The US Supreme Court's 1977 Carey decision [3] established minors' right to privacy in making decisions about use of contraceptives. In response, most states have recognized the right of teenagers to obtain reproductive counseling and contraceptive services without their parents' consent or knowledge. Many states, however, have passed laws requiring physicians to notify parents or guardians when children seek abortions, and clinicians who provide gynecological services to teens should be aware of them. The Supreme Court held in Planned *Parenthood v. Casey* (1992) [4] that a Pennsylvania law requiring parental notification, but which allowed a girl to petition for a judicial bypass of this requirement, was constitutional. Minors may obtain family planning assistance without parental consent or knowledge under federal statutory provisions (the Social Security Act and the Family Planning Services and Population Research Act of 1970).

Sexually Transmitted Diseases

Most states allow minors to obtain treatment for STDs without parental consent or knowledge, although state laws vary in the ages at which this may occur and in post-treatment notification requirements (to parents or guardians and/or public health officials).

Outpatient Substance Abuse and Mental Health Counseling

In most states, statutes expressly allow adolescents above a certain age (usually 12–14 years) to obtain information about and treatment for substance abuse without their legal custodian's consent; states vary about whether a clinician may or must inform the parent/guardian after contact with the minor has occurred. A minority of states expressly allow minors to obtain some forms of mental health treatment without the custodian's consent, and in many states, laws governing provision of medical care to emancipated or mature minors would apply to physicians rendering psychiatric care.

Of course, the *legality* of treating an adolescent without parental consent does not mean that treatment without parental involvement is *advisable*. While respecting an adolescent's legal rights and emotional needs for privacy, clinicians should also recognize that parental involvement is usually crucial to the success of a child's therapy. Figuring out what and how to tell parents about what is going on in therapy is an important clinical aspect of most psychotherapeutic work with a teenage patient.

Psychiatric Hospitalization and Civil Commitment

The laws and rules concerning psychiatric hospitalization of minors vary considerably between states. US constitutional law [5–7] gives adults a panoply of judicial protections and procedural rights before they undergo nonconsensual hospitalization. In *Parham v. J.R.* (1976 [8]), however, the Supreme Court decision held that children do not have the same constitutional rights. According to *Parham*, it is constitutionally permissible for minors to be involuntary hospitalized without judicial review if the child's legal custodian consents, the treating clinicians concur, and the clinicians periodically review the need for continued inpatient treatment.

States may grant their citizens additional rights beyond those guaranteed by the federal constitution, however, and many states have enacted laws that accord children avenues for protesting admission or seeking release once hospitalized. In some states, these laws closely resemble adults' protections against involuntary hospitalization (e.g., right to notice, a hearing, and attorney representation); in other states, the avenues for relief are not as formal as those available to adults. Clinicians who treat children as psychiatric inpatients thus must be aware of how their state's statutes or case law requirements affect procedures for involuntary psychiatric hospitalization; unlike most pediatric hospital treatment, the parent's or guardian's consent to inpatient treatment may not suffice.

Confidentiality of Records and Communications

The question of how to afford minors appropriate confidentiality in psychotherapy requires psychiatrists to recognize and sort through potential conflicts among treatment goals, ethical principles, state law, and federal law.

Intrafamilial Issues

Although some states that permit minors to consent to treatment also prohibit release of a minor's records without the child's consent, the minor's legal custodian usually decides who may have access to the minor's medical records. In theory, this implies that parents have broad rights to review information about their children's psychiatric treatment.

Despite parents' legal prerogatives, authorities who write about children's psychotherapy believe that mental health clinicians have ethical obligations that go beyond what the law allows or requires. For children and adults, the American Psychiatric Association's *Principles of Medical Ethics* [9] tells psychiatrists to reveal only information that 'is relevant to a given situation' and deemed 'usually unnecessary' to reveal '[s]ensitive information such as an individual's sexual orientation or fantasy material,' even if psychiatrists have received a broader authorization. The *Principles* also recommend that psychiatrists exercise 'careful judgment' about including parents or guardians in a child's treatment, while simultaneously assuring the child's 'proper confidentiality.'

Although these recommendations seem contradictory, they only reflect the competing obligations that psychiatrists face in their work with children. The following paragraphs outline a scheme for balancing a child's needs for privacy with the therapeutic obligation to speak with parents/guardians and third parties involved in the child's daily life.

Ground Rules

At the outset of treatment, the clinician should agree with the child and parents/guardians about how the clinician will handle the child's communications and keep adults informed. Exactly what and how the therapist informs adults will vary depending on the format and goals of treatment. For example, the therapist-to-parent communication in the family-centered treatment of a seven-year-old with encopresis will be very different from the communication to adults about therapy with 16-year-old who is dealing with issues of sexual identity. In all cases, however, minors should know that their parents or guardians must receive information about certain features of treatment, such as prescription of psychotropic medication (for which the adults must give consent), emergencies (e.g., possible suicide or behavior that threatens life and limb), the times of the child's appointments, and whether the child has attended appointments.

The Role of Confidentiality

Most published discussions of this topic emphasize precautions to protect the child's privacy and to limit disclosure to only absolutely necessary information. While these emphases reflect valid clinical concerns, they run the risk of being misunderstood by the naive therapist, to the detriment of a child patient's treatment. Confidentiality is not an end in itself; it serves therapy's larger goal of enhancing and respecting a patient's autonomy.

Value of Communication

Adolescents may object to the therapist's telling parents uncensored details of their sex lives, and psychiatrists may have to remind overly curious parents of their children's need for privacy. Yet, almost all minors *want* therapists to help them communicate with the adults in their lives. Thus, a psychiatrist can often say to a minor patient, 'Now that we see what's bothering you, how should we help your parents understand this?' When the psychiatrist and minor patient discuss what to tell adults, how the adults will be told, and who will say it, the patient learns that his psychiatrist respects his thoughts, feelings, and personhood. The minor patient also gets to communicate with adults in a way that enhances autonomy, and learns that adults are separate individuals who can provide support without compromising autonomy. A clinician's awareness of the autonomy-enhancing aspects of communication to parents is important whether the communication deals with an urgent issue (e.g., a suicide threat) or merely important but nonpressing material about developments in ongoing therapy.

Promoting Autonomy

A psychiatrist who is treating a minor in individual psychotherapy should seek the child's explicit permission before revealing information to a parent or guardian. If information must be disclosed despite the child's wishes (again, for example, a threat of suicide), the child deserves prior notice of the disclosure and an opportunity to discuss the matter with the therapist. The clinician can further convey respect for the objecting child's autonomy by explaining why the communication must take place, and by describing how the communication will include only that information necessary to allow adults to respond appropriately to the child's needs.

HIPAA and Extrafamilial Disclosures

Rules about protecting information, releasing information, and what an authorization form must contain vary from state to state, and have recently been affected by the (perhaps misnamed) Health Insurance Portability and Accountability Act (HIPAA) of 1996 [10]. In August 2002, the US Department of Health and Human Services issued the 'Privacy Rule' to implement HIPAA's requirements concerning handling of 'protected health information' (PHI). The Privacy Rule governs use and disclosure of individuals' PHI by so-called 'covered entities,' i.e., entities affected by the

Rule. The Rule also sets standards for helping individuals understand their privacy rights and control use of their health information. The following discussion is adapted from a summary prepared by the Department of Health and Human Services [11].

Covered Entities

Under the Privacy Rule, 'covered entities' are health plans, health care clearing houses, and health care providers (including doctors and hospitals) that transmit health information in electronic form, for example, by electronically filing insurance claims or referral authorizations. The Rule governs handling and release of any 'individually identifiable health information' that deals with that person's physical or mental health, providing the person with health care, or paying for the person's health care.

Disclosures

A major purpose of the Privacy Rule is to define and limit the circumstances in which covered entities may use or disclose an individual's PHI. A covered entity must disclose PHI to patients when they ask to see their own records or inquire about disclosures to others. Covered entities are allowed to disclose PHI for other reasons consistent with professional ethics. Examples of such reasons include obtaining payment, emergency situations, situations where the individual gives verbal consent (e.g., to discuss care with a relative), and writing a prescription that a pharmacist fills.

Covered entities also may disclose PHI without the individual's authorization when required by law to do so (e.g., pursuant to a statute or court order); they may also give information to police to permit criminal investigations. Covered entities also are allowed to report child abuse and certain communicable diseases, and they may release work-related PHI information so that employers can comply with state or federal law. Also permitted are *Tarasoff*-type disclosures to law enforcement agencies or other third parties to prevent harm.

In cases where disclosure is not permitted by the privacy rule, covered entities must get an individual's written authorization to release PHI. Authorization forms must use simple language, and should state what specific PHI will be disclosed, who will disclose and receive the PHI, the expiration date, and the patient's right to revoke the authorization. A covered entity must get the patient's or legal custodian's permission to disclose psychotherapy notes unless: (1) the notes are being used for training (e.g., resident supervision); (2) the covered entity is being sued by the patient; (3) a *Tarasoff*-type breach of confidentiality is needed; (4) lawful oversight of the therapist; or (5) to assist lawful activities of a coroner or medical examiner. (For purposes of HIPAA, the term 'psychotherapy notes' refers to records that document or analyze private counseling sessions and that are kept separate from the rest of the medical record. Records about medication, the frequency or times of counseling sessions, types of therapy, test results, diagnosis, functional status, treatment plans, symptoms, prognosis, and progress to date are not included within the HIPAA definition of 'psychotherapy notes.')

Patients' Rights

The Privacy Rule requires that patients receive notice of each covered entity's privacy practices, including ways in which PHI is used and disclosed, the patient's right to complain if privacy is violated, and a point of contact for more information or to make complaints. Except in emergencies, covered entities must make good faith efforts to get a patient's written acknowledgment that he/she received the privacy practices notice and must document reasons for failing to get that acknowledgment.

Patients also have the right to review their medical records, with these exceptions: psychotherapy notes, information compiled for legal proceedings, and certain laboratory results. Covered entities also may refuse a patient access if doing so might harm the patient or someone else, though patients are entitled to have such denials reviewed for a second opinion.

Patients have the right to request corrections in their medical records if their records are inaccurate or incomplete. Covered entities must make reasonable efforts to provide any corrected record to persons whom the patient believes needs the information to other person who might need the information. A covered entity may deny the patient's request for a correction, but must give the patient a written explanation and allow the patient to place a statement of disagreement in the record.

Patients have a right to find out to whom their PHI has been released over the previous six years. There are many exceptions to this rule, however, including disclosures: for treatment, payment, or health care operations; to persons involved in an individual's health care; for payment for health care; pursuant to an authorization.

Administrative Requirements

Covered entities must create written privacy policies and procedures for implementing the Privacy Rule. They must designate a privacy official responsible for developing and implementing privacy policies and procedures, and a contact person or office that receives complaints and gives patients information about their privacy practices. Covered entities must train their staff members on privacy policies and procedures so that they may carry out their functions, and must apply appropriate sanctions against staff members who violate policies, procedures, or the Privacy Rule. Finally, covered entities must develop reasonable procedures and safeguards to prevent improper use or disclosure of PHI. Examples of such safeguards include shredding documents that contain PHI before discarding them and keeping medical records in a locked area.

HIPAA and Parents

The Privacy Rule acknowledges that parents usually are the legal representatives of their minor children, and that parents may therefore access medical records on behalf of their minor children. When a parent is not the minor's representative, the Privacy Rule defers to state and other laws concerning the rights of parents to access and control PHI. Where state and other law are silent about parental access, covered entities may deny a parent access to the minor's health information when the decision to deny access is made by a licensed health care professional utilizing professional judgment.

Penalties

Covered entities may have to pay civil penalties of $100 per failure to comply with a Privacy Rule requirement. Such penalties may not be imposed if there was a reasonable cause for the failure, the failure did not involve willful neglect, and the covered entity corrected the violation within 30 days of learning about the violation. HIPAA provides for possible criminal sanctions as well: an individual who knowingly obtains or discloses PHI may be fined $50 000 and receive up to one years' imprisonment.

Comment

Long before HIPAA, psychiatrists were sensitive and cautious about responding to outsiders' requests for information. In child psychiatric practice, legitimate but informally tendered requests for information about treatment will come from noncustodial parents or extrafamilial third parties (teachers, lawyers, courts, community agencies). Many states have laws that give noncustodial parents the same access to records as custodial parents enjoy. In the absence of an emergency, however, the psychiatrist should obtain the legal custodian's *written* authorization for the disclosure before releasing information to other parties. The author's practice is to obtain the child's verbal permission as well, and, for children old enough to understand the procedure, to have children sign the consent form along with their parents or guardians. In general, a document authorizing release of records should comply with HIPAA guidelines. In many jurisdictions, the form must state explicitly whether the disclosure may include information about drug or alcohol treatment, HIV/AIDS, and other conditions. Any state laws that are contrary to the Privacy Rule are preempted by the federal requirements, which means that the HIPAA rules will apply.

Child Abuse and Neglect

Background

Following the 1962 publication of Kempe and colleague's landmark article, 'The Battered Child Syndrome,' [12] physicians and other health care professionals lobbied legislatures across the country to require mandatory reporting of child abuse to state authorities. As a result, laws in every state command physicians and various other professionals who know or suspect that a child is being or has been abused or neglected to report their belief to a law enforcement office or the appropriate local social service agency.

Most states base their definition of neglect and abuse on wording in the federal Child Abuse Prevention and Treatment Act of 1974 [13]. This law defines abuse as 'the physical and mental injuring, sexual abuse, negligent treatment or maltreatment of a child under the age of 18 by a person who is responsible for the child's welfare . . .' The obligation to report overrides the clinician's ordinary confidentiality obligations, and clinicians who make good-faith reports are immune from civil liability stemming from the reports.

Despite the nondiscretionary nature of state reporting requirements, mental health professionals who work with families may hesitate to report abuse to a social service or law enforcement agency. A professional might believe, for example, that making a report would be detrimental to the child or would disrupt therapy that will address the problem. Empirical evidence, however, suggests that although reporting abuse may temporarily injure a therapeutic relationship, it can lead to a subsequent strengthening of the treatment alliance. Moreover, in most states, practitioners who do not report suspected or known abuse may face criminal prosecution and civil liability for damages stemming from their failure to report.

Signs of Physical Abuse

Child psychiatrists typically learn about abuse through a child's or adult's verbal reports, perhaps during discussions about parents' disciplinary practices or their responses when angry with a child. Many childhood behaviors and parental characteristics have been associated with abuse and/or neglect [14]. These suspicion-creating signs are nonspecific, however, and (out of fairness to parents) should not be occasions for reporting abuse to authorities unless they are confirmed by verbal reports.

Pediatricians, especially those working in emergency settings, are more likely than psychiatrists to encounter children with physical injuries that are suggestive of child abuse. These include:

- bruises or welts in nonbony areas with shapes that suggest the object was used to inflict them;
- cigarette burns;
- burns caused by immersion in hot water, which have sharp demarcation lines and appear on extensor surfaces of the limbs and torso;
- lacerations involving the anus or genitalia;
- spiral fractures of the lower limbs (caused by twisting), multiple fractures in several stages of healing, or periosteal elevation;
- head injuries such as linear skull fractures in infants, subdural hematomata and retinal hemorrhages (caused by blows or shaking), jaw fractures, and scalp injuries (hemorrhages or missing hair caused by hair-pulling);
- abnormal vaginal flora and cultures positive for sexually transmitted diseases.

Encountering these injuries or findings obliges evaluating clinicians to rule out physical or sexual abuse. The likelihood that abuse has caused a physical injury is heightened by parental explanations that are inconsistent with the nature of the injury (e.g., a statement that a fall caused a welt that is shaped like an extension cord). Clinicians need to be aware, of course, that scientific controversy surrounds what kinds of physical findings are convincing evidence of abuse [15,16].

Interviewing Children for Suspected Sexual Abuse

Alleged sexual abuse is an increasingly common and contentious complaint encountered by psychiatrists in clinical contexts and forensic situations (e.g., child custody evaluations). The legal system may address this issue through criminal prosecution of an alleged perpetrator and/or through protective action by juvenile or family court. Clinicians who participate in sexual abuse investigations must recognize that they potentially will face complex legal issues involving the nature and presentation of courtroom evidence

[17–19], and potentially vigorous cross-examination by the party that opposes their position.

The American Academy of Child and Adolescent Psychiatry has promulgated guidelines for evaluating such children [20], to which readers who undertake such efforts are referred. Key elements of the evaluation process are establishing rapport, establishing the child's ability to recognize and report only the truth, allowing the child to give an uninterrupted report of the alleged abusive event, and avoiding leading questions. Interviewing children is just one portion of an evaluation of alleged sexual abuse, however. The full process of such an evaluation also involves receiving the request for an evaluation (which may come from a parent, attorney, or court), clarifying the social/legal situation (e.g., a divorcing couple battling for custody), and finding out what questions must be addressed. The child psychiatrist must then decide whether to accept the case (which includes deciding that one has the requisite expertise and emotional fortitude). If the case is accepted, the psychiatrist must then arrange to receive available appropriate records and establish conditions of the evaluation (who will be seen, appointment times, and payment procedures).

From a clinical standpoint, evaluating psychiatrists must take special precautions to assure that they remain objective, and must recognize their vulnerability to bias that might influence their evaluation procedures or conclusions [20]. They should document their findings appropriately, and should make sure that their opinions have a rational basis and are informed by the growing scientific literature in this area. To avoid contaminating the findings from a clinical interview with information obtained from external sources (e.g., parents or documents), some writers [17] suggest that evaluative functions be divided. In this approach, an 'intake professional' takes a history from adults and secures available documentation, and a 'child interviewer' – who knows little about the case other than the child's name and age – obtains the child's story. Although this approach is not used universally and is not always practicable, it illustrates the types of measures that thoughtful commentators recommend to assure objectivity in sexual abuse assessments, especially when preschoolers are involved.

Child interviewers encounter several pitfalls on their way to completing evaluations. They can be tempted to adopt a therapeutic, rather than an evaluative, attitude. Seemingly innocuous comments ('I'm sorry this happened to you') convey a value judgment that may contaminate a well-meant assurance or praise for talking about events risks encouraging a child whose immaturity limits ability to distinguish fact from fantasy to produce nonfactual material. Many readers will be familiar with notorious cases in which evaluators' and prosecutors' conscious or unconscious agendas led them to grosser interviewing errors: asking leading questions, asking the same question repeatedly until the desired answer is given, introducing information that the child has not himself uttered ('I know someone touched you; please tell me who?'), refusing to accept children's initial denials of abuse, or reinforcing children for 'good' (accusation-confirming) answers.

Some experts in this area [17] recommend that clinicians interview a child more than once to gauge the consistency of responses and to allow the child to become comfortable enough with the interviewer to reveal sensitive information. A combination of 'free play' and 'structured' interview techniques may let evaluators assess cognitive and developmental ability, level of sexual knowledge (which may be inappropriately high in abused children), and information specific to the allegation. Use of anatomically-detailed dolls, once considered valuable tools in evaluating abused children, is a source of scientific and legal controversy, and for preschoolers may be ill-advised [21]. Written notes are the most common form of documentation for such interviews, but audiotaping and videotaping allow interviewers more freedom to concentrate on their interaction with the child. Tapes also can provide evidence that a child's accusatory statements were not obtained through leading or contaminating interview techniques.

Termination of Parental Rights

US law and tradition grant parents very broad discretion in how they rear their children. In *Smith v. OFFER* (1977) [22], the US Supreme Court held that parents have a 'constitutionally recognized liberty interest' in maintaining custody of their children 'that derives from blood relationship, state law sanction, and basic human right.' This interest is not absolute, however, and is counterposed by the state's *parens patriae* duties to protect citizens who cannot fend for themselves.

The state may take steps to limit or end parent–child contact and make children eligible for permanent placement or adoption when the parents have: (1) abused, neglected, or abandoned their children; (2) become incapacitated in their ability to parent; (3) refused or been unable to remedy serious identified problems in caring for their children; or (4) experienced a severe breakdown in their relationship with their children (e.g., due to a lengthy prison sentence). Cognizant that severing the parent–child relationship is a dismal and serious measure, the Supreme Court held in *Santosky v. Kramer* (1982) [23] that a court may terminate parental rights only if the state shows by clear and convincing evidence that a parent has failed in one of these four ways. Most state statutes also contain provisions for parents to relinquish parental rights voluntarily.

Courts and child welfare agencies are guided by two complimentary federal laws governing cases in which parents' capacities to care for their children come into question. Passed in 1984, the Family Preservation and Support Services Act [24] requires states, as a condition of receiving federal funds, to make 'reasonable efforts' to obviate the need to remove a child from his home, or, once a child has been removed, to reunite the child with his family. The Adoption and Safe Families Act (ASFA) of 1997 [25] explicitly recognizes that reunification is not always advisable, and stresses that, 'while reasonable efforts to preserve and reunify families are still required, the child's health and safety is the paramount concern in determining what efforts at reunification should be made.' Moreover, no such efforts need be made in certain circumstances, including those in which a parent has: committed a felony assault that caused serious injury to the child or sibling; killed or tried to kill a sibling; engaged in egregious mistreatment (including abandonment, torture, chronic abuse or sexual abuse); or had parental rights to a sibling terminated involuntarily. ASFA also requires that safety of children in foster care be considered during case planning, and allows 'dual planning' (continuation of efforts at family reunification family occurring with efforts to place a child with a legal guardian or to arrange an adoption).

Child psychiatrists may become involved with this issue as evaluators of parents who have come to a domestic court's attention. Termination requires a finding that a parent's actions or condition makes him/her unable to care for his/her child and unlikely to become able in the future. Therefore, the court may request a clinician's assessment of an adult's capacity to parent, the relationship between the adult and child, and the child's special emotional needs. In doing such assessments, clinicians may discover that a psychiatric disorder is an important factor impairing parenting capacity. Courts will then need to know whether the psychiatric disorder is amenable to treatment, the time course of such treatment, and the parent's expected competence following treatment. In doing these evaluations, clinicians should remember that their focus is the adequacy of parents, and not the comparative benefits of remaining with a parent versus an available alternative placement.

Disabled Children

Access to Education

Since passage in 1975 of the Education for All Handicapped Children Act [26], all states must provide disabled children aged 3–21 years a free public education in the least restrictive setting that is appropriate to the child's needs. Fifteen years later, Congress passed the Individuals with Disabilities Education Act (IDEA), which it amended in 1997 [27], giving states an affirmative responsibility to locate children who need special services and to inform parents about availability of special education programs. Because of this requirement, it is now difficult for schools to ignore referrals for assessment from psychiatrists, psychologists, and teachers who identify a student who may be 'a child with a disability.' As used in the IDEA [20 U.S.C. §1401(3)(A)], this term means a child 'with mental retardation, hearing impairments (including deafness), speech or language impairments, visual impairments (including blindness), serious emotional disturbance, orthopedic impairments, autism, traumatic brain injury, other health impairments, or specific learning disabilities; and who, by reason thereof, needs special education and related services.'

Children identified as disabled must undergo reevaluation at least every three years, and must have a written Individualized Education Program (IEP). Under Federal law, IEPs must describe: (1) the child's present levels of educational performance; (2) measurable annual goals for enabling the child to be involved and progress in school; (3) the special services to be provided to the child; (4) the extent of the child's participation in regular classes; (5) any modifications in or exceptions from participating in state- or district-wide proficiency testing; (6) projected date for the beginning of the services; (7) for teenagers, plans for transitional services to more advanced studies (e.g., advanced-placement courses or a vocational education); and (8) how progress will be measured and how parents will be informed about progress [20 U.S.C. §1414(d)(1)(A)]. Federal law also requires that an IEP be crafted by an 'IEP Team' that includes: (1) the disabled child's parents; (2) the child's regular education teacher (if the child is in regular classes); (3) a special education teacher; (4) a representative of the local educational agency can provide or supervise specially designed instruction; (5) someone who can interpret the instructional implications of evaluation results; (6) at parents' or the agency's discretion, other individuals with special expertise concerning the child; and (7) whenever appropriate, the child himself [20 U.S.C. §1414(d)(1)(B)]. Once signed by parents and school personnel, the IEP becomes a legal contract whose conditions are enforceable through administrative hearings or state or federal court rulings.

Mental health professionals may be asked for their ideas either while an IEP is being crafted or during litigation surrounding fulfillment of an IEP's condition or the requirements of the IDEA itself. The precise limits of a school system's responsibilities under the IDEA are matters of constant litigation. One recurring common issue is the school system's financial obligations for special (and often costly) services – including counseling or psychological services – within or outside the regular school setting.

Other commonly-litigated issues deal with expulsion of disabled children, which courts have construed as a change in education placement. Federal law states that disabled children may be suspended for no more than 10 consecutive school days without triggering an IEP meeting. (An exception occurs if the child is carrying weapons or drugs, in which cases suspensions up to 45 days are permitted). A key issue in cases of serious misbehavior that might warrant lengthy suspensions or expulsion is whether the misbehavior a manifestation of the child's disability. If not, a school may require the disabled child to submit to any disciplinary procedure the school would use with a nondisabled child. However, because federal law entitles all children to a free, appropriate public education, even those children suspended or expelled must receive education in 'an alternative setting.'

If a child's misbehavior *is* deemed a manifestation of his disability, the IEP must reevaluate his placement, determine whether additional supportive measures are needed, and develop or revise a behavioral intervention plan. This plan should include measures for monitoring progress in reducing the child's misbehavior. Parents have rights to appeal school decisions with which they disagree, including mediation and formal hearings.

Mental Retardation

The American Psychiatric Association's diagnostic manual [28] defines mental retardation as a disorder with age of onset before age 18 years, characterized by '[s]ignificantly subaverage intellectual functioning' along with 'concurrent deficits or impairments in adaptive functioning' that affect daily activities, such as communication, caring for oneself, school performance, and workplace functioning. Mental retardation is subclassified as 'mild' (roughly, IQ = 50–55 to 70), 'moderate' (IQ = 35–40 to 50–55), 'severe' (IQ = 20–25 to 35–40), and 'profound' (IQ below 20–25).

Most persons with mental retardation fall into the 'mild' or 'moderate' categories, and it is persons with these levels of disability who are most likely to come to the law's attention and be evaluated by psychiatrists in forensic contexts. Legal issues frequently addressed in the evaluation of retarded children and adolescents include their need for involuntary hospitalization due to risk of harm to self or others, the ability of a retarded child to serve as a witness or stand trial in juvenile or criminal court, the ability of parents to care for them, and their needs for special educational provisions under the IDEA. Following *Atkins v. Virginia* [29], a 2002 US Supreme Court decision outlawing execution of retarded persons, a mental health clinician's determination about a youthful defendant's level of mental functioning can have life-or-death implications [30].

When they evaluate retarded children – or for that matter, any child with low intelligence or disabilities that impair communication or verbal comprehension – in a legal context, psychiatrists face special challenges. Although the legal questions are often not fundamentally different from those asked concerning minors with normal intelligence, forensic evaluations of retarded children must frequently take into account the complex interaction of mental retardation, coexisting mental illness, developmental immaturity, and simple ignorance arising from limited exposure to social expectations and legal proceedings.

Mentally retarded children are more likely than normal children to arrive at evaluations with little understanding of why they are seeing the psychiatrist, and are therefore more likely to feel frightened, overwhelmed, or perplexed. Complex and confusing legal processes only add to these feelings. The psychiatrist may need to take additional time to help the child understand his/her situation, to explain what the evaluation will consist of and why it is occurring, to gain his/her assent, and establish interpersonal rapport. The psychiatrist also should take extra care to make sure that the child understands questions and should make special allowances for limitations in communication. Obtaining factual background information from external sources – parents, schools, and medical records – is an important feature of most child psychiatric evaluations, but becomes even more critical when the evaluee has unusually limited communication or comprehension skills.

Children as Plaintiffs and Witnesses

Psychic Trauma

Although they are accustomed to thinking of legally-involved children in juvenile or domestic court proceedings, mental health professionals may be asked to evaluate children who are plaintiffs in what the law terms 'tort actions.' In a tort action, one party (the plaintiff) sues another party (the defendant) in civil court, usually alleging that the defendant's willful or negligent behavior caused damages for which the plaintiff should receive compensation (i.e., cash). When the alleged tortious act is intentional – e.g., in an action alleging emotional harm stemming from sexual misconduct with a minor – the plaintiff must show that the defendant's intentional behavior caused the injury. In a negligence suit – e.g., a medical malpractice suit or an action alleging injury stemming from a car accident – the plaintiff must show that the defendant owed the plaintiff a 'duty of care' (i.e., had a recognized social obligation to behave prudently), breached the duty through the negligent act, and thereby caused the plaintiff harm. These legal principles are the same for children as for adults. One difference involves the statute of limitations, i.e., the time after discovery of the injury during which the plaintiff may sue. Because minors are technically incompetent, the statutory limit does not begin to run until a child reaches majority.

Many issues and pitfalls in evaluating tort plaintiffs are similar for children and adults. In both cases, the evaluating psychiatrist is expected to conduct a thorough, objective examination of the plaintiff. Often, the evaluation will include devotion of considerable time to gathering and reviewing documents and information from third-party observers. The psychiatrist's goal is to learn whether the plaintiff has an emotional problem, the connection between the allegedly tortious act and the plaintiff's problem, the extent and impact of the impairment on the plaintiff's functioning, and the prognosis for recovery. In contrast to adults, however, evaluating and formulating opinions about children requires the psychiatrist to consider and comment about the effects of normal developmental trends on the injury. The psychiatrist also must attempt to weigh the impact of an emotional problem on educational attainment and subsequent psychosocial development.

It is beyond the scope of this chapter to describe the legal and clinical steps in such evaluations and in preparing for trial. Readers seeking article-length introductions to these topics will find several excellent resources available [31–33].

The Child as Witness

Children may need to testify in civil cases where they are plaintiffs, in domestic cases involving contested custody determinations, in juvenile court proceedings where they are defendants, or in criminal trials where they have witnessed allegedly illegal behavior. Although young children were once viewed as incompetent, Rule 601 of the Federal Rules of Evidence now states a presumption that '[e]very person is competent to be a witness.' Many states have similar rules; in the rest, only children above a certain age are presumed competent.

Competence to be a witness entails a capacity to observe, remember, and recount events and to understand the obligation to tell the truth. Though a child meets a jurisdiction's test for presumed competence, a judge may investigate a child's capacity before allowing him to testify. The judge may do this either by questioning the child in chambers or by having a mental health professional evaluate the child and submit a sealed report to the judge. Clinicians preparing such reports must address whether the child has a mental disorder or defect and whether that condition affects the powers needed to be a witness.

A child's *credibility* as witness is related to, but distinct from, his competence, and is influenced by age-appropriate developmental limitations and the way that the child is questioned. Children have limited powers of free recall, and therefore will not do well if asked open-ended questions requiring lengthy, organized response. Between the ages of 5 and 10 years, retrieval strategies become better developed, and children become able to give longer, discursive accounts of events. Pre-latency children are quite suggestible, and their interlocutors must take care to avoid contaminating or influencing their responses by asking leading questions. Young children also lack the ability to describe event times or sequences accurately, and they may not have achieved other concrete operational milestones such as conservation. They thus may have difficulty identifying or recognizing a defendant who was casually dressed and had a beard at the time of an offense but who has shaved and put on a suit for the trial. Child psychiatrists can assist court personnel by helping them understand these limitations and teaching them about how to ask questions (e.g., use simple words in short sentences; avoid pronouns and passive voice).

Children may need special accommodations to testify effectively and to not be intimidated by the courtroom context. Such accommodations include having a support person present, alterations in the scheduling and timing of testimony, and special considerations concerning admissibility of evidence, particularly in criminal cases involving sexual abuse. Several state laws allow children to testify via videotape or closed-circuit television. Although the 6th Amendment establishes a defendant's right to confront witnesses, the US Supreme Court held in *Coy v. Iowa* (1987) [34] that 'individualized findings that . . . particular witnesses needed special protection' might justify deviation from the customary requirement of face-to-face testimony. In a 1990 case (*Maryland v. Craig*) [35], the Supreme Court let stand a sexual assault conviction based on a six-year-old's closed-circuit television testimony, holding that the purpose of the confrontation clause – insuring that evidence is reliable and subject to potentially rigorous cross-examination – was addressed by the closed-circuit arrangement. The Supreme Court's 1992 *White v. Illinois* decision [36] upheld a conviction in which a four-year-old child's statement made immediately after a sexual assault and later repeated to physicians was used as evidence against the defendant. Ordinarily, such a statement would be disallowed as 'hearsay,' but the Court found that the particular circumstances provided 'substantial guarantees of its trustworthiness.'

Divorce and Child Custody

Background

Between 1950 and 1979, the US per capita divorce rate doubled; over the next two decades, the per capita rate declined by about a quarter, but the marriage rate fell, too. Though several other countries have higher percentages of marriage that end in divorce, the US still has the world's highest per capita divorce rate. Recent US Census Bureau projections suggest that half of couples who marry at child-bearing age will divorce, and an estimated two-thirds of divorcing couples have minor children. Other estimates suggest that a child born to married parents currently has a 40–50% chance of seeing his parents divorce before he reaches adulthood.

Because parental divorce is a potent risk factor for a child's needing mental health services, a disproportionate fraction of the children seen for psychiatric treatment come from families where once-married parents no longer live together. About 20% of divorcing parents dispute custody, and to help decide this issue, courts frequently obtain the consultation of mental health professionals. Child psychiatrists are thus very likely to be involved, either as therapist or custody evaluator, with children who are the focuses of custody disputes.

Historically, courts' resolution of these disputes has reflected the larger society's views about parental roles and functions. Before the nineteenth century, children

– like wives – were deemed the property of adult men, and were awarded to fathers after divorce. From the nineteenth century through the first two-thirds of the twentieth century, regard for the importance of maternal attention during a child's 'tender years' led to a strong presumption favoring placement with the mother. Currently, every state directs its courts to assign custody based on a 'best interests of the child' model most famously articulated by the Iowa Supreme Court in *Painter v. Bannister* (1966) [37]. The Uniform Marriage and Divorce Law, a model statute adopted by many states, directs courts to consider the wishes of the child(ren) and parents, interactions and relationships between the children and parents, siblings, and other involved persons, the child(ren)'s adjustment to school, home, and community, and the mental and physical health of all those involved. Courts are *not* to consider parental conduct (e.g., homosexuality or cohabitation) that does not affect the parent–child relationship.

Courts may award divorcing parents joint *legal* custody, in which both parents retain shared responsibility for major decisions affecting their child(ren), even when the child(ren) will live primarily with one parent. Since the late 1980s, many states have adopted legislation directing courts to view joint custody as the preferred arrangement for children of divorcing parents. The success of these arrangements varies with each parent's self-esteem, capacity to empathize, and respect for the bond between the child(ren) and the ex-spouse. Research suggests that children's outcomes depend less on the legal custody arrangements than the predivorce psychological functioning of parents and the postdivorce hostility between them. Continued, regular contact with the noncustodial parent is also associated with better postdivorce emotional adjustment.

Divorce *mediation* is a process that parents sometime use (and which, in some states is legally mandated) to reach a settlement without going to trial. Here, the divorcing parties meet without counsel, but with a neutral person (typically, a lawyer or mental health professional who has undergone special training in divorce mediation) to examine areas of contention systematically. The goal of the process is to produce a voluntary agreement about issues such as property division and custody arrangements. This process offers the potential for helping families avoid lengthy litigation and developing a plan to which sides will adhere. However, mediation is often unsuccessful – especially if it is imposed on parties who are already antagonistic toward each other – and it can be negatively affected by the limitations of the mediator (e.g., bias, inexperience, lack of 'clinical' skills).

Collaborative law, a relatively recent development, provides another avenue for parents who want to try to work out a divorce agreement. Like mediation, collaborative law is a form of 'alternative dispute resolution,' but unlike mediation, parents have the advantage of retaining and consulting with individual counsel throughout the negotiation process. Typically, the process begins with a written four-way agreement involving the two parents and their two lawyers (who usually must have special training in collaboration) stating that they will not go to court before making every possible effort to negotiate a resolution. The agreement also has a disqualification provision saying that the lawyers who represent parents during collaboration may not represent them if the parents later take their dispute to court. Parents and their attorneys then engage in informal discussions, trying to resolve all issues. If the parents and their lawyers cannot resolve all matters this way, the collaboration process ends, and both parents must retain new attorneys for court proceedings.

Thus, under the collaborative law approach, parents do not relinquish their rights to court proceedings. However, collaborative lawyers have no incentive to encourage unreasonable, accusatory, or belligerent positions that might require court proceedings to resolve, nor do they reap the financial benefits of lengthy discovery processes or preparing and attending hearings. Instead, collaborative attorneys have an incentive to facilitate settlement of differences. As for parents, if collaboration fails, they both suffer the disadvantage (and expense) of having to hire new attorneys, which reduces the incentive to argue, accuse, and threaten ('I'll see you in Court!'). The experience of collaboration may also help the parent-clients communicate better, which would benefit their children following the divorce.

Involvement in Divorce Proceedings

Because divorce is so common, and because undergoing divorce is a common reason for seeking psychiatric treatment, clinicians stand a high likelihood of becoming involved in the legal proceedings of divorcing parents. It is unwise for a therapist who has been seeing a divorcing parent in individual treatment to attempt to do a custody evaluation: the therapist's obligations to the patient and greater familiarity with one side of the matter would preclude objectivity in the evaluation, while making an honest, objective appraisal of both parents might interfere with effective therapy for the patient who is in treatment.

Even without serving as a custody evaluator, a child psychiatrist may have records subpoenaed and be called to testify in disputed custody cases. In such situations, clinicians should not release records or reveal information about patients without the patients' express written consent, unless the court commands them to do so. Courts regard the need to resolve legal issues as a higher priority than preserving doctor–patient confidentiality. A judge who finds that a psychiatrist has information needed to help decide what is in a child's best interest may therefore order the psychiatrist to produce records or testify despite a parent's objections. Clinicians must comply with such orders or risk being held in contempt of court.

Juvenile Courts and Juvenile Delinquency

Background

A 'juvenile delinquent' – in the noncolloquial use of the term – is a minor (in most states, someone less than 18 years old) who has committed an act that would be a crime were it committed by an adult. Besides dealing with delinquent children, juvenile courts have jurisdiction over children who are 'unruly' (i.e., who have committed prohibited but noncriminal acts such running away or being truant), and also children who have been found dependent, neglected, or abused and are thus entitled to state protection.

Juvenile courts form the vertex of a cultural funnel into which our society pours many problems affecting children and families, particularly those problems that stem from or are caused by America's extraordinarily high level of violence. American children and adolescents – especially, but not exclusively, those who live in impoverished conditions – are exposed to, are victims of, and commit violence far out of proportion to their representation in the population. US children spend more time watching television than they spend in school, and they view a staggering amount of violence on television – 280 000 violent acts by age 18 years, according to Comstock and Strasburger [38]. The proliferation of new media – especially video games and the Internet – offer children new, often graphic opportunities for exposure to violence. Many urban children witness knifings, shootings, and killings before they enter first grade, and each year, millions of children witness domestic violence. According to the National Center for Injury Prevention and Control, more than 877 700 persons aged 10–24 years were injured by violent acts in 2002, with about 8% of these injuries requiring hospitalization [39]. Homicide is the second leading cause of death among all young people in this age group; for young African–Americans, it is the leading cause of death [40]. During the latest US survey on the subject, one-sixth of school students reported carrying a weapon (such as a gun, knife, or club) one or more times during the month preceding the survey, and one-third reported being in a physical fight [41].

In the last third of the twentieth century, lethal violence by US juveniles escalated steadily and alarmingly until the 1990s. Between 1984 and 1994, the number of US juvenile homicide offenders nearly tripled, and the number of juvenile killings with firearms quadrupled [42]. After peaking in 1994, the juvenile arrest rate declined significantly. In 2002, there were 2.26 million arrests of young people for all crimes. These included 91 000 arrests for index violent crimes (murder, forcible rape, robbery, and aggravated assault), the lowest level since 1980 and about half the 1994 peak level. Though the once-feared 'epidemic' of youth crime had subsided somewhat by the beginning of the twenty-first century, youths still account for roughly 15% of all arrests for violent crimes [43]. Moreover, confidential self-reports of violent behavior suggested no decrease in the rates at which juveniles actually commit violent acts, with roughly three in 10 high school seniors reporting having committed a violent act in the past year [44].

Juvenile Justice System

Until juvenile courts were established in most states in the early twentieth century, minors were subject to prosecution in the same fashion as adults, though from the mid-nineteenth century onward they might be housed separately once found guilty [45]. Juvenile courts' mission since then has reflected a social–parental role that mixes the urge to punish with a belief that delinquency implies that a child needs treatment and rehabilitation. Although juveniles now enjoy many of the formal legal protections accorded to adults accused of crimes, juvenile courts retain their informal and less adversarial character. Juvenile courts also use social service agencies in handling cases, and they frequently rely on mental health professionals' ideas in interpreting and understanding children's circumstances and behavior.

Special Terminology
Juvenile courts typically employ a distinct (and initially confusing) terminology for their proceedings that reflects their historically therapeutic posture. The first step is often called 'intake,' at which an official (often a probation officer) decides whether a 'referral' (i.e., a report of a violation or crime) should be immediately dismissed or accepted for further action. A referral will often result in 'diversion,' i.e., a decision, again often made by a probation officer, to handle an offense using an informal (nonlegal) response, such as a referral to another agency for treatment. Juvenile courts refer to subsequent judicial proceedings as 'adjudication' (as opposed to trial) and 'disposition' (as opposed to sentencing). Post-sentencing monitoring is often referred to as 'after-care' (rather than parole or 'community control').

Dispositions available to the juvenile court include probation (sometimes conditioned on school attendance and conforming to other adolescent social norms, sometimes accompanied by requirements for restitution and community service), residential placements (for nondangerous children who can benefit from a structured, therapeutic community setting), psychiatric hospitalization (for mentally ill children), and 'training school' (a euphemism for a juvenile prison for serious and/or repeat offenders). Juvenile courts' dispositional options include a wide range of community agencies (if appropriate services are available). Unlike adult sentencing, juvenile court dispositions may reflect therapeutic needs rather than mere considerations of proportionality and just deserts, and may be directed toward people other than the offender (e.g., parents). Consistent with their original treatment-oriented posture, records of juvenile court proceedings are sealed, and conviction as a minor generally does not become part of one's adult criminal record. Federal law requires that minors be housed separately from adults before adjudication, and even those minors found delinquent of serious offenses must be held in special juvenile facilities separate from adult criminals. In 2001, more than 100 000 US teenagers – 336 per 100 000 population – were confined pursuant to court order in various facilities; 85% were boys [46].

Rights
Supreme Court rulings in the last third of the twentieth century established that minors charged with offenses in juvenile court enjoy some, but not all of the constitutional protections accorded to adults charged with crimes. *In re Gault* [47] held that minors facing juvenile court charges have certain due process entitlements under the Fourteenth Amendment, including the right to written notice of charges, *Miranda* protections, and legal representation. *In re Winship* [48]

extended the requirement for proof of guilt 'beyond a reasonable doubt' to accusations raised in juvenile courts. *Breed v. Jones* [49] interpreted the Fifth Amendment's prohibition against double jeopardy to bar prosecution of a minor in both juvenile and adult criminal court. However, juveniles are not constitutionally entitled to trial by jury in juvenile court (*McKeiver v. Pennsylvania* [50]). Also, juveniles who pose serious risk of committing another offense may be subject to pre-trial preventive detention without possibility of bail (*Schall v. Martin* [51]).

Transfer of Jurisdiction, or 'Waiver'

Over the last quarter century, as youth violence has increased and as administering punishment has replaced rehabilitation as the perceived *raison d'être* of criminal courts, both the public and legal scholars have argued for more severe and more adult-like handling of juvenile criminals. Recommended measures have included minimizing therapeutic interventions, application of a 'just deserts' punishment-oriented model, and – for repeat offenders and youths accused of violent crimes – developing was to impose sentences beyond the usual length of the juvenile court's jurisdiction. One way to make a lengthy sentence possible is for the juvenile court to transfer jurisdiction over an accused minor to an adult criminal court, where the minor would face trial and the potential for adult criminal sanctions. By the late 1990s, use of this last procedure (also called 'waiver,' 'bindover,' or 'certification') had substantially increased, because several states had given prosecutors increased discretion to file certain cases in adult court, or had mandated adult criminal court prosecution for youths accused of certain crimes [45] .

A 1966 US Supreme Court case [52] established minimal constitutional protections before a minor's transfer to adult court for prosecution, including a hearing, access to reports written for juvenile court, and statement of reasons for waiver. Beyond these basics, however, transfers of jurisdiction follow rules that vary greatly among the 46 states that allow the procedure. Usually, state laws require that a youth be above a minimum age (typically 14 years, but lower in some states), be charged with a serious felony, and that there be 'probable cause' (i.e., good reason) to believe the youth committed the act. In cases where transfer is optional, courts often must also find that the youth is not amenable to treatment or that placement in a juvenile facility would threaten the community's safety. When making this last determination, juvenile courts often request the opinion of mental health professionals, who then provide assessments and information

that can have an enormous potential impact on a young person's future.

In the 1990s, Americans became increasingly alarmed by their nation's level of violence (though they continued to delight in entertainments, sports, and firearm policies that implicitly condoned and glorified violence). Reacting to the public outcry over juvenile crime, political officeholders made evermore strident calls to hold juveniles accountable and ridiculed government-sponsored programs aimed at preventing or reducing youth violence [42]. Many state legislatures lowered the age at which youthful offenders could be tried as adults. In addition to increased use of waivers, many states modified statutes to require mandatory minimum sentences for certain violent or serious offenders. States also raised maximum ages for the juvenile court to retain jurisdiction over juvenile offenders; this permits juvenile courts to order dispositions that extend beyond the typical upper age of original jurisdiction, which in various states ranges from age 17 to 24 years. Finally, several states have created the possibility of 'blended sentences,' which allow courts to impose a combination of juvenile and adult criminal sanctions on certain minors.

Competence to Proceed with Adjudication

All jurisdictions recognize (either through judicial decision or statute) that a minor must be competent at a juvenile court hearing. Usually, competence to proceed in juvenile court is defined as is competence to stand trial for adults, in accordance with the Supreme Court's 1960 *Dusky v. US* ruling [53]. Dusky requires that an accused person have 'sufficient present ability to consult with his attorney with a reasonable degree of rational understanding' and 'a rational as well as factual understanding of the proceedings against him.' The legal and theoretical bases for requiring juveniles to be competent are summarized by Bonnie and Grisso [54], who suggest that those children whose cases remain in juvenile court may not need to have the same decision-making capacities as adult criminal court requires. Grisso [55] recommends that the question of a juvenile's competence to proceed with adjudication be raised whenever one or more of the following are the case:

- the minor is younger than 13 years old;
- the minor has a history of mental illness or mental retardation;
- the minor has a history of cognitive deficits, such as borderline intellectual functioning or a learning disability;

- current contacts with the minor suggest that he/she deviates from normal juveniles in his/her attentional abilities, memory, or capacity to recognize reality.

Despite what evaluators and judges sometimes assume, research suggests that minors' prior contact with the juvenile justice system provides little assurance that they grasp legal issues related to adjudicatory competence. Previous arrests or delinquency findings do not correlate well with juveniles' ability to appreciate legal rights, the meaning of plea bargains, or trial proceedings.

The last four decades have witnessed several attempts to create structured instruments to aid in assessing adult defendants' competence to proceed with adjudication in criminal court. Though no such instruments are widely accepted for use in assessing minors' competence in juvenile court, the past five years have seen the development of a nascent knowledge base regarding children's performance on standard adult competence measures [56], and clinicians should anticipate publication of additional research on this topic.

Competence to Waive Miranda Rights

Persons unfamiliar with the criminal justice system may not be aware that law enforcement personnel frequently make concerted efforts to obtain confessions from suspects, and that confessions frequently play a crucial role as evidence supporting a criminal conviction. In a landmark 1966 decision, *Miranda v. Arizona* [57], the US Supreme Court held that to be valid, a suspect's waiver of the rights to remain silent and to have an attorney present during questioning must be made voluntarily, knowingly, and intelligently. Psychiatrists therefore may be asked (usually by defense counsel) to evaluate whether a minor's confession was made after a competent waiver.

Among the factors that could invalidate a minor's confession are immaturity (chronological or social), low intelligence, lack of familiarity with legal processes, and the length and style of the interrogation. Although several commentators (e.g., Grisso [58]) argue that a confession made by a minor without an attorney or supportive adult present should never be admissible, courts have not adopted this position. Instead, courts are governed by the Supreme Court's ruling in *Fare v. Michael C.* (1979) [59], which includes a rebuttable presumption of a juvenile's competence to confess. *Fare* directs a trial court to consider admissibility of a confession based on 'the totality of circumstances' surrounding the confession, including the child's 'age, experience, education, background, intel-

ligence,' the child's understanding of his *Miranda* rights, and his understanding of the consequences of waiving those rights. A research-based assessment tool [60,61] can be used in evaluating *Miranda*-related competence, which allows comparison of a specific evaluee's performance with performances of children and adults.

The Insanity Defense

Insanity is a legal term implying that, at the time of an otherwise criminal act, a defendant's mental disorder or mental retardation so impaired his rationality that he should not be held responsible [62]. Seldom used in adult criminal proceedings, the insanity defense is even more rarely invoked in juvenile settings. One practical reason is that a successful defense would usually have little impact on the case's outcome: the usual disposition for minors with serious mental illness is treatment in a hospital, even when they have been adjudicated delinquent.

The insanity defense is most likely to be invoked when juveniles are tried as adults for serious offenses. States are free to define insanity as they see fit, or (as has happened in a few states), to abolish the insanity defense altogether. In states that allow an insanity defense in juvenile court, the criteria for a successful defense are the same as for adults. Most jurisdictions use a variation on one of two well-known definitions of insanity. The 'McNaghten' standard, formulated in Great Britain in response to Daniel McNaghten's 1843 insanity acquittal, allows for a successful defense only if the defendant was so mentally impaired at the time of his otherwise criminal act that he could not grasp the nature or wrongfulness of his behavior. The American Law Institute (ALI) test is a more liberal standard. It allows for an insanity acquittal if, at the time of the allegedly criminal act, the defendant's mental impairment rendered him unable to appreciate the criminality of his behavior or 'conform his conduct to the requirements of the law.'

The Child Psychiatrist in Court

Some Basic Concepts

Many problems that child psychiatrists encounter in their clinical work – abuse and neglect, need for involuntary hospitalization, custody resolution during divorce, or the effects of psychic trauma – have legal as well as treatment implications. In addition, several strictly legal issues discussed earlier in this chapter, such as competence to stand trial and legal sanity, require the special knowledge and clinical expertise of professionals who inform and help courts make legal judgments. Psychiatrists, who are socialized to seek consensus, generally find adversarial court proceedings, testifying, and (especially) being cross-examined unpleasant. Given the nature of our work, however, most psychiatrists probably cannot avoid making at-least-occasional courtroom appearances. In certain psychiatric practice settings (e.g., working at hospital where many patients undergo civil commitment), giving testimony can become a frequent feature of one's clinical work. Fortunately, many excellent books (e.g., [63–65]; October 2002 issue of *Child and Adolescent Psychiatric Clinics of North America*), articles, and continuing medical education offerings are available to help psychiatrists become more familiar and comfortable in their interactions with the legal system. The following paragraphs are intended as an introduction to the subject and as encouragement to explore more detailed treatments of the subject.

Fact Witnesses and Expert Witnesses

Courts may receive testimony from two kinds of witnesses. Fact witnesses are persons who, by virtue of personal observation, have direct knowledge about events bearing on a legal issue. Fact witnesses must confine their testimony to what they have done or directly observed. Expert witnesses are persons who, having shown to the court's satisfaction that they have specialized knowledge, are allowed to state *opinions* about issues within their areas of expertise. Physicians' specialized training and experience make them, in the eyes of courts, experts on issues related to medicine. Thus courts will allow them to testify about observed symptoms – observable facts – in a patient, plus their diagnoses, which, in the law's view, are opinions about the causes of symptoms.

Two Avenues to Becoming a Witness

As was suggested above, psychiatrists are at high risk for becoming witnesses because their clinical work is often intimately related to issues of concern to courts. However, their special expertise may lead attorneys to ask them to evaluate clients or otherwise become involved in legal matters not for any treatment purpose, but simply because psychiatric opinion is needed to obtain an appropriate legal outcome. Examples include custody determinations, personal injury litigation, and criminal issues such as competence to stand trial and insanity. Here, psychiatrists have the opportunity to use their expertise in evaluating complex emotional issues to assist the legal system in ways that often have profound effects on the lives of persons involved.

When psychiatrists are asked to give testimony about matters where their knowledge is merely the result of their having undertaken the treatment of a patient, their observations and opinions naturally will reflect the exigencies and limitations of the clinical context. In these circumstances, physicians (and the courts who hear their testimony) should expect no more than a conscientious effort to inform listeners about their clinical data and how they interpret those data. When a psychiatrist evaluates someone for the specific purpose of helping a court address a legal issue, however, the psychiatrist knows that his/her work will be used for legal and not clinical purposes, that his/her data and opinions may be sharply critiqued, and that his/her courtroom testimony may be challenged vigorously during cross-examination. This knowledge requires the evaluating psychiatrist to insure that his/her findings will reflect the efforts of an objective and thorough evaluation; that his/her written reports to court reflect careful attention to clarity, detail, and soundness of conclusions; and that any potential testimony be solidly grounded in clinical data and supported by current medical and scientific knowledge.

The Forensic Examination

Accepting a Referral

Although many referrals for child forensic evaluations come from a child's guardian ad litem or from a court, some will come from an attorney who represents one side of a case. Frequently, attorneys will not be sure what they want from the psychiatrist, and – as often happens in consultation-liaison psychiatry – the psychiatrist's first step will involve clarifying the legal purpose of, and questions to be addressed by, the evaluation.

With this accomplished, the psychiatrist should then ask himself/herself: Do I feel comfortable undertaking this evaluation? Am I being asked to render an opinion concerning a matter about which psychiatrists truly have expertise? Do I have the relevant background and experience? Do I have enough time to complete a good evaluation? Will the nature of the case let me stay objective and refrain from letting personal feelings about the issues or the persons involved intrude?

If all these questions get affirmative answers, the psychiatrist may be willing to accept the case. Before doing so, however, he/she should clarify several other issues. The psychiatrist should make sure that the attorney will permit (and hopefully assist with obtaining) access to all relevant written records (e.g., from schools, social service agencies, and medical/psychological treatment). The psychiatrist should establish the need to speak with all relevant third parties (e.g., in a custody evaluation, both parents and other adults, such as relatives and schoolteachers, with pertinent information). The psychiatrist should also learn what deadlines are operative (e.g., a hearing date), and figure out whether he/she can complete a report in the time available.

Finally, the psychiatrist should explain what his/her fees are and establish how he/she will be paid. In working with public agencies, one must often bill for services only after all work is completed. In working with private attorneys, however, requesting payment in advance is customary. Attorneys call such payment a 'retainer; advance payment should cover a substantial portion of the time that the expert expects to spend reviewing records, conducting interviews, and writing a report. Contingency fees – that is, fees dependent on the outcome of a case – compromise an expert's objectivity, and agreeing to payment on this basis is unethical for a psychiatrist.

Conducting the Evaluation

The primary goal of most clinical encounters is to relieve suffering. The usual aim of forensic evaluations, however, is to discover the truth about why a psychiatric condition developed or how it influenced behavior. Ordinarily, when a child psychiatric evaluation is conducted for treatment purposes, clinicians make the reasonable (if not always correct) assumption that informants are straightforward and honest. In forensic evaluations, where outcomes may affect substantial monetary gains or losses, custody arrangements, or incarceration, such an assumption is unreasonable and unwise. Forensic evaluators should treat their evaluees respectfully while remaining skeptical about what they hear. They must pay careful attention to detail and carefully explore implausible statements, contradictions, or inconsistencies. Whenever possible, they should compare interviewees' statements with independent observations or available records. These special requirements of a forensic evaluation often mean that the psychiatrist will spend much longer conducting interviews and reviewing documents than is ordinarily needed to arrive at a clinical diagnosis and treatment plan.

In meeting with parents and children, the forensic evaluator should begin by stating who he is, why the interview is occurring, and what will be done with information obtained. (In some situations, this information is presented in writing, but there is no ethical requirement to do this.) Evaluees should be informed of the option not to answer some questions, along with consequences of not answering (e.g., not answering may be noted in reports or testimony). Evaluees should also know that taking short breaks is permitted, and that truthful responses are expected.

Even when it seems from the situation that these matters should be obvious, forensic evaluees are frequently confused because of their mental impairments or the complexities of legal maneuvers. For example, evaluees may expect that, because they are talking to 'a doctor,' the purpose of the interview is to help them and will assume that the interview contents will remain confidential. One must make sure evaluees understand that exactly the opposite is the case. Before accepting the evaluee's verbal and/or written consent to participate, it is often useful to see if the evaluee can paraphrase the evaluator's explanation about the interview's nature, purpose, and nonconfidentiality.

The Written Report

In some cases (especially civil litigation), attorneys will request that the psychiatric expert prepare only a limited report, leaving it to opposing counsel to learn about what the expert thinks during a deposition (explained further below). In other cases, however, the expert's written report is *the* crucial product of the forensic evaluation. Because most legal issues are resolved without trial, the written report – which will be reviewed by both sides as they think about a settlement – will count far more than any potential medical testimony offered by the evaluator. Also, judges give great weight to written reports, expecting that they represent the clinician's considerations reduced to thoughtful prose, in contrast with unprepared and less reflective statements made during testimony.

The length and structure of a report will vary greatly depending on a case's circumstances and complexity, and on a retaining attorney's needs. A typical format includes: (1) an introduction stating the reason for the referral; (2) a listing of sources of information; (3) history or background information about the evaluee; (4) contents of the psychiatric interview(s), including the mental status evaluation; and (5) an 'opinion' section, in which the evaluator addresses the legal question for which the evaluation was sought.

Ideally, a report should be a stand-alone document, i.e., a document from which the reader can obtain a complete understanding of a case and the author's conclusions without reference to other documents. A report should present the all relevant information that formed the basis for the evaluator's conclusions, and should outline clearly how the evaluator used available data to reach those conclusions. In their training, physicians learn to use passive voice and a host of stock terms and phrases ('multiple' for 'many,' 'symptomatology' for 'symptoms,' 'secondary to' for 'caused by') that help them allay anxiety and cope with uncertainty. With assiduous practice, however, physicians can unlearn these bad habits and express themselves in prose that is simple, clear, and concise. Because most readers of forensic reports will be nonphysicians (i.e., judges and lawyers), psychiatrists should avoid using medical or psychiatric jargon, or explain the terms when they must. A short example: instead of writing 'he was treated with risperidone 2 mg b.i.d.,' one can write 'he took risperidone (an antipsychotic medication) 2 mg twice a day.' Experts should proofread their reports carefully. Minor errors can create misunderstanding, and opposing counsel can use them at trial to portray the expert as careless.

Child Custody Evaluations

Most child custody evaluations are requested in an especially contentious and emotionally charged context. Because these evaluations are prone to several kinds of errors that can generate angry recriminations by losing parties, authorities have developed recommendations for clinicians willing to offer courts their assistance in this area. Clinicians with little experience doing such evaluations would be well advised to obtain the consultation of a more experienced mentor. The following paragraphs provide an introduction to appropriate procedures for a custody evaluation and the reasons for those procedures. Readers who intend to do such evaluations should refer to much more detailed discussions available elsewhere [66,67].

Accepting Referrals

A clinician should not agree to do a custody evaluation concerning a child or parent whom he has treated. As was stated earlier, to do so could disrupt needed therapy, lead to violations of confidentiality, and/or undermine the objectivity of the custody assessment. A clinician should not agree to do a partisan evaluation in which only one parent is evaluated at the request of that parent's attorney. Clinicians who do such work are often viewed as potentially biased 'hired guns,' and they can offer courts little of value where parents' comparative merits, and not their mental health *per se*, are at issue. Ideally, a clinician should do an evaluation as an agent of the court (i.e., as a court-ordered expert), or failing this, as an expert accepted and agreed upon by both sides. Before the psychiatrist accepts the referral, all parties should agree to the structure of the evaluation (who will be seen, for how many sessions, and in what combinations) and to the fee arrangements (often being full payment in advance).

The Evaluation

Some evaluators prefer to begin by meeting with both parents to explain and clarify the purpose and nature of the assessment. In a subsequent series of interviews, evaluators will meet with each parent individually. The goal here is to understand the parents' reasons for wanting custody, how they themselves were raised, their reliability and consistency, their perception of themselves and the other spouse, and their disciplinary methods. Interviews with children assess levels of functioning, areas of special emotional or physical needs, attachments to each parent, and current and upcoming developmental tasks. Evaluators also make observations about parent–child interactions, often designing appointments around activities or tasks (e.g., a trip to a restaurant) where they can observe each parent's ability to get and stay organized, nurturing, and limit-setting in circumstances more natural and spontaneous than the office. Finally, and with the agreement of both parties, evaluators may speak with several 'collateral sources' – grandparents, schoolteachers, future stepparents – who may have valuable information about parental behavior.

Issues to Consider

Several issues are commonly encountered in child custody evaluations. These include continuity (which arrangements would conduce to the most stable living arrangement), major attachments (to parents, siblings, and others), children's preferences (especially for those over age 12 years), parents' attunement to special needs or handicaps (mental and physical), education opportunities, parents' mental and physical health, how well styles of parenting and discipline fit with children's emotional make-up, available social supports, religious differences between parents, and parents' ability to resolve conflicts. In addition, many child custody evaluations must take into account issues that reflect emerging social, political, and scientific developments. Such issues include parental kidnapping, gay and lesbian parents, rights of stepparents and/or grandparents, accusations of sexual molestation, and embryological technology (e.g., custody of frozen embryos).

The Report

Although written reports of custody evaluations may include diagnoses, the aim of the evaluation is not to reach a clinical diagnosis. Instead, the evaluator's report should give the court the evaluator's specific, factually-buttressed views about the child(ren)'s special needs and how those needs interact with each parent's abilities and limitations. The report, which may take the form of a letter to the court, can be structured using the previously described forensic report format. Ample use of quoted statements may help convey the evaluator's sense of the evaluees and the tone of the meetings with them. When writing reports, evaluators should expect both parents to read them and should avoid judgmental language. The report's final section (perhaps titled 'Recommendations') need not address psychiatric diagnosis, since parenting, not clinical status, is at issue. The report should include the evaluator's specific views about custody and/or visitation arrangements.

Testifying

Testifying in court is a knowledge-based performance skill at which psychiatrists can develop varying degrees of proficiency. Psychiatrists who must frequently appear in the witness chair may want to expend some time and effort toward developing their ability to give effective and persuasive expert testimony. Several publications geared toward forensic mental health professionals (e.g., [63,64]) provide suggestions about presenting oneself in court and handling the challenges, barbs, and tricks of opposing attorneys. For most child psychiatrists, however, spending extra time to develop courtroom skills is not necessary. Knowing the basics of courtroom procedure for handling experts is helpful, however.

Sequence of Testimony

The first part of an expert witness's testimony involves answering a series of attorney questions designed to establish the clinician's expertise, that is, his/her qualifications to offer opinions about his/her area of special knowledge. The next portion is termed the 'direct' examination. Here, the attorney who called the expert asks questions that, from the court's standpoint, establish the 'foundation' for the expert's testimony and opinion. During direct examination, the attorney will ask the witness to identify the person examined, to describe facts and findings, and to state and explain opinions. At certain points, the opposing attorney may object to questions, often for technical reasons related to proper legal procedure for presenting evidence. When this occurs, the witness should wait to answer until the judge rules on the objection. If the objection is overruled, the witness may answer; if the objection

is sustained, the examining attorney must withdraw the question or rephrase it in a legally acceptable way.

Cross-examination follows the conclusion of direct examination. Its ostensible purpose is to further the court's efforts to seek the truth by pointing up the flaws or limitations in the expert's direct testimony. When an attorney's cross-examination exposes genuine limitations in the expert's knowledge, the witness should acknowledge them; doing so should not reduce the expert's general credibility if the expert has done a thorough evaluation and reached sensible conclusions.

In the author's experience, it is unusual to encounter the vigorous, incisive, highly-critical cross-examination typically depicted in media depictions of trials (real or fictional). Occasionally, however, cross-examination gets nasty, insulting, or inappropriately personal. When this occurs, the witness should refrain from responding in kind (as difficult as this is); instead, the witness should respond patiently and politely, doing his/her best to explain points clearly, and keeping in mind that the judge and jury – not opposing counsel – are his/her real audience.

Following cross-examination, attorneys have the opportunity to do 'redirect' and 'recross' examinations aimed at challenging or bolstering points made during earlier direct testimony and cross-examination. Once such testimony is concluded, the judge may ask the expert a few questions. After this, the expert is 'excused.' The expert then should leave the courtroom, rather than linger to hear other witnesses' testimony.

A Few Tips

- Dress neatly in business attire. For men, this means wearing a suit and tie; for women, it means wearing a conservatively-styled suit or dress.
- Try always to maintain one's professional demeanor. It's fine to appear confident, but an error to appear smug or arrogant.
- Take time to think before giving answers, and if necessary, elaborate briefly when asked questions that seem to call for a yes or no answer but really cannot be answered properly in that fashion. It helps (if one can) to try to think about where the attorney is heading. This allows one to avoid getting trapped or boxed in by previous answers.
- Don't talk too much. If a question can be answered fully with a one-word response, do so.
- If asked about one's fees for time in court, answer the questions nondefensively.
- Recognize that cross-examination may seem vicious and personal, but it's only part of the opposing

attorney's job. Don't expect to escape the cross-examining attorney's jabs unscathed; be prepared to bleed a little bit.

- Finally, always bear in mind why one is testifying as an expert: to supply the court with information so it can decide a legal issue. Although the expert may have been retained by one side to a dispute or have an opinion about how the case should be resolved, the goal in testifying should be to explain the psychiatric findings succinctly, clearly, and honestly. Doing only this constitutes fulfillment of the psychiatrist's courtroom duty to provide information to help the judge or jury each the its best decision.

References

1. Emergency Medical Treatment and Labor Act 42 USC §1395dd (1986).
2. Bernet W: The noncustodial parent and medical treatment. *Bull Am Acad Psychiatry Law* 1993; **21**:357–364.
3. Carey v. Population Services International, 431 U.S. 678 (1977).
4. Planned Parenthood of Southeastern Pennsylvania v. Casey, 505 U.S. 833 (1992).
5. O'Connor v. Donaldson, 422 U.S. 562 (1975).
6. Addington v. Texas, 441 U.S. 418 (1979).
7. Zinermon v. Burch, 494 U.S. 113 (1990).
8. Parham v. J.R., 442 U.S. 584 (1979).
9. American Psychiatric Association: *The Principles of Medical Ethics with Annotations Especially Applicable to Psychiatry*, 2001 Edition. http://www.psych.org/psych_pract/ethics/medicalethics.cfm (accessed October 29, 2004).
10. Health Insurance Portability and Accountability Act of 1996 (Public Law 104-191).
11. United States Department of Health and Human Services, Office for Civil Rights. Summary of the HIPAA Privacy Rule (describing portions of 45 C.F.R. §160 and §164). April 11, 2003. Available at http://www.hhs.gov/ocr/hipaa/privacy.html (accessed December 8, 2004).
12. Kempe H, Silverman F, Steele B, Proegemueller, Selver H: The battered child syndrome. *J Am Med Assoc* 1962; **181**:17–24.
13. Child Abuse Prevention and Treatment Act (Public Law 93–247).
14. DeAngelis C: Clinical indicators of child abuse. In: Schetky DH, Benedek EP, eds. *Child Psychiatry and the Law*. Baltimore: Williams & Wilkins, 1992:104–118.
15. Geddes JF, Plunkett J: The evidence base for shaken baby syndrome. *Br Med J* 2004; **328**:719–720.
16. Reece RM: The evidence base for shaken baby syndrome. *Br Med J* 2004; **328**:1316–1317.
17. Quinn KM, White S: Interviewing children for suspected sexual abuse. In: Schetky DH, Benedek EP, eds. *Child Psychiatry and the Law*. Baltimore: Williams & Wilkins, 1992:119–144.
18. Brooks CM: The law's response to child abuse and neglect. In: Sales BD, Shuman DW, eds. *Law, Mental Health, and Mental Disorder*. Pacific Grove, CA: Brooks/Cole Publishing Company, 1996.
19. Leavitt WT, Armitage DT: The forensic role of the child psychiatrist in child abuse and neglect cases. *Child Adolesc Psychiatr Clin N Am* 2002; **11**:767–779.
20. Bernet W, Ayres W, Dunne JE, *et al.*: Practice parameters for the forensic evaluation of children and adolescents who may have been physically or sexually abused. *J Am Acad Child Adolesc Psychiatry* 1997; **36**(Suppl 10):37S–56S.
21. Bruck M, Ceci SJ, Francoeur E: Children's use of anatomically detailed dolls to report genital touching in a medical examination: Developmental and gender comparisons. *J Exp Psychol Appl* 2000; **6**:74–83.
22. Smith v. Organization of Foster Families for Equality and Reform (OFFER), 431 U.S. 816 (1977).
23. Santosky v. Kramer, 455 U.S. 745 (1982).
24. Family Preservation and Support Services Act (Public Law 96–272).
25. Adoption and Safe Families Act (Public Law 105–89).
26. Education for All Handicapped Children Act (Public Law 94–142).
27. Individuals with Disabilities Education Act (Public Law 101–476, amended in Public Law 105–17).
28. American Psychiatric Association: *Diagnostic and Statistical Manual of Mental Disorders, Fourth Edition, Text Revision*. Washington, DC: American Psychiatric Association, 2000.
29. Atkins v. Virginia, 536 U.S. 304 (2002).
30. Mossman D. Atkins v. Virginia: A psychiatric can of worms. *New Mexico Law Review* 2003; **33**:255–291.
31. Hoffman BF, Spiegel H: Legal principles in the psychiatric assessment of personal injury litigants. *Am J Psychiatry* 1989; **146**:164–169.
32. Schetky DH: Psychic trauma and civil litigation. In: Schetky DH, Benedek EP, eds. *Child Psychiatry and the Law*. Baltimore: Williams & Wilkins, 1992:318–329.
33. Lubit R, Hartwell N, van Gorp WG, Eth S: Forensic evaluation of trauma syndromes in children. *Child Adolesc Psychiatr Clin N Am* 2002; **11**:823–857.
34. Coy v. Iowa, 487 U.S. 1012 (1988).
35. Maryland v. Craig, 497 U.S. 836 (1990).
36. White v. Illinois, 502 U.S. 346 (1992).
37. Painter v. Bannister, 140 N.W.2d 152 (Iowa, 1966).
38. Comstock G, Strasburger VC: Deceptive appearances: Television violence and aggressive behavior. *J Adolesc Health Care* 1990; **11**:31–44.
39. Center for Disease Control: *Youth Violence: Fact Sheet (2004)*. http://www.cdc.gov/ncipc/factsheets/yvfacts.htm (accessed November 11, 2004).
40. Anderson RN, Smith BL: Deaths: leading causes for 2001. *National Vital Statistics Report* 2003; **52**(9):1–86.
41. Grunbaum JA, Kann L, Kinchen S, Ross JG, Lowry R, Harris WA, *et al.*: Youth risk behavior surveillance – United States, 2003. *MMWR* 2004; **53**(SS-2):1–100.
42. Gest T, Pope V: Crime time bomb. US News & World Report (March 25, 1996) **120**(12):28–36.
43. Snyder HN: *Juvenile arrests 2002. OJJDP Juvenile Justice Bulletin (September 2004)*. Washington DC: Office of Juvenile Justice and Delinquency Prevention http://ojjdp.ncjrs.org/ojstatbb/publications/StatBB.asp (accessed November 11, 2004).
44. Surgeon General: *Youth Violence: A Report of the Surgeon General*. Washington, DC: Department of Health and Human Services, 2001. http://www.surgeongeneral.gov/library/youthviolence/default.htm (accessed November 11, 2004).

45. Snyder HN, Sickmund M: *Juvenile Offenders and Victims: 1999 National Report.* Washington DC: Office of Juvenile Justice and Delinquency Prevention, 1999.
46. Sickmund M, Sladky TJ, Kang W: *Census of Juveniles in Residential Placement Databook, 2004.* http://www.ojjdp.ncjrs.org/ojstatbb/cjrp/ (accessed November 14, 2004).
47. In re Gault, 387 U.S. 1 (1967).
48. In re Winship, 397 U.S. 358 (1970).
49. Breed v. Jones, 421 U.S. 519 (1975).
50. McKeiver v. Pennsylvania, 403 U.S. 528 (1971).
51. Schall v. Martin, 467 U.S. 253 (1984).
52. Kent v. United States, 383 U.S. 541 (1966).
53. Dusky v. United States, 362 U.S. 402 (1960).
54. Bonnie RJ, Grisso T: Adjudicative competence and youthful offenders. In: Grisso T, Schwartz RG, eds. *Youth on Trial.* Chicago: University of Chicago Press, 2000:73–104.
55. Grisso T: *Forensic Evaluation of Juveniles.* Sarasota, FL: Professional Resource Press, 1998.
56. Grisso T, Steinberg L, Woolard J, Cauffman E, Scott E, Graham S, Lexcen F, Reppucci ND, Schwartz R: Juveniles' competence to stand trial: A comparison of adolescents' and adults' capacities as trial defendants. *Law Hum Behav* 2003; 27:333–363.
57. Miranda v. Arizona, 384 U.S. 436 (1966).
58. Grisso T. Juveniles' capacities to waive *Miranda* rights: an empirical analysis. *Calif Law Rev* 1980; 68:1134–1166.
59. Fare v. Michael C., 442 U.S. 707 (1979).
60. Grisso T: Instruments for Assessing Understanding and Appreciation of Miranda Rights. Sarasota, FL: Professional Resources Press, 1998.
61. Goldstein NES, Condie LO, Kalbeitzer R, Osman D, Geier JL: Juvenile offenders' *Miranda* rights comprehension and self-reported likelihood of offering false confessions. *Assessment* 2003; 10:359–369.
62. Moore MS: Law and psychiatry: Rethinking the relationship. Cambridge, MA: Cambridge University Press, 1984.
63. Brodsky SL: *Testifying in Court: Guidelines and Maxims for the Expert Witness.* Washington, DC: American Psychological Association, 1991.
64. Gutheil TG: *The Psychiatrist in Court: A Survival Guide.* Washington, DC: American Psychiatric Publishing, 1998.
65. Gutheil TG: *The Psychiatrist as Expert Witness.* Washington, DC: American Psychiatric Publishing, 1998.
66. Herman SP, Bernet W: Practice parameters for child custody evaluation. *J Am Acad Child Adolesc Psychiatry* 1997; 36(Suppl 10):57S–68S.
67. Bernet W: Child custody evaluations. *Child Adolesc Psychiatric Clin N Am* 2002; 11:781–804.

INDEX

Note: page numbers in *italics* refer to figures and tables. SSRI drugs are not named individually, but are all located under 'selective serotonin reuptake inhibitors' (SSRIs).